MAYO CLINIC NEUROLOGY
BOARD REVIEW

MAYO CLINIC NEUROLOGY BOARD REVIEW: BASIC SCIENCES AND PSYCHIATRY FOR INITIAL CERTIFICATION

Kelly D. Flemming, MD

Consultant, Department of Neurology

Mayo Clinic, Rochester, Minnesota

Associate Professor of Neurology

Mayo Clinic College of Medicine

Lyell K. Jones Jr, MD

Consultant, Department of Neurology

Mayo Clinic, Rochester, Minnesota

Assistant Professor of Neurology

Mayo Clinic College of Medicine

MAYO CLINIC SCIENTIFIC PRESS   OXFORD UNIVERSITY PRESS

OXFORD
UNIVERSITY PRESS

Oxford University Press is a department of the University of
Oxford. It furthers the University's objective of excellence in research,
scholarship, and education by publishing worldwide.

Oxford   New York
Auckland   Cape Town   Dar es Salaam   Hong Kong   Karachi
Kuala Lumpur   Madrid   Melbourne   Mexico City   Nairobi
New Delhi   Shanghai   Taipei   Toronto

With offices in
Argentina   Austria   Brazil   Chile   Czech Republic   France   Greece
Guatemala   Hungary   Italy   Japan   Poland   Portugal   Singapore
South Korea   Switzerland   Thailand   Turkey   Ukraine   Vietnam

Oxford is a registered trademark of Oxford University Press
in the UK and certain other countries.

Published in the United States of America by
Oxford University Press
198 Madison Avenue, New York, NY 10016

Library of Congress Cataloging-in-Publication Data
Mayo Clinic neurology board review : basic sciences and psychiatry for initial certification / [edited by]
Kelly D. Flemming and Lyell K. Jones.
  p. ; cm.
Neurology board review
Includes index.
ISBN 978–0–19–021488–3 (alk. paper)
I. Flemming, Kelly D., editor.   II. Jones, Lyell K., editor.   III. Mayo Clinic, issuing body.
IV. Title: Neurology board review.
[DNLM: 1. Nervous System Diseases—Examination Questions. WL 18.2]
RC343.5
616.80076—dc23
2014040337

Mayo Foundation does not endorse any particular products or services, and the reference to any products or services in this book is
for informational purposes only and should not be taken as an endorsement by the authors or Mayo Foundation. Care has been taken
to confirm the accuracy of the information presented and to describe generally accepted practices. However, the authors, editors, and
publisher are not responsible for errors or omissions or for any consequences from application of the information in this book and
make no warranty, express or implied, with respect to the contents of the publication. This book should not be relied on apart from
the advice of a qualified health care provider.

The authors, editors, and publisher have exerted efforts to ensure that drug selection and dosage set forth in this text are in accordance
with current recommendations and practice at the time of publication. However, in view of ongoing research, changes in government
regulations, and the constant flow of information relating to drug therapy and drug reactions, readers are urged to check the package
insert for each drug for any change in indications and dosage and for added wordings and precautions. This is particularly important
when the recommended agent is a new or infrequently employed drug.

Some drugs and medical devices presented in this publication have US Food and Drug Administration (FDA) clearance for limited
use in restricted research settings. It is the responsibility of the health care providers to ascertain the FDA status of each drug or device
planned for use in their clinical practice.

9 8 7 6
Printed in the United States of America
on acid-free paper

To my family for their patience and understanding. To the students and residents that inspire me.

Kelly D. Flemming, MD

To Amie, Katherine, Nathaniel, and Charlotte for their limitless patience and support. To the brilliant, talented residents of the Neurology Residency Program at Mayo Clinic in Rochester, Minnesota, without whom I would not have the best job in the world.

Lyell K. Jones Jr, MD

Foreword

The Department of Neurology at Mayo Clinic has a long-standing dedication to excellence in clinical neurology and values-driven care to our patients and to the education of colleagues across the career continuum, in all fields of medicine. Our ongoing dedication to education comes at a time of evolution and remarkable advances in the field and in an era of increasing subspecialization. Diagnostic imaging allows us to see more detail in a noninvasive manner, and there are few areas of the field unaffected by the tools of molecular genetics. Treatment options are increasing in number and improving in efficacy, and evidence-based management strategies have been advocated for many neurologic disorders. All these factors contribute to the excitement of being in such a dynamic specialty. There is an ongoing need for a core fund of knowledge for all providers to patients with neurologic disease. The current textbook takes the broad range of subspecialty neurology and distills a tremendous amount of information into a 2-volume text, the *Mayo Clinic Neurology Board Review*.

The current textbook is edited by 2 outstanding Mayo Clinic clinician-educators. They have sought the input of their colleagues from all neurology subspecialties and from neurosurgery, psychiatry, and neuro-ophthalmology, developing a concise review textbook of neurology. The book provides the most important information needed as one is studying for neurology board examinations or for a maintenance of certification (MOC) examination. The extensive use of superb diagrams and tables within the context of concise text provides a framework for efficient learning and attainment of information. The textbook is available as 2 separate volumes, so readers can select the material that is most relevant to them. For those in training or preparing for initial board certification examinations, the first volume nicely summarizes the basic neuroscience, neuroanatomy, and psychiatric information that will be of use for that examination. Volume 2 will provide an outstanding review of clinical neurology for those studying for their initial neurology board examination, for applicants for recertification, for advanced practice clinician colleagues in neurology, and for colleagues in fields of psychiatry, neurosurgery, physical medicine and rehabilitation, family medicine, and internal medicine.

Several other features make the book of tremendous interest. There are over 300 self-assessment questions providing the reader with feedback regarding potential areas requiring further study. For those using the book for recertification, there is an overview of the MOC process, and *American Medical Association Physician's Recognition Award Category 1 Credits* for continuing medical education and self-assessment are provided for those who are interested.

For a neurologist in training or in practice, the text will provide an excellent review for an in-service examination, for neurology boards or MOC, or as a well-written, high-level, beautifully illustrated summary of the field. For the non-neurologist, there is a wealth of information presented in a learner-friendly manner that will demystify many aspects of the evaluation and management of neurology patients, who are seen so commonly in most any field of medicine.

I congratulate Drs Flemming and Jones and all their contributing colleagues on the completion of this superb textbook. The legacy of the collective Mayo Clinic Department of Neurology, across all sites, continues as the Department enters its second century of existence—a group of colleagues with the highest level of dedication to excellence in the care of patients in clinical practice, to the education of their colleagues, and to the advancement of the field through innovative clinical and basic science research. This book is a testament to that legacy. Most importantly, this textbook will provide readers with an additional tool to solidify their knowledge base, leading to improved clinical care of patients with neurologic disorders.

Robert D. Brown Jr, MD, MPH

Consultant, Department of Neurology, Mayo Clinic, Rochester, Minnesota
John T. and Lillian Matthews Professor of Neuroscience
Professor of Neurology, Mayo Clinic College of Medicine

Preface

Neurology is an exciting and rapidly expanding area of medicine. We have designed *Mayo Clinic Neurology Board Review* to assist both physicians-in-training who are preparing for the initial American Board of Psychiatry and Neurology (ABPN) certification examination and neurologists who are preparing for recertification. Trainees and other physicians in related specialties such as psychiatry, neurosurgery, or physiatry may also find this book useful in preparation for their own certification examinations. While we have erred on the side of thoroughness, *Mayo Clinic Neurology Board Review* is not intended to replace an in-depth textbook or serve as a guide to the most current therapies. Instead, this book provides a core of essential knowledge of both basic and clinical aspects of neurology. The emphasis is on clinical knowledge related to diagnostic and therapeutic approaches to patient management. In addition, this text has an expansive array of illustrations, pathology, and radiologic images.

With this book, we have acknowledged that there are different needs for those who are taking the initial board examination and for those who are recertifying. Thus, this book is published in 2 volumes: Volume 1 covers basic sciences and psychiatry, and Volume 2 covers clinical neurology. It is intended that people taking the board examination for the first time will purchase both Volume 1 and Volume 2, whereas those recertifying may wish to buy only Volume 2. In both volumes, we have included high-yield facts and questions for your review.

This volume, which is Volume 1 of *Mayo Clinic Neurology Board Review*, contains an extensive review of the basic neuroscience, neuroanatomical, and psychiatric material required for the initial certification examination. To complete your preparation for the initial certification examination, you should also purchase and review Volume 2 (in other words, Volume 1 alone does not provide complete preparation for the initial certification). Volume 2 includes a broad overview of clinical neurology covered on the initial and recertification ABPN examinations.

Those who are preparing for the recertification examination will be aware of the multifaceted process of Maintenance of Certification (MOC). *Mayo Clinic Neurology Board Review* uniquely offers not only a navigation guide to the MOC process but actual *American Medical Association Physician's Recognition Award Category 1 Credits* for continuing medical education and self-assessment that can be applied to MOC (please see the Continuing Medical Education Information section, which begins on page xix, for further details). Readers who are interested in claiming these credits may go to www.cmestore.mayo.edu to find the corresponding self-study course and for further details on purchasing and documenting earned credits toward MOC, which have been approved for this purpose by the ABPN.

The faculty responsible for this text includes Mayo Clinic staff physicians in the Department of Neurology, the Department of Neurologic Surgery, the Department of Ophthalmology (Neuro-ophthalmology Team), and the Department of Psychiatry and Psychology at all 3 sites: Minnesota, Arizona, and Florida. We are deeply grateful to these incredibly talented experts who have provided such high-quality content. We also thank Nima Mowzoon, MD, for creating many of the wonderful illustrations and for spending countless hours gathering many of the figures that appear in this work.

We want to thank the staffs of the Mayo Clinic Section of Scientific Publications, the Mayo Clinic Division of Media Support Services, and the Mayo

School of Continuous Professional Development for their contributions. The support of Mayo Clinic Scientific Press and Oxford University Press is also greatly appreciated.

Cover images, clockwise from upper left: Figure 34.3B, visual evoked potentials; Figure 13.3 (base image), retinal nerves; Figure 9.8A, angiogram of internal carotid artery; and Figure 22.6A, default mode network rendering of normal wakefulness.

Kelly D. Flemming, MD
Lyell K. Jones Jr, MD

Contents

Contributors

Osama A. Abulseoud, MD
Senior Associate Consultant, Department of Psychiatry &
 Psychology, Mayo Clinic, Rochester, Minnesota
Assistant Professor of Psychiatry, Mayo Clinic College of
 Medicine

Eduardo E. Benarroch, MD
Consultant, Department of Neurology, Mayo Clinic,
 Rochester, Minnesota
Professor of Neurology, Mayo Clinic College of Medicine

Jyoti Bhagia, MD
Consultant, Department of Psychiatry & Psychology,
 Mayo Clinic, Rochester, Minnesota
Instructor in Psychiatry, Mayo Clinic College of
 Medicine

David F. Black, MD
Senior Associate Consultant, Department of Radiology,
 Mayo Clinic, Rochester, Minnesota
Assistant Professor of Neurology and of Radiology,
 Mayo Clinic College of Medicine

Paul W. Brazis, MD
Consultant, Department of Ophthalmology, Mayo Clinic,
 Jacksonville, Florida
Professor of Neurology, Mayo Clinic College of
 Medicine

Jeffrey W. Britton, MD
Consultant, Department of Neurology, Mayo Clinic,
 Rochester, Minnesota
Associate Professor of Neurology, Mayo Clinic College of
 Medicine

David B. Burkholder, MD
Fellow in Neurology, Mayo School of Graduate Medical
 Education, Mayo Clinic College of Medicine, Rochester,
 Minnesota

Richard J. Caselli, MD
Consultant, Department of Neurology, Mayo Clinic,
 Scottsdale, Arizona
Professor of Neurology, Mayo Clinic College of Medicine

Pablo R. Castillo, MD
Consultant, Division of Allergy and Pulmonary Medicine,
 Mayo Clinic, Jacksonville, Florida
Assistant Professor of Medicine, Mayo Clinic College of
 Medicine

Elizabeth A. Coon, MD
Fellow in Neurology, Mayo Graduate School of Medicine
Instructor in Neurology, Mayo Clinic College of Medicine,
 Rochester, Minnesota

Amy Z. Crepeau, MD
Senior Associate Consultant, Department of Neurology,
 Mayo Clinic, Scottsdale, Arizona
Assistant Professor of Neurology, Mayo Clinic College of
 Medicine

Brian A. Crum, MD
Consultant, Department of Neurology, Mayo Clinic,
 Rochester, Minnesota
Assistant Professor of Neurology, Mayo Clinic College of
 Medicine

Tamara J. Dolenc, MD
Senior Associate Consultant, Department of Psychiatry &
 Psychology, Mayo Clinic, Rochester, Minnesota
Assistant Professor of Psychiatry, Mayo Clinic College of
 Medicine

Scott D. Eggers, MD
Consultant, Department of Neurology, Mayo Clinic,
 Rochester, Minnesota
Assistant Professor of Neurology, Mayo Clinic College of
 Medicine

Kelly D. Flemming, MD
Consultant, Department of Neurology, Mayo Clinic, Rochester, Minnesota
Associate Professor of Neurology, Mayo Clinic College of Medicine

Ralitza H. Gavrilova, MD
Consultant, Department of Medical Genetics, Mayo Clinic, Rochester, Minnesota
Assistant Professor of Medical Genetics and of Neurology, Mayo Clinic College of Medicine

Jonathan Graff-Radford, MD
Fellow in Neurology, Mayo School of Graduate Medical Education
Instructor in Neurology, Mayo Clinic College of Medicine, Rochester, Minnesota

Anhar Hassan, MB, BCh
Senior Associate Consultant, Department of Neurology, Mayo Clinic, Rochester, Minnesota
Assistant Professor of Neurology, Mayo Clinic College of Medicine

David T. Jones, MD
Associate Consultant, Division of Behavioral Neurology, Mayo Clinic, Rochester, Minnesota

Lyell K. Jones Jr, MD
Consultant, Department of Neurology, Mayo Clinic, Rochester, Minnesota
Assistant Professor of Neurology, Mayo Clinic College of Medicine

Brian S. Katz, MD
Fellow in Neurology, Mayo School of Graduate Medical Education, Mayo Clinic College of Medicine, Rochester, Minnesota

Simon Kung, MD
Consultant, Department of Psychiatry & Psychology, Mayo Clinic, Rochester, Minnesota
Assistant Professor of Psychiatry, Mayo Clinic College of Medicine

Maria I. Lapid, MD
Consultant, Department of Psychiatry & Psychology, Mayo Clinic, Rochester, Minnesota
Associate Professor of Psychiatry, Mayo Clinic College of Medicine

Ruple S. Laughlin, MD
Consultant, Department of Neurology, Mayo Clinic, Rochester, Minnesota
Assistant Professor of Neurology, Mayo Clinic College of Medicine

Jacqueline A. Leavitt, MD
Consultant, Department of Ophthalmology, Mayo Clinic, Rochester, Minnesota
Associate Professor of Ophthalmology, Mayo Clinic College of Medicine

Jarrod M. Leffler, PhD, LP
Senior Associate Consultant, Department of Psychiatry & Psychology, Mayo Clinic, Rochester, Minnesota
Assistant Professor of Psychology, Mayo Clinic College of Medicine

Mary M. Machulda, PhD, LP
Consultant, Department of Psychiatry & Psychology, Mayo Clinic, Rochester, Minnesota
Assistant Professor of Psychology, Mayo Clinic College of Medicine

Kari A. Martin, MD
Consultant, Department of Psychiatry & Psychology, Mayo Clinic, Scottsdale, Arizona
Assistant Professor of Psychiatry, Mayo Clinic College of Medicine

Virginia V. Michels, MD
Emeritus Professor of Medical Genetics, Mayo Clinic College of Medicine, Rochester, Minnesota

Alex J. Nelson, MD
Fellow in Neurology, Mayo School of Graduate Medical Education, Mayo Clinic College of Medicine, Rochester, Minnesota

Mark W. Olsen, MD
Consultant, Department of Psychiatry & Psychology, Mayo Clinic, Rochester, Minnesota
Instructor in Psychiatry, Mayo Clinic College of Medicine

Brian A. Palmer, MD
Senior Associate Consultant, Department of Psychiatry & Psychology, Mayo Clinic, Rochester, Minnesota
Assistant Professor of Psychiatry, Mayo Clinic College of Medicine

Kemuel L. Philbrick, MD
Consultant, Department of Psychiatry & Psychology, Mayo Clinic, Rochester, Minnesota
Assistant Professor of Psychiatry, Mayo Clinic College of Medicine

Michael F. Presti, MD, PhD
Fellow in Neurology, Mayo School of Graduate Medical Education, Mayo Clinic College of Medicine, Rochester, Minnesota

Keith G. Rasmussen, MD
Consultant, Department of Psychiatry & Psychology,
Mayo Clinic, Rochester, Minnesota
Associate Professor of Psychiatry, Mayo Clinic College of
Medicine

Michael M. Reese, MD
Consultant, Department of Psychiatry & Psychology,
Mayo Clinic, Rochester, Minnesota
Instructor in Psychiatry, Mayo Clinic College of
Medicine

Nathan P. Staff, MD, PhD
Consultant, Department of Neurology, Mayo Clinic,
Rochester, Minnesota
Assistant Professor of Neurology, Mayo Clinic College of
Medicine

Jennifer A. Tracy, MD
Consultant, Department of Neurology, Mayo Clinic,
Rochester, Minnesota
Assistant Professor of Neurology, Mayo Clinic College of
Medicine

James C. Watson, MD
Consultant, Department of Neurology, Mayo Clinic,
Rochester, Minnesota
Assistant Professor of Neurology, Mayo Clinic College of
Medicine

Continuing Medical Education Information

Activity Description and Target Audience

This educational activity is part of a larger curriculum regarding the clinical practice of neurology; the curriculum includes several continuing medical education (CME) offerings at Mayo Clinic. This year is the first year that this educational resource will be available for CME and Maintenance of Certification (MOC) Part II credit. The resource will provide a broad-based review of the knowledge required for all neurologists in practice. There is no other review activity in the United States like this one; this Mayo Clinic offering is an innovative solution providing preparatory material and simultaneous CME and MOC credit. This activity is a comprehensive review of all aspects of neurologic disease evaluation, diagnosis, and treatment. This review is appropriate for neurologists, neurology trainees, providers in related specialties, and generalists.

Accreditation and Credit Designation Statement

Mayo Clinic College of Medicine is accredited by the Accreditation Council for Continuing Medical Education to provide CME for physicians.

Mayo Clinic College of Medicine designates this enduring material for a maximum of 32 *AMA PRA Category 1 Credits*™. Physicians should claim only the credit commensurate with the extent of their participation in the activity.

This text also features ABPN-approved self-assessment activities.

Learning Objectives

1. Demonstrate mastery of the broad medical knowledge requirements for clinical practice.

2. Demonstrate an understanding of the multifaceted MOC process.

3. Demonstrate an understanding of the concepts of medical professionalism and interpersonal and communication skills and how they apply in complex practices reflected in today's health care environments.

How to Request or Obtain Credit

Once you review the content, a post-test and evaluation are accessible online ce.mayo.edu (search: *Mayo Clinic Neurology Board Review*). Fees will apply depending on the CME or MOC desired. The Mayo School of Continuous Professional Development (CPD) requires that learners score at least 80% to pass; they are allowed 1 retake. Upon passing, a certificate of attendance and completion is awarded from the Mayo School of CPD and will be available online for your immediate receipt.

Owing to the extensive length of the book, the ability to claim credit has been divided into segments. This allows the learner to claim credit on smaller portions of the book as desired.

An individual report providing the questions, the learner's answers, the correct answers, and references to seek additional information will be provided for each participant. Comparable responses of the participants will also be provided.

Disclosures

As a provider accredited by the Accreditation Council for Continuing Medical Education (ACCME), Mayo Clinic College of Medicine (Mayo School of CPD) must ensure balance, independence, objectivity, and scientific rigor in its educational activities. The course director(s), Planning Committee members, faculty, and all others who are in a position to control the content of this educational activity are required to disclose all relevant financial relationships with any commercial interest related to the subject matter of the educational activity. Safeguards against commercial bias have been put in place. Faculty also will disclose any off-label or investigational use of pharmaceuticals or instruments that are described within this book. Disclosure of these relevant financial relationships is published so that participants may formulate their own judgments regarding the material. Disclosures are shown starting on the following page.

Commercial Support

No commercial support was received in the production of this activity.

Questions

For assistance with obtaining CME or MOC credits, contact the Mayo School of CPD (email: cme@mayo.edu).

Faculty, Planning Committee, and Provider Disclosure Summary

Mayo Clinic Neurology Board Review: Basic Sciences and Psychiatry for Initial Certification

As a provider accredited by ACCME, Mayo Clinic College of Medicine (Mayo School of CPD), must ensure balance, independence, objectivity, and scientific rigor in its educational activities. Course Director(s), Planning Committee Members, Faculty, and all others who are in a position to control the content of this educational activity are required to disclose all relevant financial relationships with any commercial interest related to the subject matter of the educational activity. Safeguards against commercial bias have been put in place. Faculty also will disclose any off-label and/or investigational use of pharmaceuticals or instruments discussed in their presentation. Disclosure of these relevant financial relationships will be published in activity materials so those participants in the activity may formulate their own judgments regarding the presentation.

Listed below are individuals with control of the content of this program who provided disclosures.

Relevant Financial Relationship(s) With Industry

Name	Nature of Relationship	Company
Bradley Boeve, MD	Clinical Trials Royalties Honoraria Scientific Advisory Board Research Support	Cephalon, Allon Pharmaceuticals, GE Healthcare Publication of book entitled *Behavioral Neurology of Dementia* American Academy of Neurology Tau Consortium National Institute of Aging and Mangurian Foundation
Bart Demaerschalk, MD	Consultant Grant Research Support	Genentech, Inc. Genentech, Inc.
Neill R. Graff-Radford, MD	Consultant Grant Research Support	Codman TauRX
B. Mark Keegan, MD	Grant Research Support	Terumo BCT
Claudia Lucchinetti, MD	Grant/Research Support Patent	NIH, NMSS NMO-IgG
Istvan Pirko, MD	Grant Research Support	PI on a basic science Independent Investigator Research Grant (IIRG) by Novartis Pharmaceuticals
Elizabeth Shuster, MD	Faculty	Prime Inc. Sep 2012 CME Prime MS Journal Club Event
Bryan Woodruff, MD	Grant Research Support	Principle investigator for Clinical Trials of Alzheimer's and Mild Cognitive Impairment Genentech and Avid

No Relevant Financial Relationship(s) With Industry

Osama A. Abulseoud, MD
Maria I. Aguilar, MD
Allen J. Aksamit Jr, MD
Vichaya Arunthari, MD
Patty P. Atkinson, MD
Kevin M. Barrett, MD
Eduardo E. Benarroch, MD
Sarah E. Berini, MD
Jyoti Bhagia, MD
Barry D. Birch, MD
David F. Black, MD
James H. Bower, MD
Paul W. Brazis, MD
Jeffrey W. Britton, MD
Robert D. Brown Jr, MD
David B. Burkholder, MD
Melinda S. Burnett, MD
Richard J. Caselli, MD
Pablo R. Castillo, MD
Elizabeth A. Coon, MD
Philippe Couillard, MD
Amy Z. Crepeau, MD
Brian A. Crum, MD
Mara Cvejic, DO
Radhika Dhamija, MBBS
Elliot L. Dimberg, MD
Tamara J. Dolenc, MD
Joseph F. Drazkowski, MD
Scott D. Eggers, MD
Eoin P. Flanagan, MB, BCh
Kelly D. Flemming, MD
Jessica P. Floyd, MD
William D. Freeman, MD
Jennifer E. Fugate, DO
Shinsuke Fujioka, MD
Jimmy R. Fulgham, MD
Ralitza H. Gavrilova, MD
Brent P. Goodman, MD
Jeremy K. Gregory, MD
Shamir Haji, MD
Anhar Hassan, MB, BCh
Sara E. Hocker, MD
Matthew T. Hoerth, MD
Mark E. Jentoft, MD
Derek R. Johnson, MD
David T. Jones, MD
Lyell K. Jones Jr, MD
Keith A. Josephs, MD
Orhun H. Kantarci, MD
Brian S. Katz, MD

Gesina F. Keating, MD
Qurat ul Ain Khan, MD
Bryan T. Klassen, MD
Neeraj Kumar, MD
Simon Kung, MD
Daniel Honore Lachance, MD
Maria I. Lapid, MD
Ruple S. Laughlin, MD
Jacqueline A. Leavitt, MD
Mark C. Lee, MD
Andrea N. Leep Hunderfund, MD
Jarrod M. Leffler, PhD, LP
Mary M. Machulda, PhD, LP
Kenneth J. Mack, MD, PhD
Patrick R. Mahoney, MD
Kari A. Martin, MD
Andrew McKeon, MB, BCh, MD
Virginia V. Michels, MD
Margherita Milone, MD, PhD
Samuel (S. Arthur) A. Moore, MD
Deena Nasr, DO
Alex J. Nelson, MD
Katherine C. Nickels, MD
Katherine H. Noe, MD, PhD
Mark W. Olsen, MD
Brian A. Palmer, MD
Kemuel L. Philbrick, MD
Alyx B. Porter, MD
Michael F. Presti, MD, PhD
Keith G. Rasmussen Jr, MD
Michael M. Reese, MD
Deborah L. Renaud, MD
Mark N. Rubin, MD
Gretchen E. Schlosser Covell, MD
Billie A. Schultz, MD
Wolfgang Singer, MD
Eric J. Sorenson, MD
Nathan P. Staff, MD, PhD
Nilufer Taner, MD, PhD
Michel Toledano, MD
Jennifer A. Tracy, MD
Joon H. Uhm, MD
James C. Watson, MD
Eelco F. Wijdicks, MD, PhD
John W. Wilson, MD
Heidi T. Woessner, MD
Lily C. Wong-Kisiel, MD
Zbigniew K. Wszolek, MD
Paul E. Youssef, DO
Kristine S. Ziemba, MD

References to Off-Label or Investigational Usage(s) of Pharmaceuticals or Instruments

Name	Manufacturer	Product/Device
David F. Black, MD	Bracco Diagnostics	Gadobenate dimeglumine—gadolinium use with power-injectors (such as MRA)
Bradley F. Boeve, MD		Dr. Boeve may have mentioned the use of several medications that are not FDA-approved for the indications that are reviewed, which may include the use of melatonin, clonazepam, cholinesterase inhibitors, carbidopa/levodopa, dopamine agonists, selective serotonin reuptake inhibitors, atypical neuroleptics, lithium, glycogen synthase kinase-3 beta inhibitors, anti-amyloid immunotherapies, putative tau-active agents, mematine, sedative/hypnotics, and psychostimulants for the management of cognitive impairment, neuropsychiatric disorders, parkinsonism, sleep disorders, and autonomic dysfunction
Melinda S. Burnett, MD		Treatment of essential tremor: generic primidone, Inderal LA, clonazepam, alprazolam, topiramate, gabapentin, thalamotomy for essential tremor; clonazepam, gabapentin, and sodium valproate for orthostatic tremor; clonazepam, sodium valproate, tetrabenazine, haloperidol, trihexyphenidyl, and carbamazepine for palatal tremor; sodium valproate, clonazepam up to 15 mg a day, piracetam, levetiracetam, zonisamide, primidone, acetazolamide, and phenobarbital for myoclonus; clonazepam and 5-hydroxytryptophan for essential myoclonus; clonazepam, sodium valproate, tetrabenazine, and gamma-hydroxybutyric acid for myoclonus-dystonia; drugs above and SSRIs for Lance-Adams syndrome
Eoin P. Flanagan, MB, BCh	Pfizer Multiple manufacturers Forest Pharmaceuticals Multiple manufacturers	• Donepezil in multiple sclerosis • Acetylcholinesterase inhibitors in vascular dementia • Memantine • Corticosteroids and long-term immunosuppressive treatments in autoimmune and paraneoplastic encephalitis
Anhar Hassan, MB, BCh		Idebenone
Keith A. Josephs, MD		• Levodopa for some patients with MSA, PSP, or CBS • Fludrocortisone or midodrine for OH in MSA • Dextromethorphan & quinidine for pseudobulbar effect in PSP • Clonazepam for myoclonus and dystonia in CBS • Botulinum toxin injections for dystonia in CBS
Simon Kung, MD		• The use of lithium and liothronine are off-label for the treatment of depression. • The use of oxcarbazepine is off-label for the treatment of bipolar disorder.
Andrea N. Leep Hunderfund, MD		• Carbidopa/levodopa, opioids, carbamazepine, and benzodiazepines off-label for restless legs syndrome. • Oral magnesium and riboflavin are off-label for migraine prophylaxis.
Andrew McKeon, MB, BCh, MD		All treatments for autoimmune neurologic disorders are off-label
Deena Nasr, MD		Tetrabenazine, rituximab, cyclosporin, azathioprine, myocophenolate mofetil, haldoperidol, chlorpromazin, pimozide
Wolfgang Singer, MD	Several generic medications	Several medications used for disorders that are rare enough that FDA-approved medications are sparse.
Eric J. Sorenson, MD		Anticholinergic medications and Botox are off-label for sialorrhea.
James C. Watson, MD	Multiple	Pharmacologic agents are used off-label for the treatment of neuropathic pain.

Section

I

Neuroscience and Neuroanatomy

Eduardo E. Benarroch, MD,

editor

Cerebrovascular Anatomy and Pathophysiology[a]

KELLY D. FLEMMING, MD

Introduction

The cerebrospinal vasculature originates at the aortic arch. The right brachiocephalic divides into the right common carotid and subclavian artery. The left common carotid and left subclavian arteries arise directly from the aortic arch. The 2 common carotid arteries bifurcate into the internal and external carotid arteries. The *anterior circulation* of the brain includes the distal branches from the internal carotid artery, including the anterior and middle cerebral arteries. The vertebral arteries arise off the subclavians and join at the pontomedullary junction to form the basilar artery. The vertebrobasilar system and distal branches are commonly known as the *posterior circulation* of the brain.

The deep and superficial veins of the brain ultimately drain into the venous sinuses and then to the jugular veins.

Reduced blood flow may result in symptoms and, potentially, irreversible damage. The penumbra is an area of low cerebral blood flow surrounding the core of ischemic damage that can be preserved if blood flow is restored in a timely manner or collateral circulation is adequate.

Cerebral and Spinal Vasculature

Cerebral Arteries and Arterial Territories

From the aortic arch arise 3 major blood vessels (from right to left): brachiocephalic (innominate), left common carotid, and left subclavian arteries (Figure 1.1). The

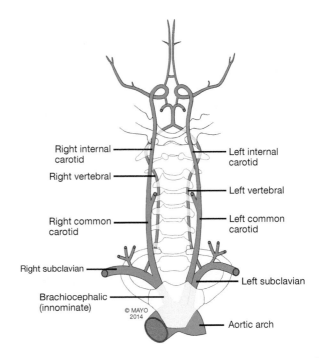

Figure 1.1 Major Arteries Supplying the Supratentorial and Posterior Fossa Levels.
(Adapted from Benarroch EE, Daube JR, Flemming KD, Westmoreland BF. Mayo Clinic medical neurosciences: organized by neurologic systems and levels. 5th ed. Rochester [MN]: Mayo Clinic Scientific Press and Florence [KY]: Informa Healthcare USA; c2008. Chapter 12, The vascular system; p. 447–88. Used with permission of Mayo Foundation for Medical Education and Research.)

---

[a] Portions previously published in Flemming KD, Brown RD Jr, Petty GW, Huston J III, Kallmes DF, Piepgras DG. Evaluation and management of transient ischemic attack and minor cerebral infarction. Mayo Clin Proc. 2004 Aug;79(8):1071-86. Used with permission of Mayo Foundation for Medical Education and Research.

Abbreviations: ACA, anterior cerebral artery; MCA, middle cerebral artery; PCA, posterior cerebral artery; PICA, posterior inferior cerebellar artery

brachiocephalic artery then branches into the right sub-clavian and right common carotid arteries. The vertebral arteries branch from their respective subclavian arteries. An anatomic variant of the arch is the bovine arch, in which there are 2 brachiocephalic arteries.

The common carotid arteries bifurcate into the internal and external carotid arteries at approximately the cervical vertebral level 3 or 4. The external carotid artery supplies the face, scalp, jaw, and base of the brain. The middle meningeal artery enters the skull at the foramen spinosum. The extracranial internal carotid artery has no branches.

The internal carotid artery is divided into multiple segments (Table 1.1). The ophthalmic segment is intradural more than 80% of the time, whereas the petrous and cavernous segments are extradural (below the dural ring). Although there are several minor branches of the intracranial carotid artery, the 3 main branches are (in order of occurrence): ophthalmic, posterior communicating, and anterior choroidal arteries (Figure 1.2 and Table 1.2).

The internal carotid artery terminates and bifurcates into the anterior artery and middle cerebral artery (MCA). The anterior cerebral artery (ACA) is composed of perforating and cortical arteries (Figure 1.3). Perforating or penetrating arteries (including the recurrent artery of Heubner and medial lenticulostriates) supply deep structures: the head of the caudate, the corpus callosum, and part of the fornix. Cortical branches, named in accordance with where they terminate, supply the medial and parasagittal aspect of the hemispheres. The 2 ACAs are connected through the anterior communicating artery.

A stroke resulting from sacrifice of the recurrent artery of Heubner during an anterior communicating

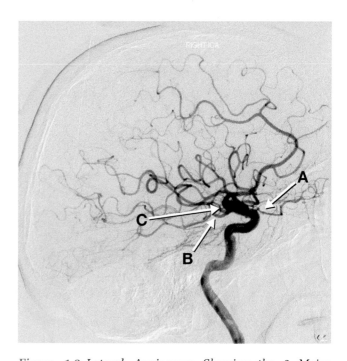

Figure 1.2 Lateral Angiogram Showing the 3 Major Branches Off the Internal Carotid Artery.
A, Ophthalmic branch. B, Posterior communicating branch. C, Anterior choroidal.

artery clipping surgery is noted in Figure 1.4. The recurrent artery of Heubner supplies part of the head of the caudate nucleus and can result in serious cognitive dysfunction because of the interconnections of the caudate head and the frontal lobe.

The MCA also has perforating and cortical branches (Figure 1.5). Perforating branches such as the lateral lenticulostriates arise from the M_1 segment (carotid

Table 1.1 • Segments of the Internal Carotid Artery

Segment	Description
Cervical	Has no branches
Petrous	Enters carotid canal of temporal bone Vidian and caroticotympanic arise from this segment
Cavernous	Traverses cavernous sinus (along with cranial nerves III, IV, VI, V1, and V2) Branches include meningohypophyseal trunk, inferolateral trunk, and capsular arteries
Clinoid	Is a small segment; no branches
Ophthalmic	Gives rise to ophthalmic artery (supplies retina) and superior hypophyseal artery
Communicating	Two branches include posterior communicating artery and anterior choroidal artery

Table 1.2 • Main Branches of Internal Carotid Artery System

Branch	Supplies
Ophthalmic	Eye (retina)
Anterior choroidal	Optic tract, posterior limb of internal capsule, cerebral peduncle, choroid plexus, medial temporal lobe, globus pallidus, lateral geniculate body
Posterior communicating	Anastomoses with posterior cerebral artery Anterior thalamoperforate branches from posterior communicating artery extend to anterior portions of thalamus

Adapted from Flemming KD. Cerebrovascular disease. In: Mowzoon N, Flemming KD, editors. Neurology board review: an illustrated study guide. Rochester (MN): Mayo Clinic Scientific Press and Florence (KY): Informa Healthcare USA; c2007. p. 435–84. Used with permission of Mayo Foundation for Medical Education and Research.

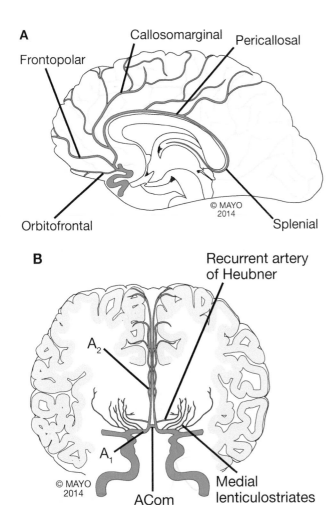

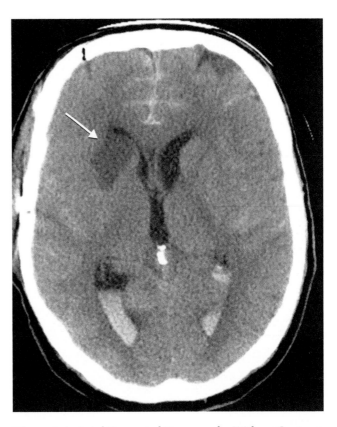

Figure 1.4 Axial Computed Tomography Without Contrast Medium Shows an Area of Hypoattenuation in the Right Caudate Consistent With a Recurrent Artery of Heubner Ischemic Stroke (arrow).
This patient had a subarachnoid hemorrhage due to an anterior communicating artery stroke, and the recurrent artery of Heubner was sacrificed during clipping of the aneurysm, thereby resulting in the stroke.

Figure 1.3 Anterior Cerebral Artery (ACA).
A, Medial aspect of cerebral hemisphere with cortical branches of ACA. B, Coronal section of cerebral hemispheres with cortical and penetrating branches of ACA. A_1 and A_2 indicate segments of ACA; ACom, anterior communicating artery.
(Adapted from Flemming KD. Cerebrovascular disease. In: Mowzoon N, Flemming KD, editors. Neurology board review: an illustrated study guide. Rochester [MN]: Mayo Clinic Scientific Press and Florence [KY]: Informa Healthcare USA; c2007. p. 435–84. Used with permission of Mayo Foundation for Medical Education and Research.)

terminus to MCA bifurcation) and supply the basal ganglia and internal capsule. The cortical branches supply the lateral aspect of the cerebral hemisphere and anterior temporal lobe, the anterior division supplies the frontal lobe, and the posterior division supplies the parietal and temporal lobes.

Several anastomoses supply the collateral circulation of the brain. The circle of Willis (Figure 1.6) is an anastomotic ring connecting the anterior (carotid) and posterior (vertebrobasilar) systems. Interestingly, only 30% to 35% of people have a full circle of Willis. Oftentimes, an A_1 ACA

(carotid terminus to anterior communicating segment), posterior communicating, or P1 (basilar terminus to posterior communicating segment) posterior cerebral artery (PCA) segment is missing. Collateral circulation also can occur through leptomeningeal collaterals and external carotid or vertebral arteries to an intracranial artery. One of the common external carotid collaterals is an anastomosis with the ophthalmic artery.

The vertebral arteries arise from their respective subclavian arteries. The cervical segment of the vertebral ascends through the transverse foramina of vertebral bodies C6 to the axis, with minor meningeal branches arising from this segment. The vertebral arteries enter the foramen magnum and pierce the dura. The intracranial (intradural) segment extends from the medulla to the pontomedullary junction (Figure 1.7). The 2 vertebral arteries join here to form the basilar artery. Commonly, 1 vertebral is dominant or larger in diameter along its entire length. Also common is seeing the intracranial vertebral end with the posterior inferior cerebellar artery

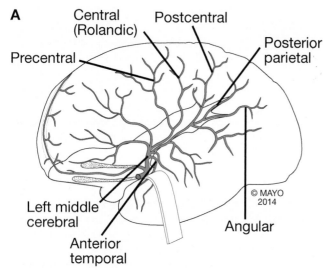

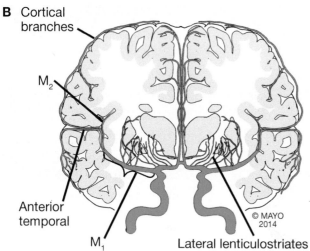

Figure 1.5 Major Branches of the Middle Cerebral Artery. A, Lateral view. B, Coronal view containing M$_1$ and M$_2$ segments.

(Adapted from Benarroch EE, Daube JR, Flemming KD, Westmoreland BF. Mayo Clinic medical neurosciences: organized by neurologic systems and levels. 5th ed. Rochester [MN]: Mayo Clinic Scientific Press and Florence [KY]: Informa Healthcare USA; c2008. Chapter 12, The vascular system; p. 447–88. Used with permission of Mayo Foundation for Medical Education and Research.)

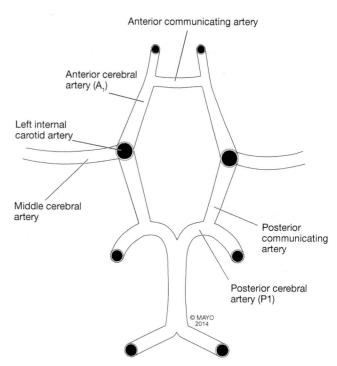

Figure 1.6 Components of the Circle of Willis.

(Adapted from Flemming KD. Cerebrovascular disease. In: Mowzoon N, Flemming KD, editors. Neurology board review: an illustrated study guide. Rochester [MN]: Mayo Clinic Scientific Press and Florence [KY]: Informa Healthcare USA; c2007. p. 435–84. Used with permission of Mayo Foundation for Medical Education and Research.)

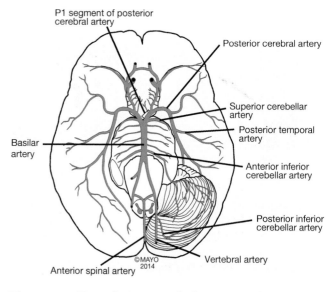

Figure 1.7 Ventral Aspect of the Brain Showing the Posterior Circulation.

(Adapted from Flemming KD. Cerebrovascular disease. In: Mowzoon N, Flemming KD, editors. Neurology board review: an illustrated study guide. Rochester [MN]: Mayo Clinic Scientific Press and Florence [KY]: Informa Healthcare USA; c2007. p. 435–84. Used with permission of Mayo Foundation for Medical Education and Research.)

and not contribute to the basilar artery as well. The branches of the intracranial vertebral arteries and their supply are noted in Table 1.3 and Figure 1.8.

The basilar artery is formed as the 2 vertebral arteries merge at the pontomedullary junction. It extends from the pontomedullary junction to the interpeduncular fossa, where it terminates by branching into the PCAs. Median and paramedian perforating branches supply their respective areas of the pons (Figure 1.8). Two long circumferential branches—the anterior inferior

Table 1.3 • Branches and Function of the Intracranial Vertebral Arteries

Artery	Supply
Anterior spinal	Midline medulla, including pyramids, and caudally to ventrolateral spinal cord
Posterior spinal	A portion of lateral medulla and caudally to posterior funiculus of spinal cord
Paramedial perforating	Paramedian aspect of medulla
Posterior inferior cerebellar	Lateral medulla, inferior aspect of cerebellum

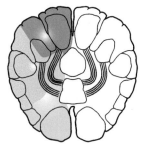 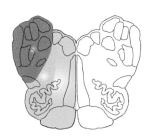

Caudal medulla   Medulla

- ▪ Posterior spinal artery
- ▪ Posterior inferior cerebellar artery
- ▫ Vertebral artery
- ▫ Anterior spinal artery

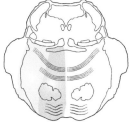 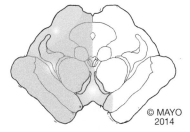

© MAYO 2014

Pons   Midbrain

- ▪ Basilar paramedian artery
- ▪ Posterior cerebral artery
- ▪ Posterior choroidal artery
- ▫ Basilar short circumferential artery

Figure 1.8 Blood Supply to the Medulla, Pons, and Midbrain.
(Adapted from Benarroch EE, Daube JR, Flemming KD, Westmoreland BF. Mayo Clinic medical neurosciences: organized by neurologic systems and levels. 5th ed. Rochester [MN]: Mayo Clinic Scientific Press and Florence [KY]: Informa Healthcare USA; c2008. Chapter 12, The vascular system; p. 447–88. Used with permission of Mayo Foundation for Medical Education and Research.)

cerebellar artery and the superior cerebellar artery—supply the lateral pons inferiorly and superiorly, respectively, and a portion of the cerebellum. The superior cerebellar artery also supplies part of the midbrain.

The PCA arises from the basilar artery. Each PCA has both perforating branches and cortical branches. Perforating branches arise from the P1 (basilar terminus to posterior communicating segment) and P2 (posterior communicating to the posterior midbrain) segments and supply the thalamus and portions of the midbrain (Figure 1.8). The cortical branches include the medial occipital artery and the lateral occipital artery. The medial occipital artery gives rise to the parietooccipital and calcarine branches, which supply the visual cortex. The lateral occipital artery gives rise to the temporal artery and supplies the inferior temporal lobe.

Blood supply to the deep structures and cerebellum are summarized in Tables 1.4 and 1.5.

The arterial vascular supply to the cortex is shown in Figure 1.9. Strokes due to hypoperfusion often result in either ACA-MCA or MCA-PCA borderzone infarctions (Figure 1.10).

Table 1.4 • Blood Supply to Basal Ganglia and Thalamus

Structure	Supply
Striatum	Lateral striate branches (MCA)
Head of caudate	Recurrent artery of Heubner (ACA)
Head of caudate, anteromedial portion	Anterior choroidal
Lateral globus pallidus	Lateral striate branches (MCA) and anterior choroidal
Medial globus pallidus	Anterior choroidal and perforating branches (PCOM)
Internal capsule Anterior limb	Lateral striate branches (MCA) and medial striates (ACA)
Genu	Internal carotid artery branches and lateral striate branches (MCA)
Posterior limb	Lateral striate branches (MCA) and anterior choroidal
Anterior thalamus	Anterior thalamoperforating branches (PCOM)
Medial thalamus	Posterior thalamoperforating branches from P1 segment PCA and tip of basilar + posterior choroidal
Lateral thalamus	Thalamogeniculate from P2 segment PCA

ACA, anterior cerebral artery; MCA, middle cerebral artery; PCA, posterior cerebral artery; PCOM, posterior communicating artery.
Adapted from Flemming KD. Cerebrovascular disease. In: Mowzoon N, Flemming KD, editors. Neurology board review: an illustrated study guide. Rochester (MN): Mayo Clinic Scientific Press and Florence (KY): Informa Healthcare USA; c2007. p. 435–84. Used with permission of Mayo Foundation for Medical Education and Research.

Table 1.5 • Blood Supply to Cerebellum

Artery	Supplies
Posterior inferior cerebellar	Inferolateral surface of cerebellum, inferior vermis (uvula and nodulus), cerebellar tonsil Lateral medulla
Anterior inferior cerebellar	Inferior surface of cerebellum, flocculus, dentate nucleus Caudal pontine tegmentum
Superior cerebellar	Medial portion supplies superior cerebellar vermis Lateral portion supplies superior hemispheres and the deep nuclei, superior medullary velum, and lateral portion of upper pontine tegmentum

Adapted from Flemming KD. Cerebrovascular disease. In: Mowzoon N, Flemming KD, editors. Neurology board review: an illustrated study guide. Rochester (MN): Mayo Clinic Scientific Press and Florence (KY): Informa Healthcare USA; c2007. p. 435–84. Used with permission of Mayo Foundation for Medical Education and Research.

Cerebral Veins and Venous Sinuses

Venous drainage occurs from pial venous plexuses that form within the brain and drain into larger cerebral veins. These cerebral veins travel in the subarachnoid space and empty into the dural venous sinuses after briefly passing through the subdural space. The dural venous sinuses are formed where periosteal and meningeal layers of dura mater separate, and they have no valves. Clinically important venous sinuses include superior sagittal, inferior sagittal, straight (rectus), transverse, and sigmoid sinuses (Figure 1.11).

The cavernous sinus is composed of a network of venous channels and is situated on either side of the sella turcica with several interconnecting channels. Importantly, cranial nerves III, IV, and VI and the first and second divisions of cranial nerve V also travel through the cavernous sinus. Thus, the pathologic conditions of the cavernous sinus, such as fistula and thrombosis, may result in diplopia, face numbness, and visual changes. Visual changes are due to the fact that the superior and inferior ophthalmic veins drain into the cavernous sinus, which then drains into the

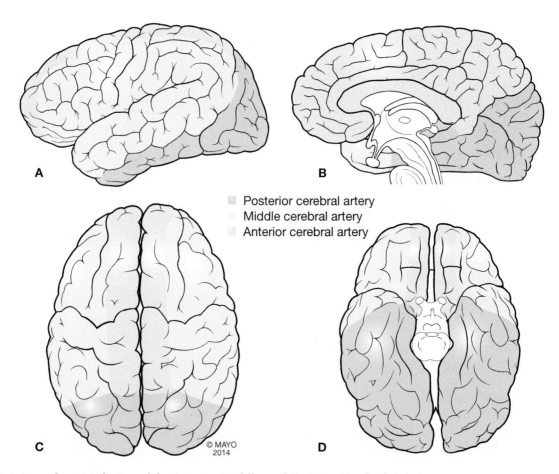

Posterior cerebral artery
Middle cerebral artery
Anterior cerebral artery

© MAYO 2014

Figure 1.9 Vascular Distribution of the Anterior, Middle, and Posterior Cerebral Arteries.
A, Lateral view. B, Medial view. C, Superior view. D, Inferior view.
(Adapted from Benarroch EE, Daube JR, Flemming KD, Westmoreland BF. Mayo Clinic medical neurosciences: organized by neurologic systems and levels. 5th ed. Rochester [MN]: Mayo Clinic Scientific Press and Florence [KY]: Informa Healthcare USA; c2008. Chapter 12, The vascular system; p. 447–88. Used with permission of Mayo Foundation for Medical Education and Research.)

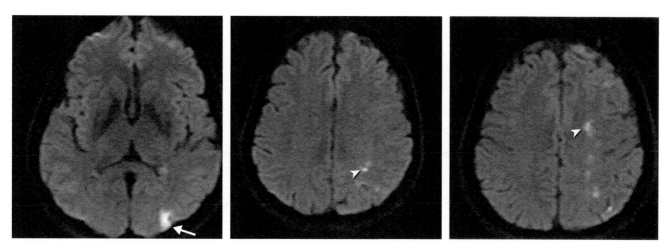

Figure 1.10 *Watershed Infarction.*
Diffusion-weighted magnetic resonance imaging scan of the brain shows a watershed infarction on the left side due to high-grade carotid stenosis. The ischemia in both the middle cerebral artery and posterior cerebral artery borderzone area (arrow) and the parasagittal ischemia (arrowheads) are suggestive of a watershed infarction.

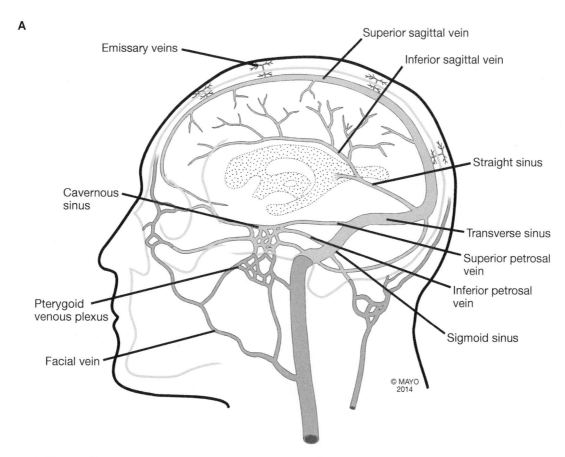

Figure 1.11 *A, Venous Sinuses. B, Magnetic resonance venogram depicting the major venous sinuses.*
(A is adapted from Flemming KD. Cerebrovascular disease. In: Mowzoon N, Flemming KD, editors. Neurology board review: an illustrated study guide. Rochester [MN]: Mayo Clinic Scientific Press and Florence [KY]: Informa Healthcare USA; c2007. p. 435–84. Used with permission of Mayo Foundation for Medical Education and Research.)

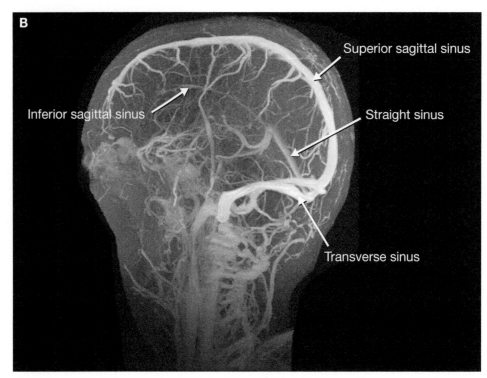

Figure 1.11 Continued

petrosal veins and finally into the transverse and sigmoid sinuses.

Deep cerebral veins drain such structures as the basal ganglia, deep white matter, and diencephalon. Figure 1.12 shows the location of the internal cerebral veins, the basal vein of Rosenthal, and the great cerebral vein of Galen.

Superficial cerebral veins drain the cerebral cortex and the superficial subcortical white matter. These veins include superior and inferior cerebral, superficial middle cerebral, superior anastomotic (Trolard), and inferior anastomotic (Labbé).

Spinal Cord Vasculature

Blood supply to the spinal cord emerges from the anterior and posterior spinal arteries (branches of the vertebral arteries) and from the spinal branches of segmental arteries. Paired anterior spinal arteries branch from vertebral arteries and join to form a single artery that descends along the anterior (ventral) aspect of the medulla and spinal cord. As the artery descends along the spinal cord, anastomotic branches from the anterior radicular arteries contribute to the vessel's continuity. The anterior spinal artery supplies the medial medulla and pyramids and the sulcal branches that enter the anterior median fissure of the spinal cord, to supply the anterior and lateral funiculi (Figure 1.13).

Paired posterior spinal arteries arise from vertebral arteries and occasionally from the posterior inferior cerebellar artery (PICA) and descend on the posterior surface of the spinal cord, medial to the dorsal roots (Figure 1.14). Similar to the anterior spinal artery, these arteries receive contributions from radicular arteries as they descend. The posterior spinal arteries supply the posterior third of the spinal cord, including the posterior columns.

Segmental and radicular arteries maintain continuity of the anterior and posterior spinal arteries at each level of the cord. The segmental arteries include the ascending cervical, intercostal, and lumbar arteries and contribute branches that further divide into anterior and posterior radicular arteries. A person may have as many as 31 pairs of radicular arteries; not every radicular artery contributes to spinal cord vascularization. The cervical cord has the most contributions. Thoracic and lumbar segments have fewer (2-4) arteries that contribute to the spinal cord blood supply, making these segments a region more vulnerable to ischemia. The blood supply to the midthoracic (T4-T6) segments is relatively tenuous and known as the *vascular watershed zone of the spinal cord*. The artery of Adamkiewicz—a large, anterior radicular artery at the level T12, L1, or L2—is a major source of blood to the lower thoracic and upper lumbar cord (Figure 1.14).

Anterolateral and anteromedian veins drain the anterior aspect of the spinal cord. The posterolateral and posteromedian veins drain the posterior cord and then drain into the radicular veins. These veins empty into the epidural venous plexus, which has longitudinal connections

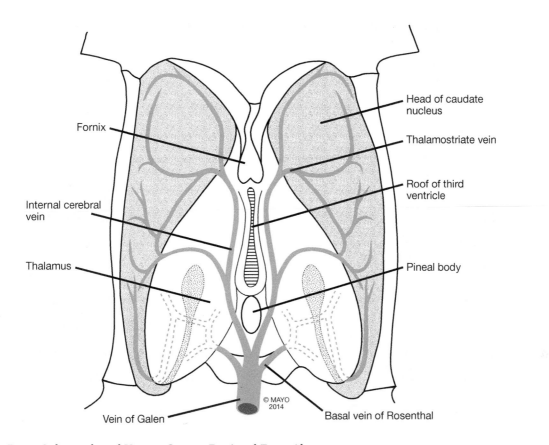

Figure 1.12 *Deep, Subependymal Venous System Depicted From Above.*
(Adapted from Flemming KD. Cerebrovascular disease. In: Mowzoon N, Flemming KD, editors. Neurology board review: an illustrated study guide. Rochester [MN]: Mayo Clinic Scientific Press and Florence [KY]: Informa Healthcare USA; c2007. p. 435–84. Used with permission of Mayo Foundation for Medical Education and Research.)

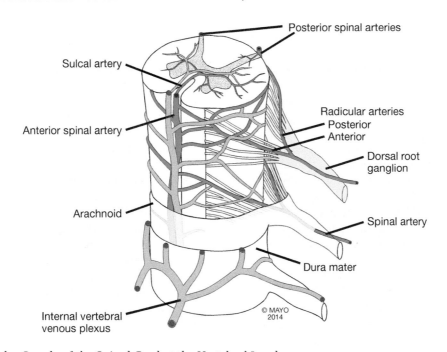

Figure 1.13 *Vascular Supply of the Spinal Cord at the Vertebral Level.*
(Adapted from Flemming KD. Cerebrovascular disease. In: Mowzoon N, Flemming KD, editors. Neurology board review: an illustrated study guide. Rochester [MN]: Mayo Clinic Scientific Press and Florence [KY]: Informa Healthcare USA; c2007. p. 435–84. Used with permission of Mayo Foundation for Medical Education and Research.)

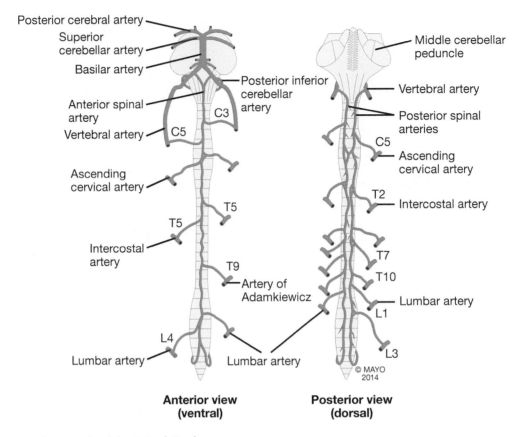

Figure 1.14 *Vascular Supply of the Spinal Cord.*
(Adapted from Flemming KD. Cerebrovascular disease. In: Mowzoon N, Flemming KD, editors. Neurology board review: an illustrated study guide. Rochester [MN]: Mayo Clinic Scientific Press and Florence [KY]: Informa Healthcare USA; c2007. p. 435–84. Used with permission of Mayo Foundation for Medical Education and Research.)

with other veins of the central nervous system (extending all the way to the brainstem region) and can drain into segmental veins and the systemic venous system.

- From the aortic arch arise 3 major blood vessels (from right to left): brachiocephalic (innominate), left common carotid, and left subclavian arteries.
- Three main branches of the internal carotid artery are (in order of occurrence) ophthalmic, posterior communicating, and anterior choroidal arteries.
- Perforating or penetrating arteries, including the recurrent artery of Heubner and medial lenticulostriates, supply the following deep structures: head of the caudate, corpus callosum, and part of the fornix.
- Cortical branches supply the medial and parasagittal aspect of the hemispheres.
- The cortical branches supply the lateral aspect of the cerebral hemisphere and anterior temporal lobe.
- The vertebral arteries arise from their respective subclavian arteries.
- Two long circumferential branches—anterior inferior cerebellar artery and superior cerebellar artery—supply

the lateral pons inferiorly and superiorly, respectively, and a portion of the cerebellum.

- Cranial nerves III, IV, and VI and the first and second divisions of cranial nerve V also travel through the cavernous sinus.
- Blood supply to the spinal cord emerges from the anterior and posterior spinal arteries, which are branches of the vertebral arteries.
- The thoracic and lumbar segments have fewer (2-4) arteries that contribute to the spinal cord blood supply, making these segments a region more vulnerable to ischemia.
- The artery of Adamkiewicz is a large, anterior radicular artery at the level T12, L1, or L2 and is a major source of blood to the lower thoracic and upper lumbar cord.

Blood-Brain Barrier

Unlike the systemic capillaries, capillaries in the brain are nonfenestrated. They are joined to other endothelial cells through tight junctions. Surrounding the endothelium is a basement membrane and a layer of astrocytic

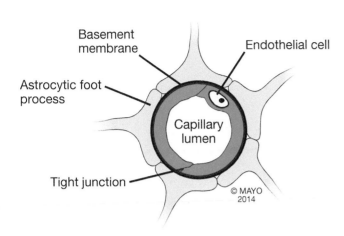

Figure 1.15 Nonfenestrated Capillary of the Central Nervous System.
Endothelial cells are joined by tight junctions that form the blood-brain barrier and are surrounded by a basement membrane and a sheath of astrocytic foot processes.
(Adapted from Benarroch EE, Daube JR, Flemming KD, Westmoreland BF. Mayo Clinic medical neurosciences: organized by neurologic systems and levels. 5th ed. Rochester [MN]: Mayo Clinic Scientific Press and Florence [KY]: Informa Healthcare USA; c2008. Chapter 4, Diagnosis of neurologic disorders: neurocytology and the pathologic reactions of the nervous system; p. 101–49. Used with permission of Mayo Foundation for Medical Education and Research.)

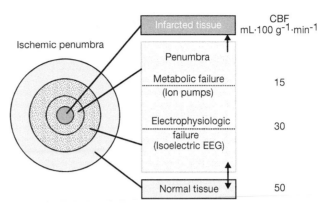

Figure 1.16 The Ischemic Penumbra.
Decreased cerebral blood flow (CBF) produces a gradient of severity of deprivation of oxygen and glucose in brain tissue. Between the area of infarction and normal tissue is an area of jeopardized brain tissue called the ischemic penumbra. *Neurons in this region have potentially reversible electrophysiologic failure due to energy deprivation but have not had the cascade leading to neuronal death. The ischemic penumbra is the target of neuroprotective treatment in ischemic stroke.*
(Adapted from Benarroch EE, Daube JR, Flemming KD, Westmoreland BF. Mayo Clinic medical neurosciences: organized by neurologic systems and levels. 5th ed. Rochester [MN]: Mayo Clinic Scientific Press and Florence [KY]: Informa Healthcare USA; c2008. Chapter 12, The vascular system; p. 447–88. Used with permission of Mayo Foundation for Medical Education and Research.)

foot processes. These barriers represent what is known as the *blood-brain barrier* (Figure 1.15).

Ischemic Stroke Pathophysiology

Principles of Cellular Injury and Vascular Biology

Normal cerebral blood flow in humans is approximately 50 to 60 mL/100 g of brain tissue per minute (Figure 1.16). When flow decreases to 20 to 40 mL/100 g per minute, neuronal dysfunction occurs; when it is less than 10 to 15 mL/100 g per minute, irreversible tissue damage occurs.

Because of extensive collateral circulation, variability exists in the perfusion changes within an ischemic lesion. The central core of the area with reduced flow often has irreversible cellular damage. Around the core is a region of decreased flow in which either the critical flow threshold for cell death has not been reached or the duration of ischemia is insufficient to cause irreversible damage. This area is called the *ischemic penumbra*. Perfusion imaging is used to quantify this penumbral region (Figure 1.17). If blood flow is not restored, the penumbra may cause permanent and irreversible damage. In addition to lack of

glucose and oxygen to the tissue, other mechanisms can contribute to this cell death. Excess glutamate release and impaired glutamate reuptake during ischemia result in elevations of calcium levels in the cytosol. Increased calcium in the cytosol then triggers release of proteases, lipases, endonucleases, and cytokines, which result in neuronal cell death.

Figure 1.18 shows the acute and subacute pathologic changes associated with ischemic infarction. In the acute phase (1 day-1 week), the gross specimen shows edema in the affected area. Microscopically, eosinophilic pyknotic neurons and neuropil vacuolation occur, often prominent at the edge of the infarction. Within 1 to 3 days, an inflammatory response is seen, followed by a mononuclear cell influx by 3 to 5 days. The mononuclear cells phagocytize dying cells.

In the subacute phase (1 week-1 month), the gross specimen shows tissue destruction and liquefactive necrosis. Infiltration of reactive astrocytes and prominent macrophages and phagocytosis are noted microscopically.

After approximately 1 month, in the chronic phase of an infarction, the affected area cavitates and has surrounding gliosis. Microscopically, a cystic cavity is noted

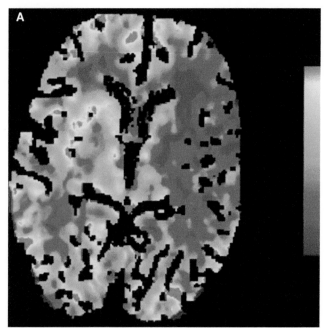

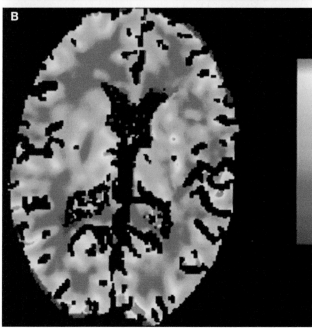

Figure 1.17 Computed Tomographic Perfusion.
A, The cerebral blood flow map reveals reduced flow in the left middle cerebral artery territory. B, The cerebral blood volume map reveals relatively normal volume (the middle cerebral artery territory is not infarcted). Taken together with the blood flow map, this perfusion sequence is suggestive of salvageable tissue in the left middle cerebral territory.

and has surrounding gliosis (Figure 1.19). Residual macrophage infiltration may also occur.

Atherogenesis

Atherosclerosis is a common cause of ischemic stroke. Atherosclerotic plaque formation requires several sequential steps that are set into motion by certain

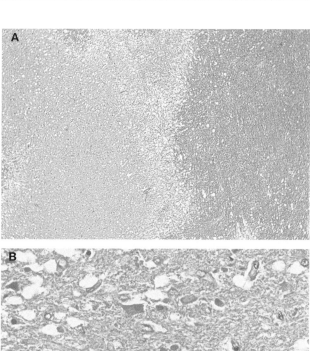

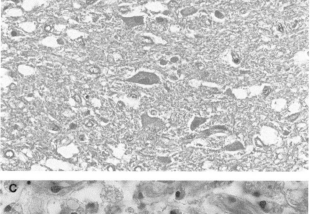

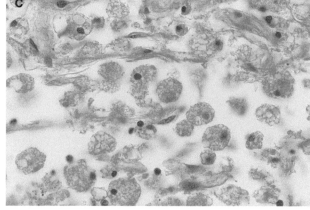

Figure 1.18 Acute and Subacute Ischemic Infarct.
In the acute stage of infarction, a clear interface often is present between the pale zone of ischemia and richly stained normal tissue. A, The edge of the infarct is marked by vacuolation of the neuropil. B, Neurons in the region of the acute ischemic event often appear pyknotic and intensely eosinophilic, appearing as little red cells. C, Foamy macrophages usually appear in the subacute stage and can persist for several months after the insult.
(Adapted from Flemming KD. Cerebrovascular disease. In: Mowzoon N, Flemming KD, editors. Neurology board review: an illustrated study guide. Rochester [MN]: Mayo Clinic Scientific Press and Florence [KY]: Informa Healthcare USA; c2007. p. 435–84. Used with permission of Mayo Foundation for Medical Education and Research.)

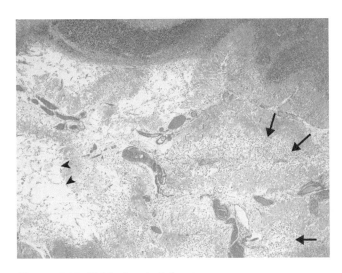

Figure 1.19 Old Ischemic Infarct.
In the chronic stage (after several weeks), liquefactive necrosis leads to cystic cavitation (arrowheads). This results from resorptive action of macrophages on damaged tissue (arrows).

(Adapted from Flemming KD. Cerebrovascular disease. In: Mowzoon N, Flemming KD, editors. Neurology board review: an illustrated study guide. Rochester [MN]: Mayo Clinic Scientific Press and Florence [KY]: Informa Healthcare USA; c2007. p. 435–84. Used with permission of Mayo Foundation for Medical Education and Research.)

triggers and risk factors, including hypertension, diabetes mellitus, obesity, chronic inflammation or infection, and an increased concentration of oxidized lipoproteins.

When endothelial cells become activated by these triggers, white cells express a cell adhesion protein. Certain adhesion molecules allow migration of white blood cells into the intima, and these monocytes transform into macrophages. The macrophages engulf lipoproteins and become *foam cells*, which can secrete mediators that allow continued accumulation of other monocytes, promote smooth muscle cell proliferation in the vessel, and change the extracellular matrix, degrading the collagenous protective structure. Over time, the plaque continually changes in response to the ongoing triggers and risk factors (lipid content, intramural hemorrhage, and calcification). Arteries may show progressive narrowing of the lumen or the endothelial integrity may become vulnerable from proliferation of metalloproteinases that degrade the plaque stability. When the plaque is unstable and ruptures, the subendothelium is exposed and platelets can adhere and aggregate, resulting in thrombus formation. Atherosclerosis is most common at arterial bifurcations, such as the branch point of the internal and external carotid arteries.

2

Meninges and Ventricles

RUPLE S. LAUGHLIN, MD; KELLY D. FLEMMING, MD

Introduction

Knowledge of the normal structure and function of the meninges and ventricular system can aid in recognizing and understanding pathologic states. This chapter reviews the meninges, ventricular system, and cerebrospinal fluid production. Clinical testing of the cerebrospinal fluid is covered in Chapter 33, "Cerebrospinal Fluid."

Meningeal Layers

Three layers of meninges cover the brain and spinal cord. They are the dura, arachnoid, and pia and function to 1) protect the underlying brain and spinal cord, 2) serve as a support framework for important arteries and veins, and 3) enclose a fluid-filled cavity important to normal function of the brain and spinal cord.

The dura mater, also called *pachymeninx*, is made of 2 layers: the periosteal layer (nearest the bone) and the meningeal layer. The dura is innervated by the fifth cranial nerve (anterior and middle fossae) supratentorially and by the vagus and cervical roots (C2 and C3) infratentorially. Arterial supply to the dura is from the branches of the external carotid artery (eg, ascending pharyngeal, middle meningeal, accessory meningeal), internal carotid artery branching off the cavernous segment, and vertebral arteries (occipital artery). The branches lie within the periosteal layer of the dura.

The 2 layers of the dura separate to form the dural venous sinuses. (See Chapter 1, "Cerebrovascular Anatomy and Pathophysiology.") The layers of meningeal dura also form septa, dividing the brain into various parts. The tentorium cerebelli overlies the cerebellum and divides the infratentorial portion of the brain from the supratentorial portion. At the tentorial notch (or incisure), the tentorium encircles the brainstem. The falx cerebri divides the 2 cerebral hemispheres.

The arachnoid lies under the dura. Arachnoid granulations are tufted protrusions of arachnoid that pass through the dura into the superior sagittal sinus; they consist of numerous arachnoid villi. In the arachnoid, cerebrospinal fluid (CSF) from the subarachnoid space is transferred to the venous system through a pressure-dependent mechanism. Between the arachnoid layer and the pia is the subarachnoid space. Blood vessels and cerebrospinal fluid run through this space, and cranial and spinal nerves exit it.

The areas where the pia and arachnoid are widely separated are known as *cisterns*. Important cisterns are cisterna magna (cerebellomedullary cistern), interpeduncular cistern, and lumbar cisterns.

The pia mater is made of 2 layers also and lies on the parenchymal surface (the brain surface). The pia and arachnoid together are referred to as the *leptomeninges*.

At the margin of the foramen magnum, the periosteal dura stops but the meningeal dura continues caudally into the vertebral canal. In the spinal cord, the meningeal dura extends to the level of the second sacral vertebra. The caudal termination of the dural sac invests the filum terminale externum to form a thin fibrous cord, the coccygeal ligament.

The spinal cord ends at the lower border of the first lumbar vertebra. Unlike the epidural space in the brain, the epidural space in the spinal cord contains fat and a venous plexus. The CSF flows in the subarachnoid space and can be accessed clinically at the level of the lumbar cistern.

- The dura mater (pachymeninx) is made of 2 layers: periosteal layer (nearest the bone) and meningeal layer.
- The dura is innervated by the fifth cranial nerve supratentorially (anterior and middle fossae) and by

Abbreviation: CSF, cerebrospinal fluid

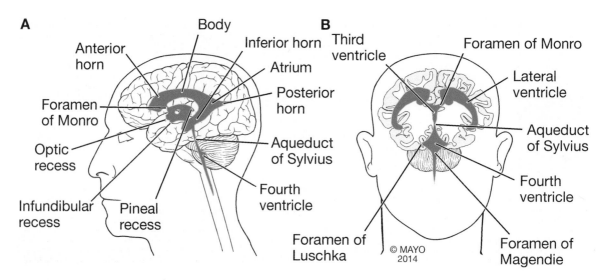

Figure 2.1 *The Ventricular System.*

A, Lateral view. B, Anterior view. The pons has been removed from panel B to show the anatomy of the fourth ventricle. (Adapted from Benarroch EE, Daube JR, Flemming KD, Westmoreland BF. Mayo Clinic medical neurosciences: organized by neurologic systems and levels. 5th ed. Rochester [MN]: Mayo Clinic Scientific Press and Florence [KY]: Informa Healthcare USA; c2008. Chapter 11, Cerebrospinal fluid: ventricular system; p. 421–46. Used with permission of Mayo Foundation for Medical Education and Research.)

the vagus and cervical roots (C2 and C3) infratentorially.

- The arachnoid is the site where cerebrospinal fluid (CSF) from the subarachnoid space is transferred to the venous system through a pressure-dependent mechanism.
- Areas where the pia and arachnoid are widely separated are known as *cisterns*.
- The pia mater has 2 layers and lies on the parenchymal surface (the brain surface).

The Ventricular System

The ventricular system is composed of the 2 lateral ventricles separated by the septum pellucidum, a midline third ventricle, and the fourth ventricle (Figure 2.1). The ventricles of the brain and the central canal of the spinal cord are lined with cuboidal epithelium, called the *ependyma*.

The blood-CSF barrier exists to allow control of certain metabolites and ions flowing into the CSF from the bloodstream. Choroidal epithelial cells connected by tight junctions line the surface of choroid plexus villi. Underneath this epithelium, a layer of collagen and fibroblasts forms a barrier between the epithelium and the blood flow.

Cerebrospinal Fluid

The epithelial cells of the choroid plexus secrete CSF. The choroid plexuses are branched structures with villous projections that extend into each of the 4 ventricles.

The process of CSF secretion involves the transport of sodium (Na^+), chloride (Cl^-) ions, and carbonic acid (HCO_3^-) from the blood and is highly dependent on the function of the Na^+-K^+/ATPase pump located in the apical membrane of the choroid plexus. In addition, a smaller percentage of CSF is made by blood vessels lining the ventricular walls.

CSF fills the ventricle of the brain, the spinal canal, and the subarachnoid space. This circulation of CSF is perpetuated by pulsations of the choroid plexus and the motion of the cilia on the ependymal cells. CSF flows from the lateral ventricles through the foramen of Monro into the third ventricle and through the aqueduct of Sylvius into the fourth ventricle. Here, it leaves the ventricles medially through the foramen of Magendie or laterally through the foramens of Luschka and moves into the subarachnoid space. Next, CSF flows over the entire surface of the brain, as well as the spinal cord.

Carbonic anhydrases are speculated to have a role in CSF production. These enzymes catalyze the formation of HCO_3^- from water and carbon dioxide. They are not directly involved in ion transport. Inhibiting carbonic anhydrase (eg, with the drug acetazolamide) reduces CSF production, likely secondary to carbon dioxide accumulation in cerebral tissue.

In humans and at any time, the total volume of CSF within the structures outlined above is about 150 mL, of which 75 mL is in the cranial cavity. However, CSF is produced at a rate of 0.35 mL/minute, or approximately 600 mL/day. This difference in the quantity made and the quantity present is possible because of active absorption of CSF by arachnoid granulations within the superior sagittal

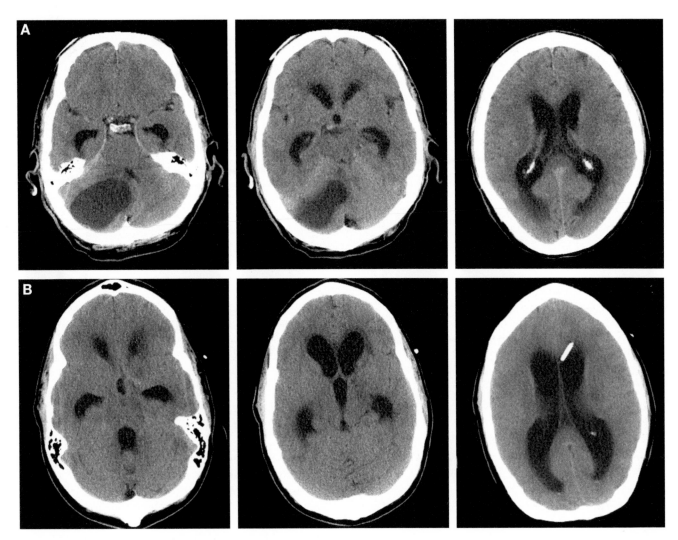

Figure 2.2 *Computed Tomography in Hydrocephalus.*
Row A, Obstructive hydrocephalus due to a cystic mass, with pressure on the fourth ventricle. Third and lateral ventricles are enlarged. Row B, Nonobstructive or communicating hydrocephalus. The lateral, third, and fourth ventricles are enlarged. An external ventricular drain is visible in the left lateral ventricle.

sinus. These granulations act as 1-way valves between the subarachnoid spaces and the dural sinuses. As a result, an average person's entire CSF volume turns over about 4 times daily.

CSF absorption is directly linked to intracranial pressure. In steady states, its rate equals CSF formation, where the normal resting pressure of CSF is typically between 150 and 180 mm H_2O. Its normal range is from 65 to 200 mm H_2O (the equivalent of 5–15 mm Hg). Of note, 1 mm Hg equals 1.36 cm H_2O.

The role of human CSF is to 1) provide buoyancy for the brain, 2) provide an excretory function (because the brain lacks a lymphatic system), 3) serve as an intracerebral transport mechanism (of neuroendocrine-stimulating hormones, for example), and 4) maintain homeostasis of the central nervous system. The choroid plexus, as

well as arachnoid granulations and capillary endothelial cells in the ependymal brain lining, are lined with tight junctions that maintain the blood-brain barrier. Portions of the brain known as *circumventricular organs* are not lined with this endothelial layer, including the area postrema, subfornical, and subcommissural organs, and therefore are more subject to the effects of systemic toxins or substances. The anatomy of the blood-brain barrier is crucial because pathologic conditions can alter the integrity of this barrier, allowing direct toxicity to the brain and central nervous system structures through alteration in the CSF composition. For example, anoxia and ischemia can cause increased transmembrane permeability of potentially toxic ion species. Chemical toxins, seizures, and other metabolic states can have a similar effect.

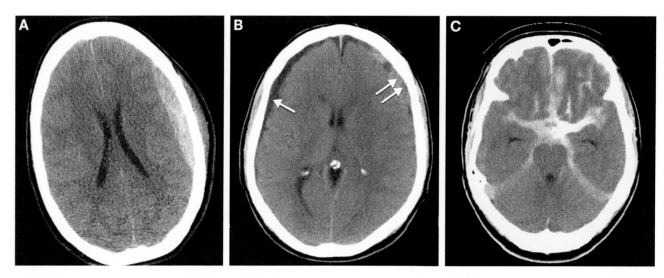

Figure 2.3 Computed Tomography of Brain Hematoma.
A, A left epidural hematoma. The lens-shaped hematoma does not cross suture lines. B, Bilateral subdural hematoma. A chronic (hypodensity on CT) subdural hematoma is visible on the right side of the brain (arrow) and a subacute (isodense on CT) subdural hematoma can be seen on the left side of the brain (double arrow). C, Hyperattenuation within the cisterns and sulci are suggestive of subarachnoid hemorrhage. The location of the subarachnoid blood shown on this scan is most suggestive of an aneurysmal subarachnoid hemorrhage.

For clinical testing of the CSF, see Chapter 33, "Cerebrospinal Fluid."

- Epithelial cells of the choroid plexus secrete CSF.
- At any given time, the total volume of CSF within the neurologic structures is about 150 mL in humans.
- The role of CSF in humans is to 1) provide buoyancy for the brain, 2) supply an excretory function (because the brain lacks a lymphatic system), 3) serve as an intracerebral transport mechanism (eg, neuroendocrine-stimulating hormones), and 4) maintain homeostasis of the central nervous system.
- The brain portions known as *circumventricular organs* are not lined with an endothelial layer, such as the area postrema, subfornical, and subcommissural organs, and therefore are more subject to effects of systemic toxins or substances.

Clinical Correlations

Hydrocephalus

Hydrocephalus results when excess CSF exists, with resultant dilatation of the ventricles. This clinical situation is most commonly due to either obstruction of the ventricular system (obstructive or noncommunicating hydrocephalus) or poor absorption by arachnoid granules (nonobstructive or communicating hydrocephalus). Obstructive hydrocephalus might result from a tumor within the ventricular system. In this type, all ventricles above the level of obstruction will be enlarged (Figure 2.2). Nonobstructive hydrocephalus might be due to meningitis or subarachnoid blood that prevents reabsorption of CSF through the arachnoid granules. This type of hydrocephalus causes enlargement of all ventricles (Figure 2.2). The differential diagnosis of the causes of hydrocephalus is in Volume 2, Chapter 70, "Malformation of the Brain, Skull, and Spine."

Types of Brain Hemorrhage

The epidural space is a potential space. The dural arteries run between the periosteal and meningeal dura, and blunt-force trauma may injure this arterial supply. The injury could result in an epidural hematoma (Figure 2.3A).

The so-called bridging veins run through the subdural space in route to draining into the venous sinuses. Head trauma may cause tearing of the bridging veins, causing a subdural hematoma (Figure 2.3B).

Subarachnoid hemorrhage commonly results from aneurysm rupture. The arteries run into the subarachnoid space and thus, when an aneurysm ruptures, it results in subarachnoid blood (Figure 2.3C).

3

Afferent System Overview

KELLY D. FLEMMING, MD; EDUARDO E. BENARROCH, MD

Introduction

The afferent, or sensory, systems include visual, auditory, somatosensory, and interoceptive (ie, pain, temperature, and visceral sensation) inputs to the central nervous system. This chapter briefly reviews principles of transduction, relay, and processing of sensory information. The dorsal column–medial lemniscal system is reviewed in more detail. However, pain, vision, olfaction, and hearing are reviewed in subsequent chapters.

General Principles of the Sensory Systems

Overview

Sensory transduction refers to the transformation of a stimulus into an electric signal. This process involves several distinct families of cation channels (Table 3.1) and associated receptor types (Figure 3.1). The change in cation influx during the transduction process elicits a receptor (or generator) potential that results in depolarization of the afferent axon. The only exceptions are the photoreceptors (rods and cones), in which light closes a cyclic

Table 3.1 • Cation Channels Involved in Sensory Transduction

Cation Channel	Type of Receptor
Degenerin/epithelial Na⁺	Mechanoreceptors
Cyclic nucleotide gated	Photoreceptors, olfactory, taste
Transient receptor potential	Pain, temperature

Abbreviation: Na⁺, sodium ion.

nucleotide-gated channel, results in hyperpolarization, and interrupts tonic release of glutamate to the target bipolar cells.

Several general features are characteristic of all afferent systems (Box 3.1).

Transduction

The intensity of the sensory stimulus results in a receptor potential whose amplitude is proportional. Intense stimuli result in receptor potentials of larger amplitude. These large-amplitude responses generate threshold action potential faster than small-amplitude responses. Thus, stimulus intensity is encoded by the firing frequency of the afferent axon. Slowly adapting receptors maintain action potential discharge as long as stimulus remains. Rapidly adapting receptors signal brief changes triggered by either onset or termination of the stimuli.

Receptor Field Organization

Most sensory pathways are modality specific and topographically organized. The receptive field of a peripheral or central sensory neuron is defined by the population of peripheral sensory receptors that can influence its activity. In general, receptive fields have a center-surround organization (Figure 3.2). This center-surround organization reflects a mechanism of lateral inhibition within each relay nucleus. Strong stimuli activate a restricted population of projection neurons and, via inhibitory interneurons, prevent relay of weaker stimuli by the surrounding projection neuron.

Thalamic Relay

All sensory pathways are excitatory and use L-glutamate as their neurotransmitter. Except for the olfactory system,

Abbreviation: GABA, γ-aminobutyric acid

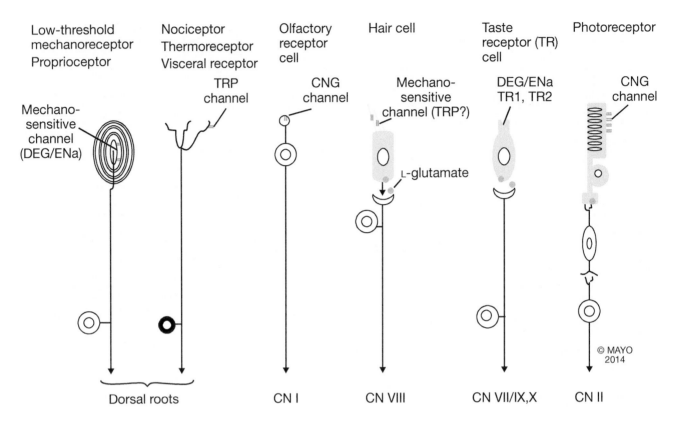

Figure 3.1 Overview of Sensory Receptors.

The receptor molecules responsible for sensory transduction belong to several distinct families of cation channels, including the degenerin/epithelial Na⁺ channel (DEG/ENa), the cyclic nucleotide-gated (CNG), and the transient receptor potential (TRP) channel families. Somatosensory and olfactory neurons are the first neurons of the sensory pathway and contain the receptor molecules in their peripheral processes. Photoreceptors, hair cells, and taste receptor (TR) cells are specialized cells to receive a synapse from a primary afferent terminal and release L-glutamate at these synapses, depolarizing the primary afferent. CN indicates cranial nerve. (Adapted from Benarroch EE. Basic neurosciences with clinical applications. Philadelphia [PA]: Butterworth Heinemann/Elsevier; c2006. Chapter 13, Relay of exteroceptive information: somatosensory, visual, and auditory systems; p. 345-90. Used with permission of Mayo Foundation for Medical Education and Research.)

sensory pathways project to modality-specific relay nuclei of the thalamus (Figure 3.3). The thalamocortical neurons project from these nuclei to layer 4 of the primary sensory cortical areas. In that same cortical column receiving thalamocortical input, layer 6 neurons project back to the thalamic relay nucleus. Thalamocortical and corticothalamic neurons also project collaterals to the reticular nucleus of the thalamus, which sends γ-aminobutyric acid (GABA) ergic inputs to the relay nuclei and serves as a gate for sensory information. In addition, each relay nuclei, together with the intralaminar thalamic nuclei, contain neurons that project diffusely to layer 1, providing for synchronized activity of spatially separate neuronal networks located in functionally related columns and receiving and processing the same type of sensory input.

Cortical Organization

The primary somatosensory, visual, and auditory cortices are characterized by a prominent layer 4 (granular layer).

Each sensory area receives topographically organized, submodality-specific projections from their respective thalamic relay nuclei. The thalamocortical neurons project to layer 4, which then projects to layers 2 and 3 in the same vertical column, or *functional unit*. Neurons within each functional unit receive input from the same thalamocortical neurons. Activation of a column is associated with inhibition of surrounding columns through GABAergic basket

Box 3.1 • Common Features of Sensory Systems
Stimulus coding
Receptive field properties
Topographic representation of receptive fields
Parallel channels for subcortical relay (thalamus)
Cortical control of sensory relay
Parallel pathways for sensory processing

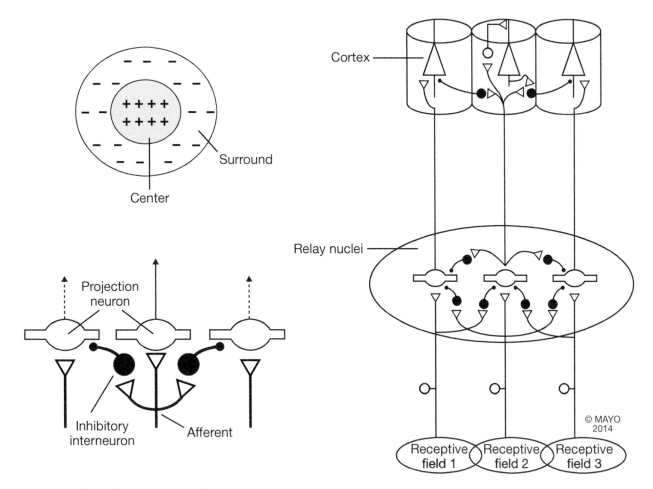

Figure 3.2 *Relay of Exteroceptive Information.*
At each relay station of the sensory systems, including the thalamus, the receptive fields have a center-surround organization, which depends on mechanisms of lateral inhibition. The afferent excites the projection neuron and the inhibitory interneuron; the interneurons activated by the most active afferent restrict, through feed-forward and feedback mechanisms, the activity of surrounding neurons receiving weaker stimuli.
(Adapted from Benarroch EE. Basic neurosciences with clinical applications. Philadelphia [PA]: Butterworth Heinemann/Elsevier; c2006. Chapter 13, Relay of exteroceptive information: somatosensory, visual, and auditory systems; p. 345–90. Used with permission of Mayo Foundation for Medical Education and Research.)

cells. This lateral inhibition is important for spatial discrimination and direction selectivity of cortical sensory neurons. Columns with similar properties are interconnected with each other over widespread areas of cerebral cortex.

Serial Processing of Sensory Organization

Serial or *hierarchical processing* refers to a propagation of sensory information from primary areas to higher-order association areas. It also may refer to information coming from association areas that modulate lower levels of information. For example, sensory information reaching the primary sensory area is then processed in unimodal sensory association areas. Through such processing, increased complexity of features can allow better representation of the whole object (eg, I feel an object vs I feel an object with a triangular shape, hard surface, and sharp edges moving along my hand).

Unimodal sensory association areas then project to heteromodal sensory association areas in the parietal and lateral temporal cortices (Figure 3.4). The neurons in these heteromodal areas respond to specific combinations of visual, somatosensory, and auditory features. Cortical organization in the cortex is discussed in Chapter 21, "Cortex Topography and Organization."

- Stimulus intensity is encoded by the firing frequency of the afferent axon.
- *Sensory transduction* refers to the transformation of a stimulus into an electric signal.
- Most sensory pathways are modality specific and topographically organized.

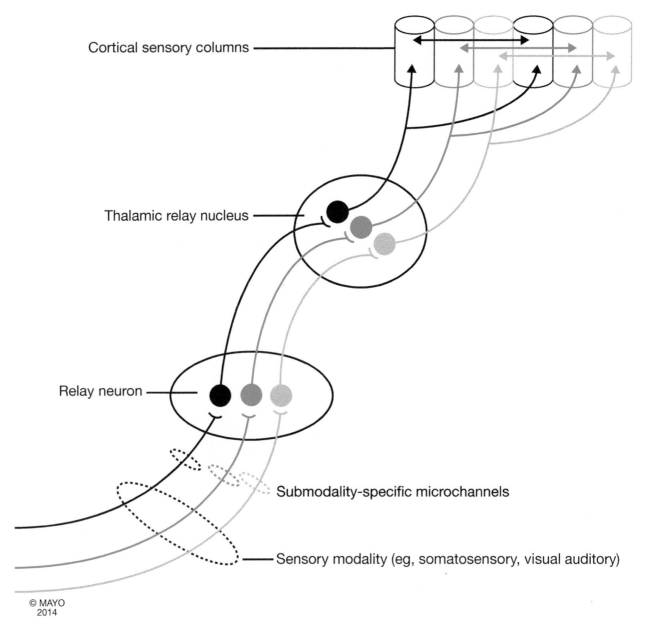

Cortical sensory columns

Thalamic relay nucleus

Relay neuron

Submodality-specific microchannels

Sensory modality (eg, somatosensory, visual auditory)

© MAYO
2014

Figure 3.3 Submodality-Specific Relay.
Each primary sensory area receives topographically organized, submodality-specific projections from the corresponding thalamic relay nucleus and subcortical relay neurons.
(Used with permission of Mayo Foundation for Medical Education and Research.)

- All sensory pathways are excitatory and use L-glutamate as their neurotransmitter.
- Except for the olfactory system, sensory pathways project to modality-specific relay nuclei of the thalamus.
- Each sensory area receives topographically organized, submodality-specific projections from their respective thalamic relay nuclei.
- *Serial* or *hierarchical processing* refers to a propagation of sensory information from primary areas to higher-order association areas.

Parallel Processing of Sensory System: The Dorsal and Ventral Streams

The dorsal stream of the sensory system is involved in visuospatial processing and contains neurons that respond to object location and movement and project to the posterior parietal cortex (Figure 3.5). This information is important for visuospatial orientation (the "where" of the object). Different subsets of posterior parietal cortex neurons project to neurons in the premotor cortex. These interconnections are important in the initiation of movements

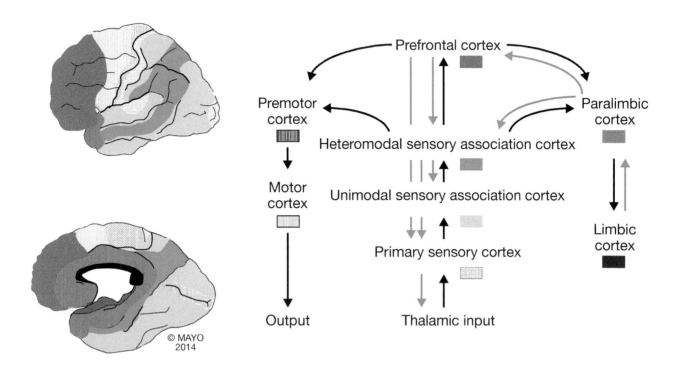

Figure 3.4 *Functional Cytoarchitectonics of the Cerebral Cortex.*
There is a hierarchical and parallel processing of sensory information in the cerebral cortex. Sensory information reaching the primary sensory areas is processed first in the unimodal sensory association areas. Serial processing by neurons in unimodal areas that respond with increased complexity to combinations of features (eg, edges, shapes, direction of movement), which allow representation of the whole object (perception). Each unimodal sensory association area projects to heteromodal sensory association areas in the posterior parietal cortex and lateral temporal cortex. Neurons in these heteromodal areas respond to specific combinations of visual, somatosensory, and auditory features. These heteromodal association areas connect with the prefrontal, and premotor cortex or, via paralimbic areas, with the amygdala and hippocampus (limbic areas).
(Used with permission of Mayo Foundation for Medical Education and Research.)

such as saccades, reaching, and grasping under visual guidance.

The ventral stream involves neurons of the lateral temporal cortex that are important in the identification of objects, including such features as shape and color (the "what" of the object). Connections of these neurons by the superior and lateral temporal gyrus and temporal pole, with the dominant language network, hippocampus, and amygdala, are essential for object and face recognition, symbolic representation and naming (language), and an emotional reaction to the object.

The heteromodal sensory areas also are connected reciprocally with the dorsolateral prefrontal cortex and paralimbic areas.

Overview of Sensory Pathways

An overview of the sensory pathways is noted in Figure 3.6. The special somatic afferent systems (vestibular, auditory, and visual) are covered in Chapter 5, "Special Somatic Sensory Afferent Overview." Pain receptors and central

pathways are reviewed in Chapter 4, "Peripheral and Central Pain Pathways and Pathophysiology." Olfaction is covered in Chapter 13, "Cranial Nerves I and II."

Dorsal Column–Medial Lemniscal System

Receptors

The dorsal column–medial lemniscal system receives input from low-threshold skin mechanoreceptors (tactile discrimination), muscle spindles in the fingers (stereognosis and fine motor control), and proprioceptors (muscle spindles and joint receptors in large joints) that regulate posture, gait, and reaching movements. In this system, submodality neurons—those that respond to inputs from tactile receptors and those that receive inputs from proprioceptors—remain segregated at the levels of the dorsal column nuclei, ventral posterior complex of the thalamus, and primary somatosensory cortex (S1). The receptors and their features are noted in Table 3.2.

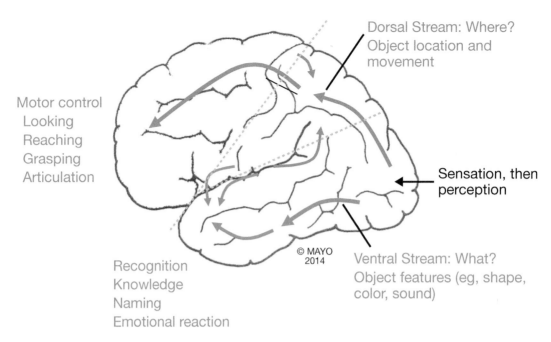

Dorsal Stream: Where?
Object location and
movement

Motor control
Looking
Reaching
Grasping
Articulation

Sensation, then
perception

© MAYO
2014

Ventral Stream: What?
Object features (eg, shape,
color, sound)

Recognition
Knowledge
Naming
Emotional reaction

Figure 3.5 Parallel Processing in Dorsal and Ventral Streams of Sensory Information. The dorsal stream is involved in visuospatial processing and contains neurons that respond to object location and movement and project to the posterior parietal cortex. This information is critical for visuospatial orientation ("where"). The ventral stream involves neurons of the lateral temporal cortex that progressively extract specific features, such as combinations of shapes and colors, that are necessary for object identification ("what").

(Used with permission of Mayo Foundation for Medical Education and Research.)

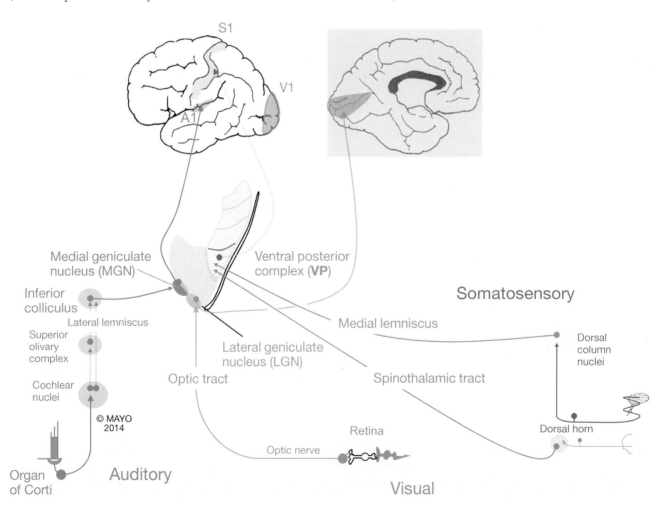

S1

V1

A1

Medial geniculate
nucleus (MGN)

Ventral posterior
complex (**VP**)

Somatosensory

Inferior
colliculus

Lateral lemniscus

Medial lemniscus

Dorsal
column
nuclei

Superior
olivary
complex

Lateral geniculate
nucleus (LGN)

Cochlear
nuclei

© MAYO
2014

Optic tract

Spinothalamic tract

Retina

Dorsal horn

Optic nerve

Organ
of Corti

Auditory

Visual

Figure 3.6 Overview of Exteroceptive Pathways (Classical).

(Used with permission of Mayo Foundation for Medical Education and Research.)

Table 3.2 • Types of Sensory Receptors

Receptor	Stimulus	Function	Receptive Field, mm	Adaptation
Meissner corpuscle	Dynamic skin deformation	Touch; edge contour; Braille-type stimuli	3–5	Moderately rapid
Merkel disk	Points, corners, edges	Touch; perception of texture and form	2–3	Slow
Ruffini end-organ	Static forces (skin stretch)	Proprioception (hand and finger position)	15–25	Slow
Pacini corpuscle	Sensitive to mechanical and vibratory stimuli	Vibration	Large	Rapid

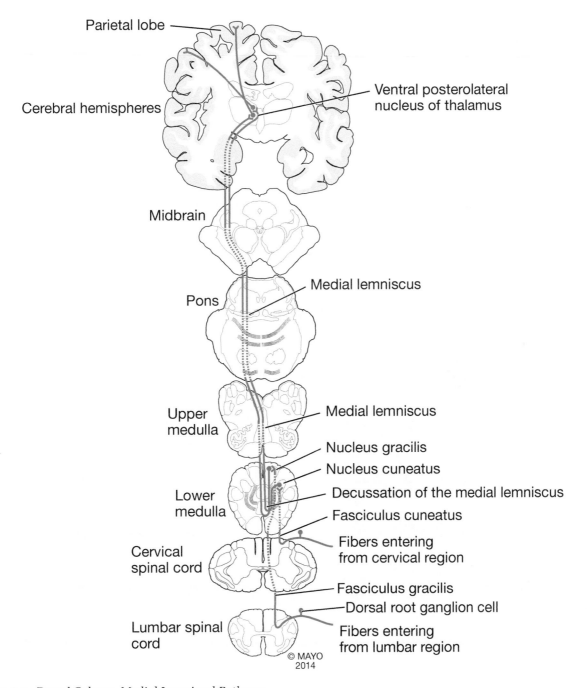

Figure 3.7. Dorsal Column–Medial Lemniscal Pathway.
Conscious proprioception and discriminative sensation.
(Adapted from Benarroch EE, Daube JR, Flemming KD, Westmoreland BF. Mayo Clinic medical neurosciences: organized by neurologic systems and levels. 5th ed. Rochester [MN]: Mayo Clinic Scientific Press and Florence [KY]: Informa Healthcare USA; c2008. Chapter 7, The sensory system; p. 217–64. Used with permission of Mayo Foundation for Medical Education and Research.)

Central Pathways

The dorsal column–medial lemniscal pathway functions to carry conscious proprioception, fine touch, and vibration (Figure 3.7).

The cells of origin for the dorsal column–medial lemniscal pathway are in the dorsal root ganglion of the spinal nerves. Sensory information from the lower extremities enters the fasciculus gracilis by way of the dorsal root ganglion. Information ascends medially and ipsilaterally in the fasciculus gracilis. Sensory information from T6 and above enters the fasciculus cuneatus and ascends ipsilaterally. Information ascends to the level of the caudal medulla, where neurons in the fasciculus cuneatus and gracilis synapse with their respective nuclei. From the second-order neuron, axons sweep forward and cross or decussate and become the medial lemniscus. The medial lemniscal fibers rise to the ventroposterior thalamus, where they synapse again. The third-order neurons from the ventroposterior group of the thalamus ascend to the primary sensory cortex.

4

Peripheral and Central Pain Pathways and Pathophysiology

EDUARDO E. BENARROCH, MD; JAMES C. WATSON, MD;
KELLY D. FLEMMING, MD

Introduction

Pain is an unpleasant sensory experience that may be associated with actual or potential tissue damage. Perception of pain includes the sensory-discriminative (intensity and location), cognitive (bodily sensation), and affective-emotional (suffering) aspects. Pain is a complex integration of anatomic pathways, including dorsal root ganglion (DRG) nociceptive neurons, dorsal horn neurons, spinothalamic and spinobulbar pathways, the thalamus, the cortex, and local modulation. Peripheral and central sensitization may occur after tissue injury.

This chapter reviews the peripheral and central processing of pain and concludes with discussion of pain pathophysiology.

Pain Receptors

Somatosensory receptors contain the receptor molecules in their peripheral processes. A nociceptor is a peripheral sensory receptor that encodes a noxious stimulus. Small neurons from the DRG terminate in free nerve endings in skin, muscle, and viscera. They may be either myelinated (Aδ) or unmyelinated (C) axons. These axons project to the dorsal horn and use glutamate. They may be further classified regarding their physiologic response: polymodal (response to mechanical, thermal, and chemical stimuli), mechano-cold response (C-MC), and mechano-insensitive Aδ response (MIA). They also may be subdivided into peptidergic (containing substance P or calcitonin gene-related peptide and expressing the TrkA receptor for nerve growth factor) and nonpeptidergic (containing P2X3 receptors and expressing Ret receptor for glial cell line–derived neural factor). Nociceptors express specific ion channels (Table 4.1 and Figure 4.1). Dysfunction of select channels has been noted to change pain perception (Table 4.2).

Nociceptors may undergo sensitization in the clinical setting of injury or inflammation (because of cytokines, chemokines, growth factors, and autocoids). This sensitization is due to plastic changes in the expression and function of cation channels. Sensitization may result in reduced threshold for activation, increased response to noxious stimuli, and decreased adaptation (see the Pain Pathophysiology section).

Table 4.1 • Cation Channels Important in Pain Transmission

Ion Channels	Examples
Voltage-gated Na⁺	Nav1.7, Nav1.8, Nav1.9
TRP	TRPV1, TRPA1
ASICs	ASIC 1-3
Receptors for ATP and serotonin	P2X, 5HT3

Abbreviations: ASIC, acid-sensing ion channel; ATP, adenosine triphosphate; TRP, transient receptor potential; TRPA1, transient receptor potential subfamily A type 1; TRPV1, transient receptor potential vanilloid type 1.

Abbreviations: AMPA, α-amino-3-hydroxy-5-methyl-4-isoxazole propionic acid; ATP, adenosine triphosphate; C-MC, mechano-cold response; DRG, dorsal root ganglion; IL, interleukin; MIA, mechano-insensitive A-delta response; NMDA, N-methyl-ᴅ-aspartate; WDR, wide dynamic range

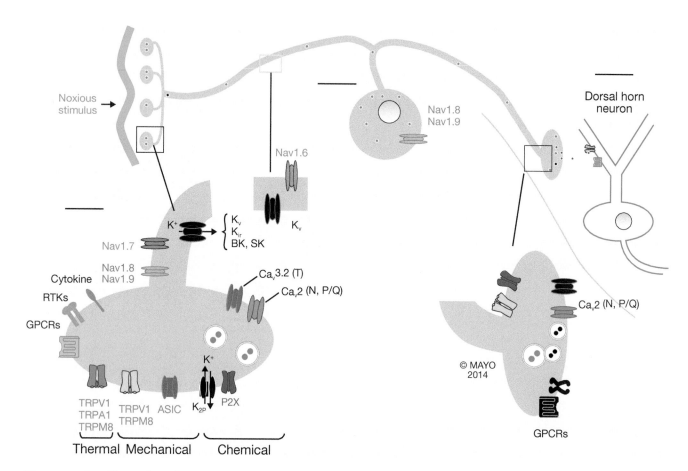

Figure 4.1 Ion Channels and Receptors in Nociceptors.
ASIC indicates acid-sensing ion channel; BK, BK voltage-gated potassium channel; GPCR, G-protein-coupled receptor; P/Q, P/Q voltage-gated calcium channel, P/Q type; RTK, receptor tyrosine kinase; SK, small conductance calcium-activated potassium channel.
(Used with permission of Mayo Foundation for Medical Education and Research.)

Table 4.2 • Channelopathy Disorders Associated With Change in Pain Perception

Disorder (Mutation)	Channel	Clinical Features
Inherited erythromelalgia, familial erythromelalgia (AD *SCN9A*)	Nav1.7	Attacks of burning pain and redness in distal extremities, triggered by mild warmth and exercise
Paroxysmal extreme pain disorder (AD *SCN9A*)	Nav1.7	Episodic lower body (rectal), ocular, and jaw pain associated with flushing and other autonomic manifestations
Channelopathy-associated insensitivity to pain (AR *SCN9A)*	Nav1.7	Inability to sense pain
Familial episodic pain syndrome (AD *TRPA1*)	TRPA1	Episodic upper-body pain triggered by fasting, cold, or stress

Abbreviations: AD, autosomal dominant; AR, autosomal recessive; TRPA1, transient receptor potential subfamily A type 1.
Adapted from Waxman SG. Channelopathic pain: a growing but still small list of model disorders. Neuron. 2010 Jun 10;66(5):622–4. Used with permission.

- Small neurons from the dorsal root ganglion (DRG) terminate in free nerve endings in skin, muscle, and viscera.
- These small neurons may be either myelinated (Aδ) or unmyelinated (C) axons.
- Nociceptors express specific ion channels.

Dorsal Horn

Pain signaling from the DRG neurons enters the spinal cord and terminates in Rexed laminae of the dorsal horn. Input from C and Aδ terminates in lamina I and II, and low-threshold mechanoreceptors (tactile) and Aβ extend

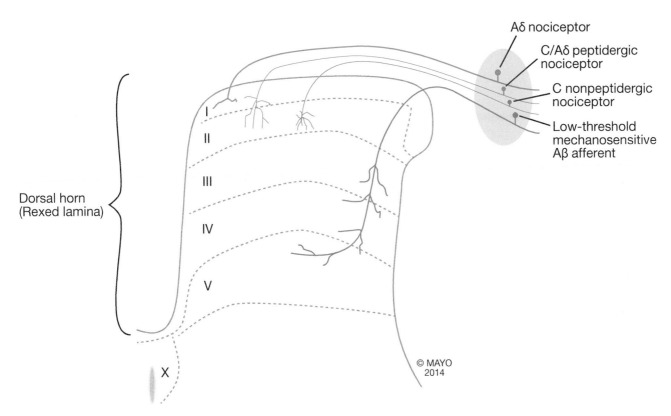

Figure 4.2 *Relay of Nociceptive Information to the Dorsal Horn.*
Aβ indicates, A-beta myelinated; Aδ, A-delta myelinated; C, unmyelinated.
(Used with permission of Mayo Foundation for Medical Education and Research.)

from lamina II to lamina V (Figure 4.2). Lamina I, III, and V project centrally via the spinothalamic tract. Other targets of pain signaling include the periaqueductal gray, lateral parabrachial nucleus, ventrolateral medulla, and nucleus of the solitary tract. Lamina II (substantia gelatinosa) contains local excitatory and inhibitory interneurons. Lamina V contains wide-dynamic-range (WDR) neurons.

Local circuitry is complex in the dorsal horn. Importantly, both local (interneurons) and descending (descending monoaminergic) central influences affect the transmission of pain.

- Pain signaling from the DRG neurons enters the spinal cord and terminates in Rexed laminae of the dorsal horn.
- Lamina I, III, and V project centrally via the spinothalamic tract.
- Lamina II (substantia gelatinosa) contains local excitatory and inhibitory interneurons.

Central Pain Pathways

Nociceptive or pain systems may be divided into lateral (sensory-discriminative) and medial (motivational-affective

and cognitive-evaluative) components (Table 4.3). Neurons from the dorsal horn cells project in the spinothalamic tract (Figure 4.3). This tract is anterolateral in the spinal cord and travels laterally in the brainstem. It terminates in various aspects of the thalamus. For the lateral system (sensory-discriminative), a synapse occurs in the ventral posterolateral nucleus. From there, third-order neurons travel to the primary (S1) and secondary (S2) somatosensory cortex (Figure 4.4).

Other neurons of the spinothalamic tract terminate in the ventral medial nucleus and then project to the insular cortex. This pathway is important in the experience of pain as a bodily sensation (cognitive-evaluative; also called *interoceptive*). Finally, some pain fibers project to the mediodorsal nucleus of the thalamus. In this pathway, third-order neurons from the mediodorsal thalamus project to the anterior cingulate gyrus. This component is responsible for the affective-emotional (suffering) aspect of pain and the arousal response associated with a painful stimulus.

Spinobulbar neurons are pain fibers that terminate in various subcortical structures, including the parabrachial nucleus, the nucleus of the solitary tract, the

Table 4.3 • Central Components of Pain Perception

System	Cell of Origin	Second-Order Neuron	Third-Order Neuron (Thalamus)	Cortex Termination	Function
Lateral	DRG	Dorsal horn	VPL	S1, S2	Sensory-discriminative
Medial	DRG	Dorsal horn	VMpo	Insula	Interoceptive (bodily sensation)
Medial	DRG	Dorsal horn	Mediodorsal	Anterior cingulate	Affective-emotional (suffering)

Abbreviations: DRG, dorsal root ganglion; S1, primary somatosensory cortex; S2, secondary somatosensory cortex; VPL, ventral posterolateral; VMpo, ventromedial posterior.

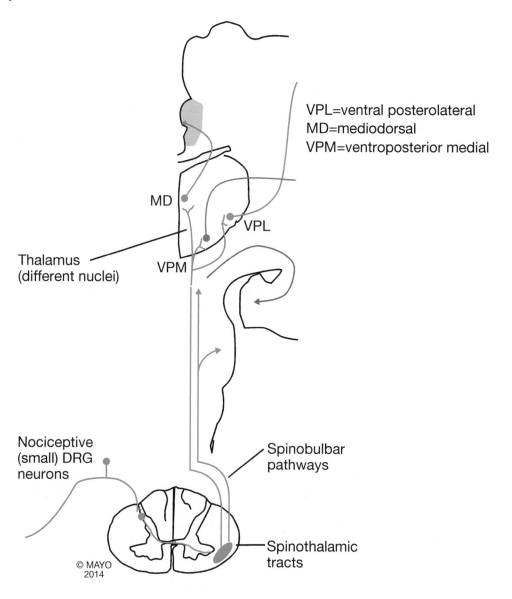

VPL=ventral posterolateral
MD=mediodorsal
VPM=ventroposterior medial

Figure 4.3. Nociceptive System.
Lamina I neurons project primarily via the contralateral lateral spinothalamic tract to the VPM. The VPM in turn projects to the insular cortex and the ventrocaudal portion of the nucleus, which projects to the anterior cingulate cortex. The VPM is continuous with the ventromedial parvocellular nucleus, which receives viscerosensory inputs from the parabrachial nucleus. The parabrachial nucleus relays taste and general visceral information from the nucleus of the solitary tract. Neurons of lamina V and the intermediate gray matter receive innocuous and nociceptive stimuli and project via the anterior spinothalamic tract to the VPL and ventroposteroinferior nuclei, which relay this information to the primary and secondary somatosensory cortex, respectively. Spinothalamic inputs from laminae VII and VIII terminate in the central lateral nucleus, which projects mainly to the striatum. DRG indicates dorsal root ganglion.
(Used with permission of Mayo Foundation for Medical Education and Research.)

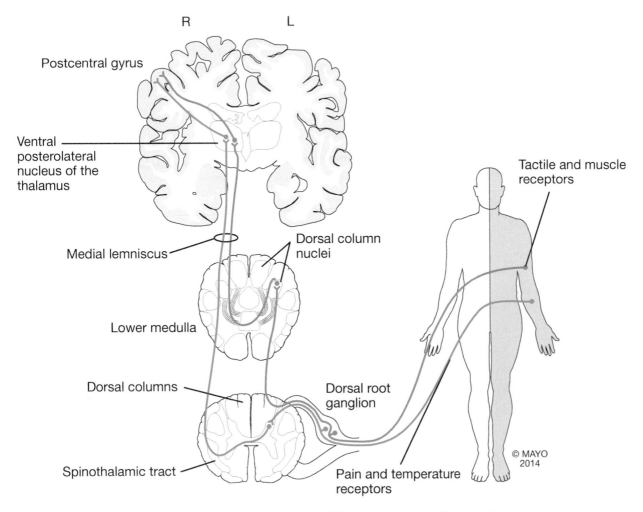

R L

Postcentral gyrus

Ventral posterolateral nucleus of the thalamus

Tactile and muscle receptors

Medial lemniscus

Dorsal column nuclei

Lower medulla

Dorsal columns

Dorsal root ganglion

Spinothalamic tract

Pain and temperature receptors

© MAYO 2014

Figure 4.4 *Sensations of Discriminative Touch, Vibration, and Proprioception and Pain and Temperature.*
Diagram of the pathway for discriminative touch, vibration, and proprioception (red) and for pain and temperature (green) of the left arm. First-order neurons are large and small dorsal root ganglion neurons. Large-diameter afferents for touch and proprioception ascend ipsilaterally in the left dorsal column at the cervical level (fasciculus cuneatus) and synapse on second-order neurons in the lower medulla (nucleus cuneatus). Axons from second-order neurons decussate and ascend in the right (contralateral) medial lemniscus to synapse in the ventral posterolateral nucleus of the thalamus, which projects to the primary sensory area in the postcentral gyrus. Small-diameter afferents for pain and temperature synapse on second-order neurons in the dorsal horn of the spinal cord. Axons of these second-order neurons decussate in the ventral white commissure and ascend as the spinothalamic tract in the contralateral ventrolateral quadrant. This tract joins the medial lemniscus and terminates in the ventral posterolateral nucleus and other nuclei in the thalamus. L indicates left; R, right.
(Adapted from Benarroch EE, Daube JR, Flemming KD, Westmoreland BF. Mayo Clinic medical neurosciences: organized by neurologic systems and levels. 5th ed. Rochester [MN]: Mayo Clinic Scientific Press and Florence [KY]: Informa Healthcare USA; c2008. Chapter 7, The sensory system; p. 217–64. Used with permission of Mayo Foundation for Medical Education and Research.)

periaqueductal gray, and the hypothalamus. These fibers also help elicit emotional, arousal, endocrine, and autonomic responses to pain, as well as pain modulation.

- Nociceptive or pain systems may be divided into lateral (sensory-discriminative) and medial (motivational-affective and cognitive-evaluative) components.

Pain Pathophysiology

After a severe peripheral nerve injury with tissue inflammation, various changes occur at both the peripheral and central nervous system levels and amplify the pain signal. These changes may lead to persistent pain even after resolution of the peripheral nerve injury.

A number of overlapping mechanisms lead to an increase in peripheral nociceptor activation and nociceptive afferent input into the dorsal horn. This increase is referred to as *peripheral sensitization*. The number of sodium (not calcium) and heat-sensitive transient receptor potential vanilloid type 1 channels increases at the site of injury and at the DRG, which lowers the threshold for activation (ie, increases sensitivity) of nociceptors and leads to ongoing peripheral nociceptive input via repetitive firing of nociceptive DRG neurons. With inflammatory processes (such as those seen in herpes zoster [shingles]), the skin strata eventually thins, dermal papillae widen, and a shift occurs toward a predominance of thin unmyelinated or thinly myelinated pain fibers. With these morphologic changes at the peripheral nociceptor level, nociceptive signaling can persist even after resolution of the process that damaged the peripheral nerve. This hypothesis is referred to as the *irritable nociceptor theory*.

Sensitization (or a lower threshold for activation) of central pain pathways is induced by the constant barrage of peripheral nociceptive afferent input. At the time of injury, a repeated but constant level of nociceptive input elicits a progressive increase in the degree of action potential firing in dorsal horn neurons. This increase is termed *windup* and depends on the ongoing peripheral nociceptive input. It resolves when the nociceptive signal is interrupted. Central sensitization involves changes (plasticity) within the central pain transmission pathways and the pathway components, leading to an increased gain (sensitivity) of the nociceptive system. These functional changes in central circuits can distort, amplify, and spatially magnify the sense of pain beyond the presence, intensity, spatial distribution, or duration of a particular peripheral painful or nonpainful stimulus.

With increased peripheral nociceptor firing, there is an increased release of glutamate (the excitatory neurotransmitter of the central nervous system) and an activation and proliferation of the dorsal horn glial cells—the astrocytes and microglia. Activation of microglia occurs early in an acute nerve injury, even without axonal loss or cell death. Astrocyte activation occurs later and is associated with axonal loss. When activated, the dorsal horn glial cells release pronociceptive neuropeptides, including substance P, calcitonin gene–related peptide, tumor necrosis factor α, interleukin (IL)-1β, nitric oxide, arachidonic acid, brain-derived neurotrophic factor, adenosine triphosphate, prostaglandins, and excitatory amino acids. All of these changes lead to increased dorsal horn sensitivity to nociceptive input and increased excitability of nociception transmission. Therefore, glial cells are important in contributing to central sensitization in the dorsal horn.

In addition to the activation of glial cells in the dorsal horn, the bolstered peripheral nociceptive input induces a cascade of changes that occur in the surface expression of *N*-methyl-D-aspartate (NMDA) and α-amino-3-hydroxy-5-methyl-4-isoxazole propionic acid (AMPA) receptors of WDR neurons. The WDR neurons integrate somatosensory input from A-β fibers and nociceptive input from thinly myelinated A-δ and unmyelinated C fibers. WDR neurons sit in the Rexed lamina V of the dorsal horn. In continuous nociceptive input, activation occurs in second messenger phosphorylation cascades, such as of calmodulin kinase II, protein kinase C, and extracellular signal-regulated kinase. These phosphorylation changes cause translocation of NMDA and AMPA receptors from intracellular stores to the synaptic membrane of WDR neurons. This translocation increases the sensitivity (ie, reduces the firing threshold) of WDR neurons to glutamate. In the clinical setting of this increased sensitivity, the normally nonpainful stimuli (via A-β fibers) can induce activation of central pain pathways (spinothalamic tract) through these sensitized integrative WDR neurons. Clinically, pain induced by a nonpainful stimulus is called *allodynia*. Similarly, the sensitivity of the system is shown in an exaggerated painful response to a normally painful stimulus (a pinprick), called *hyperalgesia*. Clinical evidence of allodynia or hyperalgesia, or both, indicates that central sensitization has occurred.

All of these sensitization processes represent a progressive, but plastic, process that is reversible in its early changes and requires ongoing nociceptive input for its maintenance. However, it is characteristic that after changes of central sensitization have occurred, and even with resolution of peripheral nociceptive input, the central changes can persist and be slow to resolve.

- *Peripheral sensitization* is an increase in peripheral nociceptor activation and nociceptive afferent input into the dorsal horn.
- *Windup* occurs at the time of injury, when repeated but constant-level nociceptive input elicits a progressive increase in the degree of action potential firing in dorsal horn neurons.
- Allodynia (pain induced by a nonpainful stimulus) and hyperalgesia (exaggerated painful response to normal painful stimulus) are phenomena of central sensitization of pain.

5 Special Somatic Sensory Afferent Overview[a]

SCOTT D. EGGERS, MD; EDUARDO E. BENARROCH, MD;
JACQUELINE A. LEAVITT, MD

Introduction

The special somatic afferent systems include vestibular, auditory, and vision. Vestibular and auditory afferent information is received by cranial nerve VIII, which then projects to central pathways. Cranial nerve II carries afferent visual information to central pathways.

This chapter reviews the receptors and structural components of these special somatic afferent systems. Clinical disorders related to the vestibular and auditory systems as well as vision are discussed in Volume 2, Section VIII, "Clinical Disorders of the Cranial Nerves and Brainstem."

Auditory

Receptors

The ossicular chain (malleus, incus, and stapes) within the air-filled middle ear serves as a transformer that bridges the impedance mismatch between sound vibrations in air on the large tympanic membrane and the resulting vibrations onto the small stapes footplate. Movement of the stapes footplate and underlying oval window produces vibration of endolymph fluid within the inner ear. The hair cells of the cochlea's organ of Corti rest on a basilar membrane and are stimulated by a specific sound frequency (lower-frequency sound at the cochlear apex). Thus, the inner ear is the transducer that converts the mechanical vibratory energy of sound into auditory nerve impulses, which are carried from the spinal ganglion to the dorsal and ventral cochlear nuclei at the pontomedullary junction.

Auditory Nerve

The auditory nerve (cranial nerve VIII) carries the transduced sound from the cochlear ganglia to the ipsilateral cochlear nuclei. After leaving the cochlea, the nerve fibers travel through the internal acoustic canal in the temporal bone to reach the lower pons in the cerebellopontine angle.

Central Pathways

Monaural information (about sounds at one ear) is transmitted in contralateral pathways to the inferior colliculus. Binaural information (about differences between sounds at both ears) is transmitted via the superior olivary complex.

Cochlear nerves from the cochlear ganglion synapse in cochlear nuclei on the ipsilateral side at the pontomedullary junction (Figure 5.1). The ventral cochlear nucleus is tonotopically organized with the low frequencies ventral and the high frequencies dorsal. After synapsing in the cochlear nuclei, there are at least 4 parallel pathways through the brainstem. With such redundancy in the system, a unilateral lesion above the level of the cochlear nuclei does not result in hearing loss.

Fibers from the ventral cochlear nucleus are transmitted ventral to the inferior cerebellar peduncle to form the trapezoid body. These fibers either terminate in the contralateral superior olive or ascend to the contralateral lateral

[a] Portions previously published in Mattox DE. Assessment and management of tinnitus and hearing loss. Continuum: Lifelong Learn Neurol. 2006 Aug;12(4):135–50. Used with permission.
Abbreviations: SCC, semicircular canal; VOR, vestibuloocular reflex

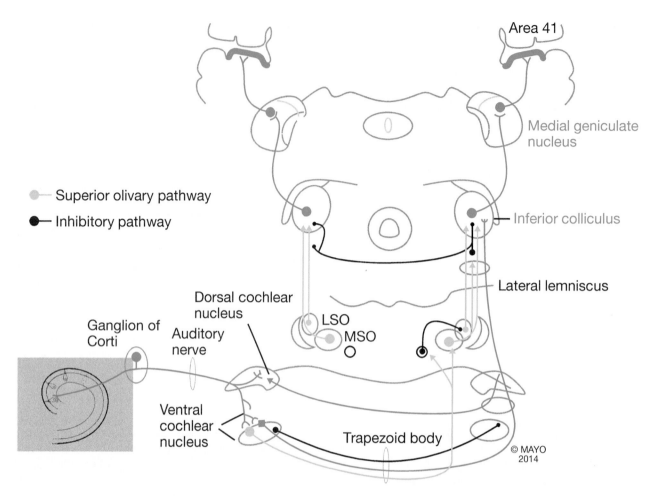

Figure 5.1 *Auditory Pathway. LSO indicates lateral superior olive; MSO, medial superior olive.*
(Used with permission of Mayo Foundation for Medical Education and Research.)

lemniscus. The superior olive contains 2 nuclei, the lateral and medial superior olivary nuclei. The superior olive is an important structure where information from both ears converges and is important for sound localization. The superior olive projects to the lateral lemniscus.

Fiber projections from the dorsal cochlear nucleus travel dorsal to the inferior cerebellar peduncle as the posterior acoustic stria and cross in the pons before joining the lateral lemniscus. These fibers are important in the monaural pathway.

The lateral lemniscus is an ascending fiber tract that terminates in the inferior colliculus. It also contains 2 nuclei, the anterior and posterior. The anterior nucleus projects to the inferior colliculus as part of the monaural pathway. The posterior nucleus, which receives information from the superior olive, also terminates in the inferior colliculus carrying information about the binaural pathway. Because additional connections are made with nuclei located within the lateral lemniscus, the inferior colliculus receives second-, third-, and fourth-order axons.

Ascending fibers terminate in the inferior colliculus. Fibers projecting to the central nucleus of the inferior

colliculus are tonotopically arranged and destined for the ventral medial geniculate body. Fibers in the paracentral regions play a role in integration of sensory input and with connections to the superior colliculus and reticular formation. Information from the inferior colliculus projects to the medial geniculate body.

The medial geniculate body lies medial to the lateral geniculate body and lateral to the pulvinar nucleus of the thalamus. There are 3 main subdivisions of the medial geniculate body. The ventral division receives tonotopic input from the inferior colliculus (central nucleus). This ventral division projects to the primary auditory cortex. The dorsal and medial divisions receive less precise organized fibers from the pericentral inferior colliculus and project to areas around the primary auditory cortex (auditory association, temporoparietal association areas, amygdala).

The primary auditory cortex (A1; Brodmann area 41) is located in the Heschl gyrus and has tonotopic arrangement. The auditory association cortex (A2; Brodmann area 42) is located in the second transverse temporal gyrus and planum temporale.

Clinical manifestations of dysfunctions of cranial nerve VII or the auditory pathway are reviewed in Chapter 9, "Brainstem and Cranial Nerves Part II: The Pons," and clinical disorders affecting cranial nerve VIII or the brainstem are discussed in Volume 2, Section VIII, "Clinical Disorders of the Cranial Nerves and Brainstem."

- The hair cells of the cochlea's organ of Corti rest on a basilar membrane and are stimulated by a specific sound frequency (lower-frequency sound at the cochlear apex).
- The auditory nerve (cranial nerve VIII) carries the transduced sound from the cochlear ganglia to the ipsilateral cochlear nuclei.
- The superior olive is an important structure where information from both ears converges and is important for sound localization.
- The lateral lemniscus is an ascending fiber tract that terminates in the inferior colliculus.
- Information from the inferior colliculus projects to the medial geniculate body.
- The primary auditory cortex (A1; Brodmann area 41) is located in the Heschl gyrus and has tonotopic arrangement.

Vestibular

Receptors

The bony labyrinth represents the part of the petrous portion of the temporal bone that houses the membranous vestibular labyrinth and cochlea (Figure 5.2). Perilymph bathes the membranous labyrinth within. Each membranous labyrinth contains endolymph (resembling intracellular fluid) and consists of 3 semicircular canals (SCCs) for sensing rotation and 2 otolith organs for sensing translation, tilt, and gravity.

The vestibular receptor cells are hair cells, each possessing many stereocilia and 1 large kinocilium, all arranged to optimally transduce mechanical shearing forces in a specific orientation into electrochemical impulses. Hair cells normally exhibit spontaneous symmetrical baseline firing, resulting in resting vestibular tone. Head movements or position changes may cause deflection of stereocilia toward the kinocilium, resulting in depolarization (stimulation), or deflection away from the kinocilium, causing hyperpolarization (inhibition).

The horizontal (lateral), anterior (superior), and posterior SCCs lie orthogonal to one another, allowing these angular accelerometers to detect all head rotations by some combination of canal stimulation. Each SCC has an ampulla (enlargement) containing a septum called the crista ampullaris, from which hair cells extend their cilia into a saillike cupula that attaches along the wall of the ampulla. Head rotation causes relative movement of endolymph within the canal, which bends the cupula and the embedded hair cells to cause either an excitatory or inhibitory response depending on the direction of movement. A push-pull arrangement means that SCCs act in working pairs during head rotation (eg, when the right posterior canal is excited, the left anterior canal is inhibited).

The elliptoid-shaped utricle and saccule (oriented perpendicular to one another) are referred to as otolith organs because their maculae (specialized sensory epithelium) are made up of calcium carbonate crystals called otoconia embedded in a gelatinous elastic matrix, into which the cilia of hair cells project. Because the crystals have a specific gravity higher than that of the surrounding endolymph fluid, the otolith organs become capable of reacting to linear accelerations including gravitational pull. The relatively heavy macula causes deflection of the stereocilia embedded within it during head translation.

Vestibular Nerve

The vestibulocochlear nerve is formed by the union of the vestibular nerve and the more anteriorly located cochlear nerve. The superior division of the vestibular nerve carries fibers from the anterior and lateral SCCs and the utricle. The inferior division innervates the posterior SCC and the saccule. The Scarpa ganglion contains bipolar ganglion cells of first-order vestibular neurons.

The vascular supply to the labyrinth parallels its innervation. The internal auditory (labyrinthine) artery, usually a branch of the anterior inferior cerebellar artery, supplies the labyrinth by further branching into anterior and posterior vestibular arteries and the main cochlear artery.

Central Pathways

Vestibular input and nuclei are important for control of eye movement and posture relative to angular and linear acceleration of the head and body. Thus the vestibular nuclei project to the ocular motor system, the spinal cord (medial and lateral vestibulospinal tracts), and to the cortex via the thalamus (conscious awareness of motion and spatial orientation). Visual and somatosensory inputs are centrally integrated to facilitate spatial orientation and postural control.

Vestibuloocular Connections

The basic 3-neuron arc of the vestibuloocular reflex (VOR) consists of the vestibular ganglion and nerve, vestibular nuclei, and ocular motor nuclei. The function of the VOR is to generate compensatory conjugate eye movements in the opposite direction of head movement and thereby maintain a stable direction of gaze and clear vision.

To generate the rotational VOR, the vestibular nuclei send excitatory and inhibitory signals to specific ocular motor nuclei to activate yoked pairs of extraocular muscles (and inhibit their antagonists), thereby moving both

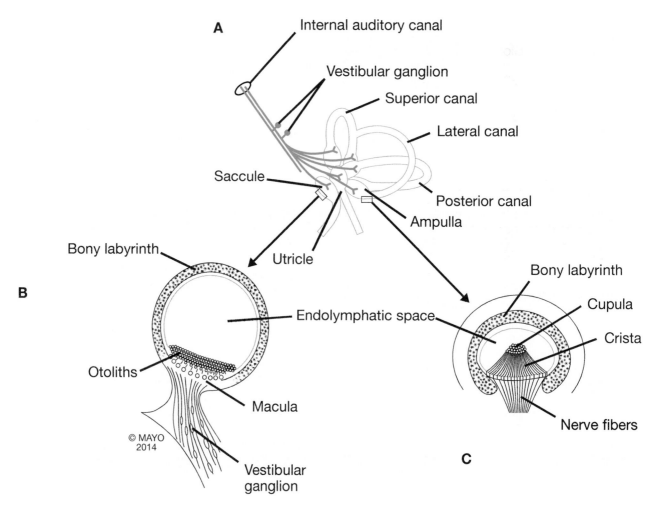

Figure 5.2 *Vestibular Receptors. A, Nerve supply to vestibular receptors (utricle, saccule, and semicircular canals). B, Macula of utricle and saccule. C, Ampulla of semicircular canals.*

(Adapted from Benarroch EE, Daube JR, Flemming KD, Westmoreland BF. Mayo Clinic medical neurosciences: organized by neurologic systems and levels. 5th ed. Rochester [MN]: Mayo Clinic Scientific Press and Florence [KY]: Informa Healthcare USA; c2008. Chapter 15B, The posterior fossa level: cerebellar, auditory, and vestibular systems; p. 633–67. Used with permission of Mayo Foundation for Medical Education and Research.)

eyes in the same plane but opposite direction as the SCC being stimulated (Figure 5.3). For example, activation of the right horizontal SCC by rightward head rotation stimulates the left abducens nucleus and the medial rectus subnucleus of the right oculomotor nucleus so that the left lateral rectus and right medial rectus produce conjugate leftward eye movements. The eye movements elicited by vestibular stimulation constitute the vestibular slow phase eye movements. However, sustained vestibular stimulation in an awake person leads to nystagmus quick phases opposite the slow phase direction (toward the side of vestibular stimulation). The nystagmus direction is named according to quick phase direction. Likewise, sudden unilateral inhibition or loss of vestibular function leads to slow phase eye movements toward the side of the lesion and contralesionally directed nystagmus quick phases.

Connections from the otolith organs mediate eye movements in response to linear acceleration as well as the ocular torsion that occurs with sustained head tilt. Lesions along this pathway from the medulla to the midbrain can produce the ocular tilt reaction.

The vestibulocerebellum (flocculi, tonsils, nodulus) receives vestibular inputs, both directly from the labyrinth and from the vestibular nuclei via the inferior cerebellar peduncle, that are important for calibrating the VOR to changing visual requirements and regulating smooth pursuit and eccentric gaze holding (see Chapter 12, "Supranuclear Ocular Motor Systems").

Clinical manifestations and clinical disorders affecting the vestibular system are discussed in Chapter 9, "Brainstem and Cranial Nerves Part II: The Pons" and Volume 2, Chapter 48, "Clinical Neurotology."

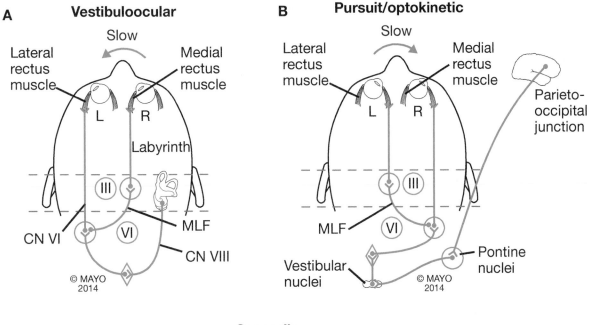

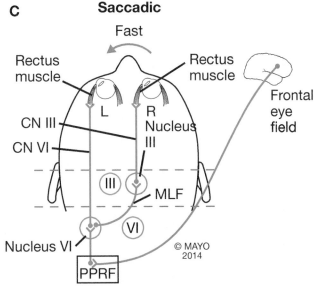

Figure 5.3 *Three Systems for Lateral Gaze. A, Vestibuloocular reflex. B, Pursuit/optokinetic system. C, Saccadic system. CN indicates cranial nerve; MLF, medial longitudinal fasciculus; PPRF, pontine paramedian reticular formation.*
(Adapted from Benarroch EE, Daube JR, Flemming KD, Westmoreland BF. Mayo Clinic medical neurosciences: organized by neurologic systems and levels. 5th ed. Rochester [MN]: Mayo Clinic Scientific Press and Florence [KY]: Informa Healthcare USA; c2008. Chapter 15B, The posterior fossa level: cerebellar, auditory, and vestibular systems; p. 633–67. Used with permission of Mayo Foundation for Medical Education and Research.)

- The semicircular canals detect angular acceleration of the head movements.
- The otolith organs, the utricle and saccule, respond to linear acceleration and gravitational pull.
- Vestibular input and nuclei are important for control of eye movement and posture relative to angular and linear acceleration of the head and body.
- Vestibular nuclei project to the ocular motor system, the spinal cord (medial and lateral vestibulospinal tracts), and to the cortex via the thalamus (conscious awareness of motion and spatial orientation).
- Activation of the right horizontal semicircular canal by rightward head rotation stimulates the left abducens nucleus and the medial rectus subnucleus of the right oculomotor nucleus so that the left lateral rectus and right medial rectus produce conjugate leftward eye movements.

- The vestibulocerebellum (flocculi, tonsils, nodulus) receives vestibular inputs that are important for calibrating the vestibulooocular reflex to changing visual requirements and regulating smooth pursuit and eccentric gaze holding.

Vision

Receptors

The retina is composed of multiple layers (Figure 5.4). There are 5 types of neurons (ganglion, amacrine, bipolar, horizontal, receptor cells) and 1 type of glial cells (Muller cells) in the retina. Receptor cells in the outer layers sense light and information flows from the outer layers to inner layers and eventually to the central pathways via the ganglion cells.

There are 4 parallel channels in the visual processing system (Table 5.1). The classic photoreceptor system includes rods (95%) and cones (5%) and serves the function of image formation and mediates conscious visual perception. Uniquely, these photoreceptors hyperpolarize to light stimuli compared to other receptors in the sensory system. The second system consists of melanopsin synthesizing intrinsically photosensitive retinal ganglion cells that detect environmental brightness (irradiance) at a subconscious level. This system has a major role in light entrainment of circadian rhythms and pupillary light response.

Sensory Transduction

Transduction of light to electric impulses involves receptor cells in the outer layer. Photons are absorbed by

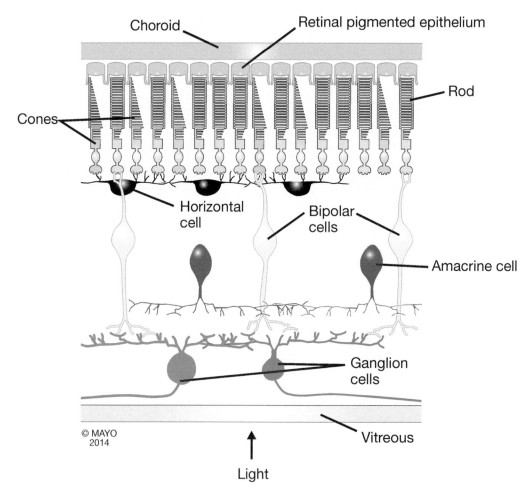

Figure 5.4 The Main Cell Groups in the Retina Are the Photoreceptor Cells, Bipolar Cells, Ganglion Cells, Horizontal Cells, and Amacrine Cells. These cells are stratified in well-demarcated layers. The photoreceptor cell layer, the outermost layer, is bound by retinal pigmented epithelium. The ganglion cell layer, the innermost layer, is adjacent to the vitreous humor. Light has to travel across the inner layers to reach the photoreceptor cells in the outer layer.

(Adapted from Benarroch EE, Daube JR, Flemming KD, Westmoreland BF. Mayo Clinic medical neurosciences: organized by neurologic systems and levels. 5th ed. Rochester [MN]: Mayo Clinic Scientific Press and Florence [KY]: Informa Healthcare USA; c2008. Chapter 16A, The supratentorial level: thalamus, hypothalamus, and visual system; p. 669–99. Used with permission of Mayo Foundation for Medical Education and Research.)

Table 5.1 • Four Parallel Channels in Visual Processing

	Image-Forming Pathways			Non–Image-Forming Pathways
Pathway	P (parvicellular)	K (koniocellular)	M (magnocellular)	Melanopsin
Photoreceptor	Cones (S and M)	S cones	Rods	Ganglion cell
Photopigment	Photopsin	Photopsin	Rhodopsin	Melanopsin
Response to light	Hyperpolarization	Hyperpolarization	Hyperpolarization	Depolarization
Information conveyed	Color Low contrast and temporal	Contrast shape	Achromatic Movement High contrast and high temporal sensitivity	Luminance
Relay	Lateral geniculate body	Lateral geniculate body	Lateral geniculate body	Suprachiasmatic nucleus Pretectal nucleus Lateral geniculate body
Target	Occipital lobe	Occipital lobe	Occipital lobe	
Post processing	Ventral stream (what)	Ventral stream (what)	Dorsal stream (where)	
Function	Visual acuity Color vision Depth perception Object identification	Color vision	Object location and motion	Circadian entrainment by light Pupillary light response

photopigments in the outer segments. Transduced information is passed by synapses from receptor cells to bipolar cells and from bipolar cells to ganglion cells. The characteristics of the synapse between receptor cells and bipolar cells determine whether the associated ganglion cells respond by increasing (on-response) or decreasing (off-response) firing rate. If the synapse is inhibitory, the ganglion cell is an "on-center" cell; if the synapse is excitatory, it is an "off-center" cell. The postsynaptic membrane of the bipolar cell determines whether the synapse is excitatory or inhibitory.

The antagonistic surround field is the result of lateral inhibition by horizontal cells. Receptor cells in the field that surrounds the ganglion cell contact horizontal cells through excitatory synapses. Horizontal cells transmit the information laterally to the central field, where they make inhibitory contact with receptor cells.

The receptor field is an area of the retina where a stimulus will evoke an electric response. The visual field of a cell is the corresponding region in visual space. Ganglion cells have a circular receptor field with either an on-center (excitatory center, inhibitory surround) or an off-center (inhibitory center, excitatory surround) configuration. Ganglion cells fire action potentials at a constant background rate in the dark. When light is shone on the center of a ganglion cell and it is an on-center cell, there will be an increase in action potential firing. If it is an off-center cell, there will be a decrease. Light shining on the surround aspect of the individual ganglion cell type has the opposite effect. If light falls on both center and surround, no change in action potential firing rate is noted.

Retina

Axons of the ganglion cells from the rods and cones ultimately project to the lateral geniculate nucleus. The retinal nerve fiber layer originating from the ganglion cells has a specific pattern within the retina as it coalesces to form the optic disc. Retinal nerve fibers forming the optic nerve travel through the optic canal.

Central Pathways and Visual Cortex

The optic nerves come together at the optic chiasm. Nasal fibers cross at the chiasm, whereas temporal fibers remain ipsilateral. The fibers continue in the optic tract synapsing in the lateral geniculate bodies. Ganglion cell axons from each eye project to distinct layers, or laminae. The contralateral nasal retina projects to laminae 1, 4, and 6. The ipsilateral temporal retina projects to laminae 2, 3, and 5. Within each layer, an orderly map of the retina is maintained: peripheral retina projects to anterior lateral geniculate body; foveal retina projects to posterior lateral geniculate body. There is reciprocal input from the visual cortex to the lateral geniculate body.

Visual fibers extend posteriorly but split so that the upper-field fibers pass through the temporal lobes (via Meyer loop) and the inferior-field fibers pass through the parietal lobes.

Ultimately, visual information is interpreted in the primary visual cortex, or striate cortex (Brodmann area 17), which spans the area surrounding the calcarine fissure. The lateral geniculate neurons project primarily to layer IV of the striate cortex. The primary visual cortex gets the name *striate cortex* from the stria of Gennari, a large myelinated band of fibers projecting to layer IV. There is retinotopic representation in the striate cortex. There is a disproportionate area of the cortex dedicated to the central 5 degrees of vision at the fovea. See also Chapter 13, "Cranial Nerves I and II" for review of the central pathway and Volume 2, Chapter 45, "Neuro-ophthalmology: Visual Fields" for discussion of disorders of the visual field.

Visual Cortex Connections

The visual cortex projects to other cortical areas, including visual association areas (areas 18 and 19; peristriate cortex), posterior parietal cortex, and the frontal eye fields. In addition, the visual cortex projects to subcortical structures, including superior colliculus, pulvinar and lateral geniculate body (thalamus), and the claustrum. Parallel pathways originating with cone cells ultimately project to the inferior temporal cortex in the ventral stream ("what" pathway). Parallel visual processing pathways originating with rod cells ultimately project to the posterior parietal cortex in the dorsal stream ("where" pathway).

- Receptor cells in the outer layers of the retina sense light and information flows from the outer layers to inner layers and eventually to the central pathways via the ganglion cells.
- Ganglion cells have a circular receptor field with either an on-center or an off-center configuration.

6 Peripheral Nerve, Neuromuscular Junction, and Muscle Anatomy

JENNIFER A. TRACY, MD

Introduction

After exiting the spinal cord, individual nerve roots coalesce to form plexi and peripheral nerves. These nerves innervate muscle and skin. Clinical localization requires a working knowledge of this anatomy. By evaluating the distribution of muscle weakness, sensory loss (Figure 6.1), and reflexes, it is often possible to localize lesions and focus a differential diagnosis.

This chapter reviews the anatomy of the peripheral nerves, neuromuscular junction, and muscle. The autonomic nervous system is discussed in Chapter 19, "Autonomic Nervous System."

Peripheral Nerve Anatomy

Spinal Nerve Roots

The spinal nerve roots consist of dorsal and ventral roots that extend from the spinal cord. The dorsal root ganglion contains a bipolar neuron that is the sensory nerve cell body. It is extraspinal, located along the dorsal root before the dorsal and ventral roots combine to form the spinal root at each level. There are 8 cervical spinal nerve roots, 12 thoracic, 5 lumbar, 5 sacral, and 1 coccygeal on each side. They exit the spinal canal via intervertebral foramina as spinal nerves. Spinal nerves provide sensory cutaneous innervation, with a cutaneous area innervated by a single spinal nerve referred to as a *dermatome*. Diagrams are provided as "dermatome maps," but it is important to remember that there is actually considerable overlap of dermatomal supply (Figure 6.1).

Cervical and Brachial Plexus

Spinal nerves ultimately form various plexi. The C1-C4 motor roots comprise the cervical plexus and provide innervation to the neck muscles, diaphragm, and lower trapezius. The C5-T1 nerve roots continue to form the brachial plexus (Figure 6.2). The upper trunk of the brachial plexus is made up of the C5-C6 nerve roots, the middle trunk is an extension of the C7 nerve root, and the lower trunk consists of the C8-T1 nerve roots. Each trunk then divides into anterior and posterior divisions, with the anterior divisions of the upper and middle trunks forming the lateral cord, the posterior divisions of all 3 trunks becoming the posterior cord, and the anterior division of the lower trunk becoming the medial cord.

Peripheral Nerves of the Upper Extremity

The cords divide into named peripheral nerves (Table 6.1). The main branches of the lateral cord are the musculocutaneous nerve (motor supply to coracobrachialis, biceps brachii, and brachialis; sensory supply via lateral cutaneous nerve of the forearm) and a contribution to the median nerve (motor supply to pronator teres, flexor carpi radialis, palmaris longus, and flexor digitorum superficialis). The main branches of the medial cord are the ulnar nerve (motor supply to flexor carpi ulnaris and flexor digitorum profundus [digits 4, 5], then motor supply to abductor digiti minimi, first dorsal and palmar interosseous muscles, adductor pollicis, flexor pollicis brevis, third and fourth lumbricals, opponens digiti minimi, and flexor digiti minimi; sensory supply through palmar cutaneous, dorsal cutaneous branches, and digital nerves) (Figure 6.3) and a contribution to the median nerve (flexor digitorum superficialis; motor supply to anterior interosseous nerve muscles: flexor digitorum profundus [digits 2, 3], flexor pollicis longus, pronator quadratus; to abductor and flexor pollicis brevis, opponens pollicis, and first and second lumbricals; sensory supply to palmar cutaneous branch and palmar digital nerves), as well as the medial cutaneous

A Anterior

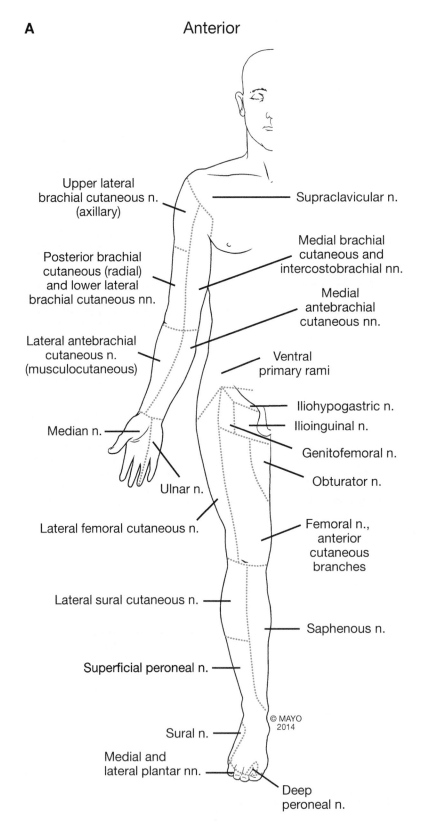

Upper lateral brachial cutaneous n. (axillary)

Supraclavicular n.

Medial brachial cutaneous and intercostobrachial nn.

Posterior brachial cutaneous (radial) and lower lateral brachial cutaneous nn.

Medial antebrachial cutaneous nn.

Lateral antebrachial cutaneous n. (musculocutaneous)

Ventral primary rami

Iliohypogastric n.

Ilioinguinal n.

Median n.

Genitofemoral n.

Obturator n.

Ulnar n.

Lateral femoral cutaneous n.

Femoral n., anterior cutaneous branches

Lateral sural cutaneous n.

Saphenous n.

Superficial peroneal n.

© MAYO 2014

Sural n.

Medial and lateral plantar nn.

Deep peroneal n.

Figure 6.1 Cutaneous Innervation Map.
A and B, Sensory distribution mapped by peripheral nerve. C, Sensory distribution mapped by dermatome. Total distribution of dermatomes is depicted alternatively in the right and left halves to best illustrate total distribution of innervation of each nerve root.

(Adapted from Kilfoyle DH, Jones LK, Mowzoon N. Disorders of the peripheral nervous system. Part B: Specific inherited and acquired disorders of the peripheral nervous system. In: Mowzoon N, Flemming KD, editors. Neurology board review: an illustrated study guide. Rochester [MN]: Mayo Clinic Scientific Press and Florence [KY]: Informa Healthcare USA; c2007. p. 799–845. Used with permission of Mayo Foundation for Medical Education and Research.)

(continued on next page)

B

Posterior

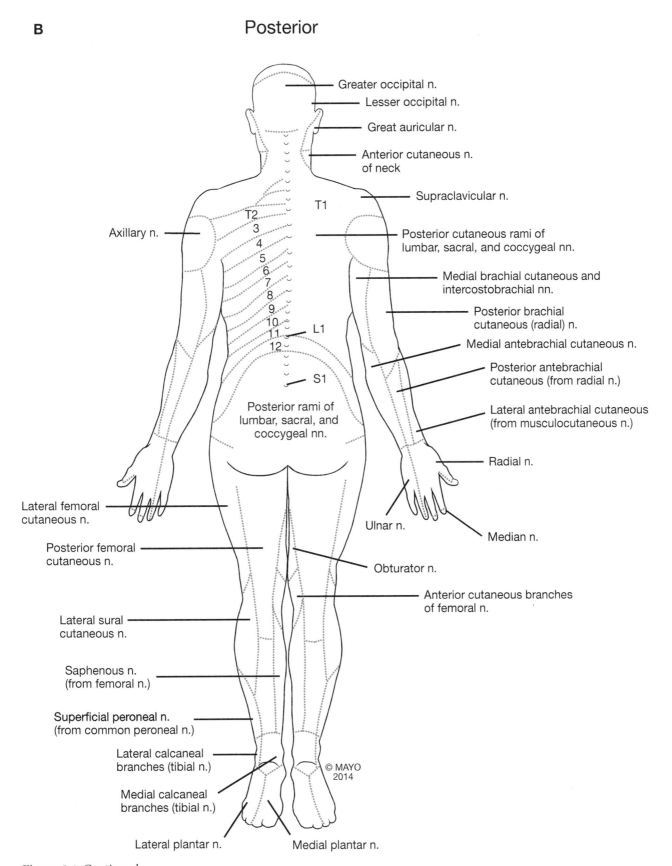

Figure 6.1 Continued.

C

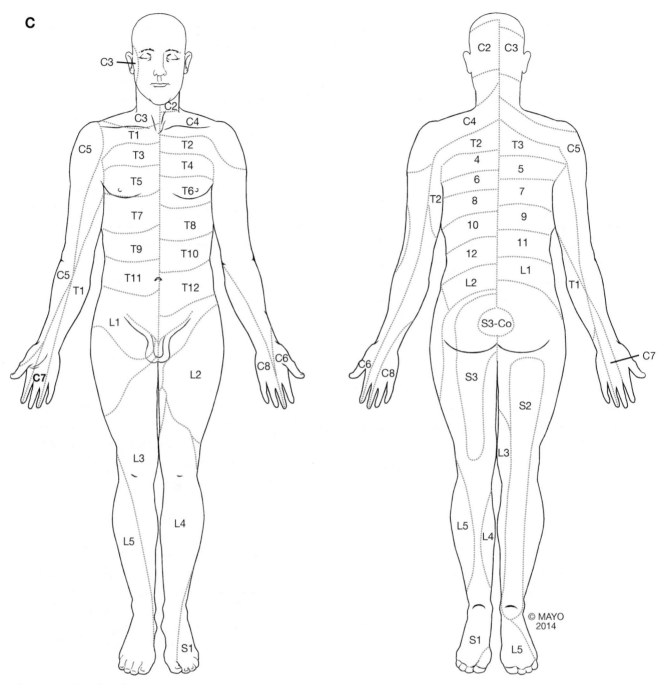

Figure 6.1 Continued

nerves of the arm and forearm (Figure 6.4). The main branches of the posterior cord are the axillary nerve (motor innervation to deltoid and teres minor; sensory innervation to upper lateral cutaneous nerve of the arm) (Figure 6.5) and radial nerve (motor innervation to triceps, brachioradialis, extensor carpi radialis longus and brevis, and anconeus, then splitting off into the superficial radial sensory branch and the motor-only posterior interosseous nerve, which innervates multiple muscles, including the supinator, extensor carpi ulnaris, and finger extensor muscles)

(Figure 6.5). Other sensory innervation from the radial nerve is via the posterior and lower lateral cutaneous nerves of the arm and the posterior cutaneous nerve of the forearm.

Important early branches off nerve roots before the initiation of the brachial plexus include the dorsal scapular nerve, which extends directly from the C5 nerve root and participates in innervation of rhomboid muscles; a branch from C5 which contributes to the phrenic nerve; and the long thoracic nerve (from roots C5-C7), which innervates

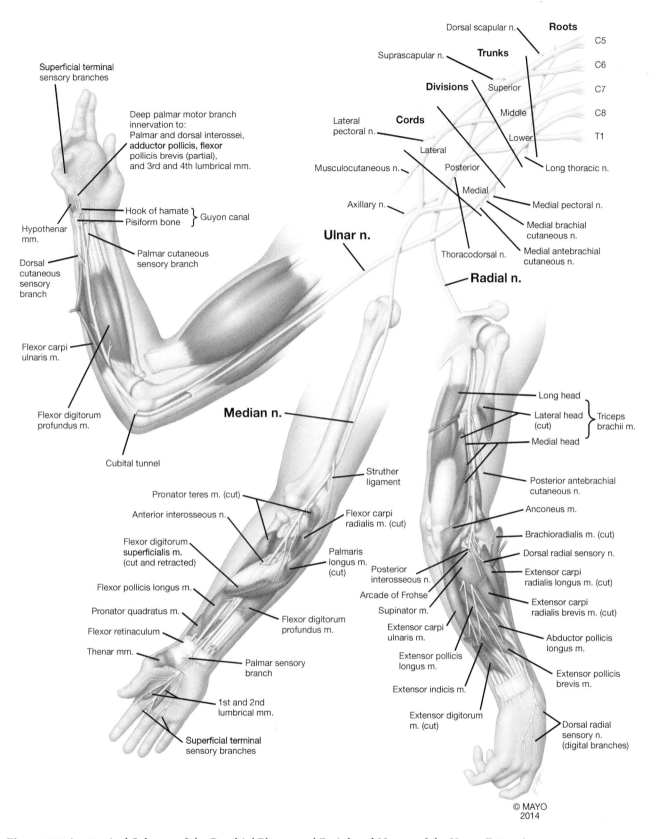

Figure 6.2 *Anatomical Schema of the Brachial Plexus and Peripheral Nerves of the Upper Extremity.*
Note the claw hand deformity of ulnar neuropathy, thenar muscle atrophy of median neuropathy at the wrist, and wristdrop of radial neuropathy.

(Adapted from Kilfoyle DH, Jones LK, Mowzoon N. Disorders of the peripheral nervous system. Part A: Anatomy of the peripheral nervous system and classification of disorders by localization. In: Mowzoon N, Flemming KD, editors. Neurology board review: an illustrated study guide. Rochester [MN]: Mayo Clinic Scientific Press and Florence [KY]: Informa Healthcare USA; c2007. p. 777–97. Used with permission of Mayo Foundation for Medical Education and Research.)

Table 6.1 • Muscle Innervation of the Upper Extremity and Trunk

Muscle	Nerve Roots	Trunk	Cord	Nerve
Diaphragm	C3-C5	...	...	Phrenic
Rhomboids	C4, C5	...	...	Dorsal scapular
Serratus anterior	C5-C7	...	...	Long thoracic
Supraspinatus	C5, C6	Upper	...	Suprascapular
Infraspinatus	C5, C6	Upper	...	Suprascapular
Deltoid	C5, C6	Upper	Posterior	Axillary
Biceps brachii	C5, C6	Upper	Lateral	Musculocutaneous
Triceps	C6-C8	Upper/middle/lower	Posterior	Radial
Pronator teres	C6, C7	Upper/middle	Lateral	Median
Flexor carpi radialis	C6, C7	Upper/middle	Lateral	Median
Flexor carpi ulnaris	C8, T1	Lower	Medial	Ulnar
Flexor digitorum superficialis	C7, C8, T1	Middle/lower	Lateral/medial	Median
Flexor digitorum profundus	C7, C8, T1	Middle/lower	Lateral/medial	Median (2,3) (anterior interosseous); ulnar (4,5)
Flexor pollicis longus	C7, C8, T1	Middle/lower	Lateral/medial	Median (anterior interosseous)
Extensor digitorum	C7, C8	Middle/lower	Posterior	Radial (posterior interosseous)
Extensor indicis proprius	C7, C8	Middle/lower	Posterior	Radial (posterior interosseous)
Abductor pollicis brevis	C8, T1	Lower	Medial	Median
Abductor digiti minimi	C8, T1	Lower	Medial	Ulnar
First dorsal interosseous	C8, T1	Lower	Medial	Ulnar

the serratus anterior. Important branches off the upper trunk include the suprascapular nerve, which innervates the supraspinatus and infraspinatus, and a branch to the subclavius muscle.

Thoracic Level Nerves

Thoracic nerve roots extend out along trunk musculature, providing motor innervation (hence local outpouching of muscle that can be seen in thoracic radiculopathies) and sensory cutaneous innervation (Figure 6.1C).

Lumbar Plexus and Peripheral Nerves of the Lower Extremity

Muscle innervation of the lower extremity is outlined in Table 6.2. The L1-L3 and most of the L4 nerve roots comprise the lumbar plexus (Figure 6.6). Prior to plexus formation, the L1 nerve gives off the iliohypogastric, ilioinguinal, and, with a contribution from L2, the genitofemoral nerve. L2 and L3 give rise to the lateral femoral cutaneous nerve. The L2-L4 roots via the plexus break off into an anterior division, which becomes the femoral nerve (motor innervaton to the iliopsoas, quadriceps, and sartorius and sensory innervation as the intermediate and medial cutaneous nerves of the thigh and the saphenous nerve) (Figure 6.7).

A posterior division becomes the obturator nerve (motor supply to obturator externus, gracilis, adductor longus, and adductor brevis muscles [note that the adductor magnus is supplied by both obturator and sciatic nerves]); there is also a cutaneous branch mediating sensation to the medial thigh.

A remaining part of the L4 nerve that does not enter the lumbar plexus joins with the L5 nerve root to form the lumbosacral trunk. The lumbosacral trunk, S1-S3, and part of S4 become the sacral plexus (Figure 6.6). The main branch off this plexus is the sciatic nerve (providing motor supply to hamstring muscles and part of the nerve supply to the adductor magnus), which branches near the popliteal fossa into the common peroneal and tibial nerves (Figure 6.8). The common peroneal nerve divides near the fibula into the deep peroneal and superficial peroneal nerves. The deep peroneal nerve provides motor innervation to the tibialis anterior, the extensor hallucis, the digitorum longus and brevis, and the peroneus tertius and sensory innervation to the sides of and space between the great and second toe. The superficial peroneal nerve provides motor innervation to the peroneus longus and brevis and sensory innervation to the distal anterolateral leg and dorsum of the foot (Figure 6.9). The tibial nerve gives motor innervation to the gastrocnemius, soleus, flexor

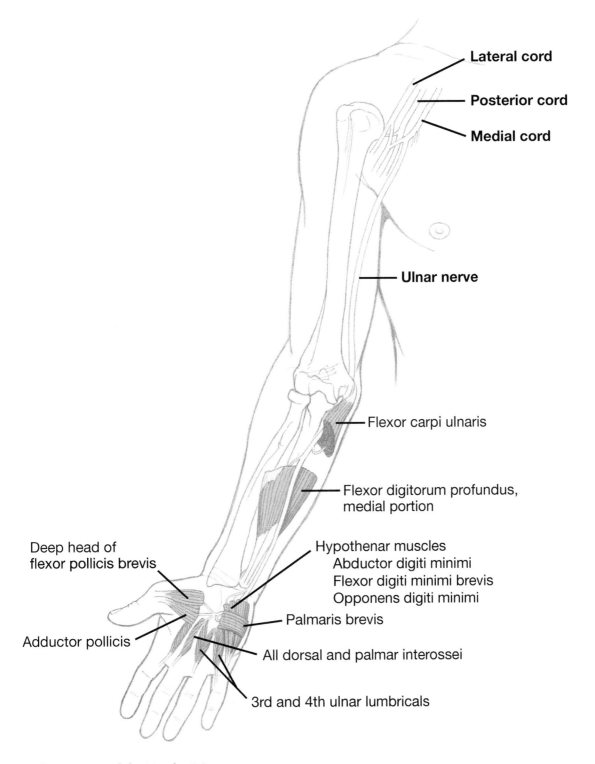

Lateral cord

Posterior cord

Medial cord

Ulnar nerve

Flexor carpi ulnaris

Flexor digitorum profundus, medial portion

Deep head of flexor pollicis brevis

Hypothenar muscles
Abductor digiti minimi
Flexor digiti minimi brevis
Opponens digiti minimi

Palmaris brevis

Adductor pollicis

All dorsal and palmar interossei

3rd and 4th ulnar lumbricals

Figure 6.3 *Ulnar Nerve and the Muscles It Innervates.*
(Adapted from Rosse C, Gaddum-Rosse P. Hollinshead's textbook of anatomy. 5th ed. Philadelphia [PA]: Lippincott-Raven; c1997. Used with permission.)

digitorum longus, posterior tibialis, and flexor hallucis longus. The sural nerve comes off the tibial nerve and gives sensory innervation to the lateral foot. The tibial nerve ultimately divides into the medial and lateral plantar nerves. The medial plantar nerve gives motor supply to the abductor hallucis, flexor hallucis brevis, and flexor digitorum brevis and sensory supply to the medial sole of the foot. The lateral plantar nerve gives

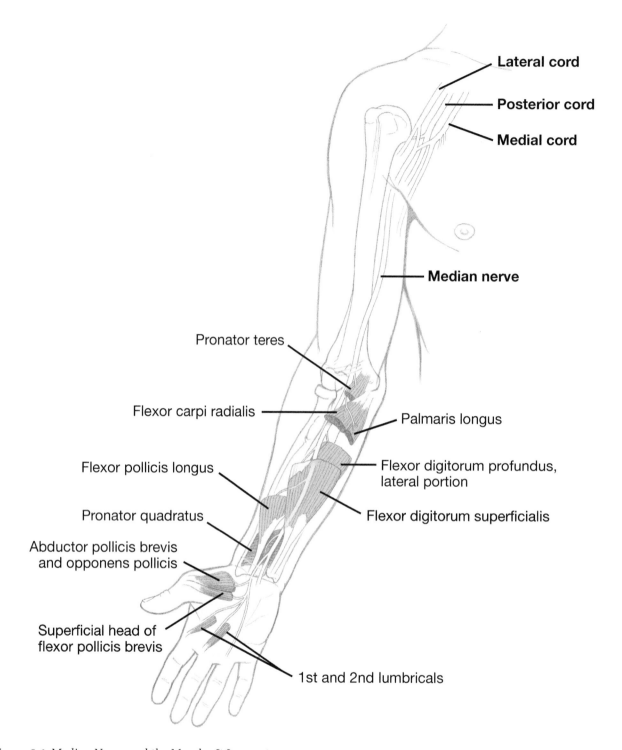

Figure 6.4 Median Nerve and the Muscles It Innervates.
(Adapted from Rosse C, Gaddum-Rosse P. Hollinshead's textbook of anatomy. 5th ed. Philadelphia [PA]: Lippincott-Raven; c1997. Used with permission.)

motor supply to the abductor digiti minimi, among other muscles of the foot, and provides sensory innervation to the lateral sole of the foot.

Other important nerves include the superior gluteal nerve, which is derived primarily from L5 (but also L4 and S1) and supplies the gluteus medius, gluteus minimus, and tensor fasciae latae, and the inferior gluteal nerve, arising from primarily the S1 (but also L5 and S2) nerve roots, supplying the gluteus maximus. These muscles are particularly important in electromyography when the question

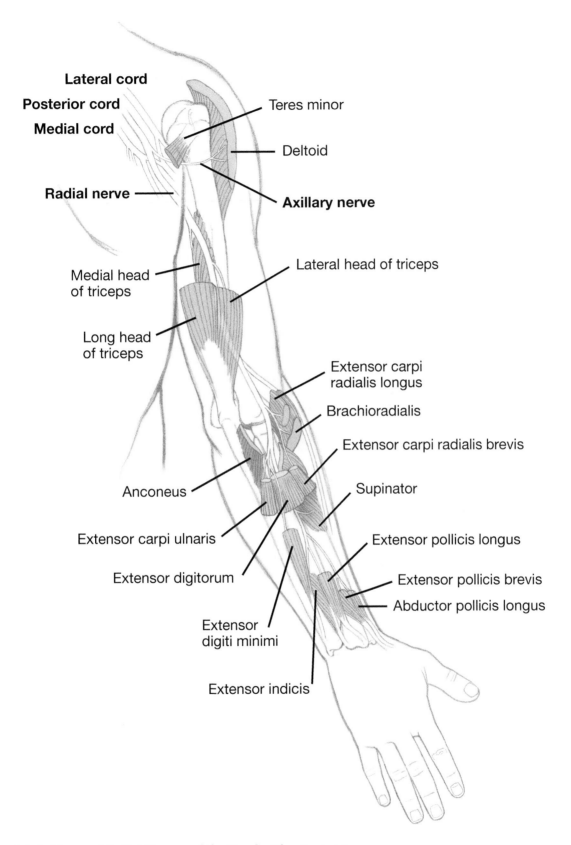

Figure 6.5 *Axillary and Radial Nerves and the Muscles They Innervate.*
(Adapted from Rosse C, Gaddum-Rosse P. Hollinshead's textbook of anatomy. 5th ed. Philadelphia [PA]: Lippincott-Raven; c1997. Used with permission.)

Table 6.2 • Muscle Innervation of the Lower Extremity

Muscle	Nerve Roots	Nerve
Iliopsoas	L2-L4	Femoral
Adductor longus	L2-L4	Obturator
Vastus medialis	L2-L4	Femoral
Vastus lateralis	L2-L4	Femoral
Rectus femoris	L2-L4	Femoral
Gluteus medius	L4, L5, S1	Superior gluteal
Gluteus maximus	L5, S1, S2	Inferior gluteal
Tensor fasciae latae	L4, L5, S1	Superior gluteal
Biceps femoris (short head)	L5, S1, S2	Sciatic (peroneal division)
Biceps femoris (long head)	L5, S1, S2	Sciatic (tibial division)
Tibialis anterior	L4, L5	Deep peroneal
Medial gastrocnemius	S1, S2	Tibial
Peroneus longus	L5, S1	Superficial peroneal
Tibialis posterior	L5, S1	Tibial
Peroneus tertius	L5, S1	Deep peroneal
Abductor hallucis	S1, S2	Tibial (medial plantar)

is whether there are affected L5- or S1-innervated muscles outside of the sciatic nerve distribution.

Clinical Localization

The distribution of muscle weakness in combination with the distribution of sensory loss may allow clinical localization. A common localization question regarding the lower extremity is when a patient presents with footdrop. To distinguish whether the footdrop is related to an L5 radiculopathy versus a peroneal neuropathy, inversion (posterior tibialis) should be assessed. The posterior tibialis is an L5/tibial nerve–innervated muscle. Thus, weakness of this muscle (in addition to the anterior tibialis and peronei) suggests an L5 nerve root lesion.

In the upper extremity, weakness of the triceps, but not the brachioradialis, supinator, extensor indicis, or extensor pollicis brevis, might suggest a radial nerve injury at the spiral groove or above.

Microscopic Peripheral Nerve Anatomy

The main classes of peripheral nerve fibers are large myelinated fibers, which generally subserve motor functions and what are classically termed large fiber sensory modalities (that is, sensation to vibration, touch pressure, and proprioception), and small fibers (myelinated or unmyelinated). Small fiber sensory modalities include temperature perception and pain (including heat pain) perception.

The anatomy of nerve at a pathologic level consists of the endoneurium, perineurium, and epineurium (Figure 6.10). The endoneurium is in the main substance of the nerve, containing large and small nerve fibers. These fibers are grouped into structures called fascicles, each of which is surrounded by connective tissue referred to as the perineurium. Multiple fascicles are surrounded by the epineurium. Nerve biopsy is sometimes used as a diagnostic tool in peripheral nerve dysfunction; in most cases, biopsy is performed on a distal cutaneous sensory nerve, but in other cases of focal abnormalities, more proximal fascicular nerve biopsies have been undertaken. Nerve biopsy allows assessment of abnormalities in the fibers themselves, including in fiber density, and assessment of interstitial changes such as inflammation, edema, amyloid deposition, or vasculitis.

The inner portion of the nerve is relatively negatively charged compared to the extracellular space (approximately −70 mV); internal to the nerve are high concentrations of potassium and negatively charged proteins and other anions; the extracellular space contains high concentrations of sodium and chloride. With an action potential, sodium channels open, allowing sodium entry into the nerve, and depolarization spreads down the nerve.

In the peripheral nervous system, Schwann cells produce myelin, which is an insulating substance surrounding the axon. This allows more efficient spread of an action potential along the axon between nodes of Ranvier by a process called saltatory conduction. The term *internodes* refers to the span of myelinated axon between the nodes. Unmyelinated fibers have a slower spread of action potentials because of the lack of myelin. Repolarization occurs through sodium channel inactivation and passage of potassium ions. A sodium-potassium adenosine triphosphatase is important to establish the resting membrane potential.

Many pathologic processes can affect the peripheral nerve, resulting in dysfunction (Figure 6.11). Clinical peripheral nerve disorders are discussed in Volume 2, Section VII, Chapter 40, "Peripheral Nerve Disorders."

- There are 8 cervical spinal nerve roots, 12 thoracic, 5 lumbar, 5 sacral, and 1 coccygeal on each side.
- The C5-T1 nerve roots form the brachial plexus.
- The main branches of the lateral cord are the musculocutaneous and median nerves. The main branches of the medial cord are the ulnar and median nerves. The main branches of the posterior cord are the axillary and radial nerves.
- The dorsal scapular nerve extends directly from the C5 nerve root and participates in innervation of rhomboid muscles.
- The L1-L3 and most of the L4 nerve roots comprise the lumbar plexus.

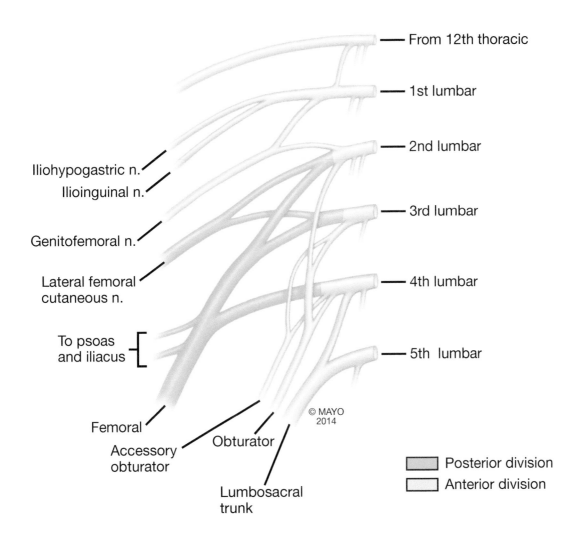

From 12th thoracic

1st lumbar

2nd lumbar

3rd lumbar

4th lumbar

5th lumbar

Iliohypogastric n.

Ilioinguinal n.

Genitofemoral n.

Lateral femoral
cutaneous n.

To psoas
and iliacus

Femoral

Accessory
obturator

Obturator

Lumbosacral
trunk

© MAYO
2014

Posterior division

Anterior division

Figure 6.6 Lumbar and Sacral Plexus.
(Modified from Hebl JR, Lennon RL, editors. Mayo Clinic atlas of regional anesthesia and ultrasound-guided nerve blockade. Rochester [MN]: Mayo Clinic Scientific Press and New York [NY]: Oxford University Press; c2010. Used with permission of Mayo Foundation for Medical Education and Research.)

- The L2-L4 roots via the plexus break off into an anterior division, which becomes the femoral nerve.
- The main branch of the sacral plexus is the peroneal and tibial nerves.

Neuromuscular Junction and Muscle Anatomy

Neuromuscular Junction

The neuromuscular junction consists of the presynaptic membrane of a motor neuron, the synaptic cleft, and the postsynaptic muscle membrane. Acetylcholine is stored in

vesicles in the presynaptic nerve terminal. When an action potential is generated within the motor neuron, a wave of depolarization travels down the axon and triggers calcium influx at the nerve terminal, with subsequent fusion of the vesicle with the presynaptic membrane and acetylcholine release into the synaptic cleft (Figure 6.12).

In normal muscles, the postsynaptic membrane has numerous junctional folds; nicotinic acetylcholine receptors are located in the crests of these folds, and voltage-gated sodium channels are clusters at the bottoms of the folds. The acetylcholine receptors consist of multiple subunits (two α, one β, one δ, and one ε in adults). Two acetylcholine molecules bind to each receptor, triggering

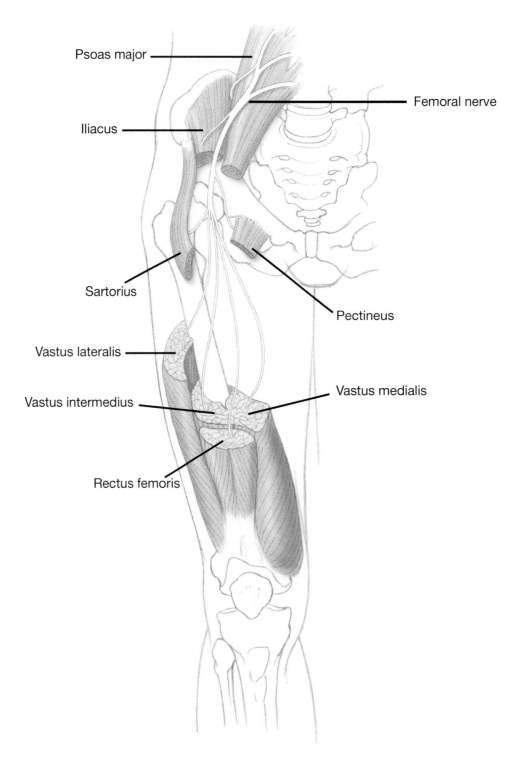

Figure 6.7 *Femoral Nerve and the Muscles It Innervates.*
(Adapted from Rosse C, Gaddum-Rosse P. Hollinshead's textbook of anatomy. 5th ed. Philadelphia [PA]: Lippincott-Raven; c1997. Used with permission.)

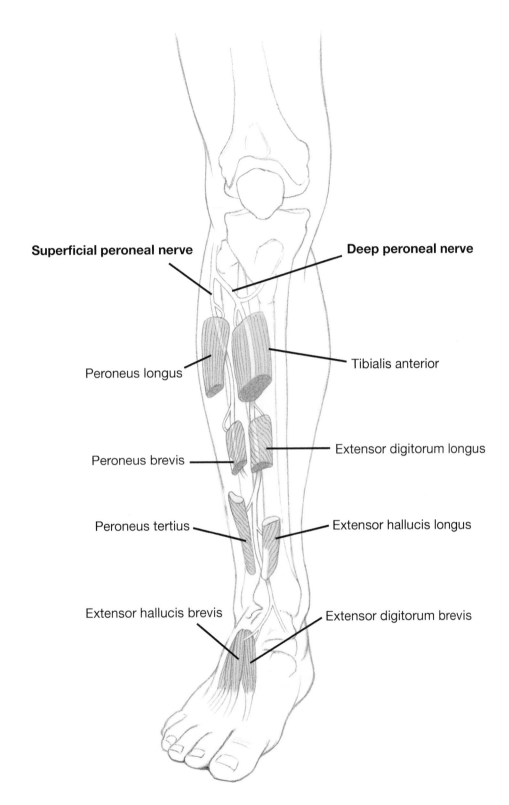

Figure 6.8 *Peroneal Nerve and the Muscles It Innervates.*
(Adapted from Rosse C, Gaddum-Rosse P. Hollinshead's textbook of anatomy. 5th ed. Philadelphia [PA]: Lippincott-Raven; c1997. Used with permission.)

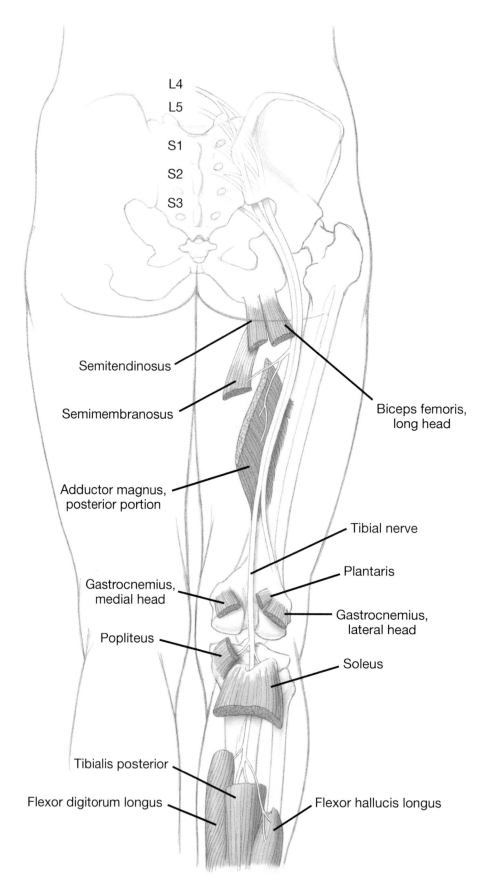

Figure 6.9 *Sciatic and Tibial Nerves and the Muscles They Innervate.*

(Adapted from Rosse C, Gaddum-Rosse P. Hollinshead's textbook of anatomy. 5th ed. Philadelphia [PA]: Lippincott-Raven; c1997. Used with permission.)

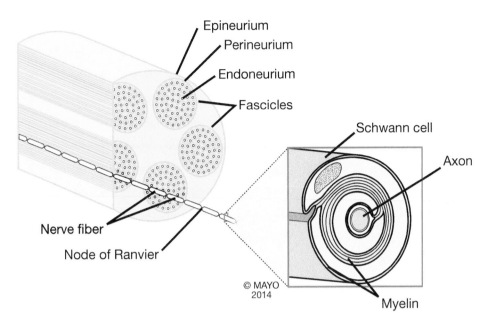

Figure 6.10 *Histologic Features of a Peripheral Nerve.*
A nerve is subdivided into fascicles by the perineurium, with multiple motor and sensory nerve fibers intermingled in each fascicle.
(Adapted from Benarroch EE, Daube JR, Flemming KD, Westmoreland BF. Mayo Clinic medical neurosciences: organized by neurologic systems and levels. 5th ed. Rochester [MN]: Mayo Clinic Scientific Press and Florence [KY]: Informa Healthcare USA; c2008. Chapter 13, The peripheral level; p. 491–546. Used with permission of Mayo Foundation for Medical Education and Research.)

what is mainly sodium influx through the receptor, leading to production of an end-plate potential. If depolarization exceeds the threshold for an action potential, the sodium channels also open, leading to muscle fiber depolarization and muscle contraction. Acetylcholine is ultimately cleaved by acetylcholinesterase in the neuromuscular junction.

Skeletal Muscle

Skeletal muscle fibers achieve contraction through components called sarcomeres (Figure 6.13). Sarcomeres are separated from each other by Z disks, which bind thin filaments composed of actin complexed with troponin and tropomyosin. Progressing from the Z disk to the middle of the sarcomere is the A band, which is made up primarily of myosin. At the center of the A band is the H zone, which is devoid of actin, and at the center of the H zone is the M line.

When an action potential is initiated, depolarization spreads along the muscle membrane. This continues down the T tubules (which are continuous with the muscle membrane), causing release of calcium into the sarcoplasm from the sarcoplasmic reticulum. This calcium binds to troponin, which exposes myosin-binding sites on actin. Myosin then binds actin (the cross-bridge), adenosine triphosphate bound to myosin is hydrolyzed, and adenosine diphosphate and inorganic phosphate are released from

myosin, causing the myosin head to flex, leading to a "power stroke." Adenosine triphosphate binds to myosin again and the cross-bridge breaks, leaving myosin to bind to the next site on actin. This repeated process causes muscle contraction as sarcomeres shorten.

Normal adult muscle, when viewed in cross section, consists of fibers approximately 30 to 80 µm in diameter with multiple peripherally located nuclei. Muscle fibers are bound by the sarcolemma, external to which is the basal lamina. The endomysium is the connective tissue between muscle fibers. The muscle itself is divided into fascicles, or groups of muscle fibers, surrounded by connective tissue referred to as the perimysium. Epimysium surrounds the muscle as a whole.

Normal muscle consists of type 1 and type 2 fibers, intermixed randomly. Type 1 fibers depend primarily on oxidative metabolism and are considered slow-twitch fibers. Type 2 fibers are considered fast-twitch fibers; type 2A fibers function well in both anaerobic and aerobic states, whereas type 2B fibers function most efficiently in an anaerobic state. Type 1 and 2 fibers can be easily differentiated by adenosine triphosphatase reactivity after incubation at acid or alkaline pH. Mitochondrial enzymes, glycogen and lipid content, myofibrillar integrity, the presence or absence of angulated fibers, vacuoles, inclusions, and some enzyme deficiencies can be readily detected under light microscopy with proper staining.

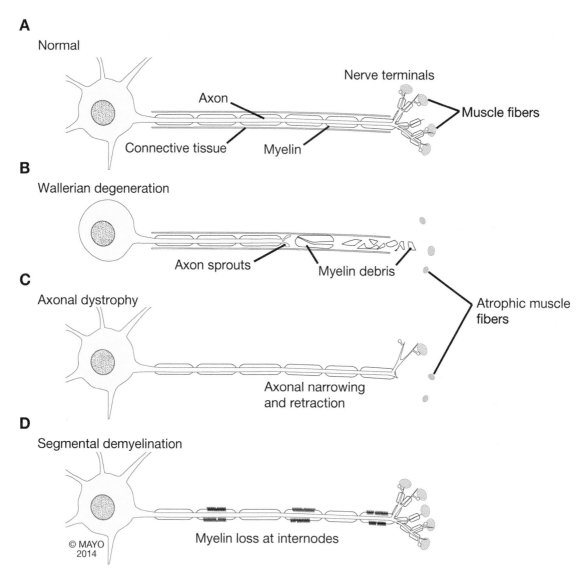

Figure 6.11 *Diagram of Pathologic Changes in Peripheral Nerve Fibers.*
A, Normal axon. B, Wallerian degeneration occurs distal to local destruction of an axon and is associated with central chromatolysis of the cell body and muscle fiber atrophy. Regeneration occurs along the connective tissue path. C, Axonal dystrophy results in distal narrowing and dying back of nerve terminals due to either intrinsic axon or motor neuron disease. D, Segmental demyelination destroys myelin at scattered internodes along the axon without causing axonal damage.
(Adapted from Benarroch EE, Daube JR, Flemming KD, Westmoreland BF. Mayo Clinic medical neurosciences: organized by neurologic systems and levels. 5th ed. Rochester [MN]: Mayo Clinic Scientific Press and Florence [KY]: Informa Healthcare USA; c2008. Chapter 13, The peripheral level; p. 491–546. Used with permission of Mayo Foundation for Medical Education and Research.)

Multiple proteins contribute to the structural integrity and proper function of the muscle fiber (Figure 6.14). Dystrophin is located on the cytoplasmic side of the muscle membrane and is important for stabilization of the membrane during contraction. The sarcoglycans (α, β, γ, and δ) are transmembrane proteins also important for stabilizing the sarcolemma. Emerin is part of the nuclear membrane, and lamin A/C is in the lamina beneath the nuclear membrane. β-Dystroglycan is located in the sarcolemmal membrane; it binds to dystrophin and also to extracellular α-dystroglycan, which in turn binds to laminin α2. Caveolin is associated with calveoli in the sarcolemmal membrane. Calpain is a protease. Dysferlin serves a membrane repair function. Myotilin is associated with the Z disk. These are but a few of the important components of normal muscle structure. Dysfunction in many of the proteins described can result in muscular dystrophies or other myopathies. There are myriad other

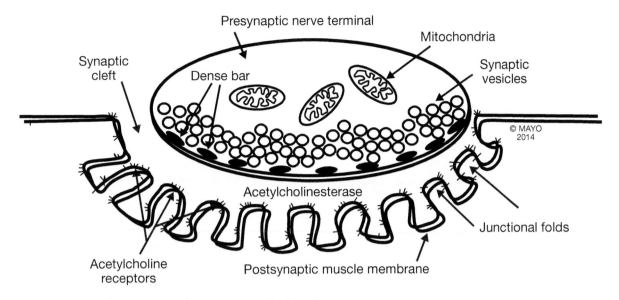

Figure 6.12 *Functional Anatomy of the Neuromuscular Junction.*
(Adapted from Boon AJ. Assessing the neuromuscular junction with repetitive stimulation studies. In: Daube JR, Rubin DI, editors. Clinical neurophysiology. 3rd ed. Oxford [UK]: Oxford University Press; c2009. p. 369–84. Used with permission of Mayo Foundation for Medical Education and Research.)

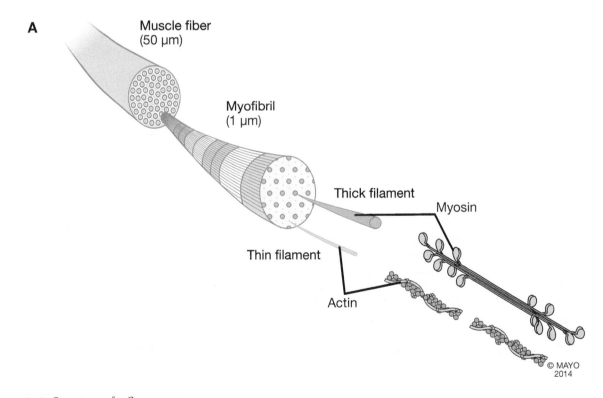

Figure 6.13 *Structure of a Sarcomere.*
A, Ultrastructure of a muscle fiber. Each fiber is made up of many myofibrils containing filaments of actin and myosin organized in bands A, I, and Z. B, Organization of protein filaments in a myofibril. A, Longitudinal section through 1 sarcomere (Z disk to Z disk) showing overlap of actin and myosin. B, Cross section through A band, where the thin actin filaments interdigitate with the thick myosin filaments in a hexagonal formation. C, Location of specific proteins in a sarcomere. C, Structure of a single muscle fiber cut longitudinally and in cross section. Individual myofibrils are surrounded and separated by sarcoplasmic reticulum. T tubules are continuous with extracellular fluid and interdigitate with the sarcoplasmic reticulum.
(Adapted from Benarroch EE, Daube JR, Flemming KD, Westmoreland BF. Mayo Clinic medical neurosciences: organized by neurologic systems and levels. 5th ed. Rochester [MN]: Mayo Clinic Scientific Press and Florence [KY]: Informa Healthcare USA; c2008. Chapter 13, The peripheral level; p. 491–546. Used with permission of Mayo Foundation for Medical Education and Research.)

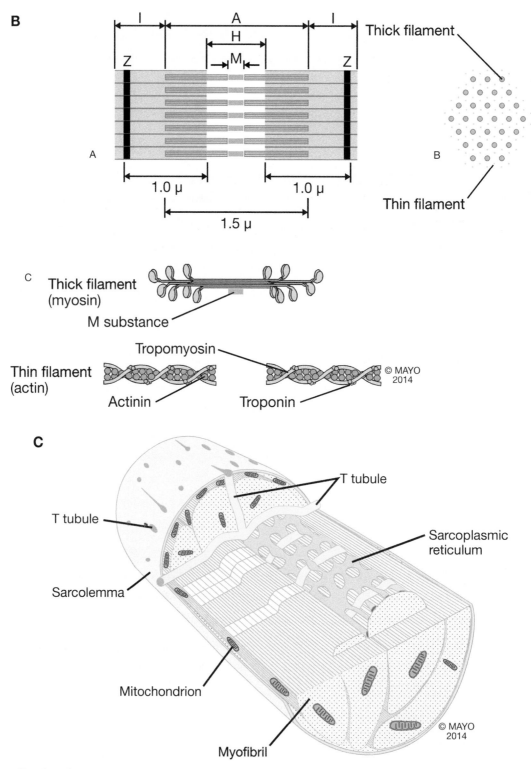

Figure 6.13 *Continued*

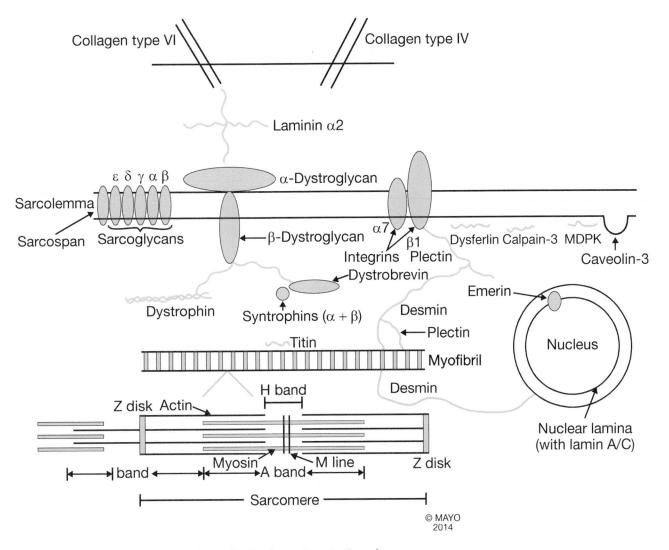

Figure 6.14 *Dystrophin-Associated Muscle Membrane Protein Complex.*
MDPK indicates myotonic dystrophy protein kinase.
(Adapted from Banwell BL. Muscular dystrophies. In: Noseworthy JH, editor. Neurological therapeutics: principles and practice. Vol 2. London [UK]: Martin Dunitz; c2003. p. 2312–27. Used with permission of Mayo Foundation for Medical Education and Research.)

causes of congenital and acquired myopathies, as well as mitochondrial and metabolic myopathies (see Volume 2, Chapter 42, "Acquired Muscle Disorders," and Chapter 43, "Inherited Muscle Disorders").

- The neuromuscular junction consists of the presynaptic membrane of a motor neuron, the synaptic cleft, and the postsynaptic muscle membrane.
- On the postsynaptic membrane, nicotinic acetylcholine receptors are located in the crests of junctional folds,

and voltage-gated sodium channels are clusters at the bottoms of these folds.
- Type 1 muscle fibers depend primarily on oxidative metabolism and are considered slow-twitch fibers.
- Type 2 muscle fibers are considered fast-twitch fibers.
- Dystrophin is located on the cytoplasmic side of the muscle membrane and is important for stabilization of the membrane during contraction.

7 Spinal Cord Anatomy

JENNIFER A. TRACY, MD

Introduction

The spinal cord begins as the cervical cord, which is just below the medulla and extends downward through the spinal canal. It then becomes the thoracic, lumbar, sacral, and coccygeal parts of the cord. The spinal cord proper ends at the lower portion of the first lumbar vertebral body in most persons where it forms the conus medullaris, followed by the filum terminale. There are enlargements at both the cervical and lumbar cord levels, which represent the innervation pathways of the upper and lower limbs, respectively.

A number of ascending and descending pathways travel in the spinal cord. These are reviewed in this chapter.

Spinal Cord Cross-sectional Anatomy

The spinal cord can be divided into white matter and gray matter. The white matter is often divided into separate funiculi (Figure 7.1). The spinal cord cross sections appear differently at each level. For example, the Clarke column is noted only at T1-L2. Fasciculus gracilis appears alone at the level of the lumbar segments, but medial to fasciculus cuneatus at the level of the cervical cord. Many ascending and descending tracts traverse the spinal cord (Figure 7.1). These tracts are discussed further later in this chapter.

The gray matter of the cord contains several types of neurons. Alpha and gamma motor neurons are present in the anterior section of the cord gray matter, referred to as the ventral horn. Alpha motor neurons supply motor innervation to skeletal muscles throughout the body. A motor unit is a single motor neuron and all the muscle fibers it supplies. Gamma motor neurons provide innervation to muscle spindles, which are stretch receptors in the muscle.

A more lateral area of gray matter from T1-L2 contains the intermediolateral cell column, which consists of sympathetic autonomic neurons at the T1-L2 level. There are parasympathetic autonomic neurons at the S2-S4 levels in the ventral horn. There are also many interneurons in the gray matter of the cord, particularly in intermediate segments of the gray matter. Another important area of spinal gray matter is the Clarke column, which is in the intermediate gray matter and contains cells that mediate information from muscle spindles and other receptors and continues into the dorsal spinocerebellar tract into the cerebellum.

Sensory neurons are present in the dorsal horn. The gray matter of the cord is separated out into Rexed laminae (I-X), in roughly a dorsal to ventral gradient with sensory neurons more dorsal (lower numbers) and motor neurons more ventral (higher numbers) and lamina X around the central canal (see also Chapter 4, "Peripheral and Central Pain Pathways and Pathophysiology").

Main Tracts: Descending

Corticospinal Tract

The corticospinal tract lies in the lateral funiculus at the level of the spinal cord (Figure 7.1). Motor neurons in layer 5 of the primary motor cortex predominantly descend as the corticospinal tract and function in executing voluntary movement (Figure 7.2). The leg fibers originate in the medial cortex, the arm and face fibers in the lateral cortex. These so-called upper motor neurons descend through the corona radiata, internal capsule, and ventral aspect of the brainstem and decussate at the caudal medulla. These axons continue as the lateral corticospinal tract in the spinal cord, ultimately synapsing on the neurons in the ventral horn gray matter. An upper motor neuron lesion at the level of the cord results in ipsilateral weakness below the level of the lesion.

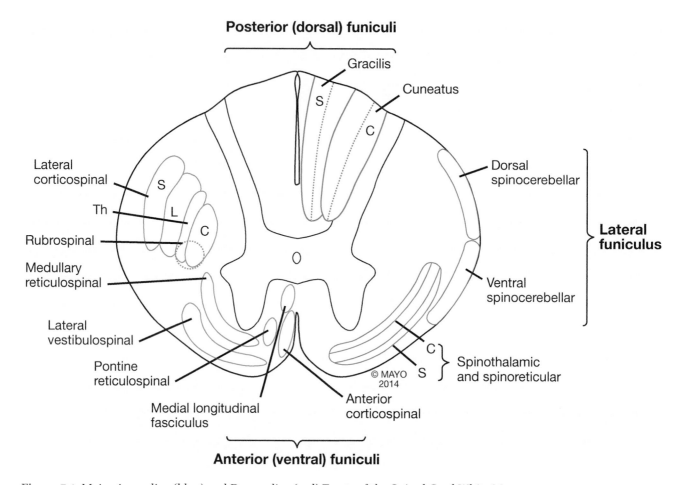

Figure 7.1 *Major Ascending (blue) and Descending (red) Tracts of the Spinal Cord White Matter. C indicates cervical; L, lumbar; S, sacral; Th, thoracic.*

(Adapted from Benarroch EE, Daube JR, Flemming KD, Westmoreland BF. Mayo Clinic medical neurosciences: organized by neurologic systems and levels. 5th ed. Rochester [MN]: Mayo Clinic Scientific Press and Florence [KY]: Informa Healthcare USA; c2008. Chapter 14, The spinal level; p. 547–94. Used with permission of Mayo Foundation for Medical Education and Research.)

Vestibulospinal Tract

The vestibulospinal tract projects from the vestibulocochlear nerve and vestibular nuclei to form the medial and lateral vestibulospinal tracts. These tracts synapse on interneurons or alpha motor neurons for maintenance of erect posture relative to head and eye motion. The medial vestibulospinal tract helps maintain head position and terminates in the cervical spine, while the lateral vestibulospinal tract projects to neurons innervating muscles in the trunk and lower extremities.

Tectospinal Tract

The tectospinal tract originates in the superior colliculus of the midbrain (Figure 7.3). The superior colliculus receives information from the oculomotor nuclei and integrates other sensory information to respond to the environment. The tectospinal tract crosses and projects to the cranial nuclei involved in extraocular movement

(oculomotor, trochlear, abducens) and the cervical spinal cord to coordinate movements of the head, neck, and eyes in response to sensory stimuli.

Rubrospinal Tract

The rubrospinal tract originates in the red nucleus in the midbrain, crosses to the opposite side, and extends primarily to the cervical spinal cord to influence flexion, primarily in the upper extremities. It descends in the spinal cord in the lateral funiculus before terminating on the anterior horn cells (Figure 7.3).

Reticulospinal Tract

The medullary and pontine reticulospinal tracts originate in the medulla and pons, respectively. These tracts are important for multiple functions but are particularly relevant for maintenance of posture during movement by suppressing reflexes that would interfere with coordinated

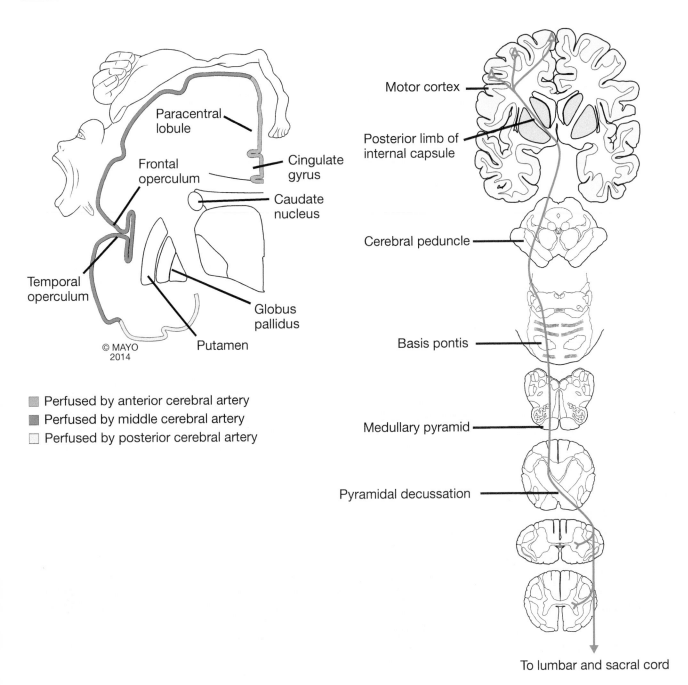

Motor cortex

Posterior limb of internal capsule

Cerebral peduncle

Basis pontis

Medullary pyramid

Pyramidal decussation

To lumbar and sacral cord

Paracentral lobule

Frontal operculum

Cingulate gyrus

Caudate nucleus

Temporal operculum

Globus pallidus

Putamen

© MAYO 2014

■ Perfused by anterior cerebral artery
■ Perfused by middle cerebral artery
□ Perfused by posterior cerebral artery

Figure 7.2 *Corticospinal Tract.*
This tract descends through the cerebral hemispheres, brainstem, and spinal cord. Some of the axons in the tract extend the entire length of the spinal cord.
(Adapted from Benarroch EE, Daube JR, Flemming KD, Westmoreland BF. Mayo Clinic medical neurosciences: organized by neurologic systems and levels. 5th ed. Rochester [MN]: Mayo Clinic Scientific Press and Florence [KY]: Informa Healthcare USA; c2008. Chapter 8, The motor system; p. 265–330. Used with permission of Mayo Foundation for Medical Education and Research.)

voluntary movement. This includes excitation of extensor muscles and inhibition of flexor muscles. The reticulospinal tracts lie in the ventral funiculus (Figure 7.2).

- The corticospinal tract lies in the lateral funiculus at the level of the spinal cord.

Main Tracts: Ascending

Fasciculus Gracilis and Cuneatus

The dorsal column–medial lemniscal system conveys information regarding vibration, joint position sense, and discriminative touch (see Chapter 3, "Afferent System

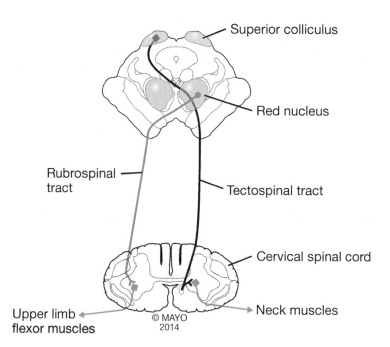

Figure 7.3 *Rubrospinal and Tectospinal Pathways (both are bilateral, but are shown unilaterally).*
The rubrospinal tract arises in the red nucleus on the opposite side and reaches the cervical spinal cord to activate flexor movements of the arm. The tectospinal tract arises in the contralateral superior colliculus and, together with the medial vestibulospinal tract (not shown), coordinates movements of the head with those of the eyes.
(Adapted from Benarroch EE, Daube JR, Flemming KD, Westmoreland BF. Mayo Clinic medical neurosciences: organized by neurologic systems and levels. 5th ed. Rochester [MN]: Mayo Clinic Scientific Press and Florence [KY]: Informa Healthcare USA; c2008. Chapter 8, The motor system; p. 265–330. Used with permission of Mayo Foundation for Medical Education and Research.)

Overview"). At the level of the spinal cord, fasciculus gracilis lies medial to fasciculus cuneatus in the dorsal funiculus. Fasciculus gracilis receives input from the dorsal root ganglion neurons from below T6. Fasciculus cuneatus receives input from the dorsal root ganglion neurons from T6 and above. This information enters the fasciculi and ascends to nucleus gracilis and cuneatus at the level of the caudal medulla where a synapse occurs with the second-order neurons. Neurons from nucleus gracilis and cuneatus project axons as the medial lemniscus to the ventroposterior lateral nucleus of the thalamus. The ventroposterior lateral neurons then project to the S1 cortex.

Spinothalamic Tract

The spinothalamic tract carries pain and temperature sensation from the body to several regions of the cortex (see Chapter 4, "Peripheral and Central Pain Pathways and Pathophysiology"). Axons from the dorsal root ganglion neurons enter the spinal cord dorsally, then synapse in the dorsal horn at or slightly above the entry level. The axons of the second-order neurons decussate (cross over) to the opposite side of the spinal cord where they ascend in the ventral funiculus as the anterior spinothalamic tract and in the lateral funiculus as the lateral spinothalamic tract.

Spinocerebellar Tract

The ventral and dorsal spinocerebellar tracts transmit information about unconscious proprioception to the cerebellum (Figure 7.4). The dorsal spinocerebellar tract originates in the Clarke column (C8-L2). This tract carries information regarding unconscious proprioception from the lower extremity and trunk. The upper extremity unconscious proprioception is carried by the cuneocerebellar tract. At the level of the spinal cord, the dorsal spinocerebellar tract courses through the lateral funiculus (Figure 7.2).

Clinical Correlations

Brown-Séquard Syndrome

Patients with a hemisection of the cord may develop Brown-Séquard syndrome. This syndrome is characterized by upper motor neuron weakness and loss of vibration/proprioception below the level of the lesion ipsilaterally and contralateral loss of sensation to pain and temperature. At the segmental level (level of the lesion), the patient may have a small area of loss of all sensory modalities (Figure 7.5).

Commissural Syndrome

Patients with syringomyelia or a central cord lesion may present with decreased sensation to pain and temperature

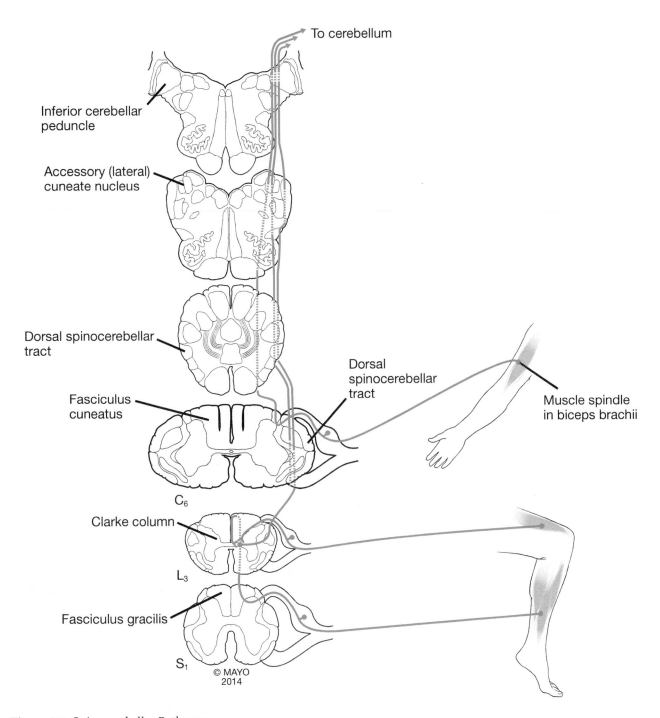

Figure 7.4 Spinocerebellar Pathways.
(Adapted from Benarroch EE, Daube JR, Flemming KD, Westmoreland BF. Mayo Clinic medical neurosciences: organized by neurologic systems and levels. 5th ed. Rochester [MN]: Mayo Clinic Scientific Press and Florence [KY]: Informa Healthcare USA; c2008. Chapter 7, The sensory system; p. 217–64. Used with permission of Mayo Foundation for Medical Education and Research.)

in a bilateral manner. At the level of the cervical cord, this is often referred to as a caped distribution. Commissural syndrome is due to interruption of the segmental crossing of the spinothalamic tract. Because a central lesion does not affect the spinothalamic tract and affects only the decussating segmental fibers, patients

have symptoms only at the level surrounding the lesion (Figure 7.6).

Anterior Spinal Artery Syndrome
The anterior spinal artery typically supplies the ventral two-thirds of the spinal cord. Ischemia of the anterior

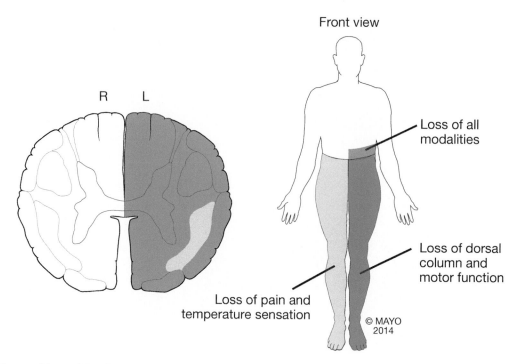

Figure 7.5 *Brown-Séquard Syndrome.*
Sensory loss produced by damage to one-half of the spinal cord by the lesion shown on the left. An ipsilateral motor deficit would also be present.
(Adapted from Benarroch EE, Daube JR, Flemming KD, Westmoreland BF. Mayo Clinic medical neurosciences: organized by neurologic systems and levels. 5th ed. Rochester [MN]: Mayo Clinic Scientific Press and Florence [KY]: Informa Healthcare USA; c2008. Chapter 7, The sensory system; p. 217–64. Used with permission of Mayo Foundation for Medical Education and Research.)

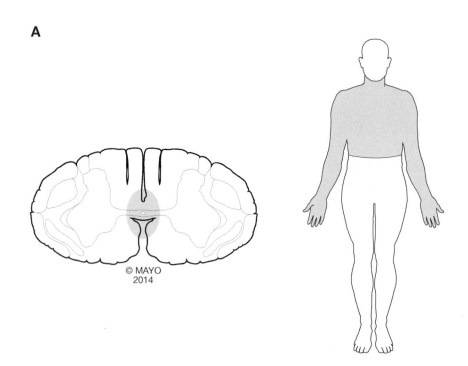

Figure 7.6 *Commissural Syndrome.*
A, Distribution of loss of pain and temperature sensation with a lesion in the location shown on the left. B, Magnetic resonance image of syringomyelia at the level of the cervical spinal cord (arrow).
(Adapted from Benarroch EE, Daube JR, Flemming KD, Westmoreland BF. Mayo Clinic medical neurosciences: organized by neurologic systems and levels. 5th ed. Rochester [MN]: Mayo Clinic Scientific Press and Florence [KY]: Informa Healthcare USA; c2008. Chapter 7, The sensory system; p. 217–64. Used with permission of Mayo Foundation for Medical Education and Research.)

B

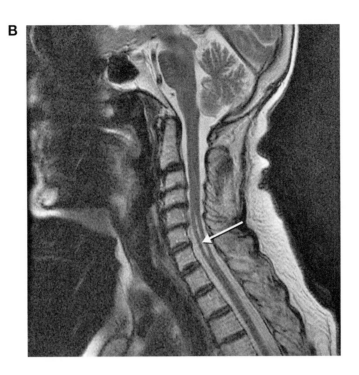

Figure 7.6 Continued.

spinal artery generally causes weakness and loss of sensation to pain and temperature below the lesion but often spares the dorsal columns.

- The dorsal column–medial lemniscal system conveys information regarding vibration, joint position sense, and discriminative touch.
- At the level of the spinal cord, fasciculus gracilis lies medial to fasciculus cuneatus in the dorsal funiculus.

- The spinothalamic tract carries pain and temperature sensation from the body to several regions of the cortex.
- Brown-Séquard syndrome is characterized by upper motor neuron weakness and loss of vibration/ proprioception below the level of the lesion ipsilaterally and contralateral loss of sensation to pain and temperature.
- Patients with syringomyelia or a central cord lesion may present with decreased sensation to pain and temperature in a bilateral manner.

Brainstem and Cranial Nerves: Overview and Medulla

8

KELLY D. FLEMMING, MD

Introduction

This chapter and the following 3 chapters will review the anatomy of the brainstem and cranial nerves. This chapter contains an overview of the cranial nerves as well as important structures at the level of the medulla. Chapter 9 discusses important structures at the level of the pons. Chapter 10 discusses important structures at the level of the midbrain. Chapter 11 discusses pathways that traverse the entire brainstem. Clinical syndromes of the brainstem and cranial nerves are discussed in Volume 2, Section VIII, "Clinical Disorders of the Cranial Nerves and Brainstem."

Overview

Cranial Nerves

There are 12 pairs of cranial nerves (numbered I through XII). Cranial nerves, like spinal nerves, contain sensory or motor fibers or a combination of fiber types. These fibers are classified by their embryologic origin or common structural and functional characteristics.

Motor

- General somatic efferent (GSE): innervate somite-derived muscles (III, IV, VI, XII)
- Special visceral efferent (SVE): innervate branchial arch–derived muscles (V, VII, IX, X, XI)

- General visceral efferent (GVE): innervate mesoderm/endoderm-derived structures; parasympathetic (III, VII, IX, X)

Sensory

- General somatic afferent (GSA): sensory information regarding sensation from body surface, joints, and mucosal membranes (V, VII, IX, X)
- General visceral afferent (GVA): sensory information from pharynx and endodermally derived structures such as the viscera (IX, X)
- Special visceral afferent (SVA): sensory information regarding taste and smell (I, VII, IX, X)
- Special somatic afferent (SSA): sensory information regarding hearing and balance and information regarding vision (II, VIII)

Table 8.1 summarizes the cranial nerves, their components, and their functions. Figure 8.1 shows the cranial nerves noted from the ventral surface of the brainstem. Figure 8.2 reviews the foramina of the skull through which cranial nerves enter and exit the skull.

The Brainstem

The brainstem is divided into the medulla, pons, and midbrain. Cranial nerves III to XII exit at the level of the brainstem. Figure 8.3 shows drawn cross sections of the brainstem.

Abbreviations: GSA, general somatic afferent; GSE, general somatic efferent; GVA, general visceral afferent; GVE, general visceral efferent; SSA, special somatic afferent; SVA, special visceral afferent; SVE, special visceral efferent; VPM, ventral posteromedial nucleus

Table 8.1 • Summary of Cranial Nerves

Cranial Nerve	Type	Ganglion/Nucleus	Function
I Olfactory	SVA	Olfactory receptor cells Olfactory bulb/tract	Sense of smell
II Optic	SSA	Retinal ganglion cells	Vision
III Oculomotor	GSE	Oculomotor nucleus	Innervates inferior, medial, and superior recti and inferior oblique muscles
	GVE	Edinger-Westphal nucleus Ciliary ganglion	Preganglionic parasympathetic to pupil and ciliary muscle
IV Trochlear	GSE	Trochlear nucleus	Innervates superior oblique muscle
V Trigeminal	SVE	Motor nucleus of V	Innervates muscles of mastication
	GSA	Trigeminal ganglion Spinal tract and nucleus of V	Ipsilateral pain and temperature sensation of face and supratentorial dura mater
	GSA	Trigeminal ganglion Principal sensory nucleus of V	Vibration, proprioception, tactile discrimination of ipsilateral face
	GSA	Mesencephalic nucleus of V	Unconscious proprioception of jaw, reflexive chewing
VI Abducens	GSE	Abducens nucleus	Innervates lateral rectus muscle
VII Facial	SVE	Facial nucleus (motor nucleus of VII) Superior salivatory nucleus Submandibular ganglion	Muscles of facial expression and stapedius muscle Innervate submandibular and sublingual glands (salivation)
	GVE	Superior salivatory nucleus (lacrimal nucleus) Pterygopalatine ganglion	Lacrimation (tearing) and nasal mucosa
	SVA	Geniculate ganglion Nucleus solitarius (rostral)	Taste buds of anterior 2/3 of tongue
	GSA	Trigeminal ganglion Spinal nucleus of V	Somatic sensation of external ear
VIII Vestibulocochlear	SSA	Vestibular ganglion Vestibular nuclei	Control posture and movement of body and eyes relative to angular and linear acceleration
	SSA	Spiral ganglion	Hearing
IX Glossopharyngeal	SVE	Nucleus ambiguus	Innervates stylopharyngeus muscle
	GVE	Inferior salivatory nucleus Otic ganglion	Innervates parotid gland (salivation)
	GVA	Inferior ganglion	Input from carotid sinus baroreceptors and carotid body chemoreceptors
		Nucleus solitarius (caudal)	Tactile input from posterior 1/3 of tongue, pharynx, middle ear, and auditory canal
	SVA	Inferior ganglion Nucleus solitarius (rostral)	Taste buds of posterior 1/3 of tongue
	GSA	Superior ganglion Spinal nucleus of V	Somatic sensation of external ear
X Vagus	SVE	Nucleus ambiguus	Innervates muscles of pharynx and larynx
	GVE	Dorsal motor nucleus of X	Preganglionic parasympathetic to viscera including heart, lungs, gastrointestinal tract
	GVA	Inferior ganglion Nucleus solitarius (caudal)	Visceral sensation
	SVA	Inferior ganglion Nucleus solitarius (rostral)	Taste buds on epiglottis, pharyngeal wall
	GSA	Superior ganglion Spinal nucleus of V	Somatic sensation of external ear
XI Spinal accessory	SVE	Cranial: nucleus ambiguus Spinal: ventral horn cells (cervical)	Innervates muscles of larynx (with X) Innervates sternocleidomastoid and trapezius muscles
XII Hypoglossal	GSE	Hypoglossal nucleus	Tongue movement

Abbreviations: GSA, general somatic afferent; GSE, general somatic efferent; GVA, general visceral afferent; GVE, general visceral efferent; SSA, special somatic afferent; SVA, special visceral afferent; SVE, special visceral efferent.

Adapted from Flemming KD. Disorders of the cranial nerves. In: Mowzoon N, Flemming KD, editors. Neurology board review: an illustrated study guide. Rochester (MN): Mayo Clinic Scientific Press and Florence (KY): Informa Healthcare USA; c2007. p. 127–62. Used with permission of Mayo Foundation for Medical Education and Research.

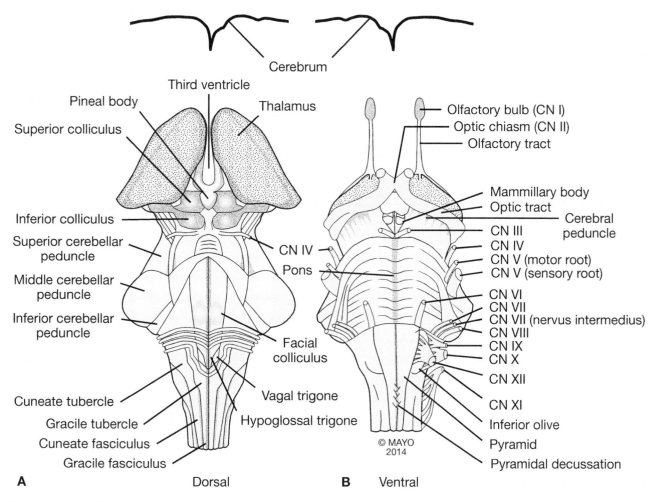

Figure 8.1 *Dorsal and Ventral Surface of the Brainstem.*
(Adapted from Benarroch EE, Daube JR, Flemming KD, Westmoreland BF. Mayo Clinic medical neurosciences: organized by neurologic systems and levels. 5th ed. Rochester [MN]: Mayo Clinic Scientific Press and Florence [KY]: Informa Healthcare USA; c2008. Chapter 3, Diagnosis of neurologic disorders: anatomical localization; p. 53–100. Used with permission of Mayo Foundation for Medical Education and Research.)

Medulla

Anatomy of the Medulla

The medulla extends from the decussation of the pyramids at the level of the caudal medulla/foramen magnum to the inferior cerebellar peduncle/striae medullares. Important structures at this level are the decussation of the pyramidal tracts, decussation of the medial lemniscus, cranial nerves IX to XII and the trigeminal nucleus of V, and nuclei including the inferior olive, nucleus ambiguus, and nucleus solitarius.

The anterior spinal artery is formed from contributions of both vertebral arteries. This artery supplies the medial portion of the medulla as well as the ventral spinal cord. The vertebral artery gives off perforating vessels to the paramedian portion of the medulla. The vertebral artery also gives rise to the posterior inferior cerebellar artery, which supplies the lateral medulla and inferior cerebellum. In the caudal medulla, the posterior spinal artery contributes to the supply of the dorsal medulla where the nucleus gracilis and cuneatus lie. The posterior spinal artery may arise from the vertebral arteries, but also commonly from the posterior inferior cerebellar artery.

Important Structures at the Level of the Medulla

Pyramidal Tracts
The corticospinal tract (see Figure 7.2 in Chapter 7, "Spinal Cord Anatomy") extends ventrally throughout the entire brainstem, with leg fibers represented lateral to arm fibers. The axons of this tract cross at the caudal medulla (level of foramen magnum) (Figure 8.3A) before descending to the spinal cord.

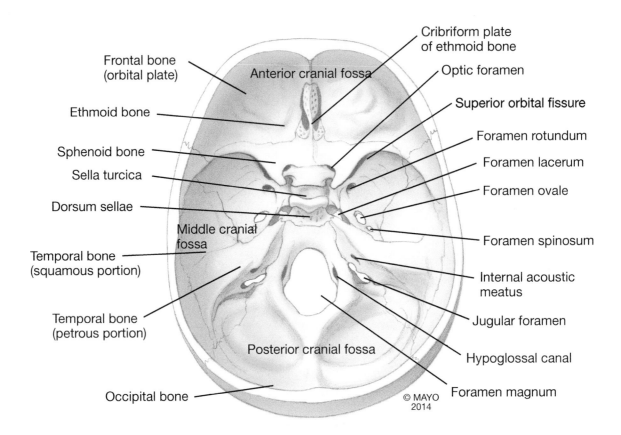

Figure 8.2 *Foramina of the Skull. Base of the skull, showing major bones and foramina.*
(Adapted from Benarroch EE, Daube JR, Flemming KD, Westmoreland BF. Mayo Clinic medical neurosciences: organized by neurologic systems and levels. 5th ed. Rochester [MN]: Mayo Clinic Scientific Press and Florence [KY]: Informa Healthcare USA; c2008. Chapter 15, Part A, The posterior fossa level: brainstem and cranial nerve nuclei; p. 595–632. Used with permission of Mayo Foundation for Medical Education and Research.)

Dorsal Columns–Medial Lemnicus

The dorsal column–medial lemniscal pathway carries joint position, vibration, and discriminative touch sensation from the limbs and body (see Figure 3.7 in Chapter 3, "Afferent System Overview"). Fibers ascend in the fasciculus cuneatus (upper body/arm) and fasciculus gracilis (lower body/leg) in the dorsal columns and synapse at their respective nuclei in the caudal medulla (Figure 8.3A).

Trigeminal Nucleus of V

Although the trigeminal nerve sensory fibers enter at the level of the pons, the trigeminal nucleus of cranial nerve V is apparent at the level of the medulla, laterally (Figure 8.3B). This structure is further discussed in Chapter 9, "Brainstem and Cranial Nerves: The Pons" with the other sensory components of V.

Inferior Olive

The inferior olive is grossly apparent in the ventral medulla (Figure 8.3B). This structure functions to compare the actual to the intended motor movement and aid in correc-

tions. Fibers from the inferior olive project to the contralateral cerebellum.

Nucleus Ambiguus

The nucleus ambiguus is located in the lateral medulla at the level of the inferior olive (Figure 8.3B). This motor nucleus has SVE and GVE components.

The SVE (motor) nucleus has components of cranial nerve IX, X, and the cranial portion of XI that innervate striated muscles derived from branchial arches 3, 4, and 5.

- Cranial nerve IX innervates the stylopharyngeus.
- Cranial nerve X innervates palatal muscles (with assistance from cranial nerve V for the tensor veli palatini), most of the pharyngeal muscles (with assistance from cranial nerve IX), laryngeal muscles, and striated muscles of the esophagus.
- Cranial nerve XI innervates laryngeal muscles (cranial portion).

Corticobulbar input is bilateral. Thus, an upper motor neuron lesion does not result in dysfunction. A unilateral

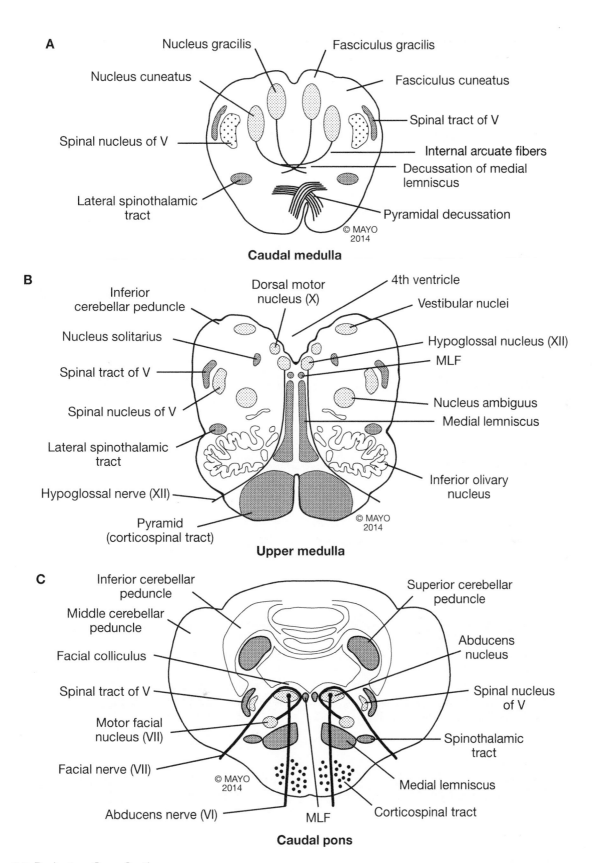

Figure 8.3 Brainstem Cross Sections.
A, Caudal medulla. B, Upper medulla. C, Caudal pons. D, Middle pons. E, Rostral pons. F, Caudal midbrain at the level of the inferior colliculus. G, Rostral midbrain at the level of the superior colliculus. MLF indicates medial longitudinal fasciculus.

(Adapted from Flemming KD. Disorders of the cranial nerves. In: Mowzoon N, Flemming KD, editors. Neurology board review: an illustrated study guide. Rochester [MN]: Mayo Clinic Scientific Press and Florence [KY]: Informa Healthcare USA; c2007. p. 127–62. Used with permission of Mayo Foundation for Medical Education and Research.)

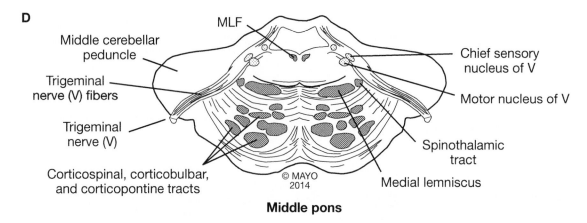

D

MLF

Middle cerebellar peduncle

Chief sensory nucleus of V

Trigeminal nerve (V) fibers

Motor nucleus of V

Trigeminal nerve (V)

Spinothalamic tract

Corticospinal, corticobulbar, and corticopontine tracts

Medial lemniscus

© MAYO 2014

Middle pons

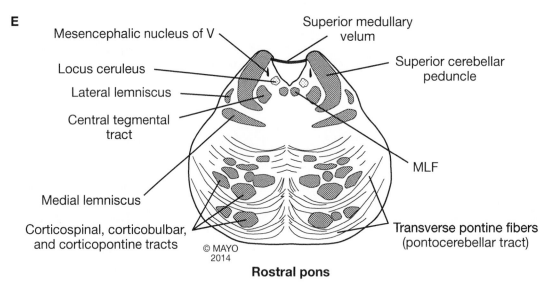

E

Mesencephalic nucleus of V

Superior medullary velum

Locus ceruleus

Superior cerebellar peduncle

Lateral lemniscus

Central tegmental tract

MLF

Medial lemniscus

Corticospinal, corticobulbar, and corticopontine tracts

Transverse pontine fibers (pontocerebellar tract)

© MAYO 2014

Rostral pons

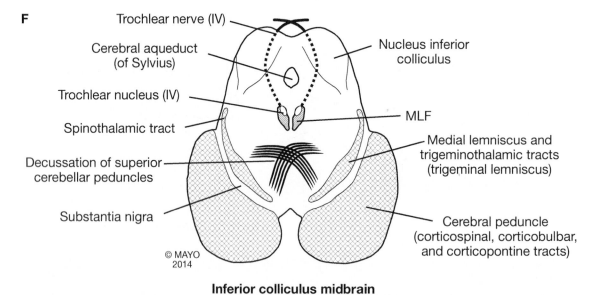

F

Trochlear nerve (IV)

Nucleus inferior colliculus

Cerebral aqueduct (of Sylvius)

Trochlear nucleus (IV)

MLF

Spinothalamic tract

Medial lemniscus and trigeminothalamic tracts (trigeminal lemniscus)

Decussation of superior cerebellar peduncles

Substantia nigra

Cerebral peduncle (corticospinal, corticobulbar, and corticopontine tracts)

© MAYO 2014

Inferior colliculus midbrain

Figure 8.3 Continued on next page

G

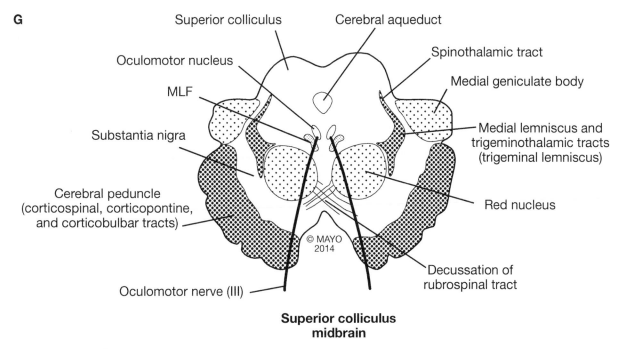

**Superior colliculus
midbrain**

Figure 8.3 Continued

lesion may result in nasal speech (palatine weakness), hoarse voice (laryngeal paralysis), and deviation of the uvula to the normal side. A bilateral lesion results in severe dysfunction—dysphagia, hoarseness, difficulty breathing (laryngeal muscle paralysis).

Vasodepressor neurons within nucleus ambiguus, along with neurons from the dorsal nucleus of cranial nerve X, play a role in maintaining blood pressure (see "Clinical Correlations" later in this chapter).

Nucleus Solitarius

This sensory nucleus runs longitudinally in the medulla. The rostral and ventral components of this nucleus have separate functions and cranial nerve involvement.

SVA fibers from cranial nerves VII (via geniculate ganglion), IX (via inferior ganglion), and X (via inferior ganglion) enter the rostral aspect of nucleus solitarius carrying information about taste sensation from the tongue, epiglottis, and pharynx (Figure 8.4). Axons from cranial nerves

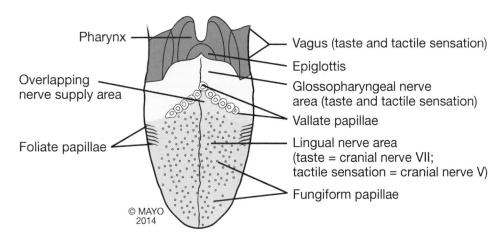

Figure 8.4 Taste Sensation.
Taste from the anterior two-thirds of the tongue (blue) is carried by cranial nerve VII. Taste from the posterior one-third of the tongue (yellow) is carried by cranial nerve IX. Taste from the epiglottis (red) is carried by cranial nerve X.
(Adapted from Flemming KD. Disorders of the cranial nerves. In: Mowzoon N, Flemming KD, editors. Neurology board review: an illustrated study guide. Rochester [MN]: Mayo Clinic Scientific Press and Florence [KY]: Informa Healthcare USA; c2007. p. 127–62. Used with permission of Mayo Foundation for Medical Education and Research.)

VII, IX, and X terminate in the rostral portion of the nucleus solitarius and ascend as the solitariothalamic tract (uncrossed) in the central tegmental tract. Axons terminate in the ventral posteromedial nucleus (VPM) of the thalamus. Axons from the VPM ascend to the ipsilateral somatosensory cortex and anterior insular cortex (Brodmann area 43).

The caudal portion of the nucleus solitarius receives GVA fibers from cranial nerves IX (via inferior ganglion) and X (via inferior ganglion). These fibers are involved in reflexive responses to GVA input (see "Clinical Correlations" later in this chapter).

- The anterior spinal artery supplies the medial portion of the medulla as well as the ventral spinal cord.
- The posterior inferior cerebellar artery supplies the lateral medulla and inferior cerebellum.
- The nucleus ambiguus has components of cranial nerves IX, X, and XI that innervate muscles of the pharynx and larynx.
- A unilateral lesion of the nucleus ambiguus may result in nasal speech (palatine weakness), hoarse voice (laryngeal paralysis), and deviation of the uvula to the normal side.
- Nucleus solitarius receives special visceral afferent (taste) input from cranial nerves VII, IX, and X as well as general visceral afferent input from cranial nerves IX and X.

Cranial Nerves IX to XII

Cranial Nerve IX (Glossopharyngeal Nerve): Anatomy, Function, Course, Dysfunction

The glossopharyngeal nerve is composed of both sensory (GVA, GSA, SVA) and motor (GVE, SVE) nerves (Table 8.1).

The parasympathetic portion of cranial nerve IX is a GVE fiber innervating the parotid gland, a salivary gland. The inferior salivatory nucleus sends preganglionic parasympathetic axons to otic ganglia. From the otic ganglia, postganglionic fibers innervate the parotid gland.

The SVE component of cranial nerve IX from nucleus ambiguus innervates the stylopharyngeus, a muscle that cannot be clinically tested in isolation.

The SVA and GVA components of cranial nerve IX enter the rostral and caudal aspects of nucleus solitarius, respectively. The GVA component of cranial nerve IX receives input from the carotid sinus baroreceptors and carotid body chemoreceptors. In addition, it receives tactile touch information from the posterior one-third of the tongue, pharynx, middle ear, and auditory canal. From there, reflexive pathways to the dorsal motor nucleus of cranial nerve X, nucleus ambiguus, and other brainstem structures occur. Taste from the posterior one-third of the tongue travels to the rostral aspect of nucleus solitarius

along with axons from cranial nerves VII and X. Fibers from nucleus solitarius then travel ipsilaterally to the VPM of the thalamus and from there to the insular cortex.

A small GSA component of cranial nerve IX comes from the external ear to the spinal nucleus and tract of V.

Cranial nerve IX exits the brainstem in the postolivary sulcus and exits the skull via the jugular foramen.

Dysfunction of cranial nerve IX may result in poor gag reflex (IX part of afferent limb), carotid baroreceptor hypersensitivity response, reduced taste, and rarely glossopharyngeal neuralgia (see "Clinical Correlations" later in this chapter).

Cranial Nerve X (Vagus Nerve): Anatomy, Function, Course, Dysfunction

Cranial nerve X (vagus nerve) is also a mixed nerve with both sensory (GSA, SVA, GVA) and motor (SVE, GVE) components (Table 8.1).

The parasympathetic portion of cranial nerve X is a GVE fiber innervating visceral organs. The dorsal motor nucleus sends preganglionic parasympathetic axons to visceral ganglia. From the visceral ganglia, postganglionic fibers innervate the individual organs. A vagal discharge may result in constriction of the bronchioles, decreased heart rate, increased blood flow, peristalsis, and increased gut secretions.

The SVE component of cranial nerve X from nucleus ambiguus innervates muscles of the pharynx and larynx.

The SVA and GVA components of cranial nerve X enter the rostral and caudal aspects of nucleus solitarius, respectively. GVA information from the viscera and aortic baroreceptors and chemoreceptors and tactile sensation from the larynx, upper part of the esophagus, and pharynx are projected to nucleus solitarius. From there, reflexive pathways to the dorsal motor nucleus of cranial nerve X, nucleus ambiguus, and other brainstem structures occur. Taste from the epiglottis and posterior pharynx travels to the rostral aspect of nucleus solitarius along with axons from cranial nerves VII, IX, and X. Fibers from nucleus solitarius then travel ipsilaterally to the VPM of the thalamus and from there to the insular cortex.

A small GSA component of cranial nerve X comes from the external ear to the spinal nucleus and tract of V.

The vagus nerve exits the jugular foramen along with cranial nerves IX and XI. It courses through the neck in the carotid sheath. The nerve enters the thorax, passing anterior to the subclavian artery on the right and anterior to the aortic arch on the left. Both nerves pass behind the roots of the lungs. The left nerve continues on the anterior side of the right nerve on the posterior side of the esophagus to reach the gastric plexus. Fibers diverge from this plexus to the duodenum, liver, biliary ducts, spleen, kidneys, and to the small and large intestine as far as the splenic flexure.

Dysfunction of cranial nerve X is variable, depending on where it is affected. In general, lesions may result in hoarseness (laryngeal muscle paralysis), dysphagia (nucleus ambiguus), baroreceptor hypersensitivity, reduced gag reflex, and reduced taste, as well as other effects.

Cranial Nerve XI (Spinal Accessory Nerve): Anatomy, Function, Course, Dysfunction

The spinal accessory nerve is an SVE motor nerve with components from the nucleus ambiguus (cranial component) and from the ventral horn cells of cervical levels I through VI (spinal component) (Table 8.1). The cranial component innervates muscles of the larynx along with cranial nerve X. The spinal component innervates the ipsilateral sternocleidomastoid and trapezius. The sternocleidomastoid functions to turn the chin to the opposite side. When both muscles contract, the 2 sternocleidomastoid muscles draw the head forward. The trapezius functions to elevate the shoulders and stabilize the scapula.

Axons from the cranial division exit the medulla from the postolivary sulcus and join the vagal nerve; axons from spinal division exit the spinal cord, ascend through the foramen magnum, and exit the skull via the jugular foramen.

A lower motor neuron lesion will result in ipsilateral shoulder droop and head tilt on the side opposite the lesion (weak ipsilateral sternocleidomastoid muscle).

Cranial Nerve XII (Hypoglossal Nerve): Anatomy, Function, Course, Dysfunction

The hypoglossal nerve is a GSE motor nerve that innervates the intrinsic and extrinsic muscles of the tongue (except the palatoglossus) (Table 8.1). Each genioglossus muscle pulls the tongue anterior and medial. When the paired genioglossi work together, the tongue protrudes forward. If one side is weak, the functional side pushes the tongue out, but it deviates toward the weak side.

Axons from the hypoglossal nucleus (Figure 8.3B) exit from the preolivary sulcus of the medulla. Axons briefly travel through the carotid sheath and exit the skull via the hypoglossal canal to innervate the genioglossus (Figure 8.5).

Corticobulbar input is unilateral and crossed. Thus, an upper motor neuron lesion results in the tongue deviating toward the side opposite the lesion. In a lower motor neuron lesion, the tongue deviates toward the side of the lesion, and associated atrophy and fasciculations may be present.

- Cranial nerve IX (glossopharyngeal nerve) is composed of both sensory and motor nerves.
- Dysfunction of cranial nerve IX may result in poor gag reflex, carotid baroreceptor hypersensitivity response, reduced taste, and rarely glossopharyngeal neuralgia.
- Cranial nerve X, like cranial nerve IX, is a mixed nerve with both sensory and motor components.
- The vagus nerve exits the jugular foramen along with cranial nerves IX and XI.

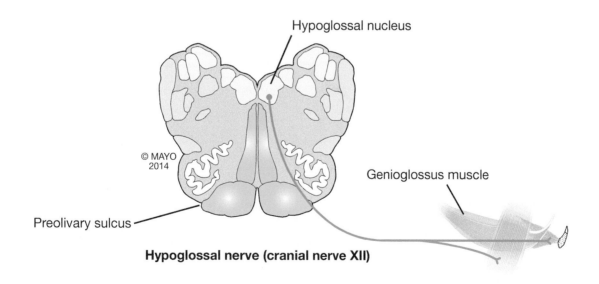

Hypoglossal nerve (cranial nerve XII)

Figure 8.5 Origin, Course, and Distribution of the Hypoglossal Nerve.

(Adapted from Benarroch EE, Daube JR, Flemming KD, Westmoreland BF. Mayo Clinic medical neurosciences: organized by neurologic systems and levels. 5th ed. Rochester [MN]: Mayo Clinic Scientific Press and Florence [KY]: Informa Healthcare USA; c2008. Chapter 15, Part A, The posterior fossa level: brainstem and cranial nerve nuclei; p. 595–632. Used with permission of Mayo Foundation for Medical Education and Research.)

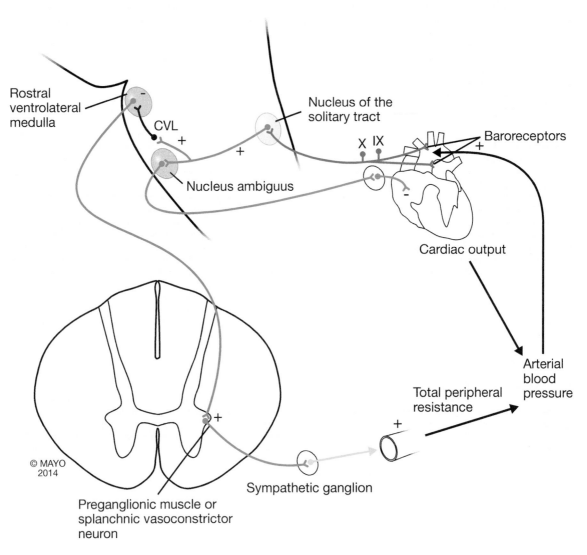

Figure 8.6 *Baroreceptor Reflex.*
The baroreceptor reflex is a critical buffering mechanism that prevents fluctuations of arterial blood pressure, thus rapidly adjusting total peripheral resistance and cardiac output. The carotid sinus and aortic baroreceptors provide excitatory input to the nucleus of the solitary tract through the glossopharyngeal (IX) and vagus (X) nerves, respectively. This baroreceptor input increases in response to an increase in arterial blood pressure, thus activating neurons in the nucleus of the solitary tract. These neurons send excitatory axons directly to nucleus ambiguus (resulting in vagal-mediated bradycardia) and indirectly send inhibitory input via caudal ventrolateral medulla (CVL) to rostral ventrolateral medulla (resulting in inhibition of sympathetic vasomotor activity, which leads to vasodilatation). The result is a decrease in arterial blood pressure. In contrast, in response to a decrease in arterial blood pressure, as with standing, baroreceptor activity decreases, leading to sympathetically mediated vasoconstriction and tachycardia.

(Adapted from Benarroch EE, Daube JR, Flemming KD, Westmoreland BF. Mayo Clinic medical neurosciences: organized by neurologic systems and levels. 5th ed. Rochester [MN]: Mayo Clinic Scientific Press and Florence [KY]: Informa Healthcare USA; c2008. Chapter 9, The internal regulation system; p. 331–83. Used with permission of Mayo Foundation for Medical Education and Research.)

- In general, lesions of cranial nerve X may result in hoarseness, dysphagia, baroreceptor hypersensitivity, reduced gag reflex, and reduced taste, as well as other effects.
- A lower motor neuron lesion of cranial nerve XI will result in ipsilateral shoulder droop and head tilt on the side opposite the lesion (weak ipsilateral sternocleidomastoid muscle).
- An upper motor neuron lesion of cranial nerve XII results in the tongue deviating toward the side opposite the lesion. In a lower motor neuron lesion of cranial nerve XII, the tongue deviates toward the side of the

lesion, and associated atrophy and fasciculations may be present.

Clinical Correlations

Baroreceptor Reflex

The carotid sinus reflex (Figure 8.6) involves both cranial nerves IX and X as well as nucleus ambiguus and nucleus solitarius. Increased blood pressure stimulates pressure receptors (baroreceptors) in the wall of the carotid sinus. Impulses are sent via the glossopharyngeal nerve (GVA fibers) to the caudal aspect of the solitary nucleus. Second-order neurons in this nucleus project through the reticular formation interneurons to the dorsal motor nucleus of X, nucleus ambiguus, hypothalamus, and ventrolateral medulla. The result of activating the dorsal motor nucleus of X and the cardiovagal neurons in nucleus ambiguus is slowing of the heart rate. There is also a signal sent from nucleus solitarius to the ventrolateral medulla (a sympathetic region of the medulla). This signal results in changes in tone of blood vessels in the muscles. Finally, signals sent to the hypothalamus may result in changes in overall blood volume (through antidiuretic hormone). Patients with a hypersensitive carotid sinus reflex may present with recurrent syncope.

Glossopharyngeal Neuralgia

Glossopharyngeal neuralgia is a rare condition. Irritation of the glossopharyngeal nerve may result in throat pain in addition to episodes of syncope related to the carotid sinus reflex. See also Volume 2, Chapter 53, "Secondary Headache Disorders."

Gag Reflex

Touching the posterior pharynx results in a gag response. The afferent limb of this reflex is cranial nerve IX (GVA fibers). The efferent limb of this reflex is via cranial nerve X (SVE—nucleus ambiguus).

* Irritation of the glossopharyngeal nerve may result in throat pain in addition to episodes of syncope related to the carotid sinus reflex.

9 Brainstem and Cranial Nerves: The Pons

KELLY D. FLEMMING, MD; PAUL W. BRAZIS, MD

Introduction

The pons extends from the pontomedullary junction to an imaginary line drawn from the exit of cranial nerve IV. Dorsal to the pons lies the cerebellum. The cerebellum receives information and projects information back to the brainstem through the inferior, middle, and superior cerebellar peduncles. Important structures at this level include corticospinal tracts, corticopontocerebellar fibers travelling through the middle cerebellar peduncle, the cerebellum, and cranial nerves V through VIII.

Blood supply to the pons is from the basilar artery and its perforating vessels (see Chapter 1, "Cerebrovascular Anatomy and Pathophysiology").

Important Structures of the Pons

Corticospinal Tracts/ Corticopontocerebellar Fibers

Corticospinal tracts remain ventral throughout the brainstem. At the level of the pons, crossing corticopontocerebellar fibers are also present ventrally. Thus, patients with a lesion in the ventral pons may present with an ataxic hemiparesis.

Cerebellum

Cerebellar anatomy and function are discussed in Chapter 18, "Cerebellum." The large middle cerebellar peduncle allows afferent information into the cerebellum and is prominent at the level of the pons (see Chapter 8, "Brainstem and Cranial Nerves: Overview and Medulla"). Predominantly efferent information exits the superior cerebellar peduncle. This peduncle crosses at the level of the midbrain.

Cranial Nerves V to VIII

Cranial Nerve V (Trigeminal Nerve)

Cranial nerve V has 4 components: 3 sensory components (general somatic afferent [GSA]) and 1 motor component (special visceral efferent [SVE]) (Table 9.1). The sensory nuclei of cranial nerve V receive information from 3 separate divisions: the ophthalmic (V1), maxillary (V2), and mandibular (V3) (Figure 9.1). The cell body for the sensory division of cranial nerve V is the trigeminal ganglion (also known as the gasserian ganglion or semilunar ganglion), which lies in the Meckel cave within the middle cranial fossa.

Table 9.1 • Components of Cranial Nerve V

Type	Ganglion/Nucleus	Function
SVE	Motor nucleus	Innervate muscles of mastication
GSA	Trigeminal ganglion Spinal tract and nucleus	Ipsilateral pain and temperature sensation to face, supratentorial dura
GSA	Trigeminal ganglion Chief principal nucleus	Vibration, proprioception, tactile discrimination of ipsilateral face
GSA	Mesencephalic nucleus	Unconscious proprioception of jaw; reflexive chewing

Abbreviations: GSA, general somatic afferent; SVE, special visceral efferent.

Abbreviations: GSA, general somatic afferent; GSE, general somatic efferent; GVE, general visceral efferent; SSA, special somatic afferent; SVA, special visceral afferent; SVE, special visceral efferent; VPM, ventral posteromedial nucleus

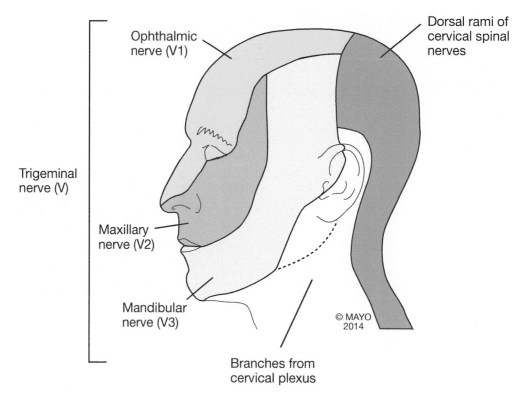

Figure 9.1 Sensory Innervation of the Face and Scalp.
The 3 divisions of cranial nerve V are ophthalmic (V1, yellow), maxillary (V2, green), and mandibular (V3, pink).
(Adapted from Flemming KD. Disorders of the cranial nerves. In: Mowzoon N, Flemming KD, editors. Neurology board review: an illustrated study guide. Rochester [MN]: Mayo Clinic Scientific Press and Florence [KY]: Informa Healthcare USA; c2007. p. 127–62. Used with permission of Mayo Foundation for Medical Education and Research.)

Spinal Tract and Nucleus of Cranial Nerve V

The trigeminal spinal tract and nucleus of cranial nerve V (GSA) carry pain and temperature sensation of the face, oral cavity, dorsum of the head, temporomandibular joint, supratentorial meninges, and teeth. Cutaneous pain and temperature receptors (C fibers) transduce information to the ganglion (first-order neuron) of cranial nerve V (trigeminal ganglion) (Figure 9.2). Sensory fibers enter the midpons and descend as the spinal trigeminal tract in the lateral brainstem. Fibers may terminate at the low portion of the pons or medulla or descend as far as C2-C3 (near zone of Lissauer) before synapsing. Fibers terminate on the spinal trigeminal nucleus, which lies medial to the tract. The axons of the second-order trigeminothalamic neurons decussate and form the anterior trigeminothalamic tract. These fibers ascend throughout the brainstem just posterior to the medial lemniscus. Fibers synapse in the ventral posteromedial nucleus (VPM) of the thalamus. From here, third-order neuronal axons terminate in the somatosensory cortex.

In addition to the path noted, some collaterals of the trigeminothalamic tract terminate in the reticular formation and alternative thalamic nuclei ("medial" pain pathways; see Chapter 4, "Peripheral and Central Pain Pathways and Pathophysiology"), and others are involved in local oral reflexes.

Dysfunction of this pathway results in ipsilateral loss of pain and temperature of the face.

Chief Sensory Nucleus of Cranial Nerve V

This GSA component of cranial nerve V functions in vibration, proprioception, and light touch/tactile discrimination of the face. Pacinian corpuscles, Merkel cells, and Meissner corpuscles of the face transduce these sensations into electrical impulses. Axons from the trigeminal ganglion enter the midpons to synapse at the chief sensory nucleus in the pontine tegmentum (Figure 9.2). Second-order neuronal axons arising from the chief sensory nucleus cross midline and ascend in the lateral brainstem to reach the VPM of the thalamus. Axons from the VPM ascend to the ipsilateral primary somatosensory cortex (Brodmann areas 3, 1, and 2). Dysfunction of this pathway results in ipsilateral loss of tactile discrimination.

Mesencephalic Nucleus of Cranial Nerve V

The mesencephalic nucleus of cranial nerve V (GSA) functions in unconscious proprioception of the jaw. Muscle

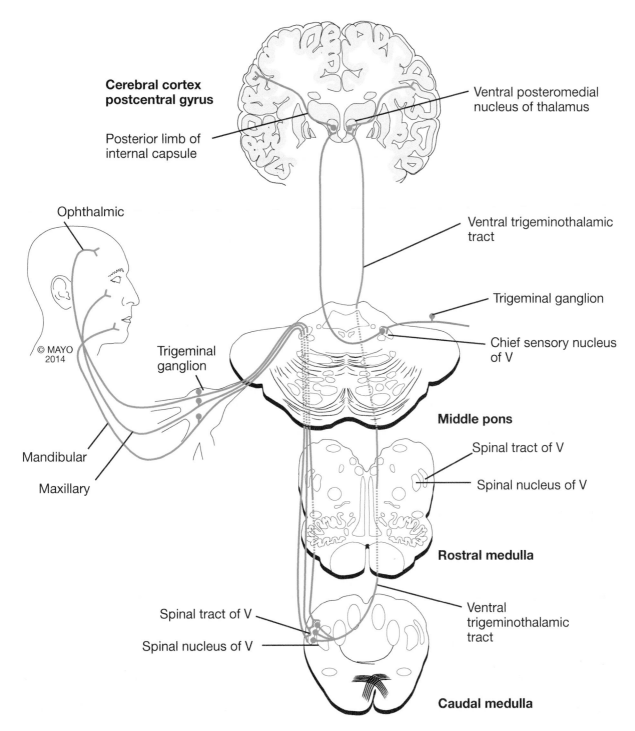

Figure 9.2 *Spinal Trigeminal Nucleus and Tract of Cranial Nerve V, Chief Sensory Nucleus of Cranial Nerve V, and Pathways.*
(Adapted from Flemming KD. Disorders of the cranial nerves. In: Mowzoon N, Flemming KD, editors. Neurology board review: an illustrated study guide. Rochester [MN]: Mayo Clinic Scientific Press and Florence [KY]: Informa Healthcare USA; c2007. p. 127–62. Used with permission of Mayo Foundation for Medical Education and Research.)

spindles in the pterygoids, masseter, and temporalis input information about force of bite and/or stretch of muscle to the mesencephalic nucleus, which forms a reflex with the motor component of cranial nerve V to adjust and control the force of bite.

This is a unique nucleus because it is within the body of the midbrain and not a ganglion cell body.

The afferent axon of this unipolar neuron enters the pons, and the cell body is located in the lower midbrain near the aqueduct. The central processes of the mesencephalic nucleus of cranial nerve V terminate within the motor nucleus of V.

Motor Component of Cranial Nerve V

Neurons of this SVE component of cranial nerve V innervate the muscles of mastication (temporalis, masseter, pterygoids). These muscles function in opening (protracting) the jaw and chewing. Cranial nerve V also innervates the anterior belly of the digastric, mylohyoid, and tensor tympani.

Axons from the motor nucleus of cranial nerve V (see Figure 8.3D in Chapter 8, "Brainstem and Cranial Nerves: Overview and Medulla") exit the brainstem laterally to travel with the V3 sensory distribution through foramen ovale to innervate skeletal muscle. There is bilateral corticobulbar input to the motor component of cranial nerve V.

An upper motor neuron lesion results in no significant weakness because of bilateral corticobulbar input. A lower motor neuron lesion results in the jaw deviating to the weak side.

Cranial Nerve VI (Abducens Nerve)

Cranial nerve VI is a motor nerve (general somatic efferent [GSE]) and innervates the ipsilateral lateral rectus, which functions to abduct the eye (Table 9.2). The paired abducens nucleus is located in the dorsal lower portion of the pons, separated from the floor of the fourth ventricle by the genu of the facial nerve (facial colliculus) (see Figure 8.3B in Chapter 8, "Brainstem and Cranial Nerves: Overview

Table 9.2 • Components of Cranial Nerve VI		
Type	Ganglion/Nucleus	Function
GSE	Abducens nucleus	Innervate lateral rectus (abduct eye)

Abbreviation: GSE, general somatic efferent.

and Medulla"). The abducens motoneurons are intermixed with internuclear neurons that send their axons across the midline to the opposite medial longitudinal fasciculus, where they ascend through the pons and midbrain to end in the third nerve nucleus. Thus, the abducens nuclear complex coordinates the action of both eyes to produce horizontal gaze (see also Chapter 11, "Brainstem: Longitudinal Brainstem").

Axons of the abducens motoneurons course ventrally in the pons. The abducens nerve then ascends along the base of the pons in the prepontine cistern and enters the Dorello canal beneath the Gruber (petroclinoid) ligament. The axons then pass through the cavernous sinus. After passing through the superior orbital fissure, the abducens nerve innervates the lateral rectus muscle (Figure 9.3).

Lesions affecting the axons of cranial nerve VI result in an ipsilateral lateral rectus palsy (poor abduction of the ipsilateral eye) (Figure 9.4A). However, lesions affecting the abducens nucleus cause not only an ipsilateral lateral rectus paresis but also an ipsilateral gaze palsy to the same side because the abducens interneurons are involved (Figure 9.4B). See also Chapter 11, "Brainstem: Longitudinal Brainstem."

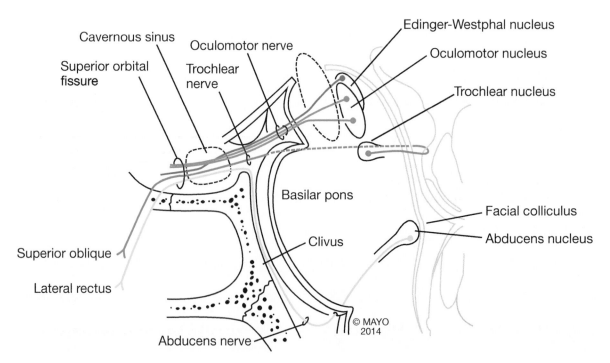

Figure 9.3 Course of Cranial Nerve VI.
(Used with permission of Mayo Foundation for Medical Education and Research.)

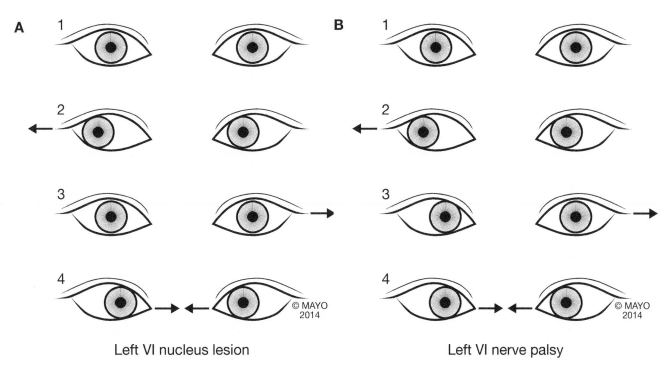

Left VI nucleus lesion   Left VI nerve palsy

Figure 9.4 Pathologic Eye Movements.
A, Left cranial nerve VI nucleus lesion. A lesion of this nucleus involves the axons innervating the ipsilateral lateral rectus muscle, but also axons that cross the midline and project through the medial longitudinal fasciculus to the neurons in the oculomotor nucleus that innervate the medial rectus muscle. The result is the inability to abduct the left eye and adduct the right eye (3). B, Left cranial nerve VI palsy. In contrast to a nuclear lesion, a left cranial nerve VI palsy results in the inability to abduct the left eye (3); however, the right eye could adduct because the medial longitudinal fasciculus is still intact.

(Adapted from Benarroch EE, Daube JR, Flemming KD, Westmoreland BF. Mayo Clinic medical neurosciences: organized by neurologic systems and levels. 5th ed. Rochester [MN]: Mayo Clinic Scientific Press and Florence [KY]: Informa Healthcare USA; c2008. Chapter 15, Part B, The posterior fossa level: cerebellar, auditory, and vestibular systems; p. 633–67. Used with permission of Mayo Foundation for Medical Education and Research.)

Cranial Nerve VII (Facial Nerve)

Cranial nerve VII has 5 components: 2 sensory (special visceral afferent [SVA], GSA) and 3 motor (general visceral efferent [GVE], SVE) (Table 9.3). Note that the GVE, SVA, and GSA fibers are collectively known as nervus intermedius.

The motor nucleus of cranial nerve VII (SVE) lies in the caudal pons (see Figure 8.3B in Chapter 8, "Brainstem and Cranial Nerves: Overview and Medulla"). The axons innervate muscles of facial expression and the stapedius muscle (functions to dampen sound). Axons sweep dorsally and around the nucleus of cranial nerve VII (facial colliculus) before exiting the pons in the cerebellar pontine angle. From here, axons enter the internal auditory meatus. Motor fibers pass through the facial canal of the temporal bone and exit the skull at the stylomastoid foramen. Before exiting the stylomastoid foramen, a small branch innervates the stapedius muscle.

Corticobulbar input to the forehead, including orbicularis oculi, is bilateral, whereas corticobulbar input to the lower part of the face is unilateral (Figure 9.5). Thus, an upper motor neuron lesion results in contralateral paralysis of the lower part of the face only. A lower motor

Table 9.3 • Components of Cranial Nerve VII

Type	Ganglion/Nucleus	Function
SVE	Facial nucleus	Muscles of facial expression and stapedius
GVE	Superior salivatory nucleus	Innervate submandibular and sublingual glands (salivation)
GVE	Lacrimal nucleus	Innervate lacrimal gland (tearing) and nasal mucosa
SVA	Geniculate ganglion Nucleus solitarius	Taste from anterior 2/3 of tongue
GSA	Trigeminal ganglion Spinal nucleus of cranial nerve V	Sensation to ear

Abbreviations: GSA, general somatic afferent; GVE, general visceral efferent; SVA, special visceral afferent; SVE, special visceral efferent.

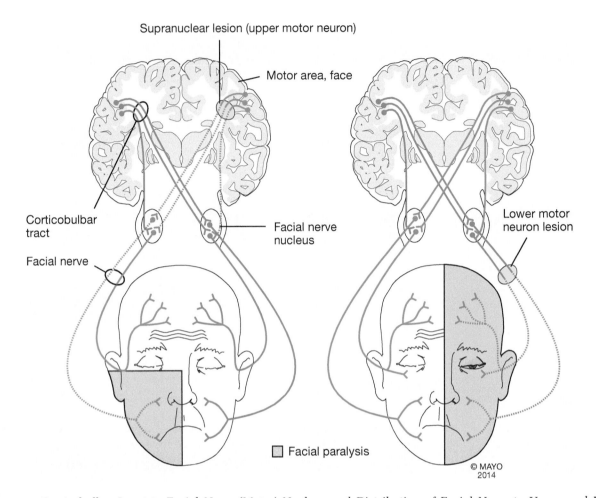

Figure 9.5 *Corticobulbar Input to Facial Nerve (Motor) Nucleus and Distribution of Facial Nerve to Upper and Lower Muscles of Facial Expression.*

Right, A supranuclear (upper motor neuron) lesion produces paralysis of the contralateral lower face. Left, A lower motor neuron lesion causes paralysis of the ipsilateral upper and lower face.

(Adapted from Flemming KD. Disorders of the cranial nerves. In: Mowzoon N, Flemming KD, editors. Neurology board review: an illustrated study guide. Rochester [MN]: Mayo Clinic Scientific Press and Florence [KY]: Informa Healthcare USA; c2007. p. 127–62. Used with permission of Mayo Foundation for Medical Education and Research.)

neuron lesion results in paralysis of the entire ipsilateral face.

Cranial nerve VII has 2 GVE components. Axons of the first originate in the superior salivatory nucleus. Preganglionic parasympathetic motor fibers exit the brainstem as part of nervus intermedius and enter the internal acoustic canal. From here, axons travel as the greater petrosal nerve, exiting the skull at the greater petrosal foramen. The axon then travels through the pterygoid canal, joining the deep petrosal nerve called the nerve of the pterygoid canal. Axons synapse in the pterygopalatine (sphenopalatine) ganglion within the pterygopalatine fossa. Postganglionic fibers are destined to synapse at the lacrimal gland (tear production) and nasal mucosa (mucous secretion). Dysfunction of this component may result in ipsilateral dry eye and nasal mucosa.

Preganglionic parasympathetic axons of the second GVE component of cranial nerve VII begin in the lacrimal nucleus. Preganglionic fibers exit the brainstem as part of nervus intermedius. Fibers enter the internal acoustic canal. Fibers continue on as the chorda tympani and then join the lingual branch of the trigeminal nerve (V3). Fibers travel near the inner surface of the jaw, where they synapse in the submandibular ganglion. Postganglionic fibers supply the submandibular and sublingual glands (salivation). Dysfunction of this component may result in reduced salivation.

The SVA fibers of cranial nerve VII carry taste from the ipsilateral anterior two-thirds of the tongue to the rostral aspect of nucleus solitarius via the geniculate ganglion. Fibers from the anterior two-thirds of the tongue travel via the ipsilateral chorda tympani to the petrous temporal bone, where the geniculate ganglion

Table 9.4 • Components of Cranial Nerve VIII

Type	Ganglion/Nucleus	Function
SSA	Vestibular ganglion Vestibular nuclei	Control posture and movement of body and eyes relative to movement
SSA	Spiral ganglion Cochlear nuclei	Hearing

Abbreviation: SSA, special somatic afferent.

lies. Axons then travel into the brainstem to synapse in the rostral part of the nucleus solitarius. From here, second-order neurons project to the ipsilateral VPM of the thalamus via the central tegmental tract. The VPM projects to the inferiormost portion of the primary sensory cortex near the insula. Dysfunction of this component may result in reduced taste from the ipsilateral anterior two-thirds of the tongue.

A small GSA component of cranial nerve VII carries tactile sensation from the external ear via the geniculate ganglion to the spinal nucleus of cranial nerve V.

Cranial Nerve VIII (Vestibulocochlear Nerve)

Cranial nerve VIII is composed of 2 types of special somatic afferent (SSA) components: vestibular and cochlear (Table 9.4).

Vestibular System

The vestibular component of cranial nerve VIII functions to control posture and movements of the body and eyes relative to the external environment. In addition, it serves to control eye movements and posture relative to linear and angular acceleration through connections to the oculomotor system and vestibulospinal tracts. There are also thalamocortical circuits such that this sensory information may also reach the level of conscious perception. This SSA component of cranial nerve VIII is discussed further in Chapter 5, "Special Somatic Sensory Afferent Overview," and Chapter 12, "Supranuclear Ocular Motor Systems."

Dysfunction of the vestibular component of cranial nerve VIII may result in vertigo, nystagmus, nausea, and imbalance. See Volume 2, Chapter 48, "Clinical Neurotology."

Auditory System

The cochlear component of cranial nerve VIII functions in hearing. The components of the external and middle ear transduce sound into electrical impulses carried by cranial nerve VIII to the cochlear nuclei. This SSA pathway is reviewed in Chapter 5, "Special Somatic Sensory Afferent Overview." Monaural information (about sounds at 1 ear) is transmitted in contralateral pathways to the inferior colliculus. Binaural information (about differences between sounds at both ears) is transmitted via the superior olivary complex; this is an important structure where information from both ears converges and is important for sound localization.

Dysfunction of the auditory component of cranial nerve VIII may result in loss of hearing if destruction is at the level of the eighth cranial nerve or at the cochlear nucleus. At the midpons or higher, unilateral destruction does not result in hearing loss. At the level of the cortex, unilateral destruction does not result in hearing loss but may impair sound localization. See Table 9.5 for more detail.

- Cranial nerve V has 4 components: 3 sensory components (GSA) and 1 motor component (SVE).

Table 9.5 • Dysfunction Due to Lesions in Auditory Pathway

Lesion	Clinical Result	Potential Causes
Cochlear nerve	Ipsilateral deafness (partial or complete), tinnitus	Trauma, infection, drugs (eg, streptomycin), AICA aneurysm, cerebellopontine angle tumors
Unilateral brainstem	Poor hearing localization (if lesion above and not involving cochlear nuclei)	Stroke, tumor, multiple sclerosis
Bilateral brainstem	Possible bilateral hearing loss if severe bilateral brainstem lesions	Stroke, tumor, multiple sclerosis
Unilateral auditory cortex	Possible difficulty localizing sound	Stroke, tumor, trauma
Unilateral dominant posterior temporal lesion or bilateral temporal lesion	Pure word deafness (auditory verbal agnosia): inability to understand spoken language despite normal hearing acuity and ability to read, write, and comprehend environmental sound	Structural lesions (stroke, tumor, trauma)
Bilateral auditory cortex	Range of disorders: cortical deafness, auditory agnosia, pure word deafness, amusia[a]	Structural lesions (stroke, tumor, trauma)

Abbreviation: AICA, anterior inferior cerebellar artery.

[a] See also Volume 2, Chapter 29, "A Review of Focal Cortical Syndromes."

- The trigeminal spinal tract and nucleus of cranial nerve V (GSA) carry pain and temperature sensation of the face.
- The chief sensory nucleus of cranial nerve V (GSA) functions in vibration, proprioception, and light touch/ tactile discrimination of the face.
- The mesencephalic nucleus of cranial nerve V (GSA) functions in unconscious proprioception of the jaw.
- Neurons of the motor component (SVE) of cranial nerve V innervate the muscles of mastication (temporalis, masseter, pterygoids).
- Cranial nerve VI is a motor nerve (GSE) and innervates the ipsilateral lateral rectus, which functions to abduct the eye.
- Lesions affecting the axons of cranial nerve VI result in an ipsilateral lateral rectus palsy.
- Lesions affecting the abducens nucleus of cranial nerve VI cause not only an ipsilateral lateral rectus paresis but also an ipsilateral gaze palsy.
- Cranial nerve VII has 5 components: 2 sensory (SVA, GSA) and 3 motor (GVE, SVE).
- The motor nucleus of cranial nerve VII (SVE) lies in the caudal pons and innervates muscles of facial expression and the stapedius muscle.

- The 2 GVE (parasympathetic) components of cranial nerve VII innervate the lacrimal glands and nasal mucosa as well as the sublingual and submandibular salivary glands.
- The SVA fibers of cranial nerve VII carry taste from the ipsilateral anterior two-thirds of the tongue to the rostral aspect of nucleus solitarius via the geniculate ganglion.
- The vestibular component of cranial nerve VIII functions to control posture and movements of the body and eyes relative to the external environment.
- The cochlear component of cranial nerve VIII functions in hearing.

Clinical Correlations of the Pons

Corneal Reflex

The corneal reflex consists of a bilateral blink after the cornea is lightly touched with a stimulus. The afferent part of this reflex is via the ophthalmic division of the trigeminal nerve (cranial nerve V1). This reflex utilizes the spinal tract and nucleus of cranial nerve V. The efferent arc of this reflex is cranial nerve VII, the facial nerve (Figure 9.6).

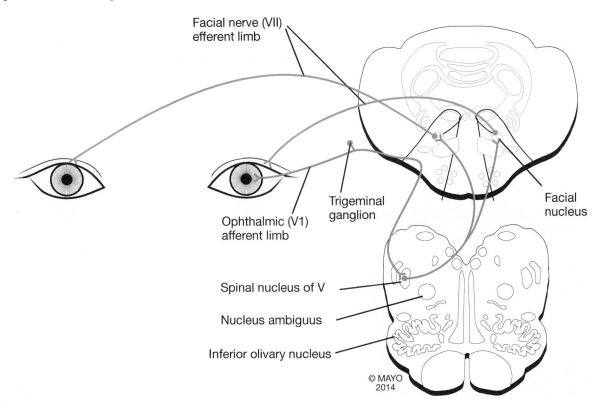

Figure 9.6 Corneal Reflex.
The afferent arm of the pathway is cranial nerve V (ophthalmic division), and the efferent arm is the facial nerve (cranial nerve VII).
(Adapted from Flemming KD. Disorders of the cranial nerves. In: Mowzoon N, Flemming KD, editors. Neurology board review: an illustrated study guide. Rochester [MN]: Mayo Clinic Scientific Press and Florence [KY]: Informa Healthcare USA; c2007. p. 127–62. Used with permission of Mayo Foundation for Medical Education and Research.)

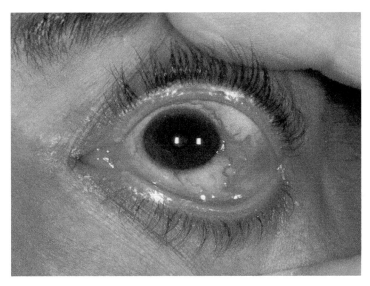

Figure 9.7 Carotid Cavernous Fistula.
This patient presented with pulsatile tinnitus. A carotid cavernous fistula may result in proptosis and arterialization of the episcleral and conjunctival veins as seen here. Any pathologic process affecting the cavernous sinus may also result in dysfunction of cranial nerves III, IV, VI, and V.

Jaw Jerk

The jaw jerk involves contraction of the masseter and temporalis muscles when the patient's lower jaw is tapped. The afferent limb of this reflex is the mandibular branch of the trigeminal nerve. These fibers enter the pons and do not have their cell body in the trigeminal ganglia. Rather, these fibers have their cell body in the mesencephalic nucleus of cranial nerve V. The efferent arc also travels with the mandibular fibers that originate in the motor nucleus of the trigeminal nerve. Lesions anywhere along this reflex arc result in depression of the ipsilateral jaw reflex, whereas bilateral supranuclear lesions result in an accentuated response.

Cavernous Sinus Syndrome

Cranial nerves III, IV, and VI traverse the cavernous sinus, as does division 1 and, in some, division 2 of cranial nerve V. The cavernous portion of the carotid artery also travels

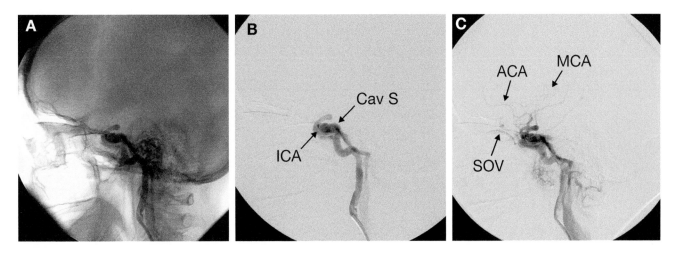

Figure 9.8 Conventional Angiogram of the Internal Carotid Artery.
A, B, and C, Sequential angiogram pictures taken seconds apart after injection of the internal carotid artery ("arterial phase") in the same patient. There is early venous shunting from the carotid cavernous segment to the cavernous sinus suggestive of a fistula. Note the diminished anterior cerebral and middle cerebral artery filling during the arterial phase due to the shunting. This represents a carotid cavernous fistula. ACA indicates anterior cerebral artery; CavS, cavernous sinus; ICA, internal carotid artery; MCA, middle cerebral artery; SOV, superior ophthalmic vein.

through the cavernous sinus, and along with it are sympathetic fibers destined to the pupillary dilator muscles and the Müller muscle of the eyelid. Patients with a cavernous sinus syndrome may have dysfunction of any of these components. In addition, patients with a cavernous sinus fistula may also have proptosis, arterialization of the episcleral and conjunctival veins (Figure 9.7) due to backfill from the cavernous sinus into the superior ophthalmic veins (Figure 9.8), and an ocular bruit.

Locked-In Syndrome

Patients with a large pontine ischemic stroke, which is often due to basilar artery occlusion, present with horizontal gaze palsy (bilateral abducens nuclear lesions) with intact vertical gaze, paralysis of the limbs (corticospinal and corticopontine fibers) and face (corticobulbar tract or the nucleus of cranial nerve VII), and inability to speak, but with preserved cognition. Communication with vertical eye movement codes (eg, look up twice for yes) helps distinguish a patient with this syndrome from a comatose patient.

Other Clinical Brainstem Syndromes

See Volume 2, Section VIII, "Clinical Disorders of the Cranial Nerves and Brainstem."

Brainstem and Cranial Nerves: The Midbrain[a]

KELLY D. FLEMMING, MD; PAUL W. BRAZIS, MD

Introduction

The midbrain (or mesencephalon) is the uppermost segment of the brainstem. This chapter reviews the important structures in the midbrain, including cranial nerves III and IV. Clinical syndromes relevant to the brainstem and cranial nerves are discussed in Volume 2, Section VIII, "Clinical Disorders of the Cranial Nerves and Brainstem."

Midbrain

Anatomy of the Midbrain

The midbrain extends from the level of the trochlear nucleus to an imaginary line drawn between the mammillary bodies and the posterior commissure. Important structures at this level include the cerebral peduncles, superior and inferior colliculi, the red nucleus, the substantia nigra, decussation of the middle cerebellar peduncle, and cranial nerves III and IV.

The blood supply differs depending on the level of the midbrain. The lower midbrain is supplied by perforators from the basilar artery and the superior cerebellar artery. The middle and upper midbrain are predominantly supplied by the posterior cerebral artery P2 segment (see Chapter 1, "Cerebrovascular Anatomy and Pathophysiology").

Important Structures of the Midbrain

Crus Cerebri

The crus cerebri are located ventrally in the midbrain. The corticospinal, corticobulbar, and corticopontine fibers traverse this structure.

Superior Colliculus

The superior colliculus (see Figures 8.1 and 8.3G in Chapter 8, "Brainstem and Cranial Nerves: Overview and Medulla") lies in the rostral midbrain dorsal to the cerebral aqueduct. The superior colliculus is a visual reflex center receiving afferent input from the retina, visual cortex, and other sensory modalities. It is the origin of the tectospinal tract, which is important for head movements in response to visual stimuli (see Chapter 7, "Spinal Cord Anatomy"). It is also an integral part of the efferent output to burst neurons involved in saccadic eye movements.

Inferior Colliculus

The inferior colliculus (see Figures 8.1 and 8.3F in Chapter 8, "Brainstem and Cranial Nerves: Overview and Medulla") lies in the caudal midbrain. Obligatory synapses in the auditory pathway occur here (see Chapter 5, "Special Somatic Sensory Afferent Overview").

Red Nucleus

The red nucleus lies in the ventral tegmentum of the midbrain. It is visible on gross pathologic specimens and on magnetic resonance imaging. The red nucleus is the origin of the rubrospinal tract. This tract originates in the red nucleus, and fibers immediately decussate to descend on the contralateral side. The tract occupies about the same position as the lateral corticospinal tract. Rubrospinal fibers terminate on ventral horn cells, but few rubrospinal fibers reach the lower cord. Therefore, the main rubrospinal influences are on flexor muscles of the upper extremities (see Chapter 7, "Spinal Cord Anatomy").

[a] Portions previously published in Brazis PW. Isolated palsies of cranial nerves III, IV, and VI. Semin Neurol. 2009 Feb;29(1):14–28. Epub 2009 Feb 12. Used with permission.

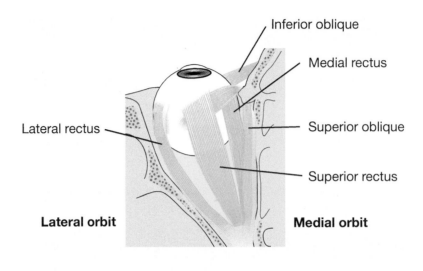

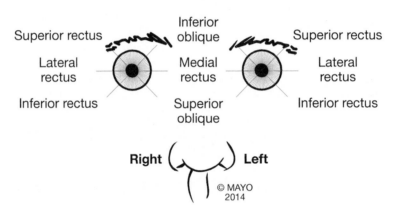

Figure 10.1 Eye Muscles.
(Adapted from Benarroch EE, Daube JR, Flemming KD, Westmoreland BF. Mayo Clinic medical neurosciences: organized by neurologic systems and levels. 5th ed. Rochester [MN]: Mayo Clinic Scientific Press and Florence [KY]: Informa Healthcare USA; c2008. Chapter 15, Part B, The posterior fossa level: cerebellar, auditory, and vestibular systems; p. 633–67. Used with permission of Mayo Foundation for Medical Education and Research.)

Substantia Nigra

The substantia nigra lies in the midbrain tegmentum just dorsal to the corticospinal tracts. The substantia nigra has important connections to the basal ganglia, which is important in motor programming. The pars compacta produces dopamine, and the pars reticulata secretes γ-aminobutyric acid as its neurotransmitter (see Chapter 17, "Basal Ganglia").

Extraocular Muscles

Each eye globe is moved by 6 muscles: 4 recti (superior, inferior, medial, and lateral) and 2 oblique (superior and inferior) (Figure 10.1). The origins and insertions and functions of each of these muscles are listed in Table 10.1.

Two muscles, both in the upper eyelid, act together to widen the palpebral fissure. Müller muscle receives

sympathetic innervation. The levator of the lid, innervated by cranial nerve III, plays the greater role in eyelid opening. Eye closure (orbicularis oculi) is effected through cranial nerve VII.

- The middle and upper midbrain are predominantly supplied by the posterior cerebral artery P2 segment.
- Two muscles widen the palpebral fissure: Müller muscle receives sympathetic innervation, and the levator of the lid, innervated by cranial nerve III, plays the greater role in eyelid opening.

Cranial Nerves III and IV

Cranial Nerve III (Oculomotor Nerve)

Cranial nerve III has both general somatic efferent and general visceral efferent components (Table 10.2). These components originate from the third nerve nuclear complex in

Table 10.1 • Functions of the Ocular Nerves

Nerve	Muscle	Normal Function		Dysfunction
		Primary Position[a]	Secondary Position[b]	
III	Medial rectus	Adduction		Eye is deviated down and out with complete paralysis of CN III (usually associated with ptosis and mydriasis)
	Superior rectus	Elevation	Intorsion	
	Inferior rectus	Depression	Extorsion	
	Inferior oblique	Extorsion	Elevation	
IV	Superior oblique	Intorsion	Depression	Limitation of downward gaze when eye is looking medially, extorsion of eye
VI	Lateral rectus	Abduction		Eye is deviated medially

Abbreviation: CN, cranial nerve.

[a] Refers to the action of the muscle when the eye is positioned in the plane of the muscle and then contracted.

[b] Refers to the action of the muscle when the eye is gazing forward in the orbit.

Adapted from Benarroch EE, Daube JR, Flemming KD, Westmoreland BF. Mayo Clinic medical neurosciences: organized by neurologic systems and levels. 5th ed. Rochester (MN): Mayo Clinic Scientific Press and Florence (KY): Informa Healthcare USA; c2008. Chapter 15, Part A, The posterior fossa level: brainstem and cranial nerve nuclei; p. 595–632. Used with permission of Mayo Foundation for Medical Education and Research.

the medial aspect of the midbrain at the level of the superior colliculus (Figure 10.2).

The Edinger-Westphal nucleus is the preganglionic parasympathetic subnucleus (general visceral efferent) of the third nerve nuclear complex and functions in pupillary constriction. Axons originating in the Edinger-Westphal nucleus synapse in the ciliary ganglion. Postganglionic fibers innervate the muscles, resulting in pupillary constriction (Figure 10.3). The pupillomotor fibers travel in the outer bundle of the third nerve complex. Thus, compressive lesions of the third nerve (eg, aneurysm) often result in a pupil-involving (pupillary dilatation due to impaired parasympathetic component) third-nerve palsy.

Four paired subnuclei containing general visceral efferent neurons innervate extraocular muscles: inferior rectus, superior rectus, medial rectus, and inferior oblique. The subnuclei for the inferior rectus, medial rectus, and inferior oblique are ipsilateral to the muscles they innervate. The subnucleus for the superior rectus is on the contralateral side. Thus, a nuclear third nerve lesion may result in an ipsilateral third nerve palsy, in addition to a contralateral superior rectus palsy.

Table 10.2 • Components of Cranial Nerve III

Component	Nucleus or Ganglion	Function
General somatic efferent	Oculomotor nucleus	Innervate medial, superior, and inferior recti and inferior oblique and levator palpebrae
General visceral efferent	Edinger-Westphal nucleus (and ciliary ganglion)	Pupillary constriction and accommodation of the lens

The central caudal nucleus of the third nerve nuclear complex lies centrally, and neurons innervate the levator palpebrae, a stimulus that aids in eye opening. Thus, a nuclear third nerve palsy also results in bilateral ptosis.

The axons of the oculomotor neurons exit ventrally. In the subarachnoid space, each third nerve passes between the superior cerebellar and the posterior cerebral arteries, courses forward near the medial aspect of the uncus of the temporal lobe, pierces the dura just lateral to the posterior clinoid process, and enters the lateral wall of the cavernous sinus (Figure 10.4). Once it reaches the superior orbital fissure, the oculomotor nerve divides into a superior division, which supplies the superior rectus and the levator palpebrae superioris, and an inferior division, which supplies the medial and inferior recti, the inferior oblique, and the presynaptic parasympathetic outflow to ciliary ganglion (sphincter pupillae muscle and ciliary muscles).

A unilateral oculomotor nerve palsy may result in ptosis, a dilated pupil, and the eye in a down (superior oblique, cranial nerve IV intact) and out (lateral rectus, cranial nerve VI intact) position (Figure 10.5). In some cases, the pupil is not involved. A unilateral oculomotor nucleus palsy will result in the same findings, in addition to contralateral ptosis and contralateral superior rectus dysfunction.

Cranial Nerve IV (Trochlear Nerve)

The trochlear nerve is purely motor (general somatic efferent). The trochlear nerve innervates the superior oblique muscle.

The trochlear nucleus lies at the level of the inferior colliculus. The nerve fascicles course posteroinferiorly around the aqueduct to decussate in the dorsal midbrain in the anterior medullary velum; they then emerge from the brainstem near the dorsal midline. After traveling on the

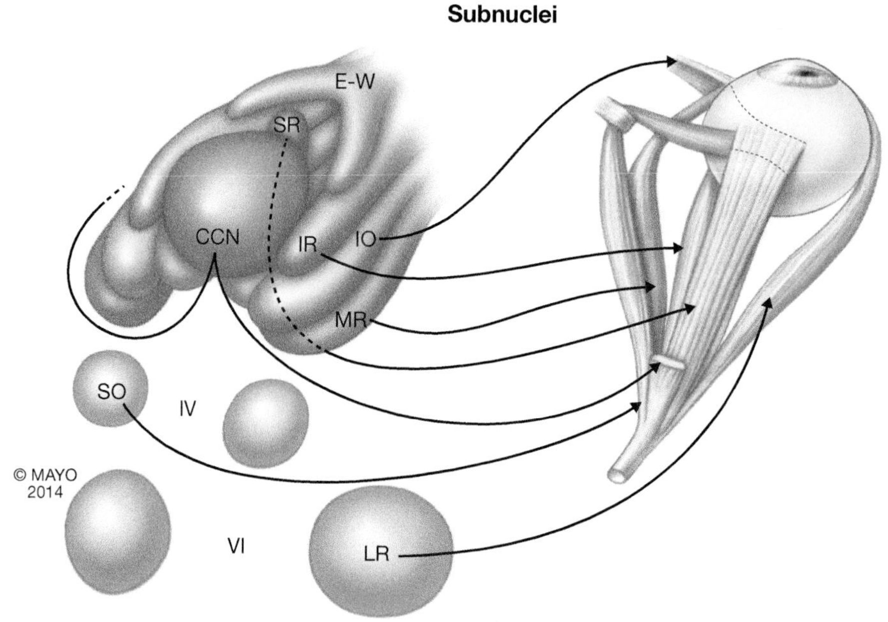

Subnuclei

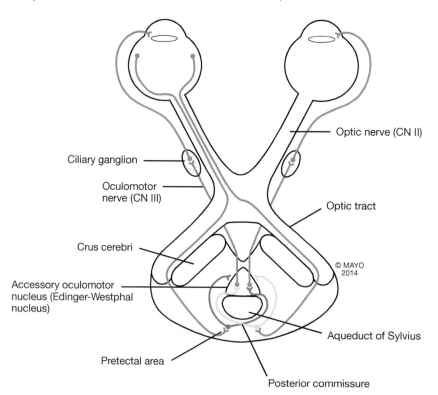

Figure 10.2 *Third Nerve Nuclear Complex.*
Each muscle innervated by cranial nerve III has a separate and distinct subnucleus within the third nerve nuclear complex. The central caudal nucleus (CCN) is midline, and a unilateral lesion of the nuclear complex could result in ptosis of both eyes. Also, superior rectus subnucleus is on the opposite side of the muscle it innervates. Thus, a nuclear third nerve lesion would result in an ipsilateral third nerve palsy in addition to a contralateral superior rectus palsy. E-W indicates Edinger-Westphal nucleus; IO, inferior oblique; IR, inferior rectus; LR, lateral rectus; MR, medial rectus; SO, superior oblique; SR, superior rectus.
(Used with permission of Mayo Foundation for Medical Education and Research.)

Figure 10.3 *Pathway of the Pupillary Light Reflex.*
The afferent arm is the optic nerve, and the efferent arm is the oculomotor nerve. CN indicates cranial nerve.
(Adapted from Benarroch EE, Daube JR, Flemming KD, Westmoreland BF. Mayo Clinic medical neurosciences: organized by neurologic systems and levels. 5th ed. Rochester [MN]: Mayo Clinic Scientific Press and Florence [KY]: Informa Healthcare USA; c2008. Chapter 15, Part A, The posterior fossa level: brainstem and cranial nerve nuclei; p. 595–632. Used with permission of Mayo Foundation for Medical Education and Research.)

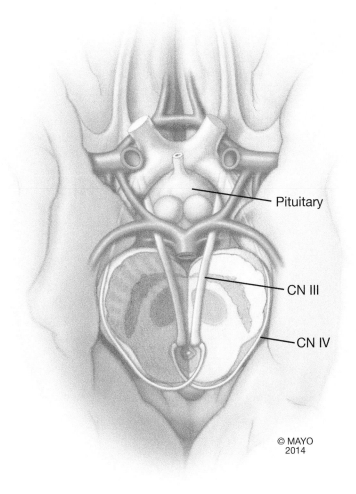

Pituitary

CN III

CN IV

© MAYO
2014

Figure 10.4 Course of Cranial Nerves III and IV.
Cranial nerve (CN) III exits ventrally and travels between the posterior cerebral artery and superior cerebellar artery before reaching the cavernous sinus. CN IV exits dorsally and crosses. It travels laterally between the posterior cerebral artery and superior cerebellar artery.
(Used with permission of Mayo Foundation for Medical Education and Research.)

undersurface of the tentorial edge, the nerve pierces the dura into the cavernous sinus along the lateral aspect (Figure 10.4). The trochlear nerve enters the orbit through the superior orbital fissure and innervates the superior oblique muscle.

Dysfunction of cranial nerve IV may result in hypertropia, excyclotropia, diplopia, and head tilt. Note that head tilt toward the abnormal side makes symptoms of diplopia worse. Recall that a lesion of the nucleus results in contralateral dysfunction. Bilateral fourth nerve

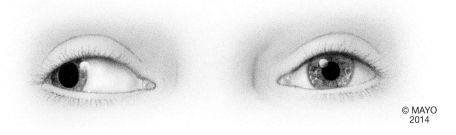

© MAYO
2014

Figure 10.5 Pupil Involving Third Nerve Palsy.
The eye is down (due to influence of the intact superior oblique innervated by cranial nerve IV) and out (due to the influence of the intact lateral rectus innervated by cranial nerve VI). The pupil is often involved in compressive lesions.
(Used with permission of Mayo Foundation for Medical Education and Research.)

palsies result in an inability to depress either eye fully in adduction.

- The Edinger-Westphal nucleus is the preganglionic parasympathetic subnucleus (general visceral efferent) of the third nerve nuclear complex and functions in pupillary constriction.
- Four paired subnuclei containing general visceral efferent neurons innervate extraocular muscles: inferior rectus, superior rectus, medial rectus, and inferior oblique.
- The central caudal nucleus of the third nerve nuclear complex lies centrally, and neurons innervate the levator palpebrae, a stimulus that aids in eye opening.
- A unilateral oculomotor nerve palsy may result in ptosis, a dilated pupil, and the eye in a down (superior oblique, cranial nerve IV intact) and out (lateral rectus,

cranial nerve VI intact) position (Figure 10.5). In some cases, the pupil is not involved. A unilateral oculomotor nucleus palsy will result in the same findings, in addition to contralateral ptosis and contralateral superior rectus dysfunction.

- Dysfunction of cranial nerve IV may result in hypertropia, excyclotropia, diplopia, and head tilt. Note that head tilt toward the abnormal side makes symptoms of diplopia worse.

Clinical Correlations

Decerebrate and Decorticate Posturing

Muscle tone is the balance between descending direct motor pathways (corticospinal tract), indirect motor

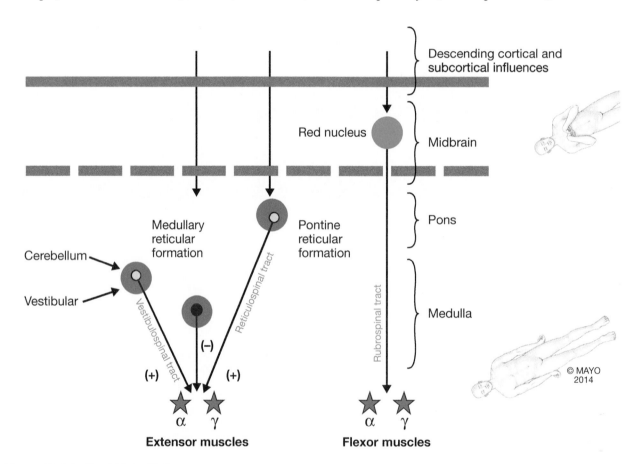

Figure 10.6 Indirect Motor Pathways.
The rubrospinal tract originates in the red nucleus at the level of the midbrain and innervates predominantly flexor muscles of the arms more than the legs. The vestibulospinal and reticulospinal tracts innervate predominantly extensor muscles in the arms and legs. Each of these indirect motor pathways receives descending input from the cortex. Working together, the direct (corticospinal tract) and indirect (vestibulospinal, reticulospinal, rubrospinal) tracts influence motor tone. A lesion about the red nucleus (heavy line) takes away the descending cortical input and the indirect pathways are unopposed. Thus, a patient would demonstrate the so-called decorticate posturing (arms flexed due to rubrospinal input and legs extended due to vestibulospinal and reticulospinal tracts remaining intact). If the lesion is below the red nucleus but above the reticular formation (dotted line), then the descending rubrospinal input is removed and only the reticulospinal and vestibulospinal tracts remain intact. This leads to decerebrate posturing (arms and legs extended).
(Used with permission of Mayo Foundation for Medical Education and Research.)

pathways (eg, reticulospinal, vestibulospinal, tectospinal, rubrospinal), and descending cortical inhibition. When descending inhibition is effected, the balance of tone is disrupted and indirect pathways may be left uninhibited. If there is a lesion at the level above the red nucleus, a patient may have decorticate posturing due to the influences of the rubrospinal (input to flexors of the upper extremity), reticulospinal (predominantly extensor influence of upper and lower extremities), and vestibulospinal tracts (predominantly extensor influence of the upper and lower extremities). If there is a lesion between the red nucleus and the medulla, a patient may have decerebrate posturing. This results because the input to flexors is removed and the patient mainly has input from the pontine reticulospinal tract and the vestibulospinal tracts (Figure 10.6).

Parkinsonism

Pathologic studies of patients with Parkinson disease show degeneration of the dopamine–producing cells of the substantia nigra (Figure 10.7). Other degenerative diseases resulting in parkinsonism show changes in the substantia nigra: progressive supranuclear palsy (pallor of substantia

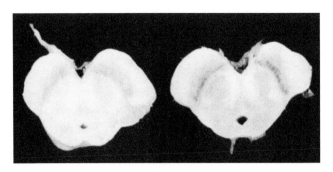

Figure 10.7 Substantia Nigra.
Left, Pallor of the substantia nigra in Parkinson disease. Right, Normal substantia nigra.
(Adapted from Okazaki H, Scheithauer BW. Atlas of neuropathology. New York [NY]: Gower Medical Publishing; c1988. p. 227. Used with permission of Mayo Foundation for Medical Education and Research.)

nigra and locus ceruleus), corticobasal-ganglionic-degeneration (intraneuronal inclusions in the substantia nigra), and multiple systems atrophy (neuronal loss in substantia nigra).

11

Brainstem and Cranial Nerves: Longitudinal Brainstem[a]

KELLY D. FLEMMING, MD; PAUL W. BRAZIS, MD

Introduction

This chapter will review pathways that are not at a single level of the brainstem, but rather involve multiple areas with supratentorial input. These include autonomic pathways, the reticular formation and chemically defined groups, and coordination of eye movements.

Autonomic Pathways of the Brainstem

The sympathetic fibers travel from the hypothalamus to the intermediolateral column in the spinal cord through the lateral brainstem. Patients with a unilateral lesion of the lateral brainstem may develop ipsilateral Horner syndrome. The ventrolateral medulla is also a sympathetic region of the brainstem. It projects to the spi-

nal cord and is involved in the innervation of blood vessels in the limbs.

Cranial nerves with parasympathetic function include III, VII, IX, and X (Table 11.1).

Other important structures in the brainstem that have interconnections with the autonomic nervous system include the pontine micturition center, parabrachial nucleus, nucleus solitarius, and periaqueductal gray (see also Chapter 19, "Autonomic Nervous System").

Reticular Formation and Chemically Defined Groups

The reticular formation has less well-defined nuclei than structures previously discussed and appears *reticulated* on pathologic examination, hence the name. The reticular

Table 11.1 • Parasympathetic Cranial Nerves

Cranial Nerve	Nucleus	Ganglion	Target	Function
III (Oculomotor)	Edinger-Westphal	Ciliary	Pupillary constrictor	Pupillary constriction and accommodation
VII (Facial)	Lacrimal Superior salivatory	Sphenopalatine Submandibular	Lacrimal gland; nasal mucosa Submandibular/sublingual glands	Tearing; mucosal secretion Salivation
IX (Glossopharyngeal)	Inferior salivatory	Otic	Parotid gland	Salivation
X (Vagus)	Dorsal motor nucleus of X Ventral nucleus ambiguus	Individual organ ganglia	Multiple organs	↓ Heart rate Bronchial constriction ↑ Gut peristalsis

[a] Portions previously published in Lee AG, Brazis PW, Mughal M, Policeni F. In: Emergencies in neuro-ophthalmology: a case based approach. Hackensack (NJ): World Scientific; c2010. Acute progressive bilateral ophthalmoplegia with mental status change; p. 59-63. Used with permission.
Abbreviations: MLF, medial longitudinal fasciculus; riMLF, rostral interstitial medial longitudinal fasciculus

Table 11.2 • Neurochemically Defined Structures of the Brainstem

Structure	Neurotransmitter	Location	Function
Locus ceruleus	Norepinephrine	Dorsal-rostral pons	Wakefulness Attention
Raphe nuclei	Serotonin	Midline at all levels of brainstem	Wakefulness Pain modulation
Ventral tegmental area	Dopamine	Ventral midbrain	Reward circuit Motivation

Table 11.3 • Omnipause, Burst, and Tonic Cells for Horizontal and Vertical Eye Movements

	Horizontal Saccade	Vertical Saccade
Omnipause neuron	Nucleus raphe interpositus	Nucleus raphe interpositus
Burst neuron	Paramedian pontine reticular formation	Rostral interstitial medial longitudinal fasciculus
Neural integrator	Nucleus prepositus hypoglossi Medial vestibular nucleus	Interstitial nucleus of Cajal
Cranial nerves	III, VI	III, IV

formation resides in the central part of the brainstem. The reticular formation is important for coordinating eye movement (eg, paramedian pontine reticular formation, rostral interstitial medial longitudinal fasciculus [riMLF]), maintaining posture (eg, reticulospinal tracts), and coordinating visceral responses (eg, blood pressure, respiration), pain regulation, arousal (eg, central tegmental tract), and the sleep/wake cycle.

In addition to the reticular formation, there are neurochemically defined nuclei within the brainstem (Table 11.2).

Coordination of Eye Movements

Reflexive and voluntary conjugate eye movements incorporate cortical, subcortical (basal ganglia, superior colliculus, pretectal region), and vestibulocerebellar (cerebellum, vestibular nuclei) input to the final common pathways of horizontal and vertical eye movements (cranial nerves III, IV, and VI, medial longitudinal fasciculus [MLF]). The final common pathways for horizontal and vertical gaze are reviewed here. Supranuclear control of eye movements is discussed in Chapter 12, "Supranuclear Ocular Motor Systems."

Final Common Pathway of Horizontal and Vertical Gaze

Cranial nerves III, IV, and VI innervate the muscles involved in eye movement. Eyes move conjugately, and eye movements are created by supranuclear input to omnipause cells, burst cells, and tonic cells (Table 11.3; Figure 11.1) related to these individual cranial nerves. Slow eye movements occur with cessation of omnipause cell firing and introduction of tonic cell firing to drive eyes to a new position and hold them there. Sudden movement of eyes is controlled by burst neurons in the pons. When the eyes change position, the omnipause cells are inhibited, the burst neurons discharge, a saccade occurs, and then the tonic and disinhibited omnipause cells hold the new position.

Horizontal Eye Movements

Horizontal eye movements involve the lateral (cranial nerve VI) and medial (cranial nerve III) recti from opposite sides to work in concert. The abducens nucleus contains 2 types of neurons: neurons innervating the ipsilateral lateral rectus and neurons innervating the contralateral third nerve subnuclei of the medial rectus (Figure 11.2). The axons of the lateral neurons are called the MLF. Burst neurons that initiate the eyes to be driven horizontally lie in the paramedian pontine reticular formation. Gaze-holding neural integrators for horizontal gaze are in the medial vestibular nucleus and the nucleus prepositus hypoglossi. Omnipause cells that inhibit burst cells are present in the raphe nuclei.

Vertical Eye Movements

Vertical eye movement involves the superior and inferior recti and the oblique muscles. The riMLF (dorsomedial to the red nucleus) contains burst neurons for both upward and downward movements and projects to motoneurons innervating depressors (inferior rectus and superior oblique) ipsilaterally, while those innervating elevators (superior rectus and inferior oblique) are probably bilateral. The gaze-holding neural integrator for vertical gaze is the interstitial nucleus of Cajal. Omnipause neurons are present in the raphe nuclei.

Commands from the riMLF for upward eye movements pass both directly and by crossing through the posterior commissure. Commands for downward eye movements pass ventral to the cerebral aqueduct. Thus, patients with upward gaze palsies often have lesions dorsal to the posterior commissure. Downward gaze palsies occur with lesions ventral to the aqueduct near the riMLF.

- Eyes move conjugately, and eye movements are created by supranuclear input to omnipause cells, burst cells, and tonic cells.

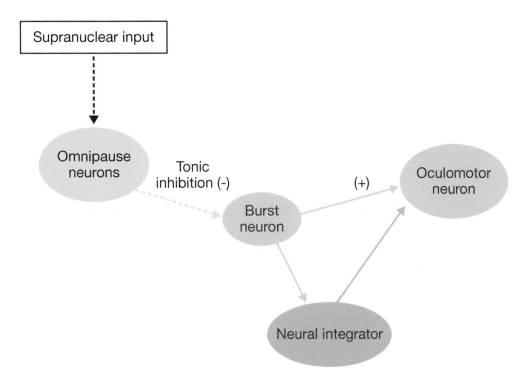

Figure 11.1 *Initiation and Maintenance of Saccades.*
The omnipause neurons tonically inhibit the burst neurons. When generating a saccadic eye movement, the omnipause cell stops firing and allows the burst neuron to fire. The burst neuron allows a rapid eye movement. Once the eyes have fixated on a target on the fovea, the neural integrator tonically fires to keep the eyes in their new position.

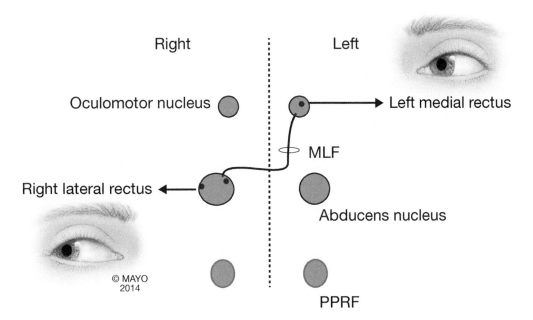

Figure 11.2 *Coordination of Horizontal Eye Movements.*
There are 2 types of interneurons in the abducens nucleus. The first type innervates the ipsilateral lateral rectus. The second sends axons to the contralateral brainstem and ascends as the medial longitudinal fasciculus (MLF) to the subnucleus of the medial rectus (cranial nerve III). PPRF indicates paramedian pontine reticular formation.

(Used with permission of Mayo Foundation for Medical Education and Research.)

- The abducens nucleus contains 2 types of neurons: neurons innervating the ipsilateral lateral rectus and neurons innervating the contralateral third nerve subnuclei of the medial rectus.

Clinical Correlations

Horizontal Conjugate Gaze Palsy

Unilateral restriction of voluntary gaze to 1 side is most often due to contralateral frontal or ipsilateral pontine damage (Figure 11.3). If the lesion is frontal, the patient generally has a hemiparesis and "looks toward the lesion," or away from the hemiparesis. The gaze palsy can be overcome with the oculocephalic maneuver or caloric stimulation. With a pontine lesion, the patient looks toward the side of the hemiparesis and the palsy cannot be overcome by oculocephalic maneuvers. Commonly with a pontine lesion, a cranial nerve VII lesion is also present, given the location of cranial nerve VII in the brainstem.

Epileptogenic lesions in the frontal eye fields may cause transient deviation of the eyes and head to the contralateral side (the patient then "looks" away from the lesion). However, in most cases, as soon as the focal seizure ceases, the patient tends to "look" to the involved side.

Acute parietal lesions may cause ipsilateral horizontal gaze deviation or preference. With right-sided lesions, there is also contralateral inattention. The latency of visually guided saccades to targets presented in either visual hemifield is increased with right-sided lesions, whereas left-sided lesions cause delay in only contralateral saccades.

Acute pathologic disorders, particularly those involving the medial thalamus, can also cause eye deviation to the side of the hemiparesis, opposite the lesion ("wrong-way eyes"). The reason for this contraversive deviation is unknown, but it may be an irritative phenomenon, because the intralaminar thalamic nuclei have a role in the production of contralateral saccades. However, some investigators have postulated that involvement of the descending ocular motor pathways from the contralateral hemisphere at the midbrain level is the most probable explanation for this phenomenon.

Vertical Conjugate Gaze Palsy

Unilateral lesions of the riMLF cause slowing of downward saccades. Bilateral riMLF lesions cause deficits of either downward saccades or downward and upward saccades.

Lesions of the posterior commissure cause vertical gaze impairment affecting all classes of vertical eye movements, especially upward gaze, with loss of vertical gaze-holding (neural integrator) function. The constellation of findings caused by lesions in this location has been variously designated as the Parinaud syndrome or dorsal midbrain syndrome. With the dorsal midbrain syndrome, all upward eye movements are impaired (although the vestibuloocular reflex and Bell phenomenon may sometimes be spared). Down-gaze saccades and smooth pursuit may be impaired, but downward vestibuloocular movements are spared. Common causes may include pineal tumors and hydrocephalus.

A sign of dorsal midbrain compression in hydrocephalic infants is a tonic downward deviation of the eyes while the retracted eyelids expose the epicorneal sclera (setting sun sign). Downbeating nystagmus may be present. The upper eyelid may be retracted, baring the sclera above the cornea (Collier tucked lid sign). The pupils are large and react poorly to light, but the near response is spared (light-near dissociation). Attempted upgaze may result in convergence-retraction nystagmus, with quick adducting-retraction jerks. This phenomenon can be elicited at the bedside by having the patient watch a downward-moving optokinetic drum.

Intranuclear Ophthalmoplegia

Clinically, this syndrome is characterized by adduction weakness on the side of the MLF lesion and monocular nystagmus of the contralateral abducting eye (Figure 11.4). However, unless the lesion is quite high, reaching the midbrain, convergence is preserved. Bilateral intranuclear ophthalmoplegia is most often seen with multiple sclerosis and ischemic lesions.

One-and-a-Half Syndrome

In these cases, there is a conjugate gaze palsy to 1 side ("one") and impaired adduction on looking to the other side ("and a half") (Figure 11.5). As a result, the only horizontal movement remaining is abduction of 1 eye, which exhibits nystagmus in abduction. The responsible lesion involves the paramedian pontine reticular formation or abducens nucleus and the adjacent MLF on the side of the complete gaze palsy. The one-and-a-half syndrome may be associated with ocular bobbing and, more often, facial nerve palsy (the eight-and-a-half syndrome). The one-and-a-half syndrome is most often caused by multiple sclerosis, neuromyelitis optica (Devic disease), infarcts, hemorrhages, trauma, basilar artery aneurysms, brainstem arteriovenous malformations, and tumors.

- Lesions of the posterior commissure cause vertical gaze impairment affecting all classes of vertical eye movements, especially upward gaze, with loss of vertical gaze-holding (neural integrator) function. The constellation of findings caused by lesions in this location has been variously designated as the Parinaud syndrome or dorsal midbrain syndrome.
- A sign of dorsal midbrain compression in hydrocephalic infants is a tonic downward deviation of the eyes while the retracted eyelids expose the epicorneal sclera (setting sun sign).

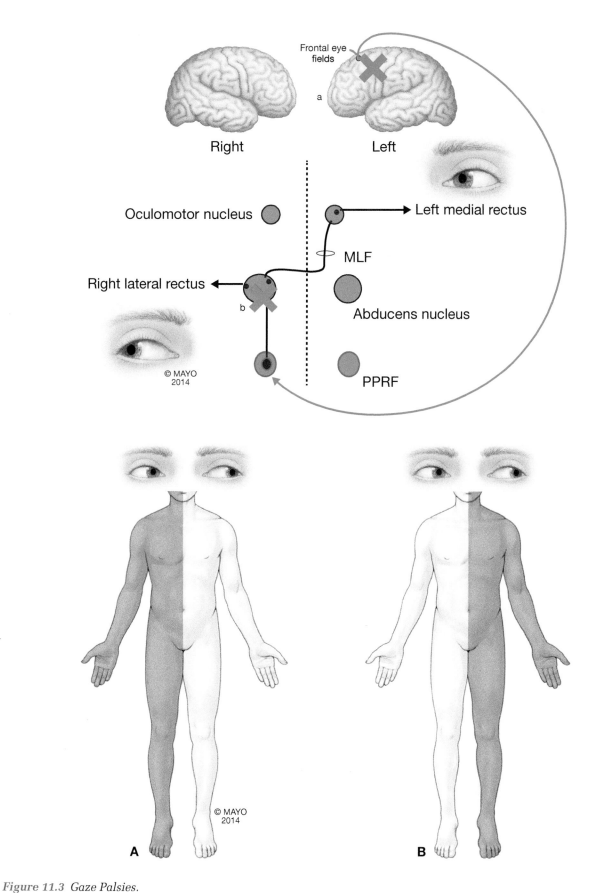

Figure 11.3 Gaze Palsies.
a, Lesion of the left frontal lobe affecting the frontal eye fields (11.3A) results in a right hemiparesis and leftward gaze deviation (11.3B). b, Lesion in the right pons (11.3A) results in a left hemiparesis and a leftward gaze deviation (11.3B). MLF indicates medial longitudinal fasciculus; PPRF, pontine paramedian reticular formation.
(Used with permission of Mayo Foundation for Medical Education and Research.)

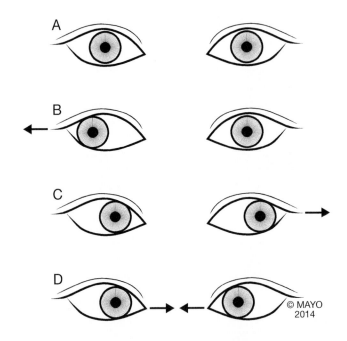

Intranuclear ophthalmoplegia

Figure 11.4. *Intranuclear Ophthalmoplegia of the Left Eye Due to a Lesion of the Left Medial Longitudinal Fasciculus.*
A, Normal primary gaze. B, When the patient is asked to look to the right, adduction of the left eye is paralyzed, associated with jerk nystagmus in the abducting eye. C, Normal gaze to the left. D, Normal convergence. Arrows indicate direction of gaze.

(Adapted from Freeman WD, Mowzoon N. Neuro-ophthalmology. In: Mowzoon N, Flemming KD, editors. Neurology board review: an illustrated study guide. Rochester [MN]: Mayo Clinic Scientific Press and Florence [KY]: Informa Healthcare USA; c2007. p. 83–126. Used with permission of Mayo Foundation for Medical Education and Research.)

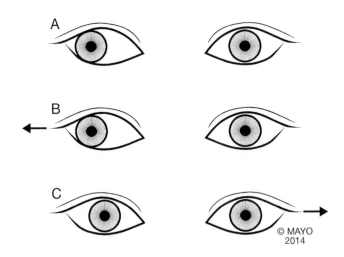

One-and-a-half syndrome

Figure 11.5. *One-and-a-Half Syndrome of the Left Eye.*
This syndrome is due to a pontine tegmental lesion involving the left abducens nucleus (or left paramedian pontine reticular formation projecting to the abducens nucleus) and medial longitudinal fasciculus (MLF) originating from the right abducens nucleus, sparing the latter. Because the left abducens nucleus gives rise to the left MLF projecting contralaterally, the lesion essentially involves the MLF bilaterally and abducens nucleus ipsilaterally. A, Exotropia of the right eye at primary gaze. B, Apparent left internuclear ophthalmoplegia on rightward gaze. C, Complete saccadic palsy on attempted leftward gaze. Arrows indicate direction of gaze.

(Adapted from Freeman WD, Mowzoon N. Neuro-ophthalmology. In: Mowzoon N, Flemming KD, editors. Neurology board review: an illustrated study guide. Rochester [MN]: Mayo Clinic Scientific Press and Florence [KY]: Informa Healthcare USA; c2007. p. 83–126. Used with permission of Mayo Foundation for Medical Education and Research.)

12 Supranuclear Ocular Motor Systems[a]

PAUL W. BRAZIS, MD; SCOTT D. EGGERS, MD

Introduction

Saccadic eye movements and nystagmus are 2 types of fast eye movements. Slow eye movements are smooth pursuit, vestibular, optokinetic, and vergence (Table 12.1). Reflexive and voluntary conjugate eye movements incorporate cortical, subcortical (basal ganglia), and vestibulocerebellar input to the final common pathways of horizontal and vertical eye movements (see Chapter 11, "Brainstem and Cranial Nerves: Longitudinal Brainstem," for discussion of the final common pathway of eye movements). This chapter reviews the anatomy and dysfunction of the supranuclear input to conjugate gaze.

The Vestibular System

Function

The function of the input from the vestibular system to the eyes is to maintain focus on an object despite head movement or rotation.

Pathophysiology

The vestibular system drives the eye in a direction opposite to the disruptive head motion (Figure 12.1). The reflex by which the vestibular system perceives head movement and makes the eyeball move in the opposite direction is called the vestibulo-ocular reflex. Thus, a horizontal vestibulo-ocular impulse originating in the horizontal canal is relayed from the ipsilateral medial vestibular nucleus to the contralateral abducens and ipsilateral medial rectus subnuclei neurons, and the eyes then deviate to the contralateral side.

Similar pathways (medial and superior) mediate vertical vestibular eye movements. Excitatory impulses from the vestibular nucleus cross in the brainstem and ascend in the medial longitudinal fasciculus (MLF) for the posterior canal projection and in the brachium conjunctivum, MLF, and ventral tegmental pathway for the anterior canal projection, synapsing in the areas of the trochlear or oculomotor nuclei where the muscles involved in the appropriate movement are represented. Stimulation of the anterior canal (eg, by downward head acceleration) excites the ipsilateral superior rectus muscle and the contralateral inferior oblique muscle, whereas stimulation of the posterior canal (eg, by upward head acceleration) excites the ipsilateral superior oblique muscle and contralateral inferior rectus muscle.

Dysfunction

The vestibulo-ocular reflex is commonly assessed in patients with coma to determine the patency of pathways through the brainstem (see Volume 2, Chapter 1, "Impaired Consciousness and Coma").

Vestibular clinical disorders are reviewed in Volume 2, Chapter 48, "Clinical Neurotology."

- The reflex by which the vestibular system perceives head movement and makes the eyeball move in the opposite direction is called the vestibulo-ocular reflex.

---

[a] Portions previously published in Brazis PW, Masdeu JC, Biller J. Localization in clinical neurology. 6th ed. Philadelphia (PA): Wolters Kluwer/Lippincott Williams & Wilkins; c2011. Chapter 8, The localization of lesions affecting the ocular motor system; p. 173-304. Used with permission.

Abbreviations: FEF, frontal eye field; MLF, medial longitudinal fasciculus; MST, medial superior temporal; MT, middle temporal; PEF, parietal eye field; PPRF, paramedian pontine reticular formation; riMLF, rostral interstitial nucleus of the MLF

Table 12.1 • Systems Controlling Conjugate Gaze

Type of Eye Movement	Main Function	Control Mechanism	Effect
Vestibular (vestibulo-ocular reflex)	Holds images steady on the fovea during brief head rotations	Semicircular canals and vestibular nuclei	Conjugate deviation of eyes opposite to direction of head rotation
Smooth pursuit	Holds image of a moving target on the fovea	Visual pathway and parieto-occipital cortex Vestibulocerebellum	Conjugated deviation toward direction of movement of object (ipsilateral to parieto-occipital cortex)
Optokinetic	Holds images of the target steady on the retina during sustained head rotation	Visual pathway and parieto-occipital cortex, vestibulocerebellum, vestibular nuclei	Maintains deviation of eyes initiated by the vestibulo-ocular reflex
Saccade	Brings the image of an object of interest onto the fovea	Frontal eye fields Superior colliculus Pontine paramedian reticular formation	Rapid conjugate deviation toward opposite side
Nystagmus quick phase	Directs the fovea toward the oncoming visual scene during self-rotation; resets the eyes during prolonged rotation	Cortical	Quick deviation toward stimulated labyrinth (vestibular) Quick deviation toward inhibited cerebellum (cerebellar)
Vergence	Moves the eyes in opposite directions (disconjugate) so that images of a single object are placed on both fovea	Unknown direct input to oculomotor neurons, likely via interneurons	Accommodation to near targets

Adapted from Benarroch EE, Daube JR, Flemming KD, Westmoreland BF. Mayo Clinic medical neurosciences: organized by neurologic systems and levels. 5th ed. Rochester (MN): Mayo Clinic Scientific Press and Florence (KY): Informa Healthcare USA; c2008. Chapter 15, Part B, The posterior fossa level: cerebellar, auditory, and vestibular systems; p. 633–67. Used with permission of Mayo Foundation for Medical Education and Research.

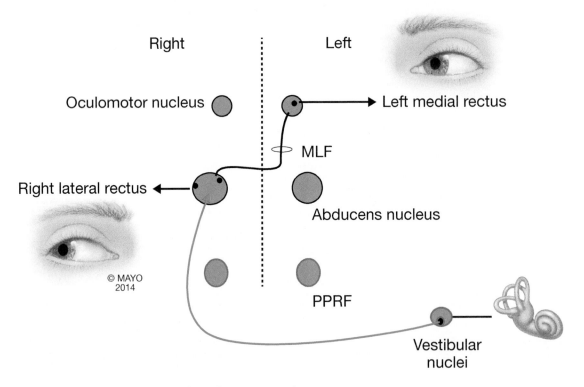

Figure 12.1 Vestibular Input to Horizontal Final Common Pathway.
Turning the head horizontally to the left results in firing of the left vestibular nuclei. The vestibular nuclei then projects to the right abducens nucleus. Thus, turning the head horizontally to the left results in the eyes deviating right. MLF indicates medial longitudinal fasciculus; PPRF, paramedian pontine reticular formation.

(Used with permission of Mayo Foundation for Medical Education and Research.)

Smooth Pursuit System

Overview

An object is seen with most detail when its image falls in the fovea, located in the posterior pole of the retina. Two ocular motor systems allow visual images to remain in the fovea: smooth pursuit, as the object moves vertically or horizontally, and vergence eye movements (convergence and divergence), as the object moves along the depth axis of the visual field, particularly as it approaches the subject. Fast-moving objects elicit quick eye movements, termed *saccades*.

Anatomy

The anatomic pathways involved in the smooth pursuit system are complex (Figure 12.2). In animals, the sensory system includes a projection from the dorsolateral geniculate nucleus to the striate cortex, which then sends fibers to the middle temporal (MT) visual area. Area MT processes

information about the speed and direction of target motion in the contralateral visual field and sends this information via an arcuate fiber bundle to the adjacent medial superior temporal (MST) area. Area MT projects contralaterally through the tapetum, major forceps, and splenium of the corpus callosum to areas MT and MST of the contralateral hemisphere. Area MST combines an internal signal of eye velocity with the motion signal from area MT. The homologues of the MT and MST in humans are probably located in the lateral occipital cortex (area 19) and the adjacent ventrocaudal aspect of Brodmann area 39 (which corresponds to the angular gyrus). Areas MT, MST, and the posterior parietal cortex all project to the frontal eye fields (FEFs).

For horizontal pursuit, the left motor system mediates smooth pursuit eye movements to the left, while the right motor system mediates movements to the right. The pathway decussates twice at the pontocerebellar level. Pontine nuclei on the side toward which the eyes move send, through the middle cerebellar peduncle, excitatory mossy fibers to granule cells of the contralateral cerebellar cortex.

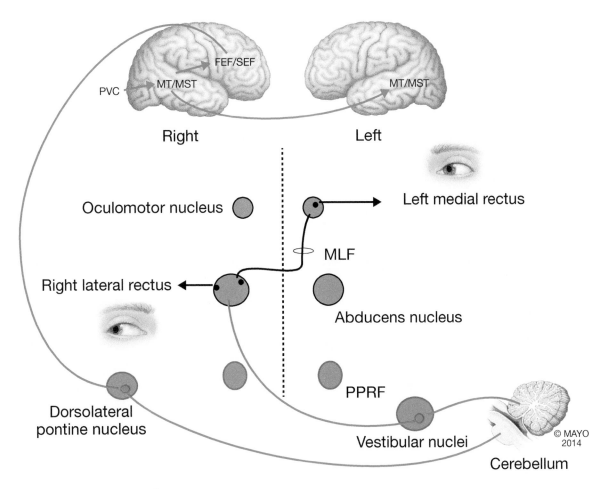

Figure 12.2 Smooth Pursuit Pathway.
FEF indicates frontal eye field; MLF, medial longitudinal fasciculus; MST, medial superior temporal; MT, middle temporal; PPRF, paramedian pontine reticular formation; PVC, primary visual cortex; SEF, supplementary eye field.
(Used with permission of Mayo Foundation for Medical Education and Research.)

The granule cells excite basket cells and stellate cells, which in turn inhibit Purkinje cells that send inhibitory projections to the ipsilateral medial vestibular nucleus. Excitatory projections from the vestibular nucleus cross the midline, ending in the opposite abducens nucleus.

Vertical pursuit signals follow a similar path and, after synapsing in the vestibular nuclei, project rostrally through the MLF and brachium conjunctivum and probably traverse the interstitial nucleus of Cajal. Upward pursuit pathways are believed to decussate in the posterior commissure, as posterior commissure lesions abolish upward pursuit, before ending in the appropriate ocular motor nuclei. Downward pursuit fibers likely descend after reaching the interstitial nucleus of Cajal and do not traverse the posterior commissure. Upward and downward smooth pursuit may be restricted by unilateral midbrain lesions.

The cerebellum plays an important role in synthesizing the pursuit signal from visual and ocular motor inputs. The dorsal vermis and fastigial nucleus may contribute mainly to the onset of pursuit, and the paraflocculus and flocculus mainly sustain the pursuit response.

Dysfunction

Smooth pursuit abnormalities occur with lesions anywhere along the course of smooth pursuit pathways. Frontal lesions may impair ipsilateral smooth pursuit, especially to targets moving in a predictable pattern. Bilateral occipital lesions abolish smooth pursuit. Parietal lesions decrease the amplitude and velocity of smooth pursuit toward the side of the lesion. Lesions occurring in a band extending from the occipito-temporal areas posteriorly, through the internal sagittal stratum, the posterior and anterior limbs of the internal capsule with adjacent striatum, to the dorsomedial frontal cortex anteriorly, cause predominantly ipsilesional pursuit deficits.

Because of the double decussation in the brainstem of the motor pursuit pathways, patients with posterior fossa lesions may have impaired ocular smooth pursuit either contralaterally or ipsilaterally. Unilateral midbrain lesions may result in ipsilateral pursuit defects, as may basal pontine lesions that damage the pontine nuclei. Unilateral cerebellar damage results in transient impairment of pursuit in the direction of the involved side, whereas bilateral damage causes permanent impairment of smooth pursuit eye movements.

- For horizontal pursuit, the left motor system mediates smooth pursuit eye movements to the left, while the right motor system mediates movements to the right.

The Saccadic System

Function

Most obvious among the eye movements are the quick refixations termed *saccades*. Their purpose is to place on the fovea objects of interest, which often have first been registered by the peripheral retina.

Anatomy

Two types of neurons are important in the generation of saccades: burst neurons and omnipause neurons in the brainstem. Excitatory burst neurons are located in the paramedian pontine reticular formation (PPRF) and lie rostral to the abducens nucleus in the dorsomedial nucleus reticularis pontis caudalis. Excitatory burst neurons project the excitatory pulse to the ipsilateral abducens nucleus (to both abducens motor neurons and internuclear neurons), a process that results in horizontal saccades. The step of innervation at the end of the saccade arises from the nucleus prepositus hypoglossi and medial vestibular nucleus that make up the neural integrator for horizontal gaze (see also Chapter 11, "Brainstem and Cranial Nerves: Longitudinal Brainstem").

Impulses from the frontal eye fields are relayed to the pontine PPRF, which coordinates both vertical and horizontal saccades. Signals for horizontal saccades proceed from the ipsilateral PPRF in the lower pons to the ipsilateral abducens nucleus and contralateral oculomotor nucleus through the MLF (Figure 12.3). Thus, the PPRF mediates a saccade to the same side of the pons but contralateral to the frontal eye field that originated the chain of command.

For vertical saccades, projections from the rostral interstitial nucleus of the MLF (riMLF) to motor neurons innervating the elevator muscles are bilateral, with axon collaterals probably crossing to the opposite side at the level of the motor neuron axons crossing within the oculomotor nucleus and not in the posterior commissure. Axons from the riMLF for depressor muscles are unilateral; thus, unilateral lesions of the riMLF will slow downward saccades but spare upward saccades. Inhibitory burst neurons for vertical and torsional saccades reside within the riMLF.

Axons from the riMLF send collaterals to the interstitial nucleus of Cajal (bilaterally for upward burst neurons and ipsilateral for downward burst neurons), which provides the step of innervation for vertical and torsional saccades (vertical neural integrator), and to the cell groups of the paramedian tracts, which project to the cerebellum.

Three different cortical areas are capable of triggering saccades: frontal eye field (FEF), parietal eye field (PEF), and supplementary eye field. The cerebral hemispheres dispatch trigger signals to omnipause neurons in the brainstem to start saccades and signals of desired saccadic amplitude and direction or of final eye position that determine the durations and directions of saccades.

The influence of the frontal (FEF) and parietal cortex (PEF) on the control of saccades appears to be via 2 parallel descending pathways (Figure 12.4). One pathway is from the FEF to the superior colliculus directly. This pathway appears to be concerned with self-generated changes in

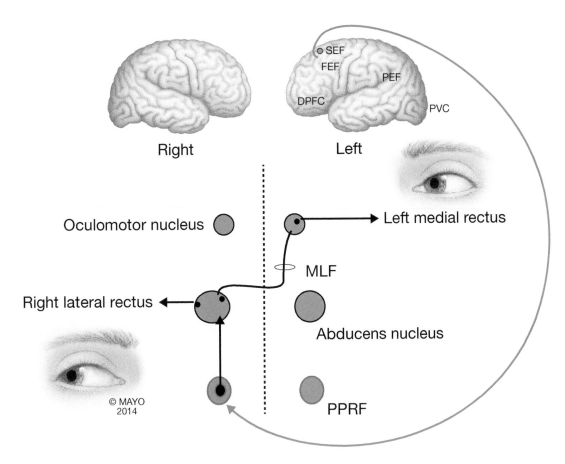

Figure 12.3 *Saccadic Eye Movement.*
DPFC indicates dorsolateral prefrontal cortex; PEF, parietal eye field. See Figure 12.2 for other abbreviations.
(Used with permission of Mayo Foundation for Medical Education and Research.)

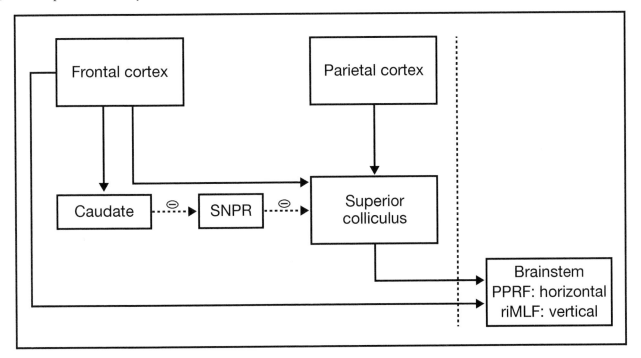

Figure 12.4 *Saccadic Eye Movement Parallel Pathways.*
PPRF indicates paramedian pontine reticular formation; riMLF, rostral interstitial nucleus of the medial longitudinal fasciculus; SNPR, substantia nigra pars reticulata.

Table 12.2 • Types of Saccadic Intrusion

Type	Description	Condition in Which It May Occur
Square wave jerks	One takes the eyes off the target and is followed after about 200 ms by a corrective saccade They may appear normally in the young and the elderly, but when larger than 1° or 2° they are pathologic	Cerebellar disease Progressive supranuclear palsy
Macrosquare wave jerks	Similar to square wave jerks but are of larger amplitude (20°–40°)	Multiple sclerosis Cerebellar hemorrhage Olivopontocerebellar atrophy Multiple systems atrophy Chiari malformation
Ocular flutter	A burst of to-and-fro horizontal saccades without an intersaccadic interval	Paraneoplastic disease (neuroblastoma) Idiopathic autoimmune disorder
Opsoclonus (saccadomania)	Similar to ocular flutter, except that in opsoclonus there are conjugate, involuntary, large-amplitude saccades in all directions Opsoclonus persists during eye closure and during sleep and is thought to be due to dysfunction of omnipause neurons that normally exert tonic inhibition on burst neurons	Brainstem disease Cerebellar disease Paraneoplastic effect with neuroblastoma or other tumors (especially small-cell lung cancer and breast cancer)

gaze related to anticipated, learned, or remembered behavior. Output from the FEF is also directed through the caudate nucleus, which projects to the substantia nigra pars reticulata. The pars reticulata projects, in turn, to the superior colliculus. The caudate inhibits the substantia nigra pars reticulata, and the pars reticulata inhibits the superior colliculus. The substantia nigra pars reticulata neurons discharge during fixation and pause; the FEF works by disinhibiting superior colliculus burst neurons that fire before and during voluntary and visually evoked saccades. Thus, the FEF has a 2-pronged excitatory effect on the superior colliculus, one direct and the other through the basal ganglia. The other pathway is directly from the PEF to the ipsilateral superior colliculus and is concerned with reorienting gaze to novel visual stimuli and, in particular, with shifting visual attention to location of new targets appearing in extrapersonal space.

Together, the FEF and superior colliculus project to the contralateral PPRF and riMLF. Each FEF or superior colliculus generates contralateral horizontal saccades, whereas vertical saccades require simultaneous activity in both FEFs or both superior colliculi. The final premotor circuits for saccades are located within the paramedian reticular formation of the pons and mesencephalon. Burst neurons in the PPRF discharge at higher frequencies just before and during horizontal saccades. These cells project in the abducens nucleus to generate horizontal saccades. Inhibitory burst neurons in the medulla provide reciprocal inhibition to the contralateral abducens nucleus. Excitatory burst neurons in the riMLF project to the ocular motor neurons to generate vertical and torsional saccades. The activity of both horizontal and vertical burst neurons is inhibited by omnipause cells in the midline of the caudal pons. These pause cells cease discharging before and during every saccade.

Dysfunction

Inappropriate saccades, or saccadic intrusions, interfere with macular fixation of an object of interest. There are several types of inappropriate saccade (Table 12.2).

- The purpose of saccades is to place on the fovea objects of interest, which often have first been registered by the peripheral retina.
- Impulses from the frontal eye fields are relayed to the pontine PPRF, which coordinates both vertical and horizontal saccades.
- Three different cortical areas are capable of triggering saccades: frontal eye field (FEF), parietal eye field (PEF), and supplementary eye field.

Convergence System

Overview

Convergence and divergence movements of the eyes bring about binocular vision. An object approaching the subject in the sagittal plane induces the near-triad reflex composed of convergence, rounding of the lens (accommodation), and constriction of the pupil (miosis).

Anatomy and Pathophysiology

The medial recti of both cranial nerve III nuclei act in concert to converge the eyes during the near response. Supranuclear input is from the peristriate cortex.

Dysfunction

Convergence insufficiency is common among teenagers and college students (especially those with an increased visual workload) but may also occur in the elderly, after mild head trauma, and with acquired cerebral lesions (especially those affecting the nondominant parietal lobe). Patients with convergence insufficiency typically complain of eyestrain and ache. After brief periods of reading, the letters blur and run together and often diplopia occurs during near work.

Parkinson disease and progressive supranuclear palsy are often associated with impaired or absent convergence.

Patients with convergence paralysis, as opposed to convergence insufficiency, often harbor a lesion of the midbrain. Other signs of midbrain damage usually are present, including impaired vertical gaze, upbeat or downbeat nystagmus, convergence-retraction nystagmus, and eyelid retraction.

- Patients with convergence paralysis, as opposed to convergence insufficiency, often harbor a lesion of the midbrain.

Nystagmus and Other Ocular Oscillations

The to-and-fro ocular movement that takes place as an individual watches the tree line when driving alongside a forest is described as optokinetic nystagmus. This type of jerk nystagmus, with a slow drift and a quick corrective component, is more common than pendular nystagmus, in which the eyes move with the same speed in both directions.

Monocular Eye Oscillations and Asymmetric Binocular Eye Oscillations

Monocular eye oscillations and asymmetric binocular eye oscillations may be due to spasmus nutans and its mimickers, monocular visual deprivation or loss, monocular pendular nystagmus, internuclear ophthalmoplegia and its mimickers, partial paresis of extraocular muscles, restrictive syndromes of extraocular muscles, or superior oblique myokymia.

Spasmus nutans is a benign syndrome characterized by a triad of head nodding, nystagmus, and abnormal head posture. This condition usually has its onset in the first year of life and remits spontaneously within 1 month to several years (up to 8 years) after onset. The sinusoidal nystagmus is often intermittent, asymmetric or unilateral, and of high frequency and small amplitude with a "shimmering" quality. The nystagmus is usually horizontal but may have a vertical or torsional component.

In all children with spasmus nutans, monocular nystagmus, or asymmetric pendular nystagmus, one must consider that the nystagmus may be due to tumor of the optic nerve, chiasm, third ventricle, or thalamus.

Dysconjugate Bilateral Symmetric Eye Oscillations

If the ocular oscillations involve both eyes to a relatively equal degree, the next step in evaluation involves determining whether the eye movements are disconjugate (the eyes moving in opposite directions) or conjugate (both eyes moving in the same direction). When the oscillations are disconjugate, the examiner should determine whether the oscillations are vertical or horizontal. Vertical disconjugate eye oscillations are usually due to see-saw nystagmus. Horizontal disconjugate eye oscillations include convergence-retraction nystagmus (nystagmus retractorius), divergence nystagmus, repetitive divergence, and oculomasticatory myorhythmia.

See-saw nystagmus refers to a cyclic movement of the eyes with a conjugate torsional component and a disjunctive vertical component: while one eye rises and intorts, the other falls and extorts; the vertical and torsional movements are then reversed, completing the cycle. Responsible lesions for see-saw nystagmus include large, extrinsic suprasellar lesions that compress the mesodiencephalon bilaterally (eg, parasellar tumors) or focal mesodiencephalic or lateral medullary brainstem lesions (eg, infarction).

Convergence-retraction nystagmus is a disorder of ocular motility in which repetitive adducting saccades, which are often accompanied by retraction of the eyes into the orbit, occur spontaneously or on attempted up-gaze saccades. Sliding an optokinetic tape downward in front of a patient's eyes may also elicit convergence-retraction nystagmus. Mesencephalic lesions affecting the pretectal region (posterior commissure) are most likely to cause this type of nystagmus, which is often associated with abnormalities of vertical gaze. Convergence nystagmus has been described without vertical gaze abnormalities in patients with dorsal midbrain stroke and in patients with Chiari malformation. Divergence nystagmus (with divergent quick phases) may occur with hindbrain abnormalities (eg, Chiari malformation) and is associated with downbeat nystagmus. Oculomasticatory myorhythmia refers to acquired pendular vergence oscillations of the eyes associated with concurrent contraction of the masticatory muscles. This distinct movement disorder has been recognized only in Whipple disease.

Binocular Symmetric Conjugate Eye Oscillations

Binocular symmetric conjugate eye oscillations (Table 12.3) may be divided into pendular nystagmus, jerk nystagmus, and saccadic intrusions. Binocular symmetric pendular conjugate eye oscillations may be due to congenital nystagmus, pendular nystagmus, oculopalatal myoclonus, spasmus nutans (discussed above), and visual deprivation nystagmus.

Table 12.3 • Types of Binocular Symmetric Conjugate Eye Oscillations

Type	Description	Causes
Congenital nystagmus	Conjugate, horizontal (even on up or down gaze)	Congenital
Acquired pendular	Wholly vertical or horizontal or both Symmetric, dissociated, or even monocular Oscillopsia disturbs visual acuity	Damage to dentatorubro-olivary pathway (eg, multiple sclerosis, tumor, or other brainstem lesion)
Oculopalatal myoclonus or tremor	Continuous, rhythmic involuntary movement of soft palate; can be accompanied by synchronous movement of other adjacent structures In some cases, associated with pendular nystagmus	Damage to dentatorubro-olivary pathway
Vestibular nystagmus	Horizontal nystagmus with the slow component toward the lesion (the opposite vestibular nuclei drive the eyes toward the diseased side) results from unilateral horizontal canal or total labyrinthine destruction. In the latter case, there is a torsional slow component causing the upper part of the globe to rotate toward the lesion side. Although constant for a particular position of gaze, the slow-phase velocity is greater when the eyes are turned in the direction of the quick component	Peripheral vestibular disease is suspected when the nystagmus is associated with subjective vertigo Central vestibular disease (eg, brainstem infarction) is suspected when associated neurologic signs and symptoms of brainstem dysfunction are present
Periodic alternating nystagmus	Eyes exhibit primary position nystagmus, which, after 90 to 120 seconds, stops for a few seconds and then starts beating in the opposite direction	Often caused by disease processes at the craniocervical junction and is thought due to involvement of the cerebellar nodulus and uvula Baclofen, a GABA-B agonist, may abolish periodic alternating nystagmus
Drug-induced nystagmus	Predominantly horizontal, predominantly vertical, predominantly rotatory, or, most commonly, mixed	Often occurs with tranquilizing medications and anticonvulsants
Downbeat nystagmus	Usually present in primary position, but it is greatest when the patient looks down (Alexander law) and to one side	May occur with cervicomedullary junction disease, midline medullary lesions, posterior midline cerebellar lesions, or diffuse cerebellar disease. May also be idiopathic (40%)
Upbeat nystagmus	Usually associated with abnormalities of vertical vestibular and smooth pursuit eye movements and with saccadic intrusions, such as square wave jerks	Damage to the ventral tegmental pathways, which may link the superior vestibular nuclei to the superior rectus and inferior oblique subnuclei of the oculomotor nuclei, may cause the eyes to glide down, resulting in upbeat nystagmus Medullary disease may cause upbeat nystagmus as may lesions of the anterior cerebellar vermis, perihypoglossal and inferior olivary nuclei of the medulla, pontine tegmentum, brachium conjunctivum, midbrain, and brainstem diffusely

Binocular symmetric conjugate jerk nystagmus may be spontaneous or induced. Spontaneous symmetric conjugate jerk nystagmus that occurs in primary position may be predominantly horizontal, predominantly torsional, or predominantly vertical. If predominantly horizontal, types include: congenital nystagmus, latent nystagmus, vestibular nystagmus, periodic alternating nystagmus, drug-induced nystagmus, and epileptic nystagmus. If the symmetric binocular jerk nystagmus is predominantly vertical, types include upbeat nystagmus and downbeat nystagmus.

Binocular Symmetric Jerk Nystagmus Present in Eccentric Gaze or Induced by Various Maneuvers

Spontaneous binocular conjugate symmetric jerk nystagmus that is induced by eccentric gaze (gaze-evoked nystagmus) includes nystagmus due to brainstem or cerebellar disease, Bruns nystagmus, drug-induced nystagmus, physiologic nystagmus, rebound nystagmus, and convergence-induced nystagmus. Downbeat nystagmus and upbeat nystagmus may occur on only downward or upward gaze, respectively.

With gaze-evoked nystagmus, the eyes fail to remain in an eccentric position of gaze but drift to midposition. The velocity of the slow component decreases exponentially as the eyes approach midposition. Usually gaze-evoked nystagmus occurs on lateral or upward gaze, less often on downward gaze. Gaze-evoked nystagmus is due to a deficient eye position signal. A "leaky" neural integrator or cerebellar (especially vestibulocerebellar) lesion may result in this type of nystagmus, which is more pronounced when the patient looks toward the lesion. Diseases of the vestibulocerebellum commonly cause gaze-evoked nystagmus, often with a downbeating component. Cerebellopontine angle tumors may cause Bruns nystagmus, a combination of ipsilateral large-amplitude, low-frequency nystagmus that is due to impaired gaze-holding, and contralateral small-amplitude, high-frequency nystagmus that is due to vestibular impairment.

Rebound nystagmus occurs in some patients with brainstem or cerebellar disease. After keeping the eyes eccentric for some time, the original gaze-evoked nystagmus may wane and actually reverse direction so that the slow component is directed centrifugally (centripital nystagmus); it becomes obvious if the eyes are returned to midposition (rebound nystagmus). Rebound nystagmus probably reflects an attempt by brainstem or cerebellar mechanisms to correct for the centripetal drift of gaze-evoked nystagmus.

Positional vertigo of the benign paroxysmal type, also known as benign paroxysmal positioning vertigo or positional nystagmus, is usually idiopathic and possibly related to degeneration of the macula of the otolith organ or to lesions of the posterior semicircular canal. It has been proposed that otoconia detached from the otoconial layer (by degeneration or trauma) gravitate and settle on the cupula of the posterior canal, causing it to become heavier than the surrounding endolymph and thus sensitive to changes in the direction of gravity (with positional change). After rapid head tilt toward the affected ear or following head extension, when the posterior semicircular canal is moved in the specific plane of stimulation, an ampullofugal deflection of the cupula occurs, with a rotational vertigo and concomitant nystagmus.

Nystagmus induced by the Valsalva maneuver may occur with Chiari malformation or perilymph fistulas. Hyperventilation may induce nystagmus in patients with tumors of the eighth cranial nerve (eg, acoustic neuroma or epidermoid tumors), after vestibular neuritis, or with central demyelinating lesions.

- Spasmus nutans is a benign syndrome characterized by a triad of head nodding, nystagmus, and abnormal head posture.
- Nystagmus induced by the Valsalva maneuver may occur with Chiari malformation or perilymph fistulas.

13 Cranial Nerves I and II

KELLY D. FLEMMING, MD; JACQUELINE A. LEAVITT, MD;
EDUARDO E. BENARROCH, MD

Introduction

Cranial nerves I and II are supratentorial, paired cranial nerves serving olfaction and vision, respectively. This chapter provides an overview of their anatomy. Clinical disorders of cranial nerves are reviewed in Volume 2, Section VIII, "Clinical Disorders of the Cranial Nerves and Brainstem."

Cranial Nerve I: Olfactory

Receptors

Cranial nerve I is a special visceral afferent nerve carrying information regarding the sense of smell. The olfactory receptors lie in the nasal cavity. Odorants activate receptors within the cilia of olfactory sensory neurons. An odorant triggers the opening of a cyclic nucleotide-gated channel. This allows a calcium influx and opening of calcium-activated chloride channels. Depolarization occurs.

Central Pathways

Axons of the olfactory receptors extend through the cribriform plate to reach the olfactory bulb and synapse on the dendrites of mitral and tufted cells (Figure 13.1). Together, these mitral and tufted cells form a glomerulus, which receives input from olfactory sensory neurons expressing the same type of odorant receptor. Mitral and tufted cells

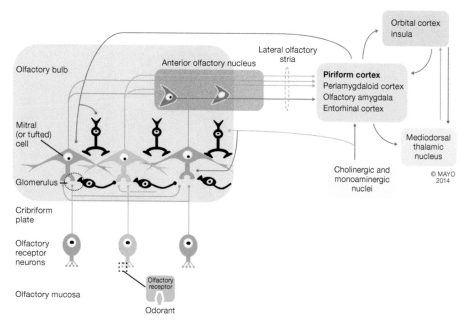

Figure 13.1 Olfactory Pathway.
(Used with permission of Mayo Foundation for Medical Education and Research.)

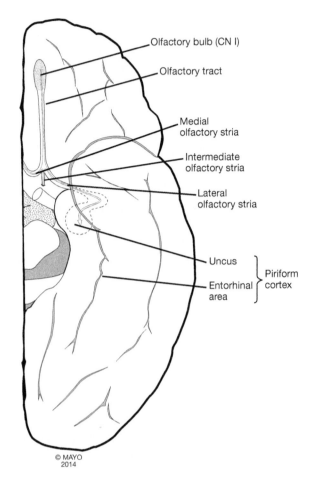

Figure 13.2 *Olfactory Cortex.*
CN indicates cranial nerve.
(Adapted from Flemming KD. Disorders of the cranial nerves. In: Mowzoon N, Flemming KD, editors. Neurology board review: an illustrated study guide. Rochester [MN]: Mayo Clinic Scientific Press and Florence [KY]: Informa Healthcare USA; c2007. p. 127–62. Used with permission of Mayo Foundation for Medical Education and Research.)

project to the olfactory cortex: anterior olfactory nucleus, piriform cortex (uncus and entorhinal cortex), and anterior cortical nucleus of the amygdala (Figures 13.1 and 13.2). Cortical areas reciprocally project back to the bulb.

The olfactory bulb and cortex also receive input from the basal forebrain, hypothalamus, and brainstem. The olfactory system interconnects with various autonomic and visceral centers via the medial forebrain bundle, the stria medullaris, and the stria terminalis.

Dysfunction may result in anosmia (lack of smell), dysosmia (distortion of smell), cacosmia (perception of bad smell), or parosmia (sensation of smell in the absence of an appropriate stimulus).

Clinical disorders associated with loss or change in olfaction are described in Volume 2, Chapter 49, "Disorders of the Cranial Nerves and Brainstem."

- Cranial nerve I is a special visceral afferent nerve carrying information regarding the sense of smell.
- Mitral and tufted cells project to the olfactory cortex: anterior olfactory nucleus, piriform cortex (uncus and entorhinal cortex), and anterior cortical nucleus of the amygdala (Figures 13.1 and 13.2).

Cranial Nerve II: Optic

Overview

The receptors and visual processing are reviewed in Chapter 5, "Special Somatic Sensory Afferent Overview." The central pathways are described here. Clinical visual field defects are described in Volume 2, Chapter 45, "Neuro-ophthalmology: Visual Fields."

Central Pathway

The visual pathway begins with the retinal photoreceptors (rods, cones), which connect to the retinal nerve fiber layer.

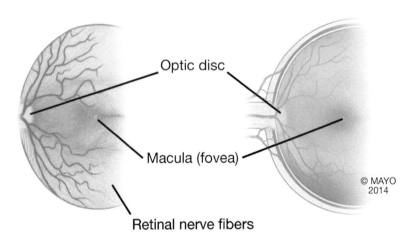

Figure 13.3 *Retinal Nerve Fibers.*
(Used with permission of Mayo Foundation for Medical Education and Research.)

The retinal nerve fiber layer has a specific pattern within the retina as it coalesces to form the optic disc. This retinal nerve fiber layer originates nasal to the macula (papillomacular bundle), and fibers nasal to the disc go directly toward the optic disc at the 3- and 9-o'clock positions. The retinal fiber layer originating temporal to the macula arches over the papillomacular bundle to enter the optic disc at the 12- and 6-o'clock positions (Figure 13.3). The optic disc has no photoreceptors, and thus it is represented by the blind spot in the temporal portion of each visual field (Figure 13.4).

Visual field information originates with the retinal photoreceptors and travels along the optic nerves to the chiasm (Figure 13.5). At the chiasm, the fibers representing the temporal fields of each eye cross to the opposite side of the chiasm so that the optic tract contains the

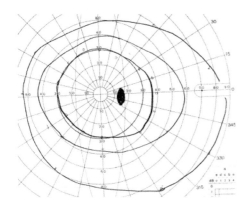

Figure 13.4 *Goldmann Visual Field, Right Eye.*
This normal visual field shows the extent of the periphery in all quadrants with 3 isopters, 3 different sizes of targets, and the normal blind spot.

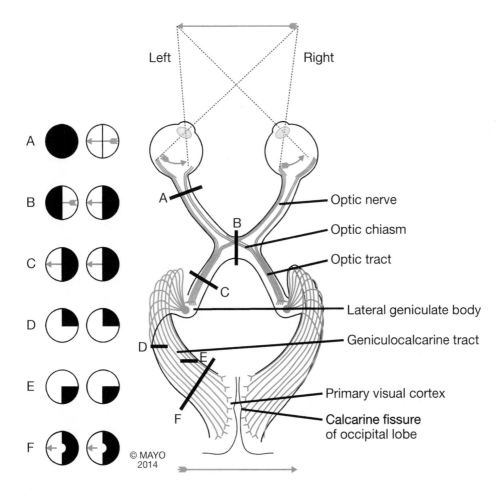

Figure 13.5 *Visual Central Pathway.*
Visual pathway as seen from the base of the brain. The visual impulses from the right half of the visual field project to the left half of each retina and to the left occipital lobe. On the left are the visual field defects (black areas) produced by lesions affecting the optic nerve (A), optic chiasm (B), optic tract (C), optic radiation in the temporal lobe (D), optic radiation in the parietal lobe (E), and occipital cortex (F).

(Adapted from Benarroch EE, Daube JR, Flemming KD, Westmoreland BF. Mayo Clinic medical neurosciences: organized by neurologic systems and levels. 5th ed. Rochester [MN]: Mayo Clinic Scientific Press and Florence [KY]: Informa Healthcare USA; c2008. Chapter 16, Part A. The supratentorial level: thalamus, hypothalamus, and visual system; p. 669–99. Used with permission of Mayo Foundation for Medical Education and Research.)

visual information from each eye representing the contralateral peripheral vision. From the optic tracts, after synapsing in the lateral geniculate bodies, the visual fibers extend posteriorly but split so that the upper field fibers pass through the temporal lobes and the inferior field fibers pass through the parietal lobes. Information is projected to the occipital cortex. Within the occipital lobes, the orientation is also stratified such that the fibers representing the superior visual fields lie inferior to the calcarine fissure and vice versa for the inferior visual fields. The fields to the right of the vertical meridian are located in the left occipital pole and vice versa for the left hemifield in each eye. There is also an orientation caudally in that the more posterior portion of the occipital cortex represents the most central or macular portion of the visual field. The most anterior component of the primary visual cortex (or striate cortex) represents the temporal crescent that has no corresponding nasal representation in the ipsilateral eye.

- Visual field information originates with the retinal photoreceptors and travels along the optic nerves to the chiasm (Figure 13.5).
- From the optic tracts, after synapsing in the lateral geniculate bodies, the visual fibers extend posteriorly but split so that the upper field fibers pass through the temporal lobes and the inferior field fibers pass through the parietal lobes.

14 Thalamus

KELLY D. FLEMMING, MD; EDUARDO E. BENARROCH, MD

Introduction

The diencephalon is composed of 4 components: 1) the epithalamus, which includes the pineal body; 2) the dorsal thalamus, which is commonly considered to be the thalamus proper; 3) the ventral thalamus, consisting of the reticular nucleus and subthalamic nucleus; and 4) the hypothalamus. This chapter focuses on the dorsal thalamus and the ventral thalamus. The hypothalamus is reviewed in Chapter 15, "Principles of Neuroendocrinology and Hypothalamic Function."

The thalamus has 3 main functions: 1) relay input from subcortical structures to the cortex, 2) control (gate) which sensory information reaches the cortex, and 3) synchronize cortical activity that relates to consciousness.

Anatomy

Figure 14.1 reviews the anatomy of the diencephalon. The thalamus extends rostrally from the mammillary bodies and optic chiasm to the pineal body. Medial to the thalamus is the third ventricle and lateral is the internal capsule.

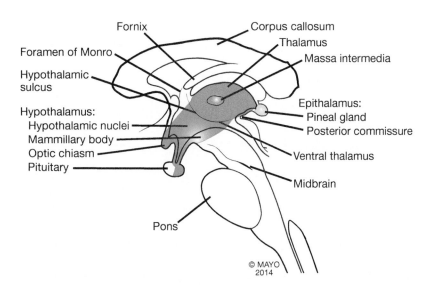

Figure 14.1 Anatomy of Diencephalon.
Diencephalon and its 4 subdivisions: thalamus (thalamus proper) (red), ventral thalamus (not pictured), hypothalamus (green), and epithalamus (yellow). The anterior pituitary (white) is not part of the hypothalamus.
(Adapted from Benarroch EE, Daube JR, Flemming KD, Westmoreland BF. Mayo Clinic medical neurosciences: organized by neurologic systems and levels. 5th ed. Rochester [MN]: Mayo Clinic Scientific Press and Florence [KY]: Informa Healthcare USA; c2008. Chapter 16, Part A, The supratentorial level: thalamus, hypothalamus, and visual system; p. 669–99. Used with permission of Mayo Foundation for Medical Education and Research.)

Abbreviation: GABA, γ-aminobutyric acid

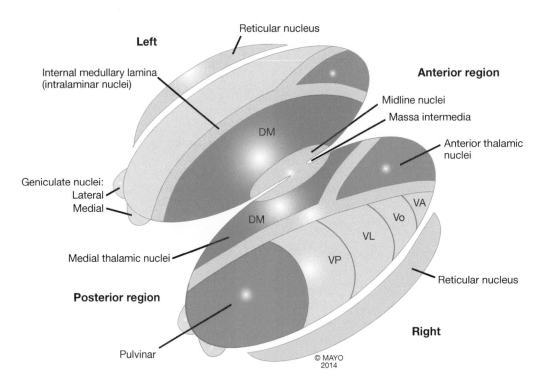

Figure 14.2 Major Regions of the Thalamus and Their Nuclei.
Nuclei are as defined by their input and output: anterior; medial (dorsomedial nucleus [DM]); lateral, including the ventral posterior (VP), ventral lateral (VL, also called ventral intermedius); ventral oral (Vo), and the ventral anterior (VA) nuclei; and posterior, corresponding to the pulvinar. The medial and lateral geniculate nuclei are located in this posterior region, just below the pulvinar. The intralaminar and midline nuclei are a functionally distinct group. The reticular nucleus corresponds to the ventral thalamus.

(Adapted from Benarroch EE, Daube JR, Flemming KD, Westmoreland BF. Mayo Clinic medical neurosciences: organized by neurologic systems and levels. 5th ed. Rochester [MN]: Mayo Clinic Scientific Press and Florence [KY]: Informa Healthcare USA; c2008. Chapter 16, Part A, The supratentorial level: thalamus, hypothalamus, and visual system; p. 669–99. Used with permission of Mayo Foundation for Medical Education and Research.)

The 2 thalami are interconnected by the massa intermedia. The thalami are further divided into individual nuclei (Figure 14.2). The reticular nucleus surrounds the dorsal thalamus (thalamus proper) and lies between the posterior limb of the internal capsule and the external medullary lamina. The blood supply to the thalamus is predominantly from the posterior circulation (Figure 14.3).

Functional Organization

Dorsal Thalamus

The dorsal thalamus or thalamus proper can be divided into 3 groups of nuclei based on function and afferent input: 1) first order relay, 2) high order relay or associative, and 3) nonspecific nuclei (Figure 14.4). The first order relay and high order relay nuclei are sometimes together known as the isothalamus. The nonspecific nuclei are sometimes referred to as the allothalamus. The main difference between the first order nuclei and the high order nuclei (association) is their afferent inputs. All nuclei of

the dorsal thalamus contain thalamocortical glutamatergic neurons that excite their cortical targets.

First order relay neurons are those that receive primary input from subcortical sensory or motor areas (anterior nucleus, ventral anterior, ventrolateral, ventral posterolateral, ventral posteromedial, medial geniculate body, lateral geniculate body) and project to primary sensory or motor areas (eg, primary somatosensory cortex) (Figure 14.5; Table 14.1). High order relay nuclei integrate cortical and subcortical information and project to high order multimodal cortex (Figure 14.6; Table 14.1). These include the pulvinar, dorsomedial, and anterior nuclei of the thalamus. Among the nonspecific nuclei, the midline nuclei (centromedian/parafascicular) project and receive inputs from the reticular formation and globus pallidus and project to the striatum or diffusely to the cortex (Table 14.1).

Ventral Thalamus (Reticular Nucleus)

The thalamic reticular nucleus is a thin layer of interconnected γ-aminobutyric acid (GABA)ergic neurons between the posterior limb of the internal capsule and the external

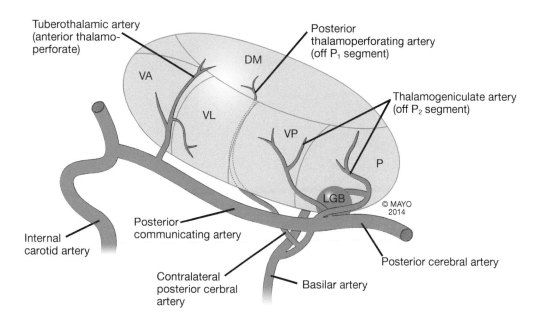

Figure 14.3 *Blood Supply to the Thalamus.*

Thalamic nuclei: DM, dorsomedial; LGB, lateral geniculate body; P, pulvinar; P_1 and P_2, segments of the posterior cerebral artery; VA, VL, VP, ventral anterior, lateral, and posterior, respectively.

(Adapted from Benarroch EE, Daube JR, Flemming KD, Westmoreland BF. Mayo Clinic medical neurosciences: organized by neurologic systems and levels. 5th ed. Rochester [MN]: Mayo Clinic Scientific Press and Florence [KY]: Informa Healthcare USA; c2008. Chapter 12, The vascular system; p. 447–88. Used with permission of Mayo Foundation for Medical Education and Research.)

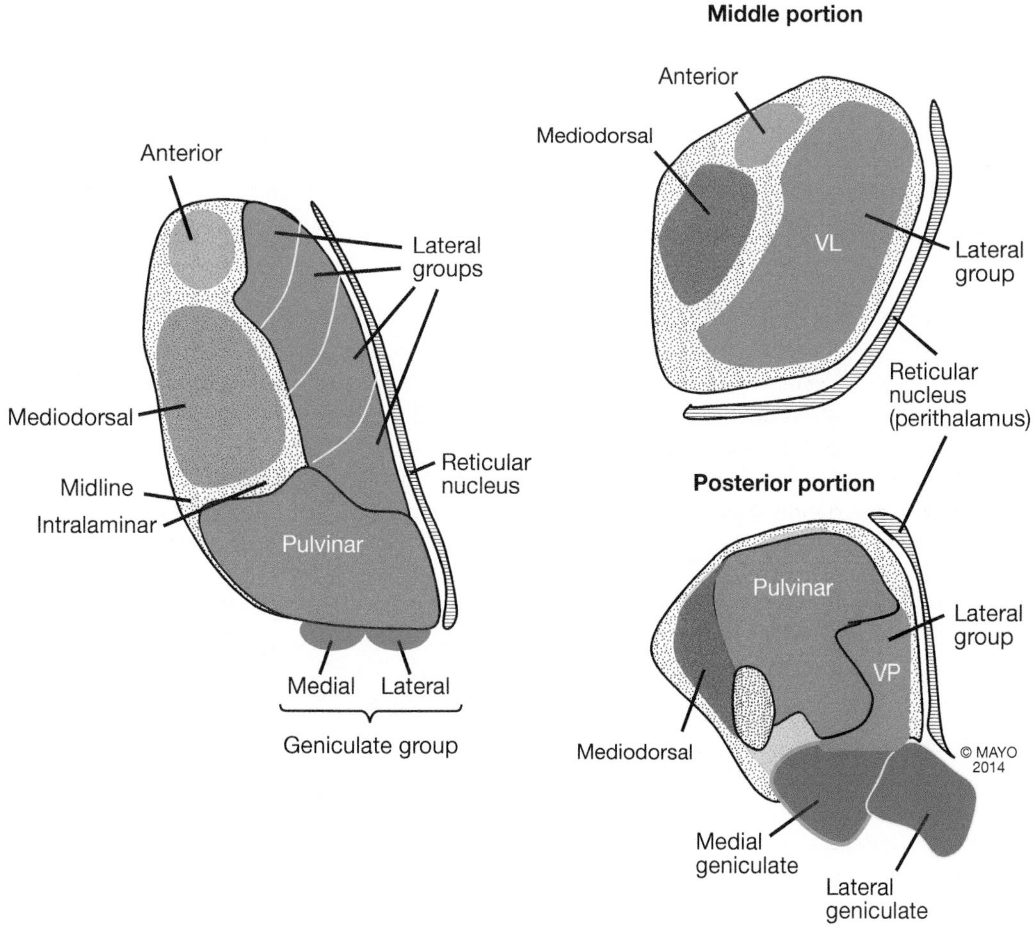

Figure 14.4 *Functional Anatomy of the Thalamus.*

VL indicates ventral lateral; VP, ventral posterior.

(Used with permission of Mayo Foundation for Medical Education and Research.)

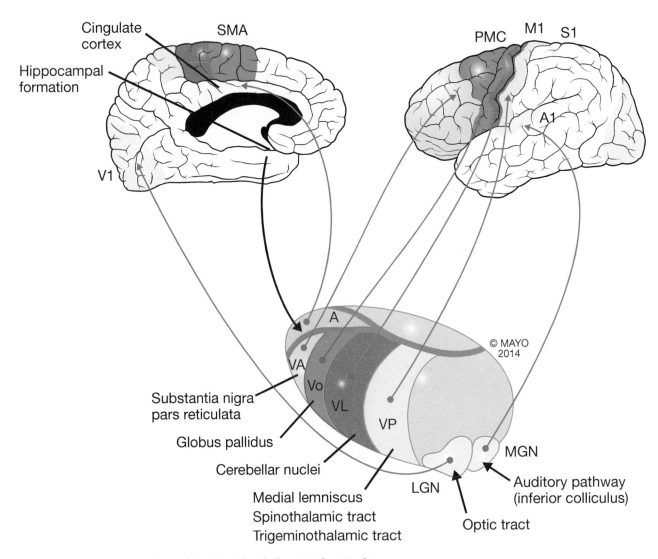

Figure 14.5 *Main Connections of the Specific Thalamic Relay Nuclei.*
The anterior (A) nuclear group receives input from the hippocampal formation via the fornix (both directly and from the mammillary bodies) and projects to the cingulate gyrus. The ventral anterior (VA) nucleus relays input from the substantia nigra pars reticulata to the prefrontal cortex and frontal eye fields; the ventral oral (Vo) relays input from the internal segment of the globus pallidus to the supplementary motor area (SMA). The ventral lateral (VL), or ventricular intermedius, relays cerebellar input to the premotor (PMC) and primary motor (M1) cortices. The ventral posterior (VP) relays input from the medial lemniscus, spinothalamic tract, and trigeminal system to the primary sensory cortex (S1). The lateral geniculate nucleus (LGN) relays retinal input to the primary visual cortex (V1), and the medial geniculate nucleus (MGN) receives auditory input from the inferior colliculus and projects to the primary auditory cortex (A1).

(Adapted from Benarroch EE, Daube JR, Flemming KD, Westmoreland BF. Mayo Clinic medical neurosciences: organized by neurologic systems and levels. 5th ed. Rochester [MN]: Mayo Clinic Scientific Press and Florence [KY]: Informa Healthcare USA; c2008. Chapter 16, Part A, The supratentorial level: thalamus, hypothalamus, and visual system; p. 669–99. Used with permission of Mayo Foundation for Medical Education and Research.)

Table 14.1 • Thalamic Nuclei Connections and Function

Nuclei	Input	Output	Function
Association nuclei			
Anterior nucleus	Mammillary bodies (via mammillothalamic tract) Medial temporal lobe (via fornix)	Posterior cingulate gyrus (via anterior limb of the internal capsule)	Limbic relay
Dorsomedial nucleus	Prefrontal cortex Substantia nigra Amygdala	Prefrontal cortex Substantia nigra Amygdala	Memory/executive function behavior Oculomotor basal ganglia circuits
Pulvinar	Sensory cortices Superior colliculus Retina	Visual association cortex Parieto-temporal occipital-association areas	Role in integration of sensory information for visual attention; visual stimulus positions
Relay nuclei			
Ventral anterior	Substantia nigra pars reticulata/ globus pallidus interna	Frontal eye fields	Oculomotor basal ganglia circuitry
Ventral posterolateral; ventral posteromedial	Lemniscal Spinothalamic Trigeminothalamic	Primary somatosensory cortex	Sensory relay to cortex
Ventrolateral			
Oralis	Globus pallidus	Supplementary motor area; premotor cortex	Motor circuitry of basal ganglia
Caudalis[a]	Cerebellum	Premotor and primary motor cortex	Cerebellar relay
Ventromedial	Spinothalamic Parabrachial nucleus	Insulary cortex	Interoceptive relays
Lateral geniculate body	Retina	Primary visual cortex	Visual relays
Medial geniculate body	Retina	Primary auditory cortex	Auditory relays
Nonspecific nuclei			
Dorsal midline	Hypothalamus Amygdala Reticular formation	Anterior cingulate Hippocampus	
Intralaminar	Globus pallidus Spinothalamic Reticular formation	Striatum Cerebral cortex	
Central group	Substantia nigra pars reticulata Superior colliculus	Putamen Primary motor cortex Frontal eye fields	

[a] Also known as ventral intermedius.

medullary lamina. Unlike thalamocortical neurons, these neurons do not project to the cerebral cortex but rather send inhibitory inputs to the thalamocortical neurons of the thalamus proper. The reticular nucleus functions to modulate, or gate, the responses of the thalamic neurons to incoming cerebral cortical input (Figure 14.7).

The GABAergic neurons of the reticular nucleus are highly coupled by gap junctions; therefore they are able to exert synchronized inhibitory activity on thalamocortical neurons. The synchronization of discharge of the reticular thalamic neurons is inhibited by reciprocal GABAergic interconnections between these cells.

The thalamus has reciprocal connections with the cerebral cortex. Corticothalamic projections to each of the dorsal thalamic nuclei send collaterals to the reticular nucleus. Thus, although it is not directly connected to the cortex, this nucleus monitors both thalamocortical and corticothalamic activity. It acts like a shield between the thalamic relay nuclei and the cortex, so that fibers passing either way between the thalamus and the cortex must go through the thalamic reticular nuclei. Nearly all thalamic efferent fibers to the cortex pass through this nuclear complex and send collaterals.

- The dorsal thalamus or thalamus proper can be divided into 3 groups of nuclei based on function and afferent input: 1) first order relay, 2) high order relay or associative, and 3) nonspecific nuclei.
- First order relay neurons are those that receive primary input from subcortical sensory or motor areas and project to primary sensory or motor areas.
- High order relay nuclei integrate cortical and subcortical information and project to high order multimodal cortex.

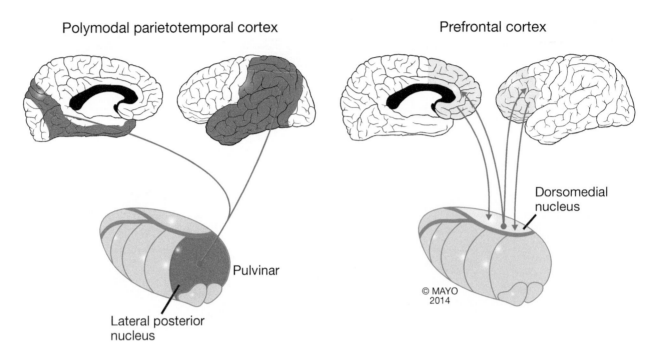

Polymodal parietotemporal cortex

Prefrontal cortex

Dorsomedial
nucleus

Pulvinar

Lateral posterior
nucleus

© MAYO
2014

Figure 14.6 Association Thalamic Nuclei.
The pulvinar (and the lateral posterior nucleus) receives input from the visual, somatosensory, and auditory cortices and projects to polymodal association areas of the posterior parietal and lateral temporal lobes. The dorsomedial (mediodorsal) nucleus has reciprocal connections with prefrontal cortex.
(Adapted from Benarroch EE, Daube JR, Flemming KD, Westmoreland BF. Mayo Clinic medical neurosciences: organized by neurologic systems and levels. 5th ed. Rochester [MN]: Mayo Clinic Scientific Press and Florence [KY]: Informa Healthcare USA; c2008. Chapter 16, Part A, The supratentorial level: thalamus, hypothalamus, and visual system; p. 669–99. Used with permission of Mayo Foundation for Medical Education and Research.)

- The thalamic reticular nucleus is a thin layer of interconnected γ-aminobutyric acid (GABA)ergic neurons between the posterior limb of the internal capsule and the external medullary lamina.
- The reticular nucleus functions to modulate, or gate, the responses of the thalamic neurons to incoming cerebral cortical input.

Firing Modes of Thalamic Neurons

Thalamocortical neurons respond to input from sensory pathways of the cortex by discharging in 1 of 2 modes: tonic or rhythmic burst (Table 14.2). These discharge modes affect the pattern on the electroencephalogram: rhythmic burst firing occurs in non–rapid-eye-movement sleep, and tonic single spike firing occurs during wakefulness or rapid-eye-movement sleep. The 2 patterns of discharge depend on multiple states: the resting membrane potential, activation of calcium channels, and the inputs (excitatory from cortex, inhibitory from reticular nucleus, ascending modulatory input from brainstem cholinergic

and monoaminergic nuclei). For example, when the resting potential of thalamic cells is relatively hyperpolarized, excitatory input activates T-type calcium channels that initiate rhythmic burst activity, leading to synchronization of the electroencephalogram (as occurs during non–rapid-eye-movement sleep).

- Thalamocortical neurons respond to input from sensory pathways of the cortex by discharging in 1 of 2 modes: tonic or rhythmic burst.

Clinical Correlations

Absence Seizures

Patients with absence seizures may display a 3-Hz spike-and-wave discharge on the electroencephalogram. Fast bursting cortical neurons may initiate these seizures via corticothalamic projections. Excitatory cortical input to the reticular nucleus of the thalamus overrides the intrinsic GABA-receptor–mediated local inhibitory mechanisms

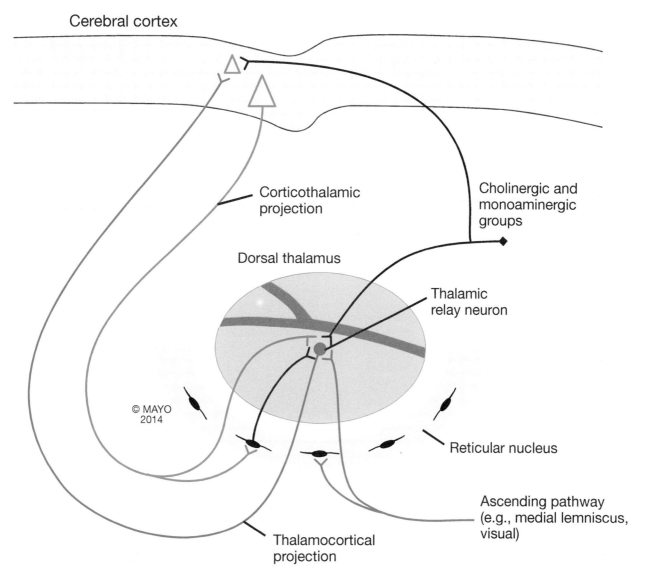

Figure 14.7 *Reciprocal Thalamocortical Interactions.*

The projection neurons of the thalamic relay nuclei receive excitatory input and send an excitatory projection to a restricted area of the cerebral cortex. Pyramidal neurons in this cortical area send a reciprocal projection to the thalamic relay nucleus and a collateral projection to the thalamic reticular nucleus. The thalamic reticular nucleus also receives an excitatory collateral projection from the thalamocortical neuron (not shown) and sends an inhibitory γ-aminobutyric acid–ergic projection to the thalamic relay neuron. The reciprocal thalamocorticothalamic interactions gate the relay of information at the level of the thalamus and control thalamocortical synchronization. These functions change during the sleep-wake cycle under the modulatory influence of cholinergic and monoaminergic neurons of the brainstem, which project to the thalamic relay and reticular nuclei as well as to the cerebral cortex.

(Adapted from Benarroch EE, Daube JR, Flemming KD, Westmoreland BF. Mayo Clinic medical neurosciences: organized by neurologic systems and levels. 5th ed. Rochester [MN]: Mayo Clinic Scientific Press and Florence [KY]: Informa Healthcare USA; c2008. Chapter 16, Part A, The supratentorial level: thalamus, hypothalamus, and visual system; p. 669–99. Used with permission of Mayo Foundation for Medical Education and Research.)

Table 14.2 • Functional States of Thalamocortical Circuits

Behavior State	Drowsiness and Non-REM (Slow-Wave) Sleep	Wakefulness and REM Sleep
TC neuron activity	Rhythmic burst firing	Tonic firing
Membrane potential of TC neuron	Hyperpolarized ($\approx$75 mV)	Depolarized ($\approx$55 mV)
Calcium channel involved	T-type	P/Q type
GABAergic influence from ReT neurons	Strong	Weak
Cholinergic influence from neurons of the PPT/LDT	Weak	Strong
Cortical (EEG) activity	High amplitude, slow (0.5-1.5 Hz), with superimposed spindles	High frequency (30-50 Hz, gamma band)
Functional implications	Memory consolidation?	Temporal binding for perceptual awareness and cognition

Abbreviations: EEG, electroencephalogram; GABA, γ-aminobutyric acid; LDT, laterodorsal tegmental nucleus; PPT, pedunculopontine tegmental nucleus; REM, rapid-eye-movement; ReT, reticular thalamic nucleus; TC, thalamocortical.

Table 14.3 • Thalamic Targets for Deep Brain Stimulation

Thalamic Nucleus	Connections	Clinical Applications
Ventrolateral or ventral intermedius	Cerebellum	Tremor
Ventral anterior	GPi/SNr	Possibly dystonia
Centromedian/ parafascicular	GPi/SNr, reticular formation, anterior cingulate	Tourette syndrome Seizures
Ventral posterior	Medial lemniscus Spinothalamic tract	Possibly central pain

Abbreviations: GPi, globus pallidus interna; SNr, substantia nigra pars reticulata.

that usually prevent synchronized reticular nucleus discharges. Excessive synchronized inhibitory input from the reticular nucleus elicits rhythmic postsynaptic inhibitory potential on thalamocortical neurons, deactivating T-type calcium channels and leading to a rebound burst of action potentials in thalamocortical cells.

Deep Brain Stimulation

The thalamic nuclei are a common target for deep brain stimulation for various conditions (Table 14.3).

15 Principles of Neuroendocrinology and Hypothalamic Function

ELIZABETH A. COON, MD; EDUARDO E. BENARROCH, MD

Introduction

The **hypothalamus is** the neural center of the endocrine system, the regulator of the autonomic nervous system, and the circadian and seasonal clock for behavioral and sleep-wake functions. The hypothalamus maintains homeostasis by integrating cortical, limbic, and spinal inputs and by affecting hormone release, temperature regulation, intake of food and water, sexual behavior and reproduction, emotional responses, and diurnal rhythms. As the link from the nervous system to the endocrine system, the hypothalamus synthesizes and secretes neurohormones that stimulate or inhibit the secretion of pituitary hormones.

This chapter reviews the basic neuroanatomy and function of the hypothalamus. Clinical disorders related to endocrine dysfunction are discussed in Volume 2, Chapter 79, "Endocrine Disease."

Anatomy and Functional Organization

The hypothalamus is located along the sides and under the floor of the third ventricle, extending from the optic chiasm and lamina terminalis anteriorly. The hypothalamus is bordered laterally by the optic tracts and posteriorly by the mammillary bodies (Figure 15.1).

Functionally, the hypothalamus and the adjacent preoptic area form a unit that is subdivided into 3 distinct longitudinal zones: the periventricular, medial, and lateral zones (Figure 15.2). The hypothalamic nuclei situated in these zones are often difficult to differentiate because

they do not have sharply delineated borders and may extend into different zones. The functions of the individual nuclei are summarized in Table 15.1 according to zones. The periventricular, medial, and lateral zones are described below.

The periventricular zone of the hypothalamus includes the suprachiasmatic nucleus, which is involved in circadian rhythms, and the magnocellular and parvocellular nuclei, which control endocrine function (see below).

The medial zone contains several nuclei that are involved in maintaining homeostasis and controlling reproduction. The medial preoptic nucleus contains thermosensitive neurons involved in thermoregulation. The medial preoptic area also contains osmosensitive neurons that receive inputs from circumventricular organs of the anterior wall of the third ventricle, such as the subfornical organ and the vascular organ of the lamina terminalis, which lack a blood-brain barrier. The circumventricular organs contain receptors for circulating peptides, such as angiotensin II and cytokines. By means of these structures, angiotensin II controls water and sodium metabolism, and cytokines trigger the febrile response. The medial hypothalamus also contains the paraventricular nucleus, which is involved not only in endocrine function but also in autonomic control and is critical in stress responses. The arcuate (infundibular), ventromedial, and dorsomedial nuclei participate in the regulation of food intake, metabolism, and reproductive function.

The lateral hypothalamus also controls food intake and the sleep-wake cycle (through orexin, also called

---

Abbreviations: CRH, corticotropin-releasing hormone; FSH, follicle-stimulating hormone; GH, growth hormone; GH-RH, growth hormone–releasing hormone; GnRH, gonadotropin-releasing hormone; LH, luteinizing hormone; TRH, thyrotropin-releasing hormone

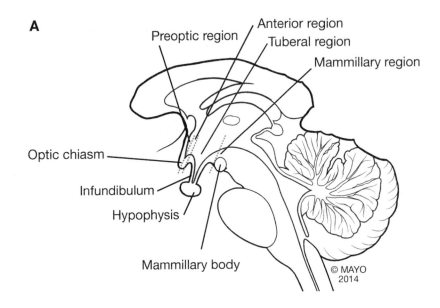

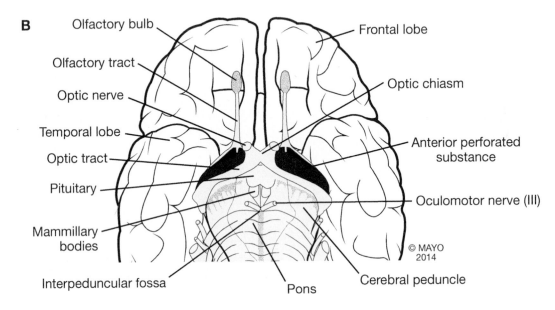

Figure 15.1 *Gross Anatomy of the Hypothalamus and Pituitary Region.*
A, Midline section shows the different regions of the hypothalamus, the pituitary gland (hypophysis) in the sella turcica, and the mammillary bodies. B, View of the base of the brain shows the optic chiasm, the pituitary, and the mammillary bodies. III indicates cranial nerve III.
(Adapted from Benarroch EE, Daube JR, Flemming KD, Westmoreland BF. Mayo Clinic medical neurosciences: organized by neurologic systems and levels. 5th ed. Rochester [MN]: Mayo Clinic Scientific Press and Florence [KY]: Informa Healthcare USA; c2008. Chapter 16, Part A, The supratentorial level; p. 669–763. Used with permission of Mayo Foundation for Medical Education and Research.)

hypocretin) and motivated behavior. Posterolateral hypothalamic neurons secrete orexin, which regulates the switch between wakefulness and sleep. This leads to reciprocal inhibitory interactions between the sleep-promoting neurons of the ventrolateral preoptic nucleus and the excitatory projections to the arousal-promoting monoaminergic and cholinergic nuclei.

Orexin neurons also stimulate food intake and are part of the reward circuit involved in drug addiction via their projections to dopaminergic neurons of the ventral tegmental nucleus.

- The periventricular zone of the hypothalamus includes the suprachiasmatic nucleus, which is involved in

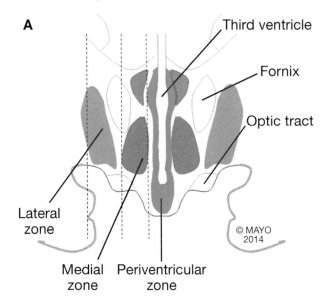

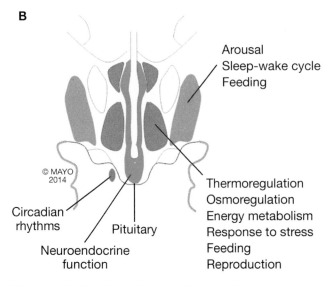

Figure 15.2 Functional Zones of the Hypothalamus.
A, The 3 functional zones are the periventricular, medial,
and lateral zones. B, The functions of the 3 zones are shown.
(Used with permission of Mayo Foundation for Medical Education
and Research.)

circadian rhythms, and the magnocellular and
parvocellular nuclei, which control endocrine
function.
- The medial zone contains several nuclei (medial
  preoptic, paraventricular, arcuate, ventromedial, and
  dorsomedial) that are involved in maintaining
  homeostasis and controlling reproduction.
- The medial hypothalamus contains the paraventricular
  nucleus, which is involved not only in endocrine
  function but also in autonomic control and is critical in
  stress responses.

Table 15.1 • Hypothalamic Nuclei

Nucleus	Function
Periventricular zone	
Suprachiasmatic	Circadian rhythms
Paraventricular (magnocellular)	Vasopressin (ADH) and oxytocin secretion
Paraventricular (parvocellular)	Response to stress
	CRH secretion
	Autonomic control
Arcuate (infundibular)	Pituitary control (eg, dopaminergic inhibition of prolactin release)
Medial zone	
Medial preoptic	GnRH secretion, sexual activity
	Thermoregulation (heat loss)
	Osmoregulation
Anterior hypothalamic	Thermoregulation (heat loss)
Supraoptic	Vasopressin (ADH) and oxytocin secretion
Dorsomedial	Thermoregulation (heat gain)
Ventromedial	Control of feeding and energy metabolism
Arcuate (infundibular)	Dual control of feeding and energy metabolism
Lateral zone	
Ventrolateral preoptic	Sleep induction
Lateral tuberal	Cortical arousal[a]
Posterolateral (orexin, also called hypocretin)	Maintenance of wakefulness
	REM sleep inhibition
	Stimulates feeding
Tuberomammillary (histamine)	Arousal

Abbreviations: ADH, antidiuretic hormone; CRH, corticotropin-releasing
hormone; GnRH, gonadotropin-releasing hormone; REM, rapid eye
movement.
[a] Unclear function.

- The lateral hypothalamus controls food intake and the
  sleep-wake cycle (through orexin, also called
  hypocretin) and motivated behavior.

Magnocellular System

Vasopressin and Oxytocin

The magnocellular system regulates the release of pituitary
hormones (oxytocin and vasopressin) by synaptic transmission. The cells of the magnocellular system of the
hypothalamus project to the posterior pituitary; together
they constitute the neurohypophysis (Figure 15.3).
Magnocellular neurosecretory cells are large-diameter
hypothalamic neurons located in the paraventricular
nucleus and the supraoptic nucleus. These neurosecretory
cells produce vasopressin and oxytocin, which are transported via axons through the stalk of the pituitary to the
posterior lobe of the pituitary where these peptides are
stored. Vasopressin and oxytocin can also be released from
dendrites into the hypophyseal portal circulation.

A

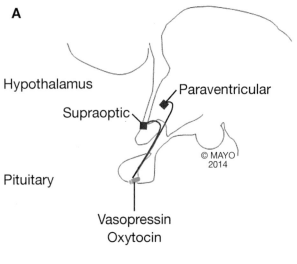

B

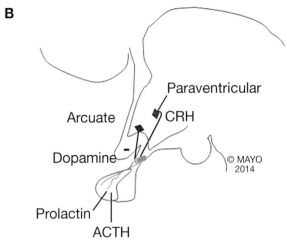

Figure 15.3 Magnocellular and Parvocellular Systems.
A, Magnocellular system. Neurons in the paraventricular
nucleus and the supraoptic nucleus produce vasopressin
and oxytocin. B, Parvocellular system. The paraventricular
nucleus produces corticotropin-releasing hormone (CRH),
which, with vasopressin, causes the pituitary to release
corticotropin (ACTH).
(Used with permission of Mayo Foundation for Medical Education
and Research.)

Vasopressin (also called antidiuretic hormone) maintains the osmolality of the blood. Vasopressin is secreted in response to an increase in plasma osmolality that is sensed directly at the supraoptic and paraventricular neurons on separate hypothalamic osmoreceptors. Vasopressin acts on vasopressin V2 receptors in the renal tubules, increasing the reabsorption of water and the concentration of the urine. Alterations in blood pressure and volume also affect vasopressin release through baroreceptors and mechanoreceptors conveyed via the vagus and glossopharyngeal nerves. The blood pressure stimulus predominates over osmolarity: Vasopressin release continues in a

hypotensive state even in the presence of low serum osmolality.

The magnocellular system also includes oxytocin, which initiates uterine contraction and ejection of milk in lactation. Oxytocin release is stimulated by distention of the cervix, labor, breastfeeding, and estrogen.

- The magnocellular system regulates the release of pituitary hormones (oxytocin and vasopressin) by synaptic transmission.
- Vasopressin (also called antidiuretic hormone) maintains the osmolality of the blood.

Parvocellular System

Neurovascular Transmission

The parvocellular system regulates pituitary hormone release by neurovascular transmission. The parvocellular system comprises small-diameter neurons in several hypothalamic nuclei in the periventricular zone. Parvocellular neurosecretory cells project to the median eminence, where their nerve terminals release peptides into the hypothalamo-hypophysial portal system (Figure 15.3). These blood vessels carry peptides to the anterior lobe of the pituitary gland, where they influence the secretion of hormones into the systemic circulation. Systemic hormones then exert negative feedback to control the secretion of the releasing hormones.

Adrenocortical Axis

The adrenocortical axis (also known as the hypothalamic-pituitary-adrenal axis) is a complex system that controls the stress response. Corticotropin-releasing hormone (CRH) is produced from the paraventricular nucleus and acts with vasopressin to release corticotropin from the pituitary (Table 15.2). Corticotropin stimulates the adrenal cortex to synthesize and release the glucocorticoid hormone cortisol. Cortisol acts at glucocorticoid receptors in the hypothalamus and anterior lobe of the pituitary to suppress production of CRH and corticotropin.

The hypothalamic cells producing CRH receive extensive input from multiple regions of the nervous system, particularly the noradrenergic pathways and limbic structures. Release of CRH from the hypothalamus is influenced by stress, physical activity, illness, and the circadian cycle.

Cushing syndrome occurs with prolonged exposure to inappropriately high levels of cortisol that result in excess levels of cortisol, corticotropin, or CRH. Prolonged administration of exogenous glucocorticoids (eg, prednisone) is the overall most common cause of Cushing syndrome. *Cushing disease* refers to a pituitary cause of Cushing syndrome. The most common cause of Cushing disease is pituitary adenoma leading to excess corticotropin

Table 15.2 • Hypothalamic Regulatory Hormones and Functions

Feature	Paraventricular Nucleus			Medial Preoptic Nucleus	Arcuate (Infundibular) Nucleus
Regulatory hormone	CRH	TRH	PRH, TRH, oxytocin	GnRH	GH-RH
Pituitary hormone	ACTH	TSH	Prolactin	LH, FSH	GH
Target	Adrenal cortex	Thyroid	Mammary glands	Ovaries, testes	Bones, liver
Effector	Cortisol	T_3, T_4	Prolactin	Females: estradiol, progesterone Males: testosterone, inhibin	Liver: IGF-1
Response	Stress response	Metabolic, protein synthesis	Lactation	Females: ovulation Males: spermatogenesis	Bone growth, glucose homeostasis
Feedback	Cortisol suppresses CRH and ACTH	T_3 inhibits TSH and TRH	Dopamine inhibits prolactin	Gonadal steroids and inhibin suppress FSH	Somatostatin inhibits GH

Abbreviations: ACTH, corticotropin; CRH, corticotropin-releasing hormone; FSH, follicle-stimulating hormone; GH, growth hormone; GH-RH, growth hormone–releasing hormone; GnRH, gonadotropin-releasing hormone; IGF-1, insulinlike growth factor 1; LH, luteinizing hormone; PRH, prolactin-releasing hormone; TRH, thyrotropin-releasing hormone; TSH, thyrotropin; T_3, triiodothyronine; T_4, thyroxine.

Adapted from Kantarci OH, Ghearing GR. Basic principles of neuroscience and neurogenetics. In: Mowzoon N, Flemming KD, editors. Neurology board review: an illustrated study guide. Rochester (MN): Mayo Clinic Scientific Press and Florence (KY): Informa Healthcare USA; c2007. p. 25–81. Used with permission of Mayo Foundation for Medical Education and Research.

production. Typical clinical features include truncal obesity with abdominal striae, thinning of the skin with easy bruising and dryness, hirsutism, osteoporosis, proximal muscle weakness, osteoporosis, and insulin resistance.

Thyroid Axis

The medial neurons of the paraventricular nucleus produce thyrotropin-releasing hormone (TRH), which stimulates the release of thyrotropin from thyrotropes in the anterior pituitary. Thyrotropin increases the synthesis of thyroid hormone and stimulates the release of thyroxine and triiodothyronine. Triiodothyronine exerts inhibitory feedback on thyrotropin and TRH. TRH also stimulates dopamine- and somatostatin-producing cells of the pituitary, leading to an inhibitory effect of somatostatin on thyrotropin.

Growth Hormone Axis

Growth hormone–releasing hormone (GH-RH) is produced in arcuate (infundibular) neurons, and its release into the hypophyseal portal system triggers growth hormone (GH) secretion from somatotropes in the anterior pituitary gland. GH-RH is released in a pulsatile manner, leading to a pulsatile release of GH.

Somatostatin, also known as growth hormone release–inhibiting hormone, is produced in the periventricular nucleus and inhibits the secretion of GH. GH enhances skeletal and muscle growth, regulates lipolysis, and has anti-insulin effects.

An excess of GH before the closure of skeletal epiphyses leads to gigantism; hypersecretion after epiphyseal closure results in acromegaly. Signs of acromegaly include soft tissue enlargement with macroglossia and hypertension, diabetes mellitus, and organ failure.

Prolactin Axis

Lactotrophic cells in the pituitary release prolactin in response to prolactin-releasing hormone, TRH, oxytocin, and several other peptides. Prolactin stimulates lactation; the hypothalamic-pituitary axis is responsible for milk production that responds to sensory stimuli from the nipples. Dopamine exerts an inhibitory effect on prolactin; clinically, this may account for galactorrhea and reproductive disorders if dopamine transport from the hypothalamus is disrupted.

Prolactin-secreting tumors (eg, prolactinomas) may clinically manifest as anovulatory infertility, amenorrhea, unexpected lactation, and sexual dysfunction in women.

Gonadotropin Axis

Cells in the medial preoptic nucleus produce gonadotropin-releasing hormone (GnRH), which affects the release of the gonadotropic hormones, luteinizing hormone (LH) and follicle-stimulating hormone (FSH). Release of FSH and LH is controlled by the frequency and size of GnRH pulses, with high-frequency GnRH pulses stimulating LH release and low-frequency GnRH pulses leading to FSH release. In females, the frequency of GnRH pulses varies during the menstrual cycle, with a large surge before ovulation; in males, GnRH is secreted at a constant frequency. In females, FSH stimulates ovarian production of estrogen. In males, LH stimulates testosterone production from the testes, and FSH stimulates testicular growth. Gonadal steroids suppress the release of FSH along with inhibin, which is released from the ovary and testis.

- The parvocellular system regulates pituitary hormone release by neurovascular transmission.
- Release of CRH from the hypothalamus is influenced by stress, physical activity, illness, and the circadian cycle.
- Cushing syndrome occurs with prolonged exposure to inappropriately high levels of cortisol that result in excess levels of cortisol, corticotropin, or CRH.
- GH-RH is produced in arcuate (infundibular) neurons, and its release into the hypophyseal portal system triggers GH secretion from somatotropes in the anterior pituitary gland.
- Somatostatin, also known as growth hormone release–inhibiting hormone, is produced in the periventricular nucleus and inhibits the secretion of GH.
- Lactotrophic cells in the pituitary release prolactin in response to prolactin-releasing hormone, TRH, oxytocin, and several other peptides.
- Dopamine exerts an inhibitory effect on prolactin.

Clinical Correlations

Diabetes Insipidus

Diabetes insipidus can be central or nephrogenic. In central diabetes insipidus, damage to the pituitary gland or stalk (or both) may result in antidiuretic hormone deficiency. This deficiency may be due to trauma, surgery, pituitary apoplexy, or infiltration of the pituitary gland (through an infectious, inflammatory, or neoplastic process). Patients often present with polyuria, nocturia, and elevated levels of serum sodium.

Hyperprolactinemia

Prolactin levels may be elevated in pituitary microadenomas and macroadenomas; however, several other conditions may result in elevated prolactin. These include pregnancy, primary hypothyroidism, postictal states, stress, and kidney or liver disease. Dopamine inhibits prolactin; thus, another cause of hyperprolactinemia is the use of dopamine receptor antagonists (eg, metoclopramide, antipsychotics, and certain antidepressants).

Hypothalamic Hamartoma

Patients with hypothalamic hamartoma may present with behavioral issues (eg, rage) in addition to gelastic seizures and precocious puberty. The medial zone of the hypothalamus is important in regulating motivated behavior (eg, defensive behavior). Thus, lesions in this region may result in behavioral dyscontrol. Hypothalamic control of sex hormones may result in precocious puberty.

16 The Limbic System

KELLY D. FLEMMING, MD; EDUARDO E. BENARROCH, MD

Introduction

The limbic "lobe" is not a well-defined lobe like other areas of the cortex. The term *limbic system* is also a misnomer because the "system" involves several cortical and subcortical structures. The cortical areas include the insular cortex, the cingulate gyrus, the parahippocampal gyrus, and the hippocampus (Figure 16.1). The subcortical structures include the amygdala, the nucleus accumbens (ventral or "limbic" striatum), the septal nuclei, the dorsomedial and anterior nuclei of the thalamus, and the hypothalamus. Brainstem components include the periaqueductal gray matter and the monoaminergic nuclei (in particular, dopaminergic neurons of the ventral tegmental area).

The general functions of the limbic system include emotional responses, behavioral arousal, motivated behavior, memory, and learning. These functions are mediated by several reciprocal interconnections among cortical and subcortical structures. From a functional standpoint, the limbic system can be conceptualized as 2 interconnected circuits (Table 16.1 and Figure 16.2). The anterior limbic circuit, centered in the amygdala, includes the insular cortex, the anterior cingulate gyrus, the orbitofrontal cortex, the nucleus accumbens, the dorsomedial nucleus of the thalamus, and areas of the hypothalamus and brainstem that control neuroendocrine and autonomic functions. The anterior limbic circuit is involved in the initiation and elaboration of emotional responses to bodily sensation (integrated in the anterior insular cortex) and control of motivated behavior (involving the anterior cingulate gyrus and the nucleus accumbens). This circuit receives strong dopaminergic influences from the ventral tegmental area.

The posterior limbic circuit includes the hippocampal formation, the entorhinal cortex, the parahippocampal gyrus, the posterior cingulate, and the retrosplenial cortex. They are interconnected via the anterior nucleus of the thalamus, receive input from the mammillary bodies, and

are strongly influenced by the cholinergic neurons of the basal forebrain, including the septal nucleus and the nucleus basalis of Meynert. The posterior limbic circuit is involved in the encoding of episodic memory (learning of autobiographical events), visuospatial memory and navigation, and, through interconnections with the frontal lobe, memory retrieval.

- The anterior limbic circuit, centered in the amygdala, is involved in the initiation and elaboration of emotional responses to bodily sensation and control of motivated behavior.
- The posterior limbic circuit, which includes the hippocampal formation, the entorhinal cortex, the parahippocampal gyrus, the posterior cingulate, and the retrosplenial cortex, is involved in the encoding of episodic memory.

Anterior Limbic Circuit

Functional Anatomy

The amygdala lies just rostral to the hippocampus, near the temporal horn of the lateral ventricle. The amygdala includes several nuclei that can be grouped into 3 functional units: 1) the basolateral amygdala (basal and lateral amygdala nuclei); 2) the corticomedial, or extended, amygdala (medial and central amygdala nuclei, the nucleus of the stria terminalis, and the adjacent basal forebrain); and 3) the olfactory amygdala. The basolateral amygdala receives information from all sensory modalities directly via the thalamus and via the cortical association areas that process visual, auditory, somatosensory, and interoceptive (pain and visceral sensation) information, including the temporal pole and insular cortex, involved in visual perception (anterior temporal lobe). The basolateral amygdala is the site of convergence of a neutral sensory stimulus (such as a sound) and an emotionally significant stimulus (such as pain); each sensory stimulus is thereby labeled with an emotional significance (Figure 16.3). The basolateral amygdala projects to the corticomedial amygdala, particularly the central nucleus, which initiates behavioral responses associated with emotion.

Several structures are important in the anterior limbic circuit and in the emotional response to sensory stimuli (Table 16.2). For example, the central nucleus projects to the hypothalamus (endocrine responses), the periaqueductal gray (pain modulation), and the brainstem nuclei involved in motor (eg, startle) and autonomic (sympathetic and parasympathetic) control. Amygdala projections to the anterior cingulate cortex, the nucleus accumbens, and the basal forebrain, either directly or via the dorsomedial nucleus, provide emotional information for behavioral arousal and motivated motor behavior. Efferent pathways from the amygdala include the stria terminalis, the ventral amygdalofugal pathway, and the stria medullaris. The activity of the amygdala is modulated by inhibitory projections from the orbitomedial prefrontal cortex, which functionally "disconnect" the basolateral amygdala from the central amygdala.

Function

The amygdala has the critical roles of providing emotional significance to sensory stimuli and initiating emotional behavior. It is involved in associative learning leading to classical conditioned responses. For humans, the most potent stimulus for activating the amygdala is seeing faces expressing fear or anger. This indicates that the amygdala is critical for social recognition and behavior. The olfactory amygdala relays olfactory inputs that may evoke emotional responses.

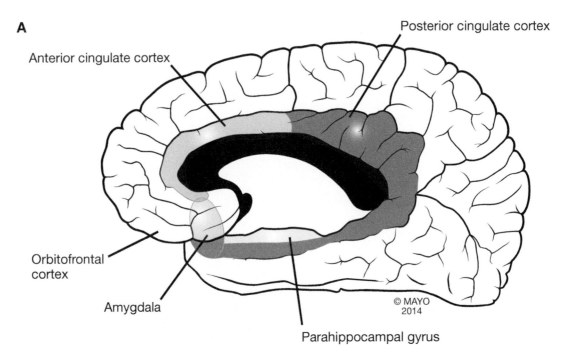

Figure 16.1 Anatomical Structures of the Limbic System.

A, Telencephalic components of the anterior (salmon) and posterior (red and yellow) limbic circuits. The anterior limbic circuit is centered in the amygdala (green) and includes the orbitofrontal and anterior cingulate cortices. These structures are interconnected with each other and the limbic striatum either directly or through the mediodorsal and midline thalamic nuclei. The posterior limbic circuit is centered in the hippocampus and includes the entorhinal cortex, the parahippocampal gyrus, and the posterior cingulate cortex. These structures are interconnected either directly or through the fornix, with a relay in the mammillary bodies and the anterior thalamic nucleus. B and C, Coronal sections through the cerebral hemispheres show the amygdala and hippocampus.

(A, Adapted from Benarroch EE, Daube JR, Flemming KD, Westmoreland BF. Mayo Clinic medical neurosciences: organized by neurologic systems and levels. 5th ed. Rochester [MN]: Mayo Clinic Scientific Press and Florence [KY]: Informa Healthcare USA; c2008. Chapter 16 Part B, The supratentorial level: telencephalon; p. 701–63. Used with permission of Mayo Foundation for Medical Education and Research. B and C, Adapted from Benarroch EE, Daube JR, Flemming KD, Westmoreland BF. Mayo Clinic medical neurosciences: organized by neurologic systems and levels. 5th ed. Rochester [MN]: Mayo Clinic Scientific Press and Florence [KY]: Informa Healthcare USA; c2008. Chapter 3, Diagnosis of Neurologic Disorders: anatomical localization; p. 53–100. Used with permission of Mayo Foundation for Medical Education and Research.)

B

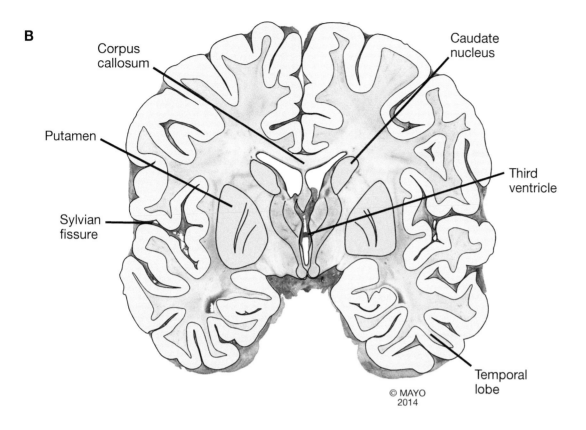

C

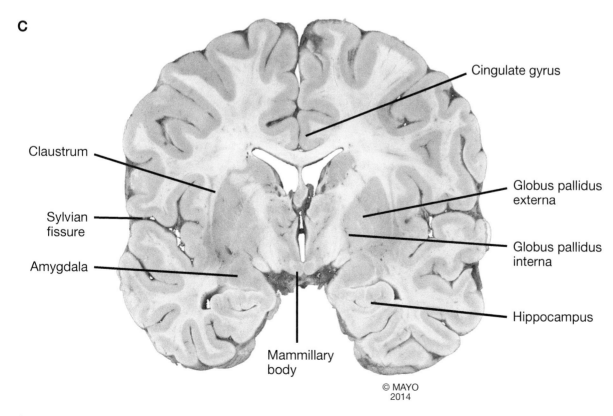

Figure 16.1 Continued.

Table 16.1 • Comparison of the Anterior and Posterior Limbic Circuits

Feature	Anterior Limbic Circuit	Posterior Limbic Circuit
Primary structure	Amygdala	Hippocampal formation
Components	Basolateral nuclear complex Corticomedial complex Olfactory amygdala	Entorhinal cortex Dentate gyrus Hippocampus proper (CA1-4 regions) Subiculum
Sensory input	Unimodal—either highly processed from cortical association areas or via direct input from the thalamus	Multimodal—from the posterior parietal (the "where" or dorsal pathway) or lateral temporal (the "what" or ventral pathway) cortex
Main receptive component	Lateral nucleus	Entorhinal cortex
Output component	Central nucleus (to hypothalamus and brainstem areas) Basal nucleus (to cortex, basal forebrain, and nucleus accumbens)	Subiculum
Subcortical efferent pathway	Stria terminalis Ventral amygdalofugal pathway	Fornix
Thalamic relay nucleus	Dorsomedial	Anterior
Cortical target	Orbitomedial prefrontal cortex Anterior cingulate cortex Insular cortex	Parahippocampal cortex Retrosplenial cortex Posterior cingulate cortex
Hypothalamic target nuclei	Preoptic Ventromedial Paraventricular Lateral hypothalamic area	Mammillary nuclei
Brainstem connections	Autonomic nuclei Periaqueductal gray Pontine reticular formation	Midbrain tegmentum
Cholinergic input from the basal forebrain	Nucleus basalis	Medial septum
Functions	Emotional behavior and emotional memory Fear	Learning and transient storage of information about facts and events
Involvement in disease	Complex partial seizures Limbic encephalitis Behavioral variant frontotemporal dementia Psychiatric disorders	Complex partial seizures Limbic encephalitis Alzheimer disease Hypoxic-ischemic encephalopathy Wernicke-Korsakoff syndrome

- The amygdala includes several nuclei that can be grouped into 3 functional units: the basolateral amygdala, the corticomedial (or extended) amygdala, and the olfactory amygdala.
- The amygdala has the critical roles of providing emotional significance to sensory stimuli and initiating emotional behavior.
- The amygdala is critical for social recognition and behavior.

Posterior Limbic Circuit

Anatomy

The hippocampal circuit includes the hippocampal formation (the dentate gyrus, the CA1-CA3 areas, and the subiculum), the entorhinal cortex, the parahippocampal cortex (including the perirhinal and posterior parahippocampal cortices), and the retrosplenial and posterior cingulate cortices.

Inputs

The hippocampal formation receives highly elaborated information from cortical association areas via the entorhinal cortex. The entorhinal cortex serves as the gateway for neocortical information reaching the hippocampus and receives input from 2 sources: 1) the perirhinal cortex, which relays information from the ventral visual lateral temporal pathway (and other sensory pathways) involved in object recognition, and 2) the posterior parahippocampal cortex, which relays information from the dorsal visual posterior parietal pathway (and other sensory pathways)

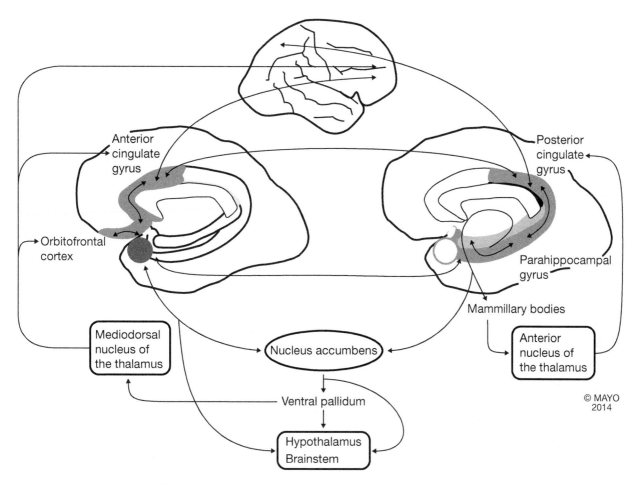

Figure 16.2 Circuits of the Limbic System.
The limbic system can be divided schematically into 2 highly interconnected circuits. The anterior limbic circuit, centered in the amygdala, is primarily involved in emotion and behavioral drive; the posterior circuit, centered in the hippocampus, is critical for declarative (explicit) memory, including autobiographical (episodic) memory, visuospatial memory, and factual (semantic) memory.

(Adapted from Benarroch EE. Basic neurosciences with clinical applications. Philadelphia [PA]: Butterworth Heinemann/Elsevier; c2006. Chapter 24, Limbic system: emotion and memory; p. 867–912. Used by permission of Mayo Foundation for Medical Education and Research.)

involved in visuospatial processing (eg, object location in space).

Intrinsic Connectivity

The entorhinal cortex conveys information to the hippocampal formation via the perforant pathway (Figure 16.4). The main termination of this pathway is in the dentate gyrus, which contains granule cells that project to the CA3 area via the mossy fiber system; pyramidal cells of the CA3 areas project to the CA1 area via the Schaffer collaterals, and CA1 neurons project to the subiculum, which provides the main output to the hippocampus. In addition to this classic trisynaptic pathway, there are direct parallel projections from the entorhinal cortex to the CA3 and CA1 areas, abundant interconnections between CA3 neurons in

different hippocampal regions, and direct output projections from CA1 neurons. All these connections are glutamatergic (excitatory) and thus provide for abundant positive feedback and feedforward circuits. This is necessary for encoding and storing information about a particular event or location (episodic memory) but also makes the hippocampus particularly susceptible to the generation of seizures and vulnerable to excitotoxicity (eg, in hypoxia).

Output

There are 2 major outputs of the hippocampal formation. One is the reciprocal connections via the subiculum to the entorhinal cortex; from there they go to the perirhinal, posterior parahippocampal, retrosplenial, and posterior cingulate cortices. A second major output is via the fornix, which

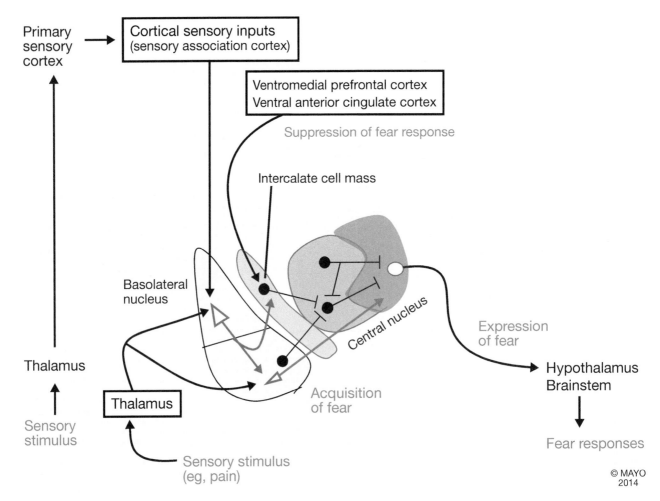

Figure 16.3 Main Connections and Functions of the Amygdala.
(Used with permission of Mayo Foundation for Medical Education and Research.)

Table 16.2 • Structures Associated With the Limbic System

Structure	Location	Function
Septal region	Anterior to the lamina terminalis	Behavior
Ventral tegmental area	Dopaminergic neurons in the ventral midbrain	Encode reward
Habenula	Near the caudal thalamus-pineal region	Projections to the midbrain sites involved in reward, arousal, and pain
Nucleus accumbens	Ventralmost aspect of the caudate and putamen convergence	Reward behavior
Basal forebrain	Rostral and ventral to the striatum	Arousal and attention toward motivated response
Raphe	Serotonergic neurons in the medial reticular formation of the brainstem	Arousal and attention
Anterior cingulate cortex	Medial cortex above the corpus callosum	Monitor behavioral drive
Anterior insula	Insular cortex	Body and emotional awareness
Orbitofrontal cortex	Frontal cortex rostral to the orbits	Decision making
Substantia innominata	Part of the basal forebrain	Encode information used in altering attention to stimuli

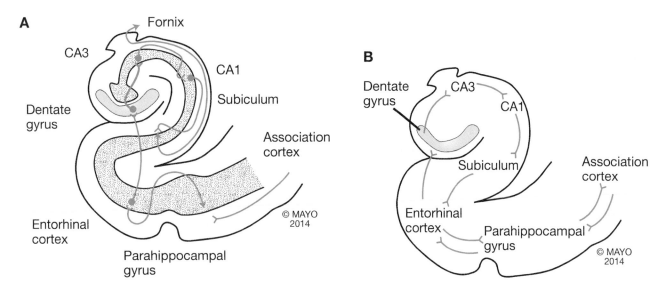

Figure 16.4 Medial Temporal Memory System.
The medial temporal memory system includes the hippocampal formation, the entorhinal cortex, and the parahippocampal region. A, Association areas of the neocortex project to the parahippocampal cortex, which projects to the entorhinal cortex. The entorhinal cortex is the gateway for entry of highly elaborated information into the hippocampus. The hippocampal formation comprises the dentate gyrus, the hippocampus proper (CA1-CA3 regions), and the subiculum. The intrinsic circuit of the hippocampal formation involves feedforward excitatory connections. Granule cells of the dentate gyrus send excitatory axons (called mossy fibers) to CA3 pyramidal neurons. CA3 pyramidal cells project via Schaffer collaterals to CA1 pyramidal neurons, which project to the subiculum. B, The neocortex, the parahippocampal gyrus, and the hippocampal formation have reciprocal feedforward and feedback connections. Association areas of the neocortex project to the perirhinal and parahippocampal cortices. These, in turn, project to the entorhinal cortex. Neurons of the CA1 region and the subiculum project back to the entorhinal cortex, which relays this input to the parahippocampal cortex, which projects to the neocortex.
(Adapted from Benarroch EE, Daube JR, Flemming KD, Westmoreland BF. Mayo Clinic medical neurosciences: organized by neurologic systems and levels. 5th ed. Rochester [MN]: Mayo Clinic Scientific Press and Florence [KY]: Informa Healthcare USA; c2008. Chapter 16 Part B, The supratentorial level: telencephalon; p. 701–63. Used with permission of Mayo Foundation for Medical Education and Research.)

includes 2 components: 1) precommissural (anterior to the anterior commissure), which contains axons from CA1 pyramidal neurons and projects to the septal area and medial prefrontal cortex, and 2) postcommissural, which contains axons from the subiculum and projects to the anterior nucleus of the thalamus. The anterior nucleus of the thalamus is a critical component of the hippocampal circuit for episodic and visuospatial memory via its connectivity to the subicular cortex, the retrosplenial cortex, and the mammillary bodies. The classic Papez circuit connects the hippocampal formation (via the fornix) to the mammillary bodies, the mammillary bodies to the anterior nucleus of the thalamus (mammillothalamic tract), and the anterior thalamic nucleus back to the parahippocampal cortex (and then to the entorhinal and hippocampal cortices) (Figure 16.5).

Function

The posterior limbic pathway is critical for learning (acquiring information), storage, and retrieval (declarative memory). Declarative memory includes episodic memory

(memory of autobiographic events), visuospatial memory (memory of places and locations), and semantic memory (memory of general facts and knowledge).

Additional information about the posterior limbic circuit is provided in Chapter 22, "Cortical Circuitry, Networks, and Function."

- The entorhinal cortex serves as the gateway for neocortical information reaching the hippocampus.
- The entorhinal cortex receives input from sensory integrative pathways for object recognition and visuospatial processing.
- The entorhinal cortex conveys information to the hippocampal formation via the perforant pathway.
- There are 2 major outputs of the hippocampus: 1) to the anterior nucleus of the thalamus via the fornix and 2) to the posterior cingulate gyrus via the subiculum and entorhinal cortex.
- The posterior limbic pathway is critical for learning (acquiring information), storage, and retrieval (declarative memory).

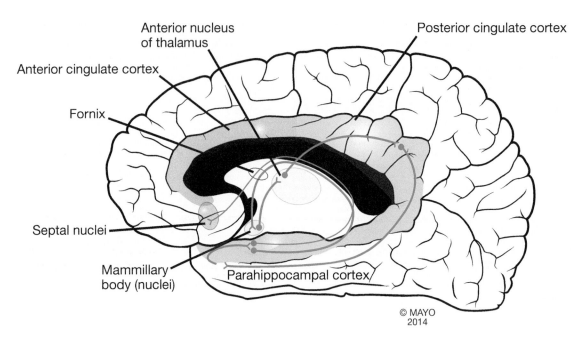

Figure 16.5 The Papez Circuit.
The hippocampal formation projects to subcortical structures through the fornix, whose axons are from pyramidal neurons of the CA1 area, particularly the subiculum. The fornix loops over the thalamus and, at the anterior commissure, divides into the precommissural fornix, containing axons from the CA1 area and terminating in the lateral septal nucleus, and the larger postcommissural fornix, containing axons from the subiculum and terminating in the mammillary body (nuclei). The mammillary body projects to the anterior nucleus of the thalamus, which conveys information to the cingulate cortex. The cingulate cortex projects back to the parahippocampal gyrus and the entorhinal cortex, and these regions project to the hippocampal formation. These cortical-diencephalic-cortical connections form the Papez circuit.
(Adapted from Benarroch EE, Daube JR, Flemming KD, Westmoreland BF. Mayo Clinic medical neurosciences: organized by neurologic systems and levels. 5th ed. Rochester [MN]: Mayo Clinic Scientific Press and Florence [KY]: Informa Healthcare USA; c2008. Chapter 16 Part B, The supratentorial level: telencephalon; p. 701–63. Used with permission of Mayo Foundation for Medical Education and Research.)

Clinical Correlations

Behavioral Variant Frontotemporal Dementia

The anterior insular and anterior cingulate cortices, which are highly interconnected components of the "salience network" and are components of the anterior limbic circuit connected with the amygdala, contain a particular type of pyramidal neuron, called a von Economo neuron, which is particularly susceptible to neurodegeneration in patients with behavioral variant frontotemporal dementia. The main manifestations are those of emotional blunting, behavioral disinhibition, lack of empathy, and other manifestations of disrupted control of emotional and social behavior.

Klüver-Bucy Syndrome

Bilateral damage to the temporal lobes affecting the amygdala may result in Klüver-Bucy syndrome, which is characterized by poor short-term memory, hypersexuality, hyperphagia, and docile behavior. This is best characterized in experimental animals, but some components can be observed in patients with behavioral variant frontotemporal dementia.

Amnesia

Deficits in recent memory (an amnestic syndrome) may occur with lesions anywhere along the posterior limbic circuit. In Wernicke-Korsakoff syndrome, due to thiamine deficiency, pathologic abnormalities are found in the mamillary bodies, dorsomedial thalamus, and ocular and vestibular nuclei, and Purkinje cell loss occurs in the cerebellum.

Pathologic Susceptibility of the Hippocampus

Various insults may affect the hippocampus, but they often do so differently. Mesial temporal sclerosis, often associated with seizures, involves the medial region of the temporal lobe and hippocampus and frequently affects the dentate gyrus. Hypoxia often occurs in patients with cardiac arrest, which preferentially affects the CA1 area of the Ammon horn. When Alzheimer disease begins, the entorhinal cortex is one of the first places affected. Hyperactivity of the hippocampus has been noted in several psychiatric disorders through functional magnetic resonance imaging studies. The CA1 region is hyperactive in schizophrenic patients, whereas the dentate and CA3 regions are hyperactive in patients with posttraumatic stress disorder.

Alzheimer Disease

Alzheimer disease is the prototypical neurodegenerative disorder affecting the posterior hippocampal circuit. Hyperphosphorylated tau pathology (neurofibrillary tangles), which is the hallmark of neuronal degeneration, occurs first in the perirhinal and entorhinal cortices and then involves the hippocampus proper, the parahippocampal gyrus, and the perirhinal and posterior cingulate cortices. These areas are the components of the posterior default network, as defined with functional neuroimaging. (See Chapter 22, "Cortical Circuitry, Networks, and Function.")

- Klüver-Bucy syndrome, due to bilateral temporal damage including the amydgala, results in poor short-term memory, hypersexuality, hyperphagia, and docile behavior.
- Deficits in recent memory (an amnestic syndrome) may occur with lesions anywhere along the posterior limbic circuit.
- Hypoxia often occurs in patients with cardiac arrest, which preferentially affects the CA1 area of the Ammon horn.

17 Basal Ganglia

JONATHAN GRAFF-RADFORD, MD; ALEX J. NELSON, MD;
EDUARDO E. BENARROCH, MD

Introduction

The basal ganglia are a group of nuclei connected by circuits that help select appropriate actions and other behaviors. They promote the sequential activation of movements or behaviors in response to stimuli. These movements become reinforced over time, eventually becoming habits. The key components of the basal ganglia include the striatum (putamen, caudate nucleus, and nucleus accumbens), globus pallidus (GP), subthalamic nucleus (STN), substantia nigra, pedunculopontine nucleus (PPN), and parts of the thalamus and cortex. The basal ganglia are critical components of parallel circuits that also involve the cortex and thalamus. They include the motor, oculomotor, associative, and limbic circuits. The anatomy and circuitry of the basal ganglia are reviewed in this chapter. Clinical movement disorders are covered in Volume 2, Section IV, "Movement Disorders."

- Basal ganglia promote the sequential activation of movements or behaviors in response to stimuli.

Anatomy

Gross Anatomy and Organization

The basal ganglia include the striatum, derived from the telencephalon, and the GP, derived from the diencephalon. The striatum includes the putamen and caudate nucleus (referred to as the dorsal striatum or neostriatum) and the nucleus accumbens (also referred to as the central or limbic striatum). The GP includes external (GPe) and internal (GPi) segments. Together, the putamen and the GP form a macroscopic structure referred to as the lenticular nucleus, which is a misnomer. Integral components of the basal ganglia circuits are the substantia nigra, including the pars reticulata (SNr) and pars compacta (SNc); the STN; and the PPN (Figure 17.1 and Table 17.1).

Vascular Supply to the Basal Ganglia

The majority of the basal ganglia is supplied by the middle cerebral artery. The lateral lenticulostriate arteries from the M1 segment supply the putamen and GP. The GP may also be served by the anterior choroidal artery (branch of the internal carotid artery). The inferior portion of the head of the caudate is supplied by the recurrent artery of Heubner, which is a branch from the A1 or A2 segment of the anterior cerebral artery. The superior (rostral) portion of the head is supplied by the lenticulostriate arteries. The tail of the caudate is supplied by the anterior choroidal artery.

- The majority of the basal ganglia is supplied by the middle cerebral artery.
- The inferior portion of the head of the caudate is supplied by the recurrent artery of Heubner, which is a branch from the A1 or A2 segment of the anterior cerebral artery.

Circuitry

Striatum

The majority of the neurons in the striatum are medium spiny GABAergic projection neurons. These neurons

---

Abbreviations: GP, globus pallidus; GPe, globus pallidus external; GPi, globus pallidus internal; PD, Parkinson disease; PPN, pedunculopontine nucleus; SNc, substantia nigra pars compacta; SNr, substantia nigra pars reticulata; STN, subthalamic nucleus; VTA, ventral tegmental area

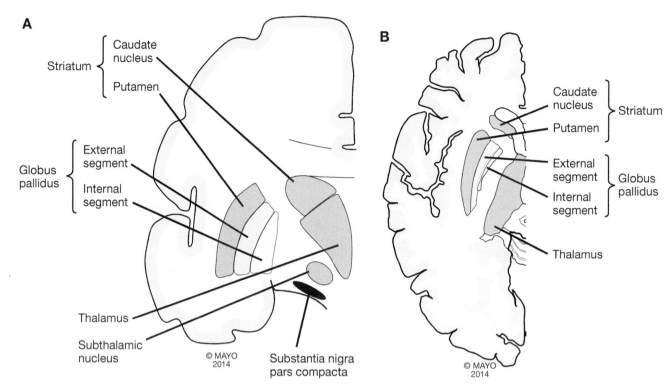

Figure 17.1 *Main Nuclei and Connections of the Basal Ganglia Circuit.*
The basal ganglia include the striatum (putamen, caudate nucleus, and nucleus accumbens [not shown]), globus pallidus (including external and internal segments), subthalamic nucleus, and substantia nigra (including pars reticulata [not shown] and pars compacta). A, Coronal section. B, Horizontal section.
(Adapted from Benarroch EE, Daube JR, Flemming KD, Westmoreland BF. Mayo Clinic medical neurosciences: organized by neurologic systems and levels. 5th ed. Rochester [MN]: Mayo Clinic Scientific Press and Florence [KY]: Informa Healthcare USA; c2008. Chapter 8, The motor system; p. 265–330. Used with permission of Mayo Foundation for Medical Education and Research.)

Table 17.1 • Interconnections of the Substantia Nigra

Component	Afferent Input	Efferent Output
Substantia nigra pars compacta (SNc)	Striatum Prefrontal cortex SNr PPN	Striatum (nigrostriatal) Globus pallidus (nigropallidal) Subthalamic nucleus PPN SNr
Substantia nigra pars reticulata (SNr)	Striatum (predominantly matrix) Subthalamic nucleus SNc	Neostriatum (nigrostriatal) Superior colliculus (nigrotectal) SNc Subthalamic nucleus Thalamus (VA, DM, VL)

Abbreviations: DM, dorsomedial; PPN, pedunculopontine nucleus; VA, ventral anterior; VL, ventrolateral.

receive glutamatergic inputs from 2 sources, the frontal lobe (including the motor, premotor, prefrontal, and anterior cingulate cortices) and the intralaminar thalamic nuclei. The majority of the medium spiny neurons occupy the "matrix" compartment of the striatum and include 2 separate populations, 1 projecting to the GPi and SNr (hereafter referred to as GPi/SNr) and the other projecting to the GPe. The striatum also contains small compartments called patches or striosomes, which contain medium spiny neurons that project to the SNc. In addition to medium spiny neurons, the striatum contains local GABAergic neurons and a population of cholinergic interneurons.

Globus Pallidus

The GPi and the SNr are the output nuclei of the basal ganglia and provide a tonic GABAergic inhibition of motor pattern generators in the motor cortex (via the ventral anterior and ventral oralis nuclei of the thalamus), the PPN (locomotor pattern generator), and the superior colliculus (saccadic pattern generator). The tonic inhibitory output of the GPi/SNr is promoted by glutamatergic inputs from the STN and inhibited by GABAergic input from the striatum. The GPe is a critical component of the intrinsic circuit of the basal ganglia. It receives inhibitory inputs from the medium spiny neurons of the striatum and excitatory input from the STN; the GPe has an inhibitory influence on the GPi/SNr, both directly and via inhibition of the STN. The

GPe also sends reciprocal inhibitory inputs to GABAergic interneurons of the striatum.

Subthalamic Nucleus

The STN receives direct excitatory inputs from the cerebral cortex and inhibitory inputs from the GPe; the STN increases activity of the GPi/SNr and the GPe (Figure 17.2). The reciprocal interactions between the STN and the GPe provide the potential for oscillatory network activity in the basal ganglia circuits and their target, via the effects on the GPi/SNr and their influence on the thalamus, and therefore, on the motor cortex.

Pedunculopontine Nucleus

The PPN receives direct inputs from the motor cortex and inhibitory inputs from the GPi. The PPN contains glutamatergic, GABAergic, and cholinergic neurons that project to the medullary and spinal cord locomotor pattern generators, to the basal ganglia (particularly the STN), and to the thalamus (particularly the intralaminar nuclei). In addition to its role as a locomotor pattern generator, the PPN promotes thalamocortical arousal.

Substantia Nigra Pars Compacta

The SNc and the adjacent ventral tegmental area (VTA) provide dopaminergic input to the basal ganglia circuits. The ventral portion of the SNc innervates the putamen, the dorsal portion of the SNc innervates the caudate, and the VTA innervates the nucleus accumbens and the medial prefrontal and anterior cingulate cortex, amygdala, and hippocampus. Neurons of the SNc and VTA have a low level of tonic activity at rest and show a burst of discharge

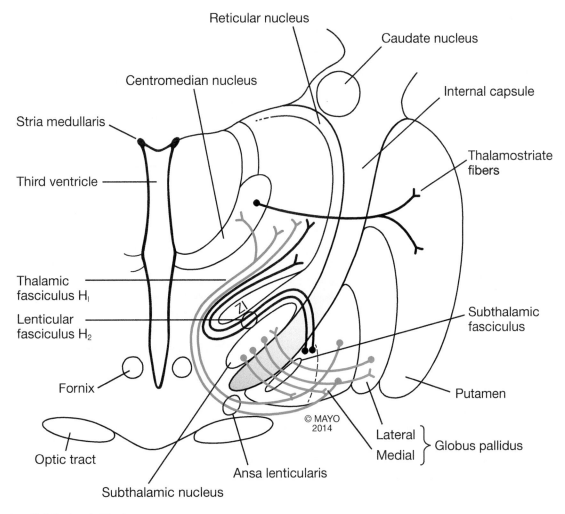

Figure 17.2 Subthalamic Nucleus.
The subthalamic nucleus receives input from the cerebral cortex and the globus pallidus externa. It projects back to the globus pallidus and to the substantia nigra pars reticulata. Neurons that project to and from the globus pallidi to the subthalamic nucleus do so in the subthalamic fasciculus. H_1 and H_2 indicate fields H_1 and H_2, respectively, in the fields of Forel. ZI, zona incerta.
(Used with permission of Mayo Foundation for Medical Education and Research.)

in response to unanticipated rewards or behaviorally salient stimuli.

- The majority of the neurons in the striatum are medium spiny GABAergic projection neurons.
- The GPi and the SNr are the output nuclei of the basal ganglia and provide a tonic GABAergic inhibition of motor pattern generators.
- The PPN is a locomotor pattern generator and promotes thalamocortical arousal.
- The SNc provides dopaminergic input to the basal ganglia.

Physiology

Parallel Basal Ganglia Circuits

The basal ganglia form part of the parallel frontal lobe-striatal-pallido-thalamocortical loops or circuit (Table 17.2). The motor circuit involves inputs from the sensorimotor cortex to the putamen, which projects to the ventrolateral GPi and GPe and the dorsolateral STN. The circuit is closed by inhibitory projections from the GPi to the ventral oralis nucleus, which in turn projects to the supplementary motor area. The motor circuit is involved in the selection of motor programs, is modulated by dopaminergic inputs from the ventral SNc, and is selectively vulnerable in disorders associated with parkinsonism. The associative circuit involves the prefrontal cortex, the

caudate nucleus, and specific portions of the GPi/SNr, GPe, and STN; this circuit controls the activity of neurons of the ventral anterior and mediodorsal nucleus of the thalamus that project to the prefrontal cortex. The associative circuit receives dopaminergic inputs from the dorsal SNc, is involved in decision making and other executive functions, and is affected in conditions such as Huntington disease. The oculomotor circuit controls saccadic eye movements and involves the frontal eye fields, caudate nucleus, SNr, and superior colliculus. The limbic circuit involves the medial prefrontal and anterior cingulate cortices, the nucleus accumbens, and the dopaminergic neurons of the VTA; this circuit is involved in emotional processing and motivated behavior and is affected in disorders such as drug addiction.

Direct and Indirect Pathways

Glutamatergic inputs from the cerebral cortex to the striatum (corticostriate input) activate 2 different subpopulations of medium spiny neurons in the striatum, 1 projecting to the GPi/SNr and the other projecting to the GPe (Figure 17.3). The activity of these medium spiny neurons depends on their transition from a "down" state, when they are silent, to an "up" state, when they fire a burst of action potentials in response to corticostriate inputs. These 2 populations of medium spiny neurons mediate a direct pathway and an indirect pathway that have opposing influence on the inhibitory output of the basal ganglia,

---

Table 17.2 • Basal Ganglia Control on Targets

Pathway	Direct	Indirect
Cortical input	Less strong	Stronger
Intralaminar thalamic input	Strong	Less strong
Medium spiny neuron involved	GABA, substance P, dynorphin	GABA, enkephalin
Receptor expression	Dopamine D_1 more than D_2	Dopamine D_2 more than D_1 Adenosine A_{2A}
Target	GPi or SNr	GPe
Effect on STN	None	Disinhibition
Effect on the tonic output of GPi/SNr	Phasic inhibition	Phasic facilitation
Effect on motor output	Phasic facilitation of a selected motor program	Phasic inhibition of competing motor programs
Main effect of dopamine	Facilitatory	Inhibitory
Main effect of acetylcholine	Inhibitory	Facilitatory
Pathologic involvement	Less affected than the indirect pathway in PD May mediate levodopa-induced dyskinesia May be primarily involved in dystonia	More susceptible in PD (presumably because of excessive compensatory cortical input and lack of dopamine D_2 receptor effect preventing calcium accumulation in dendritic spines) Earlier involvement in Huntington disease

Abbreviations: GABA, γ-aminobutyric acid; GPe, globus pallidus externa; GPi, globus pallidus interna; PD, Parkinson disease; SNr, substantia nigra pars reticulata; STN, subthalamic nucleus.

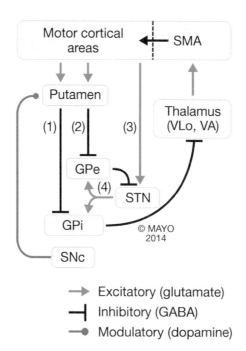

Figure 17.3 *Connectivity of the Basal Ganglia as Exemplified in the Motor Circuit of the Basal Ganglia.*
The cerebral cortex provides input to the striatum and subthalamic nucleus (STN). The putamen is a component of the striatum. Neurons of the striatum contain γ-aminobutyric acid (GABA) and project to both the external (GPe) and internal (GPi) segments of the globus pallidus and substantia nigra (projection not shown). The GPi (and the substantia nigra pars reticulata, which is not shown) contains GABAergic neurons that tonically inhibit basal ganglia targets, including the ventral oralis (VLo) nucleus, which projects to the supplementary motor area (SMA), and the ventral anterior (VA) nucleus, which projects to the prefrontal cortex. These thalamic nuclei control initiation of motor programs. The GPi also sends an inhibitory projection to the pedunculopontine tegmental nucleus (not shown), which controls muscle tone and locomotion. The STN sends an excitatory projection to both the GPe and the GPi. The STN receives direct excitatory input from the cerebral cortex and reciprocal inhibitory input from the GPe. The substantia nigra pars compacta (SNc) sends dopaminergic axons to all components of these circuits, particularly the striatum. These basal ganglia connections are organized into 3 intrinsic pathways: direct corticostriatopallidal pathway to the GPi (1), indirect corticostriatopallidal (GPe) STN pathway (2), and hyperdirect corticosubthalamic pathway (3). The direct pathway inhibits the GPi, whereas the indirect and hyperdirect pathways, via the STN, increase the activity in the GPi. Reciprocal connections between the GPe and the STN (4) sustain oscillatory activity in the basal ganglia circuits.

(Adapted from Benarroch EE, Daube JR, Flemming KD, Westmoreland BF. Mayo Clinic medical neurosciences: organized by neurologic systems and levels. 5th ed. Rochester [MN]: Mayo Clinic Scientific Press and Florence [KY]: Informa Healthcare USA; c2008. Chapter 8, The motor system; p. 265–330. Used with permission of Mayo Foundation for Medical Education and Research.)

mediated by the GPi/SNr, which exert a tonic inhibitory influence on the initiation of motor programs ("no-go" signal) (Table 17.3). The direct pathway involves medium spiny neurons that express dopamine D_1 receptors and send a direct GABAergic projection to the GPi/STN; this pathway transiently inhibits the GPi/SNr, disinhibiting their targets and promoting initiation of a selected motor program ("go" signal). The indirect pathway involves medium spiny neurons that express dopamine D_2 receptors and send an inhibitory projection to the GPe; this interrupts its inhibitory influence on the GPi/SNr directly and through inhibition of the STN. Thus, this indirect pathway prevents initiation of unselected motor programs by promoting the "stop" signal from the basal ganglia. Dopamine,

via D_1 and D_2 receptors, exerts opposite effects on medium spiny neurons of the direct and indirect pathways; D_1 receptors are excitatory and promote the "on" state on medium spiny neurons of the direct pathway; D_2 receptors are inhibitory and maintain the "off" state of medium spiny neurons of the indirect pathway. By these mechanisms, dopamine promotes the initiation and prevents excessive inhibition of selected motor programs.

Hyperdirect Pathway

In addition to the direct and indirect pathways via the striatum, a hyperdirect pathway involves direct projection inputs from the cortex to the STN. This pathway may

Table 17.3 • Parallel Pathways in Basal Ganglia Circuitry

Feature	Motor Circuit	Oculomotor Circuit	Behavior Circuits		Limbic Circuit
Level	Motor	Oculomotor	Dorsolateral prefrontal	Orbitofrontal	Medial frontal
Striatal	Putamen	Caudate (body)	Dorsal caudate (head)	Ventral caudate	Nucleus accumbens
Output	GPi SNr	SNr	GPi	GPi	Ventral pallidum
Thalamic	VL VA, CM	VA, DM	VA, DM	VA, DM	DM
Target	Motor cortex SMA PPN	Frontal eye fields Superior colliculus	Dorsolateral prefrontal cortex	Orbitofrontal cortex	Cingulate limbic
Function	Motor planning and execution; somatomotor control	Fast saccades; orientation and gaze	Executive behavior	Social behavior	Motivation

Abbreviations: CM, centromedian nucleus; DM, dorsomedial; GPi, globus pallidus interna; PPN, pedunculopontine nucleus; SMA, supplementary motor area; SNr, substantia nigra pars reticulata; VA, ventral anterior nucleus; VL, ventral lateral nucleus.

provide a "stop" signal for unselected motor programs via the excitatory input of the STN to the GPi/SNr. It may also engage the STN in burst activity that triggers abnormal synchronized oscillations in the basal ganglia–thalamocortical circuits. This activity depends on the reciprocal interactions of the STN with the GPe and GPi in the presence of an abnormal pattern of GPe activity, as may occur with dopamine deficiency.

Thalamostriate Circuit

The intralaminar thalamic nuclei (centromedian and parafascicular) provide the second glutamatergic input to the striatum. This thalamostriate input is activated in the presence of behavioral arousal ("attention" signal) and triggers activity in local cholinergic neurons, which provide a "stop" signal that interrupts ongoing motor behavior and allows new action selection.

- Glutamatergic inputs from the cerebral cortex to the striatum (corticostriate input) activate 2 different subpopulations of medium spiny neurons in the striatum, 1 projecting to the GPi/SNr and the other projecting to the GPe (Figure 17.3).

Clinical Correlations

Parkinson Disease

Parkinson disease (PD) results from the loss of dopaminergic neurons of the SNc and affects first the ventrolateral portion of the SNc targeting the putamen. Studies in experimental models provide the basis for the influential hypothesis that impaired dopamine D_1 and D_2 receptor signaling creates an imbalance between the direct and indirect output pathways of the striatum, with hypoactivity of

the D_1 receptor–activated direct pathway and hyperactivity of the D_2 receptor–inhibited indirect pathway, resulting in the motor manifestations of PD, particularly hypokinesia and bradykinesia due to relatively excessive activity of the STN-GPi/SNr circuit. Dopamine depletion also promotes abnormal entrainment of cortical and thalamic oscillations via the STN-GPe-GPi circuit, resulting in correlated, coherent, and rhythmic activity at beta and tremor frequencies both within and between the basal ganglia circuits and their targets. By disrupting this abnormal activity, high-frequency deep brain stimulation of the GPi or STN improves the levodopa-responsive manifestations of PD. Changes in synaptic plasticity at the corticostriate synapse may contribute to levodopa-induced dyskinesia. In PD, progressive loss of dopaminergic terminals leads to dysregulation of synaptic dopamine levels in response to individual doses of levodopa; this reflects the loss of regulation by the presynaptic dopamine transporter and D_2 inhibitory autoreceptors, as well as abnormal dopamine production and release from serotonergic terminals. Individual doses of levodopa elicit peak synaptic dopamine levels that trigger phasic activation of D_1 receptors, which promote long-term potentiation in corticostriate synapses on the direct pathway, mediated by glutamate acting via N-methyl-D-aspartate receptors. Amantadine, a weak N-methyl-D-aspartate–receptor antagonist, provides a sustained beneficial effect in reducing the severity of levodopa-induced dyskinesia.

Hyperkinetic Movement Disorders

Genetic and experimental studies indicate that primary dystonia reflects, either directly or indirectly, abnormal dopaminergic signaling in the striatum. The clearest indication is dopa-responsive dystonia linked to mutations that affect genes encoding proteins involved in dopamine biosynthesis. Dystonia is also elicited by D_2-receptor antagonists. The fact that reduced dopaminergic signaling in the striatum can lead to either parkinsonism or dystonia cannot be explained by the simple direct and indirect pathway model and indicates that many mechanisms may be involved, including age-dependent synaptic plasticity. This may explain why dystonia is more common in early-onset PD compared with late-onset PD.

Early selective loss of medium spiny neurons of the indirect pathway, leading to impaired GPi/SNr output, may explain the development of chorea in Huntington disease. Hemiballismus is a flailing type movement of the limbs. It generally occurs contralateral to a lesion of the STN. Reduced STN activity would remove its excitatory input to the GPi/SNr, resulting in the inability to suppress unwanted motor programs. The net result is increased movement.

- PD results from the loss of dopaminergic neurons of the SNc and affects first the ventrolateral portion of the SNc targeting the putamen.
- Hemiballismus, a flailing type movement of the limbs, is generally caused by a lesion of the STN.

18 Cerebellum

JONATHAN GRAFF-RADFORD, MD; ANHAR HASSAN, MB, BCH;
EDUARDO E. BENARROCH, MD

Introduction

The cerebellum is crucial for planning, executing, terminating, and learning movements. The cerebellum compares actual motor performance with intended motor performance; thus, it is important in the adaptation of movement and posture as well. In addition, the cerebellum contributes to cognition and behavior. The main functions of the cerebellum appear to be the timing of motor functions and other functions.

This chapter reviews the anatomy and circuitry of the cerebellum. Clinical disorders of ataxia are covered in Volume 2, Chapter 26, "Cerebellar Disorders and Ataxias."

Anatomy

The primary fissure divides the cerebellum anatomically into anterior and posterior lobes (Figure 18.1). The posterior lobe is divided from the flocculonodular lobe by the posterolateral fissure. The cerebellum may also be divided into functional zones, including the vermis (midline), paravermal region, and hemispheres (most lateral). In addition, the individual lobes may be subdivided into lobules.

The 4 deep nuclei of the cerebellum are the dentate, emboliform, globose, and fastigial nuclei. The globose and emboliform nuclei are sometimes also referred together as the interposed nuclei. Functionally, the vestibular nuclei act as deep nuclei of the cerebellum.

Three cerebellar peduncles carry information to and from the cerebellum. The middle cerebellar peduncle carries information *to* the cerebellum. The superior cerebellar peduncle carries information *from* the cerebellum. The inferior cerebellar peduncle carries both efferent and afferent information.

There are 2 motor maps in the vermis and paravermis of the cerebellum: 1 in the anterior lobe and the other in the posterior lobe. They have an inverted representation of the body (foot anterior, followed by upper limb and then face) and are mirror images of each other.

The blood supply to the cerebellum is from the posterior circulation (Figure 18.2). The posterior inferior cerebellar artery supplies the inferolateral surface of the cerebellum, including the nodulus and cerebellar tonsil. This artery also supplies the lateral medulla. The anterior inferior cerebellar artery supplies the inferior and ventral surface of the cerebellum as well as the ventral aspect of the dentate nucleus. The superior cerebellar artery supplies the superior hemispheres and vermis, the rostral aspect of the dentate nucleus, and the remaining deep nuclei. This artery also supplies some of the lateral pontine tegmentum.

- The primary fissure divides the cerebellum anatomically into anterior and posterior lobes.
- The 4 deep nuclei of the cerebellum are the dentate, emboliform, globose, and fastigial nuclei.
- Three cerebellar peduncles carry information to and from the cerebellum.
- The superior cerebellar artery supplies the superior hemispheres and vermis, the rostral aspect of the dentate nucleus, and the remaining deep nuclei.

Cerebellar Cytoarchitecture

Cerebellar Cortex

The cerebellar cortex consists of 3 layers: the molecular layer, the Purkinje cell layer, and the granular layer. The molecular layer is the most superficial layer and consists of Purkinje cell dendrites, parallel fibers of the granule cells, basket cells, and stellate interneurons (Figure 18.3). The Purkinje cell layer consists of Purkinje cells. The granular layer consists of granule cells and Golgi cells. The Purkinje cells are the main

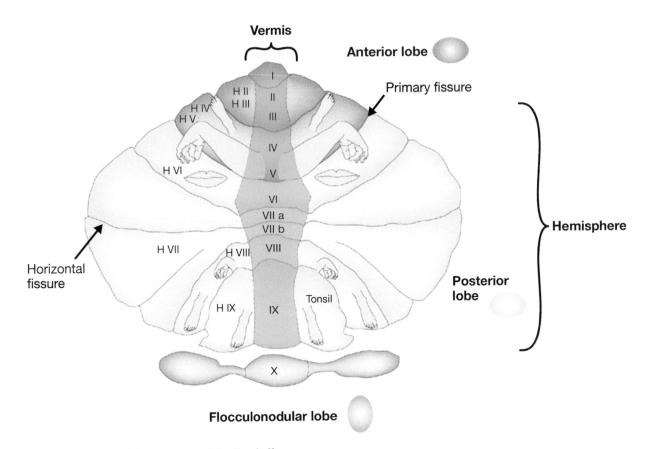

Figure 18.1 *Functional Somatotopy of the Cerebellum.*
This sketch shows representation of the arms, feet, and lips in the human cerebellum. Face representation is not indicated.
H *indicates a lobule of the hemisphere.*
(Adapted from Manni E, Petrosini L. A century of cerebellar somatotopy: a debated representation. Nat Rev Neurosci. 2004 Mar;5(3):241–9. Used with permission.)

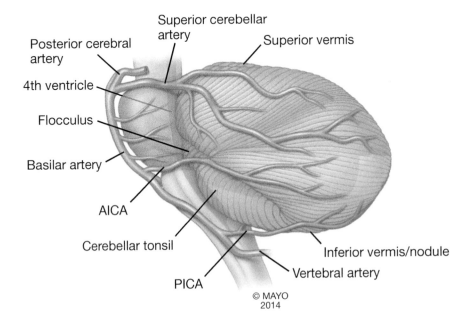

Figure 18.2 *Blood Supply of the Cerebellum.*
AICA indicates anterior inferior cerebellar artery; PICA, posterior inferior cerebellar artery.
(Used with permission of Mayo Foundation for Medical Education and Research.)

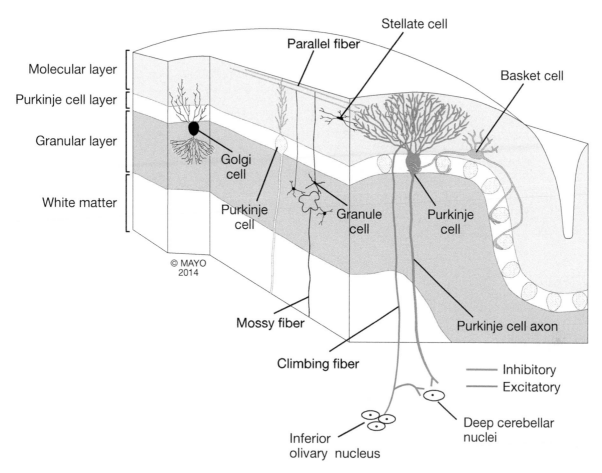

Figure 18.3 Cytoarchitecure of the Cerebellar Cortex.
Please see text for details regarding functional roles of these cell types.
(Adapted from Mowzoon N. The cerebellum and cerebellar disorders. In: Mowzoon N, Flemming KD, editors. Neurology board review: an illustrated study guide. Rochester [MN]: Mayo Clinic Scientific Press and Florence [KY]: Informa Healthcare USA; c2007. p. 377–99. Used with permission of Mayo Foundation for Medical Education and Research.)

output cells of the cerebellar cortex. All cell types in the cortex are GABAergic except the granule cells.

Cell Types

Purkinje Cells
Purkinje cells are the output cells of the cerebellar cortex and provide inhibitory input (γ-aminobutyric acid) to the deep nuclei, which provide output from the cerebellum. Purkinje cells are controlled by glutamatergic input from parallel fibers that synapse on multiple Purkinje cells, glutamatergic input from climbing fibers that synapse on a few Purkinje cells, and γ-aminobutyric acid inputs from basket and stellate cells.

Granule Cells
Granule cells, the only excitatory neurons in the cerebellar cortex, receive mossy fiber input and project to the molecular layer, where they become parallel fibers that synapse with Purkinje cell dendrites.

Golgi Cells
Golgi cells are excited by both mossy and climbing fibers. Golgi cells inhibit the granule cells.

Stellate and Basket Cells
Stellate and basket cells receive excitatory input from granule cells and provide lateral inhibition to Purkinje cells.

Afferent and Efferent Fibers

The 2 main inputs to the cerebellum are mossy fibers and climbing fibers; both are excitatory and use L-glutamate (Figure 18.4). Mossy fibers provide collaterals to the cerebellar nuclei and synapse on both granule cells and Golgi cells. Granule cells provide an ascending axon that bifurcates into parallel fibers, which traverse long distances along the folia to synapse on the dendritic spines of multiple Purkinje cells. The mossy-parallel fiber input provides constant information regarding velocity and direction of movement.

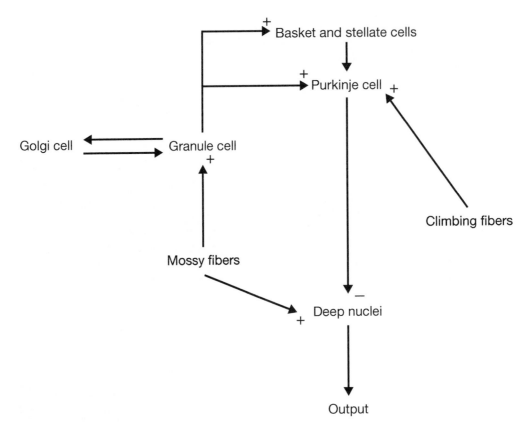

Figure 18.4 Circuitry of Cerebellar Neurons.
Plus sign indicates excitatory synapse; minus sign, inhibitory synapse.
(Adapted from Mowzoon N. The cerebellum and cerebellar disorders. In: Mowzoon N, Flemming KD, editors. Neurology board review: an illustrated study guide. Rochester [MN]: Mayo Clinic Scientific Press and Florence [KY]: Informa Healthcare USA; c2007. p. 377–99. Used with permission of Mayo Foundation for Medical Education and Research.)

Mossy fibers originate from the pontine nuclei (ponto-cerebellar pathway), spinal cord (spinocerebellar tract), vestibular nuclei (vestibulocerebellar tract), and reticular formation. Mossy fiber activation of granule cells results in simple spike Purkinje cell discharge.

Climbing fibers originate from the inferior olivary nucleus. They provide input to the deep cerebellar nuclei and Purkinje cells and regulate the response of Purkinje cells to mossy fiber input. Each Purkinje cell is in contact with 1 climbing fiber. Climbing fibers directly activate Purkinje cells, resulting in complex spike Purkinje cell discharge. The firing is phasic and provides a timing signal to Purkinje cells. Climbing fiber input may help correct errors in movement.

Cerebellar Nuclei

The cerebellar nuclei provide cerebellar output. Their output is modulated by excitatory input from collaterals of the cerebellar afferent systems and the inferior olivary nucleus, with inhibition from Purkinje cells. Each nucleus is associated with certain functions of the cerebellum (see below).

- The cerebellar cortex consists of 3 layers: the molecular layer, the Purkinje cell layer, and the granular layer.
- Purkinje cells are the output cells of the cerebellar cortex and provide inhibitory input (γ-aminobutyric acid) to the deep nuclei, which provide output from the cerebellum.
- The 2 main inputs to the cerebellum are mossy fibers and climbing fibers; both are excitatory and use L-glutamate.
- The mossy-parallel fiber input provides constant information regarding velocity and direction of movement.
- Climbing fiber input may help correct errors in movement.

Functional Subdivisions of the Cerebellum

Overview

A common scheme functionally subdivides the cerebellum into the vestibulocerebellum, spinocerebellum, and cere-brocerebellum (Figure 18.5 and Table 18.1). This scheme is based on the area of cerebellar cortex involved in a particular pathway. Each area of the cerebellum relates to specific deep nuclei and is involved in a specific function. Another scheme subdivides the cerebellum by specific functions, including motor, oculomotor, cognitive, and limbic (Figure 18.6 and Table 18.2).

Motor Circuitry for Gait and Posture

Gait is a complex interaction of the cortex, basal ganglia, indirect motor pathways, the cerebellum, and certain brainstem nuclei (pedunculopontine nucleus). The vermis of the cerebellum controls the spinal central pattern generator for gait via the reticulospinal system. This pattern generator is also under the influence of the pedunculopontine nucleus and the basal ganglia.

The medial vermis receives proprioceptive input from the limbs via the spinocerebellar tracts (Figure 18.7). In addition, it receives input from the vestibular system. The medial vermis projects to the reticular formation via the fastigial nucleus and gives rise to the reticulospinal pathways. The medial vestibular nucleus gives rise to the medial vestibulospinal tract involved in head and eye coordination. The lateral vermis projects to the lateral vestibular nucleus, which gives rise to the lateral vestibulospinal tract (important for tone and posture, especially to extensor muscles).

Motor Circuitry for Limb Movements

The medial hemisphere, or paravermal region, of the cerebellum processes proprioceptive information from the spinocerebellar neurons for unconscious proprioception (Figure 18.8). This area of the cerebellum functions in sequence activation and in coordination of agonist and antagonist muscles in multijoint movements. The paravermal cerebellum compares the actual and intended movement of limbs and then aids in correction. It does so by receiving afferent input from the motor cortex, ventral spinocerebellar tract, and dorsal spinocerebellar tract. The globose and emboliform nuclei are the deep cerebellar nuclei associated with the paravermal region. These nuclei discharge after the onset of the movement; they project to the premotor and motor cortex and provide input also to the rubrospinal neurons.

The paravermal region of the lateral cerebellum is also important in planning, initiation, and timing of specific patterns of movement. The corticopontine fibers descend from the motor cortex to the ipsilateral pontine nuclei (Figure 18.9). Here they synapse, and axons from the pontine nuclei project to the contralateral cerebellum via the middle cerebellar peduncle. Efferent information from the motor portion of the lateral cerebellar cortex is conveyed via the dorsal portion of the dentate nucleus to the contralateral ventral lateral thalamus via the superior cerebellar

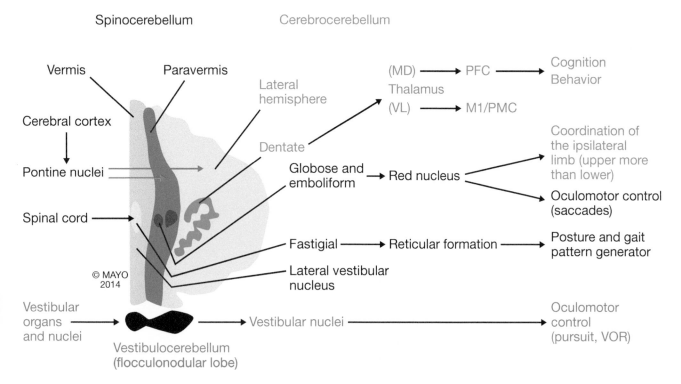

Figure 18.5 Functional Subdivisions of the Cerebellum.
M1 indicates primary motor cortex; MD, mediodorsal nucleus; PFC, prefrontal cortex; PMC, premotor cortex; VL, ventral lateral nucleus; VOR, vestibuloocular reflex.
(Used with permission of Mayo Foundation for Medical Education and Research.)

Table 18.1 • Subdivisions of the Cerebellum by Functional Region

Functional Region	Cerebellar Cortical Region	Principal Input	Deep Nucleus	Principal Destination (Target)	Function
Vestibulocerebellum	Flocculonodular lobe	Vestibular labyrinth Vestibular nuclei DLPN	Medial vestibular	Oculomotor nuclei	Vestibuloocular reflex Smooth pursuit
Spinocerebellum	Dorsal vermis	NRTP PPRF	Fastigial	PPRF (excitatory burst neurons)	Saccadic eye movements (amplitude, direction, velocity of saccades)
	Medial vermis	Labyrinth Vestibular nuclei Visual and auditory Spinocerebellar (from trunk and proximal areas of the limbs)	Fastigial	Vestibular nucleus Reticular formation	Gait Posture Tone
	Lateral vermis	Spinocerebellar (from trunk and proximal areas of the limbs)	Lateral vestibular	Reticular formation	Posture
	Paravermal region	Spinocerebellar afferents	Interposed (globose and emboliform)	Red nucleus (magnocellular) Ventral lateral thalamus Distal regions of the motor cortex	Sequence activation and coordination of skilled multijoint movements of the limbs
Cerebrocerebellum	Lateral part of hemisphere	Motor Premotor	Dentate (dorsal)	Red nucleus (parvocellular) Ventral lateral thalamus Motor (area 4), premotor cortex (area 6)	Initiation, planning, and timing of movement Motor learning
		Posterior parietal Prefrontal Temporal Cingulate	Dentate (ventral)	Posterior parietal Prefrontal Temporal and cingulate	Role in cognition, language, and limbic system

Abbreviations: DLPN, dorsolateral pontine nucleus; NRTP, nucleus reticularis tegmentum pontis; PPRF, pontine paramedian reticular formation.

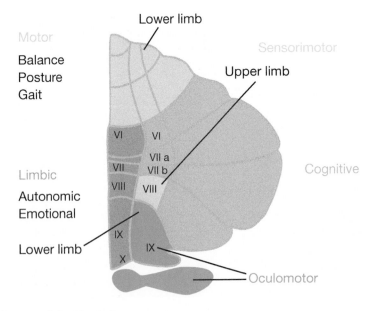

Figure 18.6 Functional Clusters of the Cerebellum.
Please see text for details.
(Adapted from Makris N, Schlerf JE, Hodge SM, Haselgrove C, Albaugh MD, Seidman LJ, et al. MRI-based surface-assisted parcellation of human cerebellar cortex: an anatomically specified method with estimate of reliability. Neuroimage. 2005 May 1;25(4):1146–60. Used with permission.)

Table 18.2 • Subdivisions of the Cerebellum by Specific Function

Subdivision	Topography	Function	Clinical Manifestation
Motor	Anterior lobe Posterior lobe	Gait, posture Multijoint movement	Ataxia Dysarthria Limb dysmetria
Oculomotor	Flocculus, paraflocculus, and nodulus Dorsal vermis and fastigial nucleus	Control of vestibular ocular reflex and smooth pursuit Control of saccades	Impaired pursuit Gaze-evoked nystagmus Saccadic dysmetria Opsoclonus
Cognitive	Posterior lobe Dentate	Executive Visuospatial Language Memory	Impaired executive function, visuospatial disorientation, verbal fluency, and visual memory
Affective (limbic)	Posterior lobe (vermal) Fastigial nucleus	Emotion, affect Autonomic	Blunted or disinhibited behavior

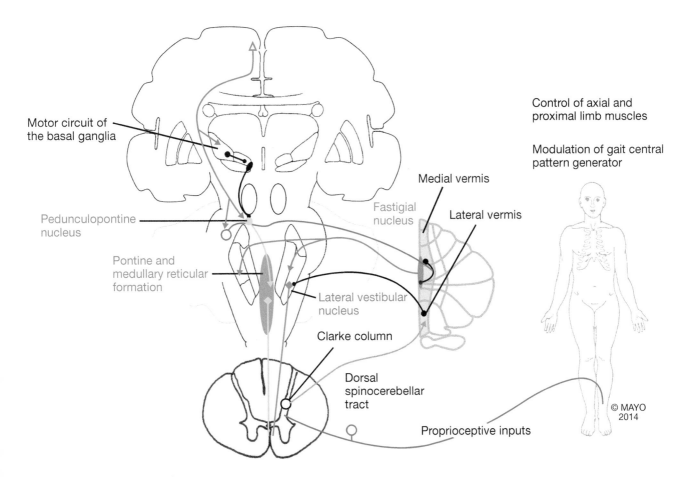

Figure 18.7 Motor Gait and Posture.
The vermis regulates the activity of brainstem nuclei controlling axial and proximal limb muscles. It receives proprioceptive and cutaneous inputs via the dorsal spinocerebellar tracts and vestibular inputs. The medial vermis, via the fastigial nucleus, projects to nuclei of origin of reticulospinal pathways involved in locomotion and medial vestibulospinal pathways involved in head-eye coordination. The lateral vermis projects directly to the lateral vestibular nucleus, which gives rise to the vestibulospinal tract, which is critical for maintenance of posture against gravity.
(Adapted from Benarroch EE. Basic neurosciences with clinical applications. Philadelphia [PA]: Butterworth Heinemann/Elsevier; c2006. Chapter 17, Basal ganglia and cerebellum: functional organization and role in control of motor and cognitive behavior; p. 513–69. Used by permission of Mayo Foundation for Medical Education and Research.)

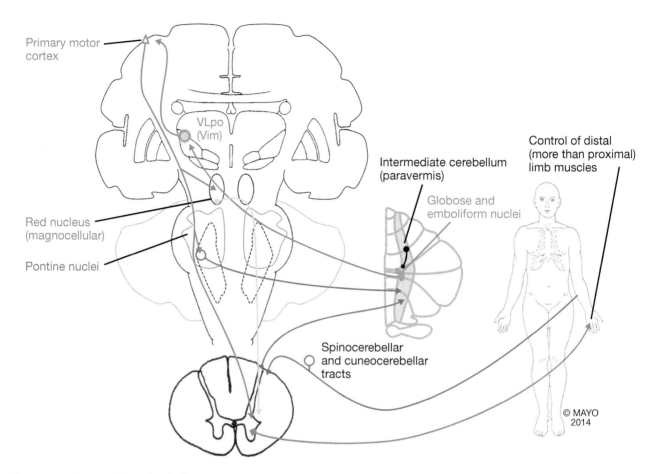

Figure 18.8 *Intermediate Cerebellum.*

The intermediate cerebellum (paravermis) receives information about the progress of limb movements from peripheral receptors via the dorsal spinocerebellar and cuneocerebellar tracts, about excitability of spinal interneurons via the ventral spinocerebellar tract, and about cortical motor commands via the pontine nuclei. It projects, via the globose and emboliform nuclei, to the magnocellular subdivision of the red nucleus, which gives rise to the rubrospinal tract, and to the posterior portion of the ventral lateral nucleus of the thalamus (VLpo), also called the ventral intermediate nucleus (Vim), which projects to motor cortical areas that give rise to the corticospinal tract. Through these connections, the intermediate cerebellum controls the motor pathways that project to the motoneurons innervating the more distal portions of the limbs and digits.

(Adapted from Benarroch EE. Basic neurosciences with clinical applications. Philadelphia [PA]: Butterworth Heinemann/Elsevier; c2006. Chapter 17, Basal ganglia and cerebellum: functional organization and role in control of motor and cognitive behavior; p. 513–69. Used by permission of Mayo Foundation for Medical Education and Research.)

peduncle. From the ventral lateral nucleus of the thalamus, axons project to the motor and premotor cortices. The dentate discharges and provides a trigger signal to the motor cortex and initiates a movement with a sensory stimulus. This stimulus allows the dentate to aid in specification of the direction, timing, intensity, and pattern of muscle use.

Ocular Motor Circuitry

The vestibulocerebellum (flocculus, paraflocculus, and nodulus) is important in the vestibuloocular reflex and smooth pursuit (Figure 18.10). (See also Chapter 12, "Supranuclear Ocular Motor Systems.") The vestibulocerebellum receives mossy fiber input from the vestibular nuclei, smooth pursuit pathway (middle superior temporal area via the dorsolateral pontine nuclei), and the nucleus prepositus hypoglossi and medial vestibular nuclei (involved in gaze holding). Efferent axons from the flocculus and paraflocculus project back to the medial vestibular nuclei and then to the cranial nerve nuclei involved in ocular movement. Dysfunction of this pathway may result in saccadic pursuit and gaze-evoked nystagmus.

The dorsal vermis of the cerebellum controls the amplitude, direction, and velocity of saccadic eye movements. The dorsal vermis receives input from the paramedian pontine reticular formation (excitatory burst neuron

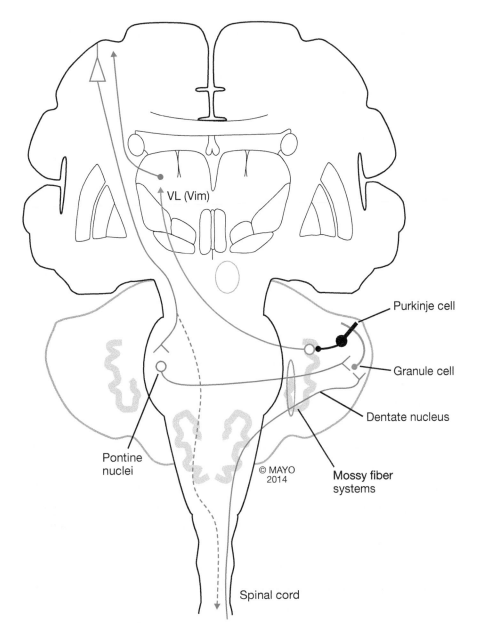

Figure 18.9 *Cortico-Pontocerebellar Pathway.*
The lateral portion of the cerebellar hemisphere receives inputs almost exclusively from the cerebral cortex via the pontine nuclei and provides the major input to the ventral lateral thalamus (VL) via the dentate nucleus. The dentate consists of 2 main territories. The dorsal, or motor domain of the dentate, targets the classic motor subdivisions of the VL, which project to the primary motor and lateral premotor cortices. The ventral portions of the dentate project to dorsal portions of the VL, which provide inputs to the prefrontal and parietal cortex. Vim indicates ventral intermediate nucleus.
(Adapted from Benarroch EE. Basic neurosciences with clinical applications. Philadelphia [PA]: Butterworth Heinemann/Elsevier; c2006. Chapter 17, Basal ganglia and cerebellum: functional organization and role in control of motor and cognitive behavior; p. 513–69. Used by permission of Mayo Foundation for Medical Education and Research.)

for horizontal saccades) and the nucleus reticularis tegmentum pontis (relay from the frontal eye fields and superior colliculus for planning saccades). Purkinje cells of the dorsal vermis discharge before the contralateral saccades and project to the fastigial nuclei. The fastigial nuclei then project axons to the contralateral brainstem premotor burst and omnipause neurons controlling saccades (Figure 18.11). Dysfunction along this pathway may result in saccadic dysmetria and sometimes opsoclonus.

Cognitive and Limbic Circuitry

There are many reciprocal interconnections of the cerebellum with areas of the cortex, particularly the prefrontal

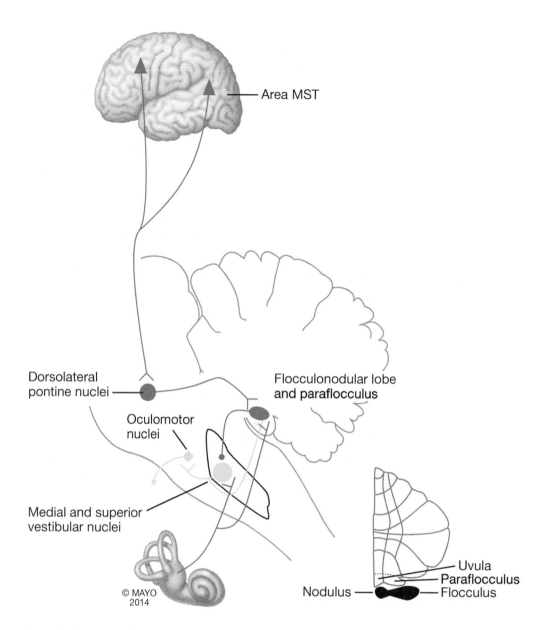

Figure 18.10 Smooth Pursuit Pathway.
The main function of the flocculonodular lobe and adjacent uvula and ventral paraflocculus (vestibulocerebellum) is the control of eye movements. The nodulus and the uvula receive vestibular inputs directly from the labyrinth or from the vestibular nuclei; inputs from the frontal eye fields and the middle temporal and middle superior temporal (MST) areas via the dorsolateral pontine nuclei; and inputs from the oculomotor control network via the nucleus prepositus hypoglossi and the nuclei of the paramedian tracts. The flocculus and paraflocculus project to the medial and superior vestibular nuclei, which control eye movements, including the horizontal and vertical vestibuloocular reflexes and smooth pursuit.
(Adapted from Benarroch EE. Basic neurosciences with clinical applications. Philadelphia [PA]: Butterworth Heinemann/Elsevier; c2006. Chapter 17, Basal ganglia and cerebellum: functional organization and role in control of motor and cognitive behavior; p. 513–69. Used by permission of Mayo Foundation for Medical Education and Research.)

cortex, as well as the parahippocampal region and the posterior parietal and superior temporal regions. Information descends via the pontine nuclei and returns via the ventral dentate to the same cortical region. In functional brain imaging studies, the lateral aspect of the posterior lobe of the cerebellum appears to be important for language, verbal working memory, spatial tasks, executive function, and emotional processing.

The limbic circuitry involves the vermis of the posterior lobe and the fastigial nucleus.

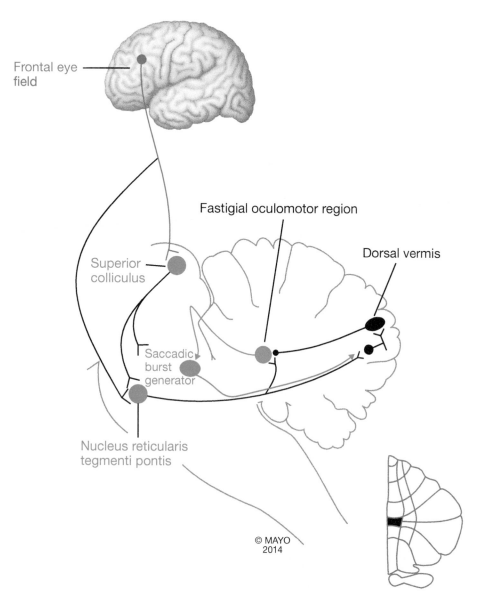

Figure 18.11 *Fastigial Nucleus and Control of Saccades.*
The posterior or dorsal vermis, via the fastigial oculomotor region, controls the amplitude, direction, and velocity of saccadic eye movements. These structures receive inputs from the pontine paramedian reticular formation, which contains the excitatory burst neurons for horizontal saccades, and from the nucleus reticularis tegmenti pontis, which relays saccadic signals from the frontal eye fields and superior colliculus. The fastigial nucleus projects to the saccadic burst generator of the brainstem via the uncinate fasciculus and controls the amplitude of ipsilateral and contralateral saccades.

(Adapted from Benarroch EE. Basic neurosciences with clinical applications. Philadelphia [PA]: Butterworth Heinemann/Elsevier; c2006. Chapter 17, Basal ganglia and cerebellum: functional organization and role in control of motor and cognitive behavior; p. 513–69. Used by permission of Mayo Foundation for Medical Education and Research.)

Cerebellar Nuclei–inferior Olivary Nucleus Interactions

The inferior olive compares intended motor commands to actual motor commands from the cerebral cortex, the brainstem nuclei, and the feedback afferent system. If the inputs do not match, an increase in firing of the inferior olivary nucleus results in an error signal. This modifies the Purkinje response to mossy fibers. The role of the inferior olive may be to provide a timing signal to the cerebellum, and the inferior olive may contribute to detection and correction of errors in motor performance.

Neurons of the inferior olivary nucleus project a low-frequency, synchronized oscillatory activity via the

Table 18.3 • Clinical Correlations of Cerebellar Dysfunction

Location of Lesion	Clinical Finding
Flocculus or paraflocculus	Saccadic dysmetria Gaze-evoked nystagmus
Dorsal vermis	Saccadic dysmetria Opsoclonus
Vermis	Gait ataxia
Cerebellar hemisphere	Limb ataxia
Cerebellar-thalamocortical loop	Tremor
Guillain-Mollaret triangle (dentate-red nucleus-inferior olive pathway)	Palatal myoclonus Essential tremor

climbing fiber system to the cerebellar nuclei (eliciting monosynaptic excitation) and the Purkinje cells (eliciting rhythmic disynaptic inhibition followed by a rebound burst discharge of the cerebellar nuclei). The cerebellar nuclei regulate the inferior olivary nucleus via 2 competing connections. They project an inhibitory GABAergic projection to the inferior olive. In addition, they project an indirect, excitatory projection via the red nucleus to the inferior olive.

- The vermis of the cerebellum controls the spinal central pattern generator for gait via the reticulospinal system.
- The medial hemisphere, or paravermal region, of the cerebellum processes proprioceptive information from the spinocerebellar neurons for unconscious proprioception. This area of the cerebellum functions in sequence activation and in coordination of agonist and antagonist muscles in multijoint movements.
- The paravermal region of the lateral cerebellum is also important in planning, initiation, and timing of specific patterns of movement.
- The vestibulocerebellum (flocculus, paraflocculus, and nodulus) is important in the vestibuloocular reflex and smooth pursuit.
- The dorsal vermis of the cerebellum controls the amplitude, direction, and velocity of saccadic eye movements.
- Cognitive information from diffuse areas of the cortex projects to the lateral cerebellum and returns to the cortex via the ventral dentate.
- The limbic circuitry involves the vermis of the posterior lobe and the fastigial nucleus.
- The inferior olive compares intended motor commands to actual motor commands from the cerebral cortex, the brainstem nuclei, and the feedback afferent system.

Clinical Correlations

Examination findings related to lesions of the cerebellum or its pathways are provided in Table 18.3. For clinical disorders resulting in cerebellar findings or ataxia, see Volume 2, Chapter 26, "Cerebellar Disorders and Ataxias."

Ataxic hemiparesis is a common manifestation of ischemic stroke and is often due to a lacunar mechanism. Patients have mild upper motor neuron weakness but moderate to severe ataxia on the weak side. While most commonly this stroke localizes to the ventral pons, the location is variable and can occur anywhere the corticospinal tract and cortico-pontocerebellar tracts entwine (Figure 18.12).

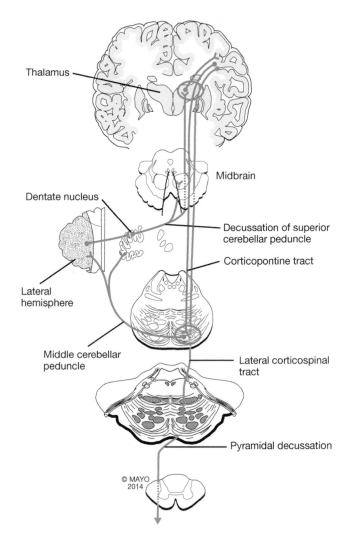

Figure 18.12 Ataxic Hemiparesis.
Ataxic hemiparesis is a clinical syndrome resulting from impairment of both the cerebrocerebellar circuit and the corticospinal tract. Where the 2 tracts are close to each other (red ovals), a lesion may result in ataxic hemiparesis. (Adapted from Mowzoon N. The cerebellum and cerebellar disorders. In: Mowzoon N, Flemming KD, editors. Neurology board review: an illustrated study guide. Rochester [MN]: Mayo Clinic Scientific Press and Florence [KY]: Informa Healthcare USA; c2007. p. 377–99. Used with permission of Mayo Foundation for Medical Education and Research.)

19 Autonomic Nervous System

JENNIFER A. TRACY, MD; EDUARDO E. BENARROCH, MD;
KELLY D. FLEMMING, MD

Introduction

The autonomic nervous system is involved in many important unconscious body functions. It aids in maintaining the internal environment and responds and adapts to the external environment. The autonomic nervous system consists of peripheral components (sympathetic and parasympathetic nerves) and central components (ventrolateral medulla, nucleus ambiguus, nucleus of the solitary tract, periaqueductal gray, anterior cingulate gyrus, insular cortex, amygdala, and hypothalamus).

This chapter briefly reviews the anatomy and functional components of the autonomic nervous system and the anatomical clinical correlations. Clinical autonomic diseases are presented in Volume 2, Chapter 44, "Autonomic Disorders."

Peripheral Autonomic System

Overview

Sympathetic and parasympathetic components of the autonomic nervous system provide balance for autonomic functions. The effects of the sympathetic nervous system depend on the target organ, but they include increased heart rate and blood pressure, increased sweating response, bronchodilatation and pupillary dilatation, and inhibition of peristalsis. In general, parasympathetic inputs produce the opposite effect of the sympathetic response (Table 19.1).

Table 19.1 • Functions of the Sympathetic and Parasympathetic Systems

Target	Sympathetic			Parasympathetic		
	Action	NT[a]	Receptor[a]	Action	NT[a]	Receptor[a]
Pupil	Dilation	NE	α_1	Constriction, accommodation	Ach	M3
Salivary gland	Variable	...	...	Stimulation	Ach	M3
Blood vessels	Constriction	NE	α_1	Dilation	NO	...
	Dilation	Epi	β			
Sweat gland	Stimulation	Ach	M3	...	...	...
Heart	Stimulation (increased heart rate)	NE	β_1	Inhibition (decreased heart rate)	Ach	M2
Respiratory tract	Bronchial dilation	Epi	β	Bronchial constriction	Ach	M3
Gastrointestinal motility	Inhibition	NE	α_2, β	Stimulation	Ach	M3
Bladder						
Detrusor	Inhibition	NE	β	Stimulation	Ach	M3
Sphincter	Contraction	NE	α_1	Relaxation	NO	
Sexual organs	Ejaculation	NE	α_1	Erection	NO	...

Abbreviations: Ach, acetylcholine; Epi, epinephrine; M, muscarinic; NE, norepinephrine; NO, nitrous oxide; NT, neurotransmitter.
[a] Postganglionic.

An overview of the peripheral autonomic structures is shown in Figure 19.1. Preganglionic sympathetic fiber neurons originate in the thoracolumbar region of the spinal cord. Preganglionic parasympathetic fibers originate in the craniosacral segments.

The efferent components include a preganglionic neuron at the level of either the brainstem (parasympathetic) or the spinal cord (sympathetic or parasympathetic). The axons of this neuron synapse in a peripheral ganglion, and the axons of the postganglionic neurons then innervate a target organ.

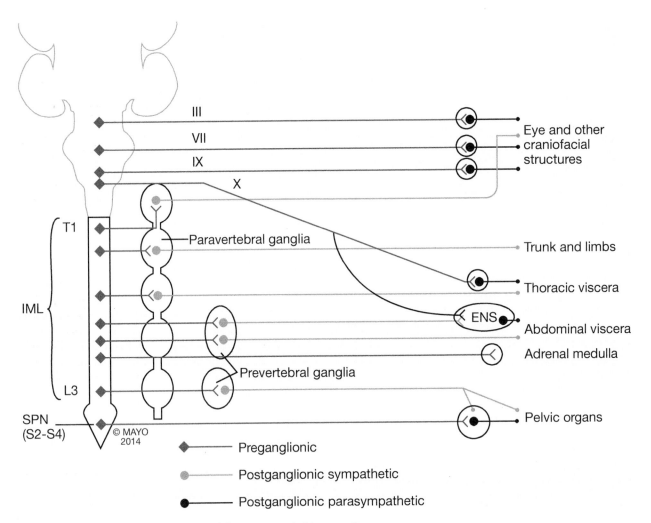

Figure 19.1 *Generalized Organization of the Autonomic Nervous System.*
The sympathetic preganglionic neurons are located at spinal cord segments T1 through L3. The preganglionic sympathetic axons are small myelinated fibers that reach the paravertebral sympathetic chain; some synapse in paravertebral ganglia at the same level or above or below the level of entry, whereas others pass through the chain to innervate the prevertebral ganglia and the adrenal medulla. The paravertebral ganglia innervate the face, trunk, limbs, and thoracic viscera; the prevertebral ganglia innervate the abdominal and pelvic viscera. The parasympathetic outflow has cranial and sacral components. Cranial parasympathetic neurons are located in the general visceral efferent column of the midbrain, pons, and medulla. Their preganglionic axons are components of the oculomotor nerve (III) innervating the eye, the facial nerve (VII) innervating the lacrimal gland, the glossopharyngeal nerve (IX) innervating the parotid gland, and the vagus nerve (X) innervating all the thoracic and abdominal viscera. The sacral parasympathetic nucleus (SPN), located at segments S2 through S4, innervates the bladder, rectum, and sexual organs. The enteric nervous system (ENS), located in the walls of the gut, controls gastrointestinal tract motility and secretion. Preganglionic and postganglionic parasympathetic neurons are cholinergic; postganglionic sympathetic neurons (except those innervating sweat glands) are adrenergic. IML, indicates intermediolateral.

(Adapted from Benarroch EE. Basic neurosciences with clinical applications. Philadelphia [PA]: Butterworth Heinemann/Elsevier; c2006. Chapter 20, Peripheral autonomic control of visceral organs; p. 679–720. Used by permission of Mayo Foundation for Medical Education and Research.)

Acetylcholine is the primary neurotransmitter at preganglionic synapses, whether sympathetic or parasympathetic, and at parasympathetic postganglionic neurons. The receptors are nicotinic. The adrenal medulla is innervated by a preganglionic sympathetic axon, and the adrenal chromaffin cells produce primarily epinephrine. Parasympathetic postganglionic axons release acetylcholine at muscarinic receptors. Norepinephrine is the main neurotransmitter of sympathetic postganglionic pathways at adrenergic receptors, with the exception of sweat glands, for which acetylcholine is the main neurotransmitter.

Both sympathetic and parasympathetic fibers also release other nonadrenergic and noncholinergic chemicals. For example, sympathetic fibers may also release adenosine triphosphate and neuropeptide Y. Parasympathetic fibers may release nitric oxide and vasoactive intestinal polypeptide.

The adrenergic receptors include α_1, α_2, β_1, and β_2 receptors. The muscarinic receptors include M1, M2, and M3 receptors.

Sympathetic

Sympathetic preganglionic neurons originate in the intermediolateral nucleus of the spinal cord, from spinal cord segments T1 through L3 (Figure 19.1). Sympathetic fibers leave the spinal cord along with the ventral roots, travel along the white rami, and either synapse at a particular level in the paravertebral sympathetic chain or form splanchnic nerves extending to the prevertebral ganglia. The paravertebral ganglia provide sympathetic innervation to most areas of the body (except for the abdominopelvic area), including the head. The prevertebral ganglia (eg, superior and inferior mesenteric ganglia, celiac ganglia) provide sympathetic innervation to the abdomen and pelvis. Preganglionic fibers also innervate medullary cells in the adrenal glands.

Parasympathetic

Parasympathetic neurons originate in brainstem nuclei and cranial nerves (oculomotor [III], facial [VII], glossopharyngeal [IX], and vagus [X]) and in the sacral cord at levels S2 through S4 (Figure 19.1 and Table 19.2).

Fibers from the oculomotor nerve (which come from the Edinger-Westphal nucleus) travel to the ciliary ganglion, which allows for pupillary constriction. Fibers from the facial nerve (arising from the lacrimal and superior salivatory nuclei) travel to the sphenopalatine and submandibular ganglia. Fibers from the glossopharyngeal nerve (arising from the inferior salivatory nucleus) supply the otic ganglion.

The vagus nerve, originating in the dorsal motor nucleus of X (caudal medulla), has widespread input to many visceral organs. The vagus nerve increases gut motility, stimulates smooth muscle relaxation of the gut, and stimulates exocrine gland secretion through the enteric nervous system. The dorsal motor nucleus of X also innervates the respiratory tract to constrict bronchi. Cholinergic neurons of the ventral aspect of the nucleus ambiguus provide preganglionic projections to the autonomic ganglia innervating the heart.

The sacral parasympathetic outflow tracts located in spinal cord segments S2 through S3 are important for sexual function and for excretory functions of the bladder and bowel.

- Preganglionic sympathetic fiber neurons originate in the thoracolumbar region of the spinal cord.

Table 19.2 • Functional Organization of the Parasympathetic Outflow

Location	Nucleus	Nerve	Ganglion	Effect
Cranial division				
Midbrain	Edinger-Westphal	CN III	Ciliary	Pupilloconstriction
				Accommodation
Pons	Superior salivatory	CN VII	Sphenopalatine	Lacrimation
			Submandibular	Salivation (submaxillary and sublingual glands)
Medulla	Inferior salivatory	CN IX	Otic	Salivation (parotid gland)
	Dorsal nucleus of the vagus	CN X	Near end organs	Bronchoconstriction
				Bronchosecretory
				Gastrointestinal peristalsis and secretion
	Ambiguus	CN X	Near end organs	Decreases heart rate and conduction
Sacral division				
Segments S2 through S4	Intermediolateral cell column	Pelvic Splanchnic	Near end organs	Emptying of bladder and rectum
				Erection

Abbreviation: CN, cranial nerve.

Adapted from Benarroch EE, Daube JR, Flemming KD, Westmoreland BF. Mayo Clinic medical neurosciences: organized by neurologic systems and levels. 5th ed. Rochester (MN): Mayo Clinic Scientific Press and Florence (KY): Informa Healthcare USA; c2008. Chapter 9, The internal regulation system; p. 331–83. Used with permission of Mayo Foundation for Medical Education and Research.

- Preganglionic parasympathetic fibers originate in the craniosacral segments.
- Acetylcholine is the primary neurotransmitter at preganglionic synapses.
- Parasympathetic postganglionic axons release acetylcholine at muscarinic receptors.
- Norepinephrine is the main neurotransmitter of sympathetic postganglionic pathways at adrenergic receptors, with the exception of sweat glands, for which acetylcholine is the main neurotransmitter.

Central Autonomic Structures and Function

Overview

Several interconnected central structures have a role in autonomic functions (Table 19.3 and Figure 19.2). These central structures aid in simulating or modulating autonomic (visceromotor) output, endocrine response, somatomotor response (sphincter, respiratory motor neurons), and pain. Descending input from the hypothalamus and brainstem aid in coordinating the sympathetic response (Figure 19.3). The parasympathetic system receives some modulatory descending input but largely responds to the internal milieu on a reflex basis.

Brainstem Autonomic Areas

Several brainstem areas mediate and modulate autonomic outputs and reflexes. These include the periaqueductal gray matter parabrachial nucleus, the nucleus of the solitary tract, the ventrolateral medulla, the dorsal motor nucleus of X, the cardiovagal portion (ventrolateral) of the nucleus ambiguus, and the medullary raphe nuclei. The carotid baroreceptor reflex that buffers fluctuations of blood pressure is initiated by baroreceptor afferent input from cranial nerve IX, which terminates in the nucleus of the solitary tract; this triggers inhibition of sympathoexcitatory neurons of the rostral ventrolateral medulla and activation of cardiovagal neurons of the nucleus ambiguus (see Chapter 8, "Brainstem and Cranial Nerves: Overview and Medulla").

Role of the Hypothalamus

The hypothalamus integrates input from the external and internal environments, including visceral and pain afferents, humoral signals (such as blood glucose level), circadian influences, and cognitive-emotional influences via the limbic systems. The hypothalamus coordinates patterns of autonomic, endocrine, arousal, and behavioral responses according to the stimulus. For example, the paraventricular nucleus provides a major output to autonomic nuclei of the brainstem and spinal cord and initiates hormonal responses (such as release of corticotropin-releasing factors) and autonomic responses (via input to autonomic nuclei in the brainstem and spinal cord) in response to internal or external stressors (Figure 19.3).

Cortical Areas Involved in Autonomic Responses

The insular cortex is folded within the sylvian fissure. This cortical area is the primary viscerosensory area and integrates visceral sensation with pain and temperature sensation, providing conscious perception of the bodily state (Figure 19.4).

The anterior cingulate gyrus is located in the medial hemisphere just above the corpus callosum and is interconnected with the insular cortex and amygdala. It is important in behavioral motivation triggered by emotionally significant stimuli, and it is involved in behavioral arousal and control of motor and autonomic output in response to emotionally or socially relevant information.

Table 19.3 • Central Components of the Autonomic Nervous System

Structure	Function
Insular cortex	Interoceptive sensation (bodily sensation); integration of visceral, pain, and temperature sensations
Anterior cingulate cortex	Modulation of autonomic output involved in goal-directed behavior
Amygdala	Providing emotional significance to sensory stimuli
Preoptic region of hypothalamus	Integration of autonomic, endocrine, and behavioral responses for homeostasis, stress response, and immune modulation
Periaqueductal gray	Integration of autonomic, somatic, and pain modulating responses
Parabrachial nucleus	Integration and relay of somatic and visceral inputs to the hypothalamus, thalamus, and amygdala
Nucleus of the solitary tract	Site for relay of taste and visceral afferents; reflexes to multiple areas
Ventrolateral medulla	Control of vasomotor tone related to blood pressure and for respiratory pattern generation
Medullary raphe	Control of sympathetic tone (vasoconstriction) to skin (important in thermoregulation)

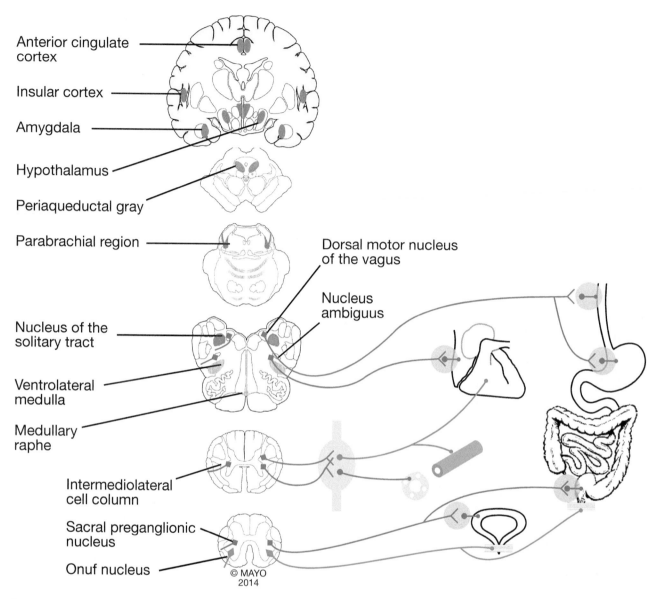

Anterior cingulate cortex

Insular cortex

Amygdala

Hypothalamus

Periaqueductal gray

Parabrachial region

Dorsal motor nucleus of the vagus

Nucleus ambiguus

Nucleus of the solitary tract

Ventrolateral medulla

Medullary raphe

Intermediolateral cell column

Sacral preganglionic nucleus

Onuf nucleus

© MAYO 2014

Figure 19.2 Central Autonomic Control Areas.
Please see text for detailed discussion of roles of important central autonomic structures.
(Used with permission of Mayo Foundation for Medical Education and Research.)

The amygdala is located just anterior to the hippocampus. It is a critical component of the anterior limbic system (see Chapter 16, "The Limbic System"). It provides emotional significance to sensory stimuli and initiates integrated responses (autonomic, endocrine, and motor) to emotion, particularly fear. For example, a sensory stimulus eliciting fear may require a fight-or-flight sympathetic autonomic response and a motor response to escape the feared stimulus.

- The hypothalamus integrates input from the external and internal environments, including visceral and pain afferents, humoral signals (such as blood glucose level), circadian influences, and cognitive-emotional influences via the limbic systems.
- The paraventricular nucleus provides a major output to autonomic nuclei of the brainstem and spinal cord and initiates hormonal responses (such as release of corticotropin-releasing factors) and autonomic responses (via input to autonomic nuclei in the brainstem and spinal cord).
- The insular cortex is folded within the sylvian fissure.
- The anterior cingulate gyrus is important in behavioral motivation triggered by emotionally significant stimuli.

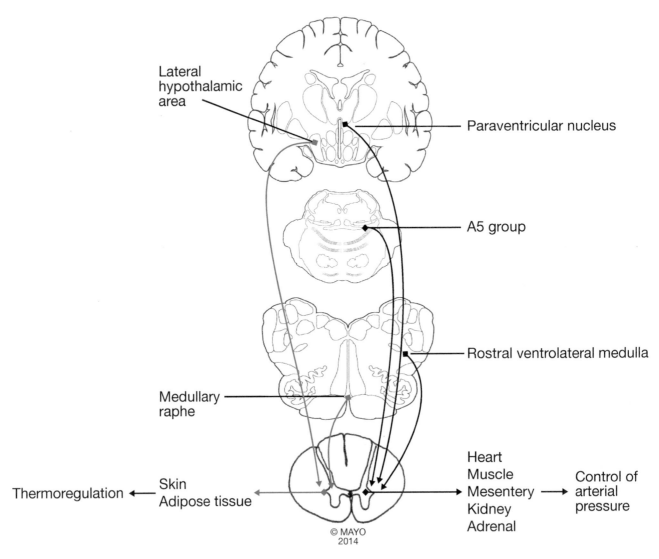

Figure 19.3 Descending Control of Sympathetic Neurons.
Please see text for details.
(Used with permission of Mayo Foundation for Medical Education and Research.)

Clinical Correlations

Horner Syndrome

Horner syndrome is characterized by miosis, ptosis, and anhidrosis unilaterally. It is due to a unilateral lesion of the sympathetic innervation. The lesion may be anywhere along the 3-neuron course (Figure 19.5). Note that internal carotid artery lesions distal to the bifurcation may result in only miosis and ptosis without anhidrosis because the sudomotor fibers to the face travel along the external carotid artery.

Urinary Bladder Function

Storage of urine in the urinary bladder requires contraction of the external sphincter, contraction of the bladder neck, and relaxation of the detrusor muscle. Bladder emptying requires contraction of the detrusor muscle with relaxation of the sphincter. This bladder control involves both sympathetic and parasympathetic output as well as somatic neurons and supratentorial input (Figure 19.6).

Parasympathetic fibers originating at spinal segments S2 through S4 project via the pelvic nerve and innervate the detrusor muscle, aiding in bladder emptying. Sympathetic fibers originating in the lower thoracic and upper lumbar segments project via the hypogastric nerve and innervate the detrusor muscle (relaxation) and the bladder neck (contraction). The sympathetic fibers thus help retain or store urine. Somatic motor neurons originating in the Onuf nucleus at sacral level S2 and S3 project through the pudendal nerves and innervate the external sphincter, helping to prevent urine outflow.

When the urinary bladder is full, afferent information travels to the periaqueductal gray matter and parabrachial

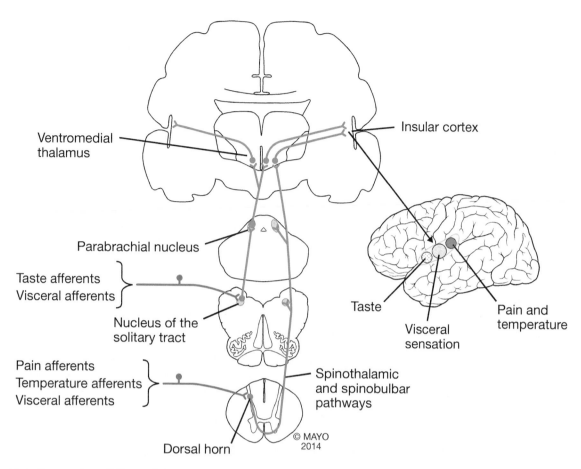

Figure 19.4 Integration of Visceral Sensory, Pain, and Temperature Information at the Level of the Insular Cortex.
The insular cortex is the primary viscerosensory cortex for taste, visceral, pain, and temperature sensations. Spinal visceral
afferents, conveying visceral sensation, relay in the dorsal horn; brainstem visceral afferents, conveying taste and visceral
sensation, relay in the nucleus of the solitary tract. Both the dorsal horn and the nucleus of the solitary tract project to the
parabrachial nucleus. All these areas cover taste, visceral, pain, and temperature sensations to the ventromedial region of
the thalamus, which projects to the insular cortex. All these sensory modalities are represented topographically in the
insula.
(Adapted from Benarroch EE. Basic neurosciences with clinical applications. Philadelphia [PA]: Butterworth Heinemann/Elsevier;
c2006. Chapter 9, The internal regulation system; p. 331–83. Used by permission of Mayo Foundation for Medical Education and
Research.)

nucleus. The periaqueductal gray matter projects to the pontine micturition center and is excitatory. The medial frontal cortex (with input from the insula) also projects to the pontine micturition center (inhibitory). The hypothalamus, insula, anterior cingulate, and lateral prefrontal cortices also are involved in the behavioral control of micturition (appropriateness of time and place for micturition). The pontine micturition center then projects to the sacral spinal cord, stimulates the coordinated activation of the sacral parasympathetic neurons innervating the detrusor muscle, and inhibits the motor neurons in the Onuf nucleus, relaxing the external bladder sphincter.

A lesion of the peripheral nerves innervating the urinary bladder may result in a flaccid bladder. This is characterized by urinary retention with overflow incontinence.

A lesion of the spinal cord may result in a spastic bladder if influence of the pontine micturition center is absent. This results in detrusor-sphincter dyssynergia (dyscoordination of the detrusor and the external sphincter). Patients often have increased urinary frequency and incontinence. An uninhibited bladder and urinary incontinence frequently result from a frontal lobe injury that damages the descending inhibition of the pontine micturition center.

Visceral Pain Referral Patterns

Visceral afferent information synapses in the dorsal horn similar to afferent fibers of the spinothalamic tract. These visceral afferents similarly cross the midline and travel near the spinothalamic tract (Figure 19.7A). Because

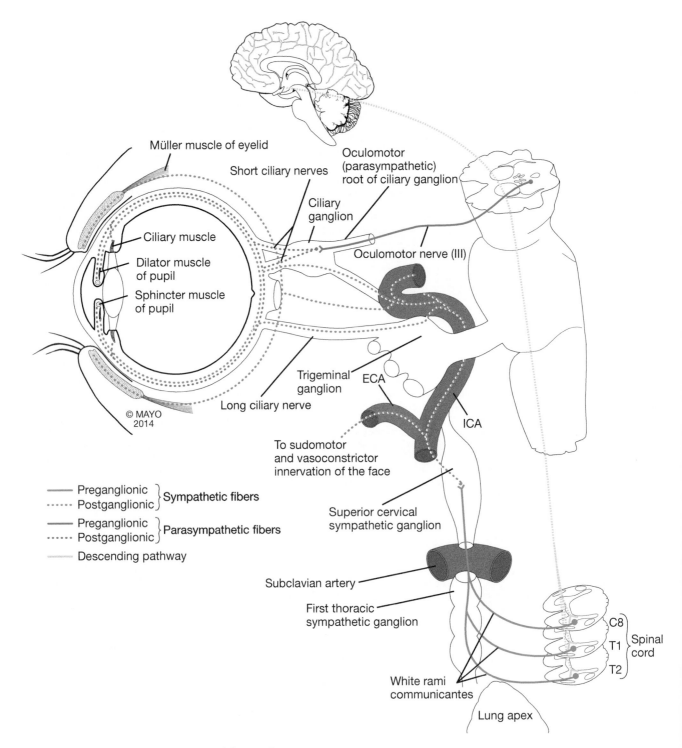

Figure 19.5 Autonomic Innervation of the Pupil.
ECA indicates external carotid artery; ICA, internal carotid artery; III, cranial nerve III.
(Adapted from Freeman WD, Mowzoon N. Neuro-opthalmology. In: Mowzoon N, Flemming KD, editors. Neurology board review: an illustrated study guide. Rochester [MN]: Mayo Clinic Scientific Press and Florence [KY]: Informa Healthcare USA; c2007. p. 83–126. Used with permission of Mayo Foundation for Medical Education and Research.)

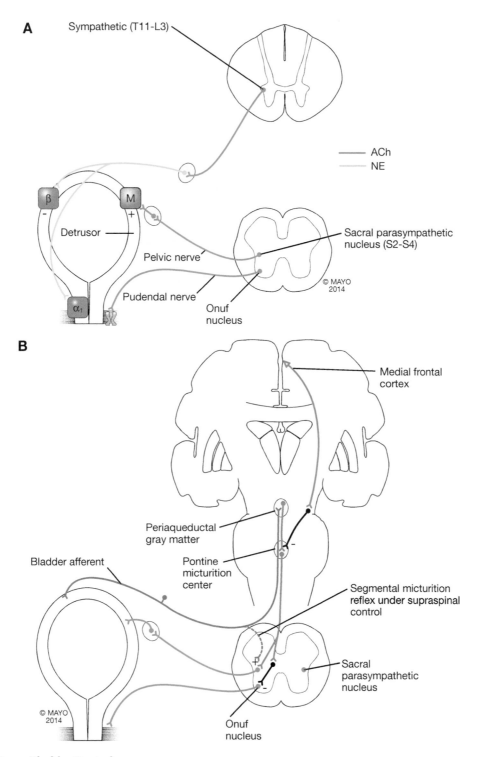

Figure 19.6 *Urinary Bladder Control.*

A, Peripheral innervation of the bladder. ACh indicates acetylcholine; α_1, α-adrenergic receptor; β, β-adrenergic receptor; M, muscarinic receptor; NE, norepinephrine. B, The normal micturition reflex involves a supraspinal pathway. The reflex is coordinated by the pontine micturition center. This region, activated by input from the bladder, contains neurons that stimulate sacral preganglionic neurons and inhibit a lateral pontine region that activates neurons in the Onuf nucleus. Thus, activation of the pontine micturition center leads to the coordinated contraction of the bladder detrusor muscle and relaxation of the external urethral sphincter muscle required for normal micturition. The excitability of the pontine micturition center is controlled by inhibitory input from the medial frontal lobe, which is the basis for the voluntary control of micturition.

(Adapted from Benarroch EE, Daube JR, Flemming KD, Westmoreland BF. Mayo Clinic medical neurosciences: organized by neurologic systems and levels. 5th ed. Rochester [MN]: Mayo Clinic Scientific Press and Florence [KY]: Informa Healthcare USA; c2008. Chapter 9, The internal regulation system; p. 331–83. Used by permission of Mayo Foundation for Medical Education and Research.)

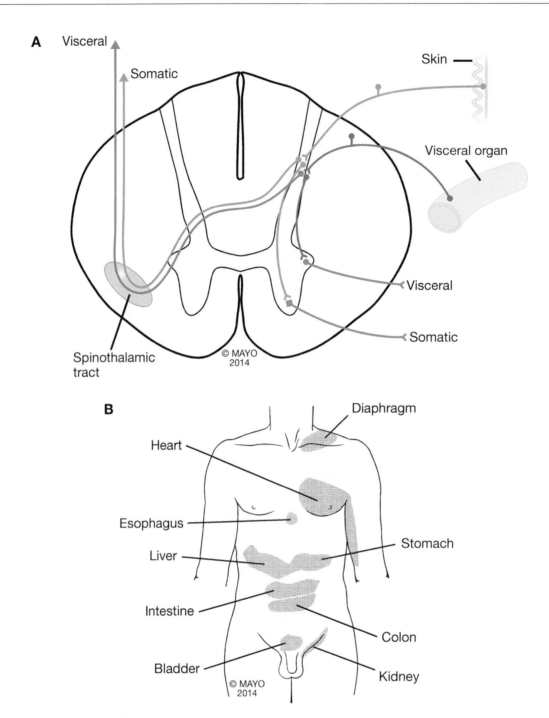

Figure 19.7 *Referral of Visceral Pain.*
A, Visceral afferents synapse with dorsal horn neurons and interneurons in the intermediate gray matter. Axons of dorsal horn neurons transmit information about visceral sensation, including visceral pain, in the spinothalamic tract. Many visceral afferents converge with somatic afferents on single dorsal horn neurons, providing the basis for referred pain. Local interneurons receiving visceral afferents project to preganglionic and somatic motor neurons and initiate segmental viscerovisceral and viscerosomatic reflexes. B, Shading indicates dermatomal areas to which visceral pain is referred.
(Adapted from Benarroch EE, Daube JR, Flemming KD, Westmoreland BF. Mayo Clinic medical neurosciences: organized by neurologic systems and levels. 5th ed. Rochester [MN]: Mayo Clinic Scientific Press and Florence [KY]: Informa Healthcare USA; c2008. Chapter 9, The internal regulation system; p. 331–83. Used with permission of Mayo Foundation for Medical Education and Research.)

visceral afferents converge with somatic afferents, patients may have referred pain from visceral organs (Figure 19.7B).

- Horner syndrome is characterized by miosis, ptosis, and anhidrosis unilaterally. It is due to a unilateral lesion of the sympathetic innervation.
- Parasympathetic fibers originating at spinal segments S2 through S4 project via the pelvic nerve and innervate the detrusor muscle, aiding in bladder emptying.

- Sympathetic fibers originating in the lower thoracic and upper lumbar segments project via the hypogastric nerve and innervate the detrusor muscle (relaxation) and the bladder neck (contraction). The sympathetic fibers thus help retain or store urine.
- The medial frontal cortex (with input from the insula) also projects to the pontine micturition center (inhibitory).
- Because visceral afferents converge with somatic afferents, patients may have referred pain from visceral organs.

Cortex: Gross Anatomy

KELLY D. FLEMMING, MD

Introduction

The cerebral cortex consists of 2 hemispheres, the left and the right. These are divided by the falx cerebri, a dural-derived structure.

The cerebral cortex receives input from a wide variety of subcortical structures, often connecting via the thalamus and from other areas of the cortex via association fibers. The cortex then projects back to wide regions of the central nervous system, including the cortex, thalamus, basal nuclei, cerebellum, brainstem, and spinal cord. The types of fibers connecting areas of the central nervous system are designated based on the regions they connect. For instance, the fibers connecting the cortex to subcortical structures are called projection fibers. The fibers connecting 1 hemisphere to the opposite hemisphere are called callosal fibers, and the fibers connecting areas within the same hemisphere are called association fibers. Fibers connecting the cortex to the thalamus are designated corticothalamic.

The cortex is further divided into lobes and functional areas. This chapter reviews the gross anatomy of the cerebral cortex. Functional organization, cortical networks, and clinical cortical syndromes are reviewed in other chapters.

Frontal Lobe

Boundaries

The central sulcus divides the frontal and parietal lobes (Figure 20.1). The primary motor cortex lies in the precentral gyrus. The inferior border of the frontal lobe is the lateral sulcus or fissure. The frontal lobe also contains a superior, middle, and inferior frontal gyrus.

Blood Supply

The lateral cortex, basal ganglia, and internal capsule are supplied by the middle cerebral artery. The medial cortex, the head of the caudate, the fornix, and anterior part of the corpus callosum are supplied by the anterior cerebral artery.

Specific Areas

Primary Motor Cortex

The primary motor cortex is located in the precentral gyrus (Brodmann area 4, M1). This cortex is idiotypic. The primary motor cortex functions in strength and dexterity of the contralateral body part. Figure 20.2 is a somatotopic representation of each body part along the cortex. Stimulation of the primary motor cortex results in contralateral movement of the represented limb. Damage to this same cortex will result in an upper motor neuron pattern of weakness contralateral to the lesion.

Supplementary Motor Area

The supplementary motor area is located at the medial aspect of the superior frontal gyrus in front of the paracentral lobule (Brodmann area 6). It is a homotypical (unimodal) area. This area functions in motor intention and initiation and motor programming for complex movements. Stimulating this area results in posturing and turning the head and eyes toward the elevated contralateral arm. Dysfunction may result in apraxia (see Chapter 23, "Focal Cognitive Syndromes").

Premotor Cortex

The premotor cortex is located on the lateral surface of the cortex just anterior to the precentral gyrus (Brodmann area 6). This is a homotypical (unimodal) area. The premotor cortex aids in motor programming. Stimulation of this area results in contralateral movements in larger muscle groups. Dysfunction results in apraxia (see Chapter 23, "Focal Cognitive Syndromes").

Frontal Eye Fields

The frontal eye fields are located in the middle frontal gyrus extending to the superior frontal gyrus. This is a

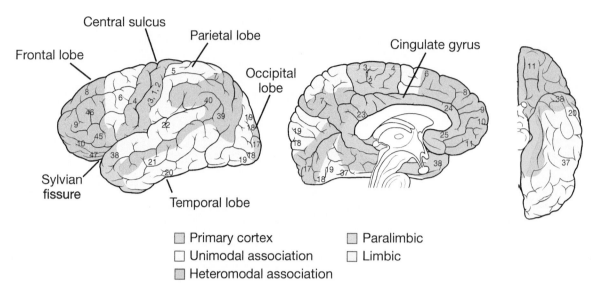

Figure 20.1 *Lobes, Cytoarchitecture, and Brodmann Areas of the Cortex.*
(Adapted from Grabowski TJ Jr, Anderson SW, Cooper GE. Disorders of cognitive function. Chapter 1, Neural substrates of cognition. Continuum Lifelong Learn Neurol. 2002 Apr;8[2]:7–40. Used with permission.)

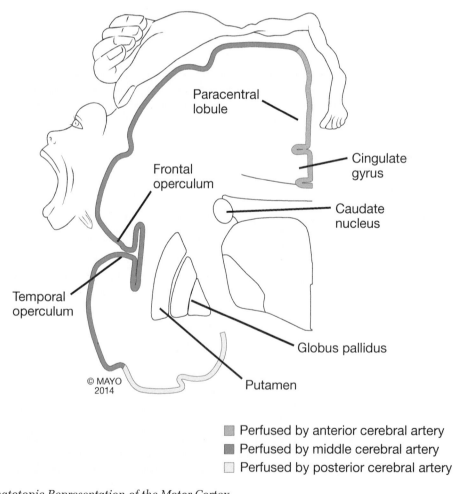

Figure 20.2 *Somatotopic Representation of the Motor Cortex.*
(Adapted from Benarroch EE, Daube JR, Flemming KD, Westmoreland BF. Mayo Clinic medical neurosciences: organized by neurologic systems and levels. 5th ed. Rochester [MN]: Mayo Clinic Scientific Press and Florence [KY]: Informa Healthcare USA; c2008. Chapter 8, The motor system; p. 265–330. Used with permission of Mayo Foundation for Medical Education and Research.)

Table 20.1 • Areas of the Prefrontal Cortex

Area	Function	Dysfunction
Orbitofrontal	Visceral and emotional activity	Disinhibition
Dorsolateral	Executive function (conceptualizing, planning, judgment, problem solving)	Poor judgment and planning Poor abstraction Difficulty with complex sequences or multitasking
Anterior cingulate	Goal-directed behavior and motivation	Apathy Reduced self-awareness

homotypical (unimodal) area of cortex. This area is responsible for voluntary conjugate movement of the eyes independent of visual stimuli. Stimulation of this area results in conjugate eye deviation to the contralateral side. A lesion in this area causes the eyes to deviate toward the side of lesion (opposite paralysis).

Prefrontal Cortex
The prefrontal cortex involves one-quarter of the entire cerebral cortex and includes the lateral, medial, and inferior surfaces of the frontal lobe in front of areas 6 and 45. It includes Brodmann areas 8 through 12, 46, and 47. This cortex is homotypical (heteromodal). The prefrontal cortex is important in the association of motivational cues with complex objects and events. In addition, it aids in integration of sensory and motor functions required in movement initiation and modulation of that response. The prefrontal cortex can be divided into 3 clinically important areas (Table 20.1).

* The primary motor cortex is located in the precentral gyrus (Brodmann area 4, M1).
* The premotor cortex is located on the lateral surface of the cortex just anterior to the precentral gyrus (Brodmann area 6).

Parietal Lobe

Boundaries

The central sulcus divides the frontal and parietal lobes (Figure 20.1). The primary sensory cortex lies in the postcentral gyrus. The posterior border of the parietal lobe is an imaginary line from the parieto-occipital sulcus to the preoccipital notch. Inferiorly, the parietotemporal boundary is roughly at the lateral fissure (sylvian).

Blood Supply

The lateral cortex is supplied by the middle cerebral artery. The medial cortex is supplied by the anterior cerebral artery.

Specific Areas

Primary Somatosensory Cortex
The primary somatosensory cortex is located in the postcentral gyrus and paracentral lobule (Brodmann areas 3, 1, 2; S1). This cortex is idiotypic and functions to receive somatosensory information from the body. The cortex has a somatotopic representation. Stimulation of this area results in contralateral tingling in the area of the body represented. A lesion of this cortex may result in contralateral numbness of the body part represented.

Somatosensory Association Cortex
The somatosensory association cortex extends from the parietal operculum into the posterior insula and includes the superior parietal lobule (Brodmann area 5 and anterior aspect of 7). This area is important for finer aspects of touch localization, synthesis of body schema, and complex somatosensory memories. A lesion of this area often results in tactile agnosia (impaired tactile recognition of objects).

Temporoparietal Area
The temporoparietal area is located at the inferior parietal lobule and area near the superior temporal sulcus, including the angular gyrus (Brodmann area 39), supramarginal gyrus (Brodmann area 40), and caudal superior parietal lobule (Brodmann area 7). This area is considered the homotypic (heteromodal) cortex. This area functions in sensorimotor integration.

* The primary somatosensory cortex is located in the postcentral gyrus and paracentral lobule (Brodmann areas 3, 1, 2; S1).

Temporal Lobe

Boundaries

The temporal lobe is separated from the frontal lobe by the lateral sulcus (Sylvian sulcus). It is composed of the superior, middle, and inferior gyri (Figure 20.1).

Blood Supply

The inferior surface of the temporal lobe is supplied by posterior cerebral artery cortical branches. The lateral surface of the temporal lobe is supplied by the middle cerebral artery.

Specific Areas

Primary Auditory Cortex
The auditory cortex is seated in the transverse gyri of Heschl (Brodmann areas 41 and 42). The primary auditory cortex is the idiotypic cortex, which functions in hearing. At the level of the cortex, a lesion does not result in hearing loss. Rather, a patient might have difficulty recognizing the

distance and direction from which sounds are coming, especially in the ear contralateral to the lesion.

Auditory Association Cortex

The auditory association cortex is located at the caudal one-third of the superior temporal gyrus near the Wernicke area. It is a homotypical (unimodal) cortex. This area functions in auditory processing.

Pure word deafness may result from a bilateral or dominant lesion of this area. A patient may have auditory agnosia for verbal material but can react to environmental sounds (not deaf) and can understand written language. A nondominant lesion may result in difficulty identifying melodies or certain sounds. See also Chapter 23, "Focal Cognitive Syndromes."

Wernicke Area

The Wernicke area is located at the superior temporal gyrus (Brodmann area 22). See Volume 2, Chapter 29, "A Review of Focal Cortical Syndromes," for further details about aphasia.

- The auditory cortex is seated in the transverse gyri of Heschl (Brodmann areas 41 and 42).
- At the level of the cortex, a lesion does not result in hearing loss. Rather, a patient might have difficulty recognizing the distance and direction from which sounds are coming, especially in the ear contralateral to the lesion.

Occipital Lobe

Boundaries

The occipital lobe is separated from the parietal lobe by an imaginary line drawn from the parieto-occipital sulcus down to the pre-occipital notch (Figure 20.1). The calcarine sulcus divides the upper and lower distributions of visual field representation.

Blood Supply

The occipital lobe is supplied by the posterior cerebral artery. The occipital pole (where macular representation exists) also has some supply from the middle cerebral artery, hence the possibility of macular sparing with vascular lesions of the occipital cortex.

Specific Areas

Primary Visual Cortex

The primary visual cortex is located along the calcarine fissure (Brodmann area 17). The cortex contains a visual representation of the contralateral field. Lesions in this region often result in a complete or partial homonymous hemianopsia (see Volume 2, Chapter 45, "Neuro-ophthalmology: Visual Fields").

Visual Association Cortex

The visual association cortex is located in the peristriate areas (Brodmann areas 18 and 19) of the occipital lobe. Some of the visual association cortex extends to the middle and inferior temporal gyri (Brodmann areas 20, 21, and 37). These are homotypical (unimodal) cortical regions. These regions function in complex visual processing, including interpretation of shape, color, size, motion, and orientation. A lesion in the occipitoparietal regions (dorsal stream; "where" pathways) may result in deficits of spatial orientation and depth perception and misjudgment of distance. A lesion of the occipitotemporal regions (ventral stream; "what" pathways) results in deficits of pattern recognition (agnosias) (see Chapter 23, "Focal Cognitive Syndromes").

- The primary visual cortex is located along the calcarine fissure (Brodmann area 17).

Insula

The insula is the portion of cerebral cortex located deeply within the lateral sulcus (Sylvian sulcus). It is part of the paralimbic group connecting the limbic cortex with the neocortex. Primary visceral sensory, taste, and pain information project to the insular cortex. The blood supply is the middle cerebral artery.

- Primary visceral sensory, taste, and pain information project to the insular cortex.

Limbic Lobe

Although, anatomically, the limbic system is not a "lobe," several anatomic structures function in circuitry together. These structures are important in memory and learning, motivation and affect, and processing autonomic information. Additional information on the limbic circuitry is provided in Chapter 22, "Cortical Circuitry, Networks, and Function," and Chapter 16, "The Limbic System."

Components of the limbic lobe include mesocortical structures (cingulate, parahippocampal gyrus, insula, orbitofrontal cortex, retrosplenial regions, and pericallosal region), allocortical structures (hippocampus and piriform/olfactory cortex), and corticoid components (amygdala, septal nuclei, and substantia innominata).

21 Cortex Topography and Organization

RICHARD J. CASELLI, MD; DAVID T. JONES, MD

Introduction

The cerebral cortex functions in a wide variety of simple and complex activities. It is made up of layers of neuronal cell bodies, hence the term *gray matter*. These layers of cell bodies are then organized into gyri (convolutions).

The cortex can be divided into functional components in several different ways. Various schemes exist and may be based on function, cytoarchitecture, topography, or Brodmann areas. The terminology can be confusing because the same area of cortex could be designated by several names. For instance, Brodmann area 17 is also called the primary visual cortex, the striate cortex, and the calcarine cortex. Brodmann designated 52 regions of the cerebral cortex based on cytoarchitecture (Brodmann areas are discussed in Chapter 20, "Cortex: Gross Anatomy.")

Another common scheme based on function and cytoarchitecture includes the following (from least complex to most complex): corticoid, allocortex (limbic), mesocortex (paralimbic), homotypic isocortex (unimodal association and heteromodal association), and idiotypic isocortex (Table 21.1 and Figure 21.1).

Cytoarchitecture and Cortical Organization

Layers of the Cerebral Cortex

The laminar organization of the cortex is the basic structural substrate of cortical functional units at the microcircuit level. The number of layers in the cortex varies by cortex type. Areas such as the hippocampus have only 3 layers, the entorhinal cortex has 3 to 5 layers, and the neocortex (idiotypic isocortex and homotypical isocortex) such as the primary motor cortex contains 6 layers.

Layers of the neocortex are defined in large part by the neuronal cell types they contain; the major distinction is between granular neurons (small, lots of dendrites, specialized for receiving input or sensory function) and pyramidal neurons (large, very long axons, specialized for output or motor function) (Figure 21.2).

Functional Connections of the Cerebral Cortex

Within the neocortex there is regional variability in the presence of these layers and their cellular composition, commonly referred to as the cytoarchitectonics of the region. Pyramidal cell layers are expanded in motor cortices (with the largest neurons in the brain, Betz cells, present in layer 5 of the precentral gyrus), and granular cell layers are expanded in sensory cortices. Isocortex itself is further specialized in primary sensorimotor areas. A primary sensorimotor cortex is monosynaptically connected to a thalamic relay nucleus: visual/lateral geniculate nucleus, auditory/medial geniculate nucleus, somatosensory/ventroposterolateral (limbs) and medial (face) nuclei, and movement/ventrolateral nucleus. Beyond these primary sensorimotor cortices are modality-specific association cortices (each contiguous with its respective primary sensorimotor cortex) and heteromodal association cortices (including the parietal and prefrontal association regions). Association areas also have thalamic inputs, but not from the relay nuclei.

In addition to thalamic connections, there are important cortical connections. For each cortical region there exists a reciprocal connection with its homologous region in the contralateral hemisphere and with its proximate network modules in the ipsilateral hemisphere. Thus, primary somatosensory cortex (postcentral gyrus) has a forward connection to primary motor cortex (precentral gyrus) and a backward connection to modality-specific somatosensory association cortex (superior parietal lobule). Modality-specific somatosensory association cortex has a forward projection to modality-specific motor

Table 21.1 • Functional Organization of the Cortex by Cytoarchitecture

Division	Description	Example
Corticoid	Least differentiated No consistent lamination	Basal forebrain (septal area, diagonal band of Broca, substantia innominata) Amygdaloid complex
Allocortex (limbic)	Three-layered structure	Piriform cortex (primary olfactory cortex) Hippocampus
Mesocortex (paralimbic)	Increase in granular neurons in layers 2 and 4 Increase in myelin Contains 3-6 layers Differentiation of layer 5 from 6	Parahippocampal gyrus Cingulate gyrus Orbitofrontal (caudal) Insula Temporal pole
Homotypic isocortex Heteromodal association	Not confined to a single modality Inputs from unimodal association areas of more than one modality Lesions with complex deficits	Prefrontal (orbitofrontal and dorsolateral prefrontal cortex) Inferior parietal lobule Posteroventral temporal lobe
Unimodal association (modality specific)	Receives input from primary sensory cortex and other unimodal areas of *same* modality Lesions result in specific deficits	Auditory association area (superior temporal gyrus) Visual association area (inferotemporal area)
Idiotypic isocortex	Well-differentiated 6 layers	Primary motor cortex (precentral gyrus) Primary sensory cortex (postcentral gyrus)

association cortex (supplementary motor area) and a backward connection to heteromodal association cortex (posterior parietal lobe). Heteromodal parietal association cortex has a forward projection to prefrontal heteromodal association cortex and a backward connection to paralimbic regions. Similar connection patterns exist for all the modal networks (vision, hearing, motor, balance, and probably more primitive sensory networks for chemoreception [eg, smell and taste]) (Figure 21.3).

The combination of cytoarchitecture, cellular components, thalamocortical and corticocortical connections, and neurochemistry defines regions within the cortical mantle as unique areas and leads to the creation of cortical maps. The most widely used is that of Brodmann. The Brodmann areas representing the primary sensorimotor areas include area 4 (primary motor cortex, precentral gyrus), areas 3, 2, 1 (primary somatosensory cortex, postcentral gyrus), area 17 (primary visual cortex), and areas 41 and 42 (primary

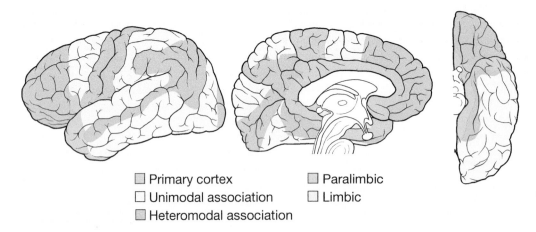

☐ Primary cortex   ☐ Paralimbic
☐ Unimodal association   ☐ Limbic
☐ Heteromodal association

Figure 21.1 Divisions of the Cortex by Cytoarchitecture.
Cytoarchitectonic subdivisions of the lateral, medial, and inferior aspects of the cerebral cortex on the basis of phylogenetic origin, differentiation of cortical layers, and connectivity patterns. Primary cortex, unimodal association cortex, and heteromodal association cortex constitute neocortex.
(Adapted from Grabowski TJ Jr, Anderson SW, Cooper GE. Disorders of cognitive function. Chapter 1, Neural substrates of cognition. Continuum: Lifelong Learn Neurol. 2002 Apr;8[2]:7–40. Used with permission.)

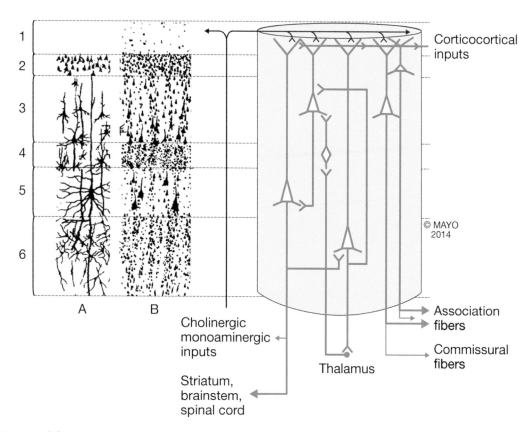

Figure 21.2 Layers of the Neocortex.

Left, Laminar structure of the neocortex as shown with Golgi (A) and Nissl staining (B). This is prototypical 6-layered cortex, as in areas of association cortex. Right, Basic excitatory connectivity pattern within a functional column of neocortex. Input from a thalamic relay nucleus terminates primarily in layer 4, which contains spiny stellate excitatory neurons that project to pyramidal neurons in layers 2 and 3. These neurons project to pyramidal neurons in layer 5, which in turn activate pyramidal neurons in layer 6. These neurons send recurrent excitatory projections to layers 2 and 3. The excitatory interactions within a column are controlled by different types of local interneurons (not shown), which also mediate lateral inhibition of surrounding columns. The apical dendrites of pyramidal cells reach layer 1, where they receive input from other cortical areas, thalamic intralaminar nuclei, and cholinergic and monoaminergic systems of the brainstem, hypothalamus, and basal forebrain. Cortical pyramidal cells give rise to extrinsic connections: layer 2 cells to intrahemispheric corticocortical association fibers, layer 3 cells to interhemispheric commissural fibers, layer 5 cells to corticostriate, corticorubral, corticopontine, corticobulbar, and corticospinal fibers, and layer 6 cells to corticothalamic fibers.

(Adapted from Benarroch EE, Daube JR, Flemming KD, Westmoreland BF. Mayo Clinic medical neurosciences: organized by neurologic systems and levels. 5th ed. Rochester [MN]: Mayo Clinic Scientific Press and Florence [KY]: Informa Healthcare USA; c2008. Chapter 16, Part B, The supratentorial level: telencephalon; p. 701–63. Used with permission of Mayo Foundation for Medical Education and Research.)

auditory cortex). Most studies using brain anatomy use the Brodmann classification scheme, and, depending on the area of inquiry, other regions are often mentioned.

Finally, although poorly understood, there is an important laterality effect such that the left hemisphere in essentially all right-handed persons and in roughly 75% of left-handed persons supports language, whereas the right hemisphere in such cases appears to be dominant for spatial skills. Handedness and language therefore appear to be related, but not absolutely. Some left-handed persons have

mixed language dominance, and a small subset are completely right hemisphere language dominant.

- The number of layers in the cortex varies by cortex type.
- The neocortex (idiotypic isocortex and homotypical isocortex) such as the primary motor cortex contains 6 layers.
- There is a hierarchical processing of information in the cerebral cortex.

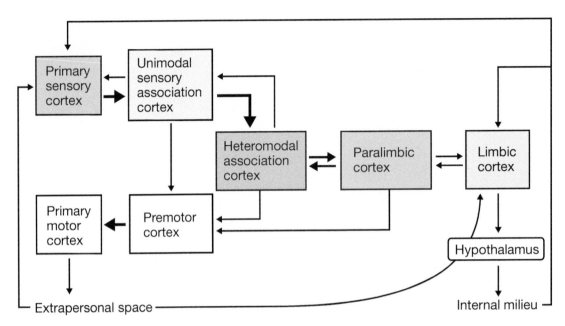

Figure 21.3. Hierarchical Processing of Information in the Cerebral Cortex.
Sensory information is processed serially from primary sensory, to unimodal sensory, to heteromodal sensory association areas in the posterior parietal and lateral temporal cortices. These areas project to both heteromodal association areas of the frontal lobe (prefrontal cortex) and paralimbic areas, which provide input to the hippocampus and amygdala. The prefrontal cortex projects to premotor areas (unimodal motor association areas), which activate primary motor cortex. Note the feedback connections between the paralimbic, heteromodal, and unimodal areas.
(Adapted from Benarroch EE, Daube JR, Flemming KD, Westmoreland BF. Mayo Clinic medical neurosciences: organized by neurologic systems and levels. 5th ed. Rochester [MN]: Mayo Clinic Scientific Press and Florence [KY]: Informa Healthcare USA; c2008. Chapter 16, Part B, The supratentorial level: telencephalon; p. 701–63. Used with permission of Mayo Foundation for Medical Education and Research.)

Anatomic Connections of the Cerebral Cortex

The cerebral cortex receives input from a wide variety of subcortical structures, often connecting via the thalamus and from other areas of the cortex via association fibers. The cortex then projects back to wide regions of the central nervous system including the cortex, thalamus, basal nuclei, cerebellum, brainstem, and cord. The types of fibers connecting areas of the central nervous system are designated based on regions they connect. For instance, the fibers connecting the cortex to subcortical structures are called projection fibers. The fibers connecting 1 hemisphere to the opposite hemisphere are called callosal fibers, and the fibers connecting areas within the same hemisphere are called association fibers. Fibers connecting the cortex to the thalamus are designated corticothalamic.

22

Cortical Circuitry, Networks, and Function

DAVID T. JONES, MD

Introduction

Functional magnetic resonance imaging has revolutionized the understanding of the functional and structural architecture of the brain and serves as the lens through which we will review this complex system. This chapter reviews cortical circuitry and networks of the cerebral cortex.

Multiscale Organization

The human brain is a complex information processing system whose proper functioning depends on the organization of its processing units. The scale of these processing units spans multiple levels from the genetic to systems level (Figure 22.1). A complete understanding of any 1 of these levels necessitates understanding each level because they are interdependent. For example, the genetic expression of a signal neuron determines the protein composition of that neuron, which, in turn, influences its firing pattern within a microcircuit. Microcircuits form local circuits that interact to form larger regional circuits and eventually influence systems-level–distributed neural networks that are more closely associated with behavioral interactions with the environment.

However, the direction of this system's causal influence also extends in the reverse direction, in that the organization of distributed neural networks changes in response to environmental inputs. Thus, the firing pattern of neurons within circuits changes, which leads to a change in the genetic expression within individual neurons in order to optimally respond to this new firing pattern. The complex interaction between these various levels is typically summarized as an interaction between genes and environment. At any point in time, it is impossible to know every piece of information necessary to fully characterize the complexity within these systems. However, general principles of this multiscale organization are emerging via interdisciplinary investigations of complex adaptive systems. This early work has shown that hierarchical, modular, and scale-free network dynamics characterize the brain's complex organization at all scales. These principles can be more easily characterized and used to understand the brain in health and disease.

A discussion of these complex network principles is beyond the scope of this chapter, but the structural, functional, and behavioral aspects of this multiscale system are reviewed in more detail. The interaction of 2 neurons is the smallest possible functional unit at the cellular level in the brain's information processing network. However, the basic structural unit supporting any 2 neurons' functional interaction extends to a supporting astrocyte and the vascular endothelium. Therefore, the basic bipartite functional unit (ie, 2 neurons) is supported by a basic tripartite structural unit (ie, neuron, astrocyte, and a vascular endothelial cell). This structural-functional relationship leads to the phenomena of neurovascular coupling that is the basis of the blood oxygenation level–dependent (BOLD) signal used in functional magnetic resonance imaging experiments. Neurovascular coupling related to this bipartite functional and tripartite structural arrangement allows for the identification of regions of the brain that are functionally connected at the systems level. These BOLD-derived functional connectivity maps are used throughout this chapter to illustrate the anatomic locations of these systems-level functional interactions. The relationship

Abbreviations: aDMN, anterior DMN; BOLD, blood oxygenation level–dependent; DMN, default mode network; pDMN, posterior DMN; vDMN, ventral DMN

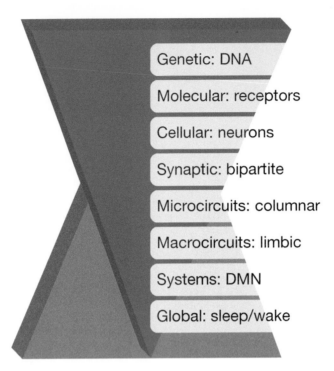

Figure 22.1 Bidirectional Hierarchical Multiscale Organization of the Brain. DMN indicates default mode network.

between the various functional and structural units across the brain's multiscale organization becomes increasingly complex at higher levels.

The laminar organization of the cortex is the basic structural substrate of cortical functional units at the microcircuit level. The cerebral cortex is composed of 6 possible cortical layers, with regional variability in the presence of these layers and their cellular composition, commonly referred to as the cytoarchitectonics of the region (see Chapter 21, "Cortex Topography and Organization").

- The basic bipartite functional unit (ie, 2 neurons) is supported by a basic tripartite structural unit (ie, neuron, astrocyte, and a vascular endothelial cell). This structural-functional relationship leads to the phenomena of neurovascular coupling that is the basis of the blood oxygenation level–dependent (BOLD) signal used in functional magnetic resonance imaging experiments. Neurovascular coupling related to this bipartite functional and tripartite structural arrangement allows for the identification of regions of the brain that are functionally connected at the systems level.

Anterior and Posterior Limbic Circuits: Emotion and Memory

The structures involved in the anterior and posterior limbic systems are evolutionarily primitive, which speaks to their critical role in fundamental aspects of behavior, with higher neocortical functions arising with the need to modulate these primitive circuits. The brain evolved only once in evolutionary history, and all subsequent organisms with nervous systems share a common ancestor. Bilaterally symmetric mobile muticellular organisms driven to interact with the extrapersonal environment first developed a primitive olfactory sensory system in order to efficiently guide movements to sources of sustenance. The circuitry involved in coordinating this driven behavior evolved into the anterior limbic circuit. The anterior limbic circuit is involved in coordinating motivational drives (eg, hunger, thirst, procreation, emotion), and complex cognitive processes and motor plans satisfy those drives through certain behaviors. This function is modulated by the current sensory information being processed in this circuit and the organism's previous experience with these inputs (ie, memory). More complex memory-related modulation of behavioral responses is accomplished through the semantic, visual-spatial, and autobiographic memory processes mediated by the posterior limbic circuit. The function of these circuits has led to the tight association of the limbic system with emotion, cognition, and memory.

The connections between the nidus of the anterior limbic circuit (ie, the amygdala) and sensory processes are bidirectional, and ongoing sensory information influences anterior limbic activity and limbic activity also influences sensory processing. This interaction is true for all major sensory domains (ie, extrapersonal, personal, and intrapersonal). There also exists a similar bidirectional interaction

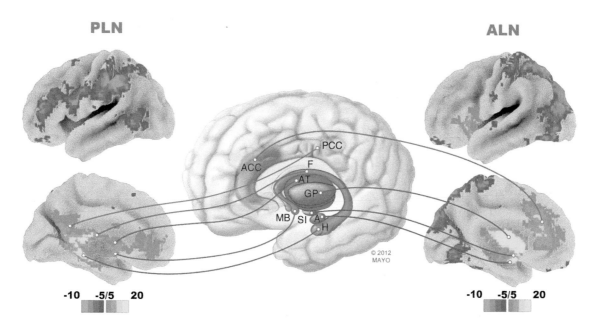

Figure 22.2 *Functional Connectivity of the Posterior and Anterior Limbic Circuits.*
Key regions of the anterior (purple) and posterior (cyan) limbic circuit are highlighted in the center illustration. These include the anterior cingulated cortex (ACC), globus pallidus (GP), substantia inominata (SI), and amygdala (A) in the anterior limbic circuit and the posterior cingulated cortex (PCC), hippocampal formation (H), fornix (F), mammillary bodies (MB), and anterior thalamic nucleus (AT) for the posterior limbic circuit. Regions of positive (yellow) and negative (blue) functional connectivity within these systems are shown on surface renderings highlighting these structures. The color bars encode the strength of connectivity, with red being the strongest and purple the weakest. ALN indicates anterior limbic circuit; PLN, posterior limbic circuit.
(Used with permission of Mayo Foundation for Medical Education and Research.)

between the amygdala and the nidus of the posterior limbic circuit (ie, the hippocampus). The information in the anterior and posterior limbic circuits is integrated not only by the reciprocal connections between the amygdala and the hippocampus but also by subcortical-cortical loops that interact in the cingulate gyrus to connect these 2 pathways via the cingulate fasciculus (Figure 22.2). The details of the posterior limbic circuit and its associated neocortical systems are discussed in detail below, followed by the neocortical associations of the anterior limbic system.

The classic circuit of Papez constitutes the major posterior limbic subcortical-cortical loop. Hippocampal outputs from the subiculum travel via the fornix to the mammillary bodies then via the mammillothalamic tract to the anterior nucleus of the thalamus, which sends efferents to the cingulate gyrus (see Chapter 16, "The Limbic System"). From here the information can be integrated with anterior circuit activity in the anterior cingulate via the cingulate fasciculus, travel to the precuneus or other posterior association cortices, or return to the hippocampus via the cingulum bundle. Lesions anywhere along this circuit may impair new memory formation for autobiographic events, semantic knowledge, or visual-spatial information. The extent to which these symptoms are present depends on how much

the posterior limbic system's interaction with particular distributed neural systems is disrupted. Symptoms related to disruption of posterior limbic-related activity are prominent in Korsakoff syndrome, typical Alzheimer dementia, and Alzheimer dementia variants such as posterior cortical atrophy.

- The anterior limbic circuit is involved in coordinating motivational drives (eg, hunger, thirst, procreation, emotion), and complex cognitive processes and motor plans satisfy those drives through certain behaviors.
- Complex memory-related modulation of behavioral responses is accomplished through the semantic, visual-spatial, and autobiographic memory processes mediated by the posterior limbic circuit.
- Lesions anywhere along the posterior limbic circuit may impair new memory formation for autobiographic events, semantic knowledge, or visual-spatial information.

Posterior Neocortical Networks

The major distributed neural networks in posterior neocortical regions support visuospatial processing and object

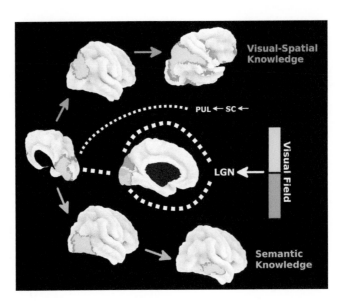

Figure 22.3 Visual Processing.
Information in the visual field is initially processed by the structures within the eye and the optic nerve, which form the optic tract. The optic tract sends the majority of this information to the lateral geniculate nucleus (LGN), which sends information to the occipital lobe via geniculostriate projections. Inferior visual field information travels dorsally through the parietal lobe via Baum's loop (upper thick-dashed line), and superior visual field information travels ventrally through the temporal lobe via Meyer's loop (lower thick-dashed line). Lesions to Meyer's loop cause a superior quadrantanopia. A minority of information from the optic tract reaches primary and secondary cortical visual processing areas via projections to the superior colliculus (SC), which then projects to the pulvinar nucleus of the thalamus (PUL) before arriving in cortical visual areas (thin-dashed line). This PUL-mediated pathway for information from the visual field may be preserved independent of damage to LGN information, which may relate to rare phenomena such as "blindsight" and Anton syndrome. The dorsal stream (blue arrows) is chiefly responsible for producing visual-spatial knowledge from visual information, and the ventral stream (pink arrows) produces semantic knowledge from visual information. Dorsal stream–related clinical correlates include the triad of Balint syndrome (optic ataxia, oculomotor apraxia, and simultanagnosia). Ventral stream–related clinical correlates include alexia, cerebral achromatopsia, prosopagnosia, and other visual agnosias. The cortical regions shown are from 7 networks of functional connectivity related to visual processing identified in 892 participants in the Mayo Clinic Study of Aging.

recognition. Traditionally, these 2 separate functions have been conceptually divided into 2 linear hierarchically organized pathways (ie, the ventral "what" and dorsal "where" streams of processing). Although this concept is unlikely to be entirely accurate, given that the dynamics supporting these functions are highly parallel, reentrant, and diffusely distributed, the linear 2-pathway model in which successively more complex properties (eg, categorical membership) are added to more rudimentary attributes (eg, shape and color) is still a useful conceptualization for relating function to neocortical regions (Figure 22.3).

Neocortical visual processing begins in the primary visual cortex area of the occipital lobe (V1 or BA 17), which contains retinotopically organized neurons receiving information from magnocellular and parvocellular pathways emanating from the ipsilateral lateral geniculate nucleus of the thalamus. These V1 neurons are sensitive to edges, movement, length, binocular disparity, luminance, and wavelength of stimulus. Modular and columnar organization of these neurons becomes preferentially sensitive to orientation, movement, stereopsis, or color.

The next step in visual processing takes place in the peristriate cortex or visual unimodal association cortex (orange and blue regions in Figure 22.3). Perception of color and motion begins in V1 and V2 and becomes progressively more developed in V4 and V5. Color and shape processing in V4 (lateral and ventral occipitotemporal cortex) serve as the relay station for the ventral object recognition processing stream, or the "what" pathway, which extends into the ventromedial and polar regions of the temporal lobe. Object location and movement processing in V5/MT (middle temporal cortex) serve as the relay station for the dorsal visuospatial processing stream, or the "where" pathway, which extends into the posterior parietal cortex and then to medial and superior parietal regions. The superior parietal and intraparietal sulcal portions of the dorsal stream (top right surface rendering in Figure 22.3) are functionally connected to the premotor cortex, and there are particularly strong connections between this region and the frontal eye fields (BA 8). This posterior-to-anterior connection is especially important to coordinate hand and eye movements directed toward the environment using visual-spatial knowledge. As a result, this system is sometimes referred to as the dorsal attention network, because hand-eye coordination and eye movements directed toward the external environment are accompanied by attentional shifts toward the external environment (see the discussion of executive networks below for more details).

- The major distributed neural networks in posterior neocortical regions support visuospatial processing and object recognition.

Anterior Neocortical Networks

The anterior limbic circuitry involved in the coordination of anterior neocortical networks includes interactions between the amygdala, limbic-basal-ganglia regions, medial dorsal nucleus of the thalamus, and the anterior cingulate cortex (Figure 22.2). The amygdala projects to the ventromedial parts of the striatum (limbic striatum), including the nucleus accumbens, medial edge of the caudate nucleus, and ventral part of the putamen. The limbic striatum projects to the ventral palladium and rostral globus pallidus. The anterior limbic-basal ganglia and the amygdala have projections to the medial dorsal nucleus of the thalamus. The medial dorsal nucleus of the thalamus, in turn, has reciprocal connections with the orbitofrontal, prefrontal, anterior cingulate, and anterior insular cortices. This pathway is the basic cortical-subcortical circuitry, which coordinates activity in the anterior neocortical networks. The dopaminergic input to the limbic basal ganglia comes from the ventral tegmental area, in contrast to the dopaminergic projections from the substantia nigra to motor and premotor-related basal ganglia structures. These striatonigrostriatal pathways form an ascending spiral pattern of connectivity that maintains a phrenotopic pattern of organization (Figure 22.4). In other words, the regions of the frontal lobe that interact with the initiation of the ascending spiral subserve cognitive processes most distal to a final behavioral motor response.

For example, primitive behavioral drives related to feeding behavior and emotions are located in the orbitofrontal cortex. They influence the selection or suppression of higher order drives related to social cognition in the dorsal prefrontal regions, which interact with the next step up in the ascending spiral. Ultimately, a behavioral response is determined after integration in anterior cingulate regions and then initiates the final output via interactions with premotor and motor regions. A disconnection between behavioral drives and motor plans may occur with lesions

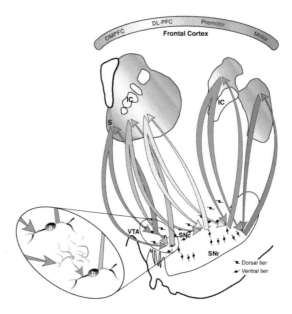

Figure 22.4 *Hierarchical Organization of the Striatonigrostriatal Pathways and Their Relationship to the Frontal Lobe.*

The a indicates the inhibitory circuit; b, disinhibitory circuit; DL-PFC, dorsolateral prefrontal cortex; IC, inferior colliculus; OMPFC, orbital and medial prefrontal cortex; S, striatum; SNc, substantia nigra pars compacta; SNr, substantia nigra pars reticulata; VTA, ventral tegmental area.

(Adapted from Haber SN, Fudge JL, McFarland NR. Striatonigrostriatal pathways in primates form an ascending spiral from the shell to the dorsolateral striatum. J Neurosci. 2000 Mar 15;20(6):2369–82. Used with permission.)

to the anterior cingulate, resulting in abulia or akinetic mutism in severe cases.

- Primitive behavioral drives related to feeding behavior and emotions are located in the orbitofrontal cortex. They influence the selection or suppression of higher order drives related to social cognition in the dorsal prefrontal regions, which interact with the next step up in the ascending spiral. Ultimately, a behavioral response is determined after integration in anterior cingulate regions and then initiates the final output via interactions with premotor and motor regions. A disconnection between behavioral drives and motor plans may occur with lesions to the anterior cingulate, resulting in abulia or akinetic mutism in severe cases.

Default Mode Network

The default mode network (DMN) is a distributed neural network comprised of heteromodal association cortices. The exact function of this system is an ongoing area of

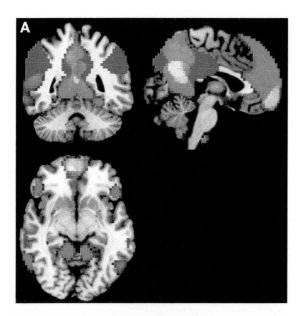

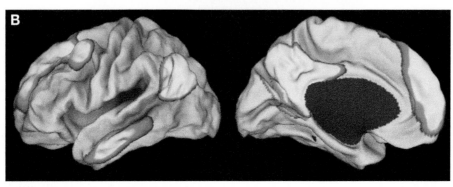

Figure 22.5 Default Mode Network (DMN).
The DMN is shown on brain-surface renderings highlighting typical regions involved in this distributed system. The regions commonly described as participating in the DMN include the posterior cingulate, precuneus, lateral parietal (angular gyrus), middle/anterior temporal, and medial prefrontal cortices.

investigation given its relatively recent discovery, but some general principles related to its function are emerging. The regions of the brain that belong to the DMN were first identified in experiments using functional neuroimaging techniques (eg, positron emission tomography and functional magnetic resonance imaging), but more recently they have been investigated using direct measures of electrophysiology (eg, magnetoencephalography, electroencephalography, and corticography). The regions first reported to belong to the DMN were identified by regions that deactivated (ie, became less metabolically active or decreased BOLD signal) during active tasks relative to a passive resting baseline. These regions include the posterior cingulate, precuneus, lateral parietal, middle/anterior temporal, and medial prefrontal cortices (Figure 22.5). These regions also show high levels of basal metabolic activity relative to the rest of the brain and maintain a high level of continuous functional connectivity. However, the magnitude and spatial arrangement of

the relationship between the functional connectivity within this system and other regions of the brain are dynamic and modulated by cognitive state. The relationship is significantly weakened in impaired states of consciousness (eg, anesthesia, coma, persistent vegetative state, and minimally conscious state) and absent in brain death (Figure 22.6).

Some theories of the function of the DMN revolve around the intrinsic baseline organization of the brain, which maintains a continuous background level of synchrony, allowing the system to optimally respond to and predict ever-changing environmental demands. This intrinsic background, or default state, is most apparent in the intrinsic organization of the DMN. Although it appears to be true that there is an intrinsic organization to the dynamic complex information processing network of the brain, it does not necessarily need to be the case that it is housed within specific heteromodal association cortices. Rather, it is likely intrinsic to the entire system as a whole.

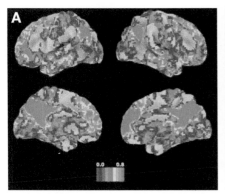 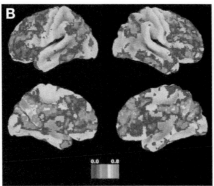 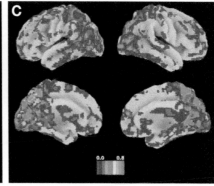

Figure 22.6 Default Mode Network (DMN) in Various States of Consciousness.
The functional connectivity within the DMN is displayed on surface renderings for a state of normal wakefulness (A),
minimally conscious state (B), and persistent vegetative state (C). The color bars encode the strength of connectivity, with
red being the strongest and purple the weakest. The connectivity within the DMN is strong in the fully conscious state and
impaired in the minimally conscious state; there is almost complete absence of the systems-level organization of the DMN
in the persistent vegetative state.

The DMN does not uniformly deactivate during all cognitive tasks. Several cognitive paradigms induced significant increases in activity in regions of the DMN. These tasks involve social cognition, theory of mind, mind wandering, autobiographic memory, and mental projection of the self into the past and future. These processes all require an integration of information that is organized by aspects of the posterior and anterior neocortical networks described above. It appears that there are multiple subsystems within the DMN that support different aspects of these cognitive functions.

A core posterior DMN (pDMN) system involving the precuneus, posterior cingulate cortex, and medial prefrontal cortex is important for the perception of integrated anterior and posterior network information and dynamically associates with many different systems. An anterior DMN (aDMN) system centered on the dorsal medial prefrontal cortex is related to mentation requiring a representation of a cognitive, emotional, or social self. A ventral DMN (vDMN), centered on posterior medial temporal lobe structures and the restrosplenial posterior cingulate cortex, is important for mnemonic processes requiring scene construction. Recalling and encoding the majority of autobiographic memories requires an interaction between the perceptual core pDMN, self-information (cognitive, emotional, or social) from the aDMN, and the mnemonic scene construction attributes of the vDMN. Neurodegenerative disease may selectively impair certain aspects of these interacting systems more than others. For example, typical Alzheimer disease has a predilection for damaging medial temporal lobe structures that relate to the impairment in posterior cingulate and temporoparietal function. This leads to a disturbance in vDMN-related mnemonic scene construction and pDMN perceptual integration that typically manifests as impaired autobiographic memory and

poor spatial navigational abilities. Executive processes mediated by other frontoparietal systems are also important for high-level integration of anterior and posterior information. These executive processes include attention and working memory, which are discussed in the next section.

- The default mode network (DMN) is a distributed neural network comprised of heteromodal association cortices.
- The DMN regions include the posterior cingulate, precuneus, lateral parietal, middle/anterior temporal, and medial prefrontal cortices (Figure 22.5).
- Theories of the function of the DMN revolve around the intrinsic baseline organization of the brain, which maintains a continuous background level of synchrony, allowing the system to optimally respond to and predict ever-changing environmental demands.
- It appears that there are multiple subsystems within the DMN that support different aspects of these cognitive functions.

Executive Networks

The executive faculty of attention involves high-level distributed neural systems biasing the ongoing lower-level processing of cognitive, affective, perceptual, and behavioral information, making certain features more likely to influence the brain's ongoing activity. Attentional processes are traditionally conceptualized as being directed by either top-down or bottom-up dynamics. Top-down influence involves attentional biasing of information processing to support the higher-order faculties related to cognitive processes such as goal-directed behavior. Alternatively, bottom-up influence involves perceptual information

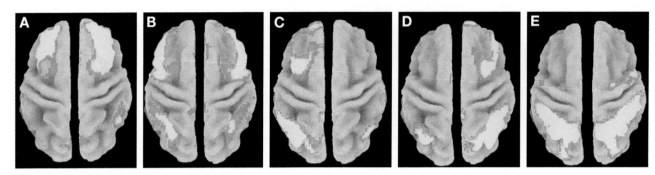

Figure 22.7 *Frontal and Parietal Networks Supporting Executive Processes.*
Shown are the salience network (A), attention network (B), left working memory network (C), right working memory network (D), and dorsal attention network (E). The cortical regions shown are from 5 networks of functional connectivity related to executive processing identified in 892 participants in the Mayo Clinic Study of Aging.

redirecting attention. The executive faculty of working memory involves sustaining certain features being biased by attentional processes for longer periods and allowing them to be manipulated by higher-order cognitive processes. Performing cognitive, affective, perceptual, and behavioral tasks optimally requires varying degrees of attentional and working memory resources. Distributed neural networks spanning heteromodal association cortices in the frontal and parietal lobes are ideally positioned to perform these executive functions for all of these various tasks (Figure 22.7).

Functional imaging experiments, in which subjects are directed to perform a particular task, activate these systems to varying degrees, depending on the informational content required for the task and the task difficulty. Hence, these regions have been referred to as the task-positive network. The regions in the task-positive network are inversely synchronized or anticorrelated with the DMN (task-negative network) if brain activity is averaged over many tasks or subjects. However, depending on the task relevance of the information within task-negative network subsystems, regions of the task-negative network and the task-positive network likely will be strongly correlated for a time.

Executive functions involving mainly perceptual processes are chiefly supported by parietal lobe structures. The intraparietal sulcus and superior parietal lobe with strong frontal eye field connections (Figure 22.7E) support attention processes related to visual-spatial and intrapersonal perceptual and behavioral activities. In contrast, the dorsal lateral prefrontal, anterior prefrontal, fronto-insular, and dorsal anterior cingulate regions (Figure 22.7A) support executive processes relating to cognitive, homeostatic, or affective activities.

- Distributed neural networks spanning heteromodal association cortices in the frontal and parietal lobes are ideally positioned to perform executive functions for cognitive, affective, perceptual, and behavioral tasks.

23 Focal Cognitive Syndromes[a]

RICHARD J. CASELLI, MD

Introduction

The neurologic results of cortical lesions reflect the structural properties of the affected region. Lesions affecting primary sensorimotor cortices result in primary sensorimotor deficits that are qualitatively all-or-nothing, such as blindness (hemianopia) and paralysis (hemiparesis). Quantitatively, though, the severity of the deficit depends on the extent of the lesion (so that a hemiparetic patient may not be completely paralyzed but simply weak). Lesions affecting modality-specific association regions result in conceptually more complex disorders that are confined to a single modality, such as nonfluent aphasia (a form of motor speech disorder reflecting the language-dominant hemisphere) or prosopagnosia (a visual disorder impairing the ability to disambiguate visually similar entities, specifically faces, reflecting the "what" visual pathway in inferotemporal cortices).

This chapter reviews clinical cortical syndromes. Clinical behavioral disorders are covered in Volume 2, Section V: "Behavioral Neurology."

Aphasia

The Boston classification (Table 23.1), first proposed in the 1960s, is still used today despite the gradual erosion of the clinically defined boundaries that distinguish the various aphasic syndromes.

Nonfluent Aphasia

Broca Aphasia

Patients with classic Broca aphasia have impaired fluency, repetition, and severe phonemic paraphasias. A phonemic paraphasia reflects the correct semantic target, but the phonemes constituting the word are wrong (eg, *helichopper* for *helicopter*). There is relative preservation of comprehension, although prepositions (and the relationship of various parts of sentences) may be impaired. In patients with Broca aphasia, the lesion is typically in the language-dominant (typically left) frontal operculum (a motor association cortex), also known as the Broca area or as Brodmann areas 44 and 45 (Figure 23.1).

Transcortical Motor Aphasia

Transcortical motor aphasia resembles Broca aphasia except that repetition is preserved. This is usually due to damage surrounding the Broca area in a vascular watershed zone.

Fluent Aphasia

Wernicke Aphasia

Classic Wernicke aphasia results from a lesion in the language-dominant posterior superior temporal gyrus (auditory association cortex adjacent to the primary auditory cortex), which is called the Wernicke area or Brodmann area 22 (posterior portion) (Figure 23.1). Wernicke aphasia is characterized by impaired comprehension, impaired repetition, and agrammatic, semantic, and phonemic paraphasias. Patients with semantic paraphasias use the wrong word, but typically the word is within the correct category or is a supraordinate term. For example, *wrench* is an intracategorical semantic error for *pliers; tool* or *thing* is a supraordinate term.

Transcortical Sensory Aphasia

Transcortical sensory aphasia resembles Wernicke aphasia but is typically less severe, and repetition is preserved. This is usually due to damage surrounding the Wernicke area or the watershed zone (vascular mechanism).

---

[a] Portions previously published in Caselli RJ. Creativity: an organizational schema. Cogn Behav Neurol. 2009 Sep;22(3):143–54. Used with permission.

Abbreviation: VTA, ventral tegmental area

Table 23.1 • Major Aphasia Syndromes of the (Usually) Left Hemisphere

Type of Aphasia	Fluency	Comprehension	Repetition	Naming	Localization
Broca	Severe	Mild	Severe	Phonemic errors	Frontal operculum (Broca area)
Wernicke	Intact	Severe	Severe	Semantic errors	Posterior superior temporal (Wernicke area)
Conduction	Intact or mild	Intact or mild	Severe	Varies	Arcuate fasciculus or insula
Global	Severe	Severe	Severe	Severe	Entire MCA territory
Transcortical motor	Severe	Intact	Intact	Phonemic errors	Frontal lobe watershed area
Transcortical sensory	Intact	Severe	Intact	Semantic errors	Parietal lobe watershed area
Isolation of the speech area	Severe	Severe	Intact	Severe	MCA watershed area
Anomic	Intact	Intact	Intact	Semantic errors	Anterior temporal cortex (not part of the Boston classification) Inferior parietal lobe (Boston classification)

Abbreviation: MCA, middle cerebral artery.

Conduction Aphasia

Conduction aphasia results from damage to the insula and underlying white matter (arcuate fasciculus). Affected patients have impaired repetition with preserved fluency and comprehension.

Anomic Aphasia

Anomic asphasia is characterized by impaired naming with preserved fluency, comprehension, and repetition. It occurs as a primary defect, not as the residual of a more severe form of aphasia (naming is impaired in essentially all aphasic syndromes, but it occurs less commonly in isolation). Localization in the language-dominant anterior temporal lobe is the most frequent cause overall. This type of aphasia is most often seen as a degenerative syndrome (as a subtype of frontotemporal lobar degeneration or semantic variant frontotemporal dementia). Within the Boston classification, inferior parietal lesions are thought to cause anomic aphasia, typically within the

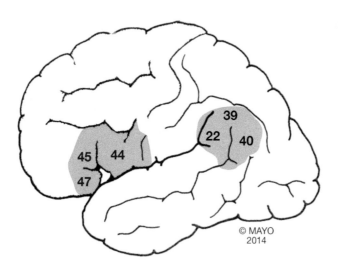

© MAYO 2014

Figure 23.1 *Localization of Broca Aphasia and Wernicke Aphasia.*
Both the Wernicke area (gray shading) and the Broca area (red shading) are functionally heterogeneous. The Wernicke area is a convergence zone that connects word forms, word meanings, and association between words with other knowledge about objects and concepts. The Broca area contains separate regions involved in semantic, syntactic, and phonologic processing and in articulation.

(Adapted from Benarroch EE. Basic neurosciences with clinical applications. Philadelphia [PA]: Butterworth Heinemann/Elsevier; c2006. Chapter 25, Cortical networks for object recognition, language, attention, and executive control of behavior; p. 913–51. Used by permission of Mayo Foundation for Medical Education and Research.)

context of other deficits of the angular gyrus or Gerstmann syndrome.

Global Aphasia

Global aphasia results in severe impairment of all language functions, including fluency, comprehension, and repetition. The transcortical equivalent is isolation of the speech area, another watershed infarction-based lesion sparing the arcuate fasciculus so that patients echo what they hear without comprehension and offer little spontaneous or fluent output.

Alexia and Agraphia

Surface Dyslexia

Patients who have surface dyslexia lose whole-word recognition and must sound out words (particularly irregular words such as *yacht*). The process is similar to the way a child first learns to read.

Phonologic Dyslexia

Patients who have phonologic dyslexia lose the ability to sound out words and must read at the whole-word level. They have difficulty reading nonwords (eg, *floink*) and distinguishing between visually similar words (eg, *tablet* and *table*). Localization is commonly the area of the superior temporal gyrus, inferior parietal lobe, and supramarginal gyrus.

Deep Dyslexia

A patient with deep dyslexia reads or speaks with categorically relevant semantic errors (eg, *castle* for *knight*).

Aphasic and Apraxic Agraphia (and Micrographia)

Patients with aphasic or apraxic agraphia or micrographia have difficulty writing and spelling. Aphasic agraphia is primarily a language disorder in which spelling is often impaired even without writing. Apraxic agraphia is primarily a spatial or movement disorder in which spelling may be preserved when spoken, yet the patient cannot correctly write the letters.

Alexia Without Agraphia

Alexia without agraphia was initially described as a disconnection syndrome in a patient with a lesion damaging the left occipital lobe (causing a right homonymous hemianopia and thus allowing no direct connection within the left hemisphere between visual and comprehension regions) and corpus callosum (thus disconnecting the right visual cortex from the left hemisphere comprehension area). This is the classic description. However, this syndrome is probably more commonly produced by a lesion affecting the left (language-dominant) inferior temporal cortex (the "what" pathway in the verbal hemisphere; Brodmann area 37).

Alexia with agraphia is far more common. It reflects a more pervasive language deficit and is most often associated with the left inferior parietal lobe as part of Gerstmann syndrome, but it may occur without its other elements.

Subcortical Aphasia

Aphasia may develop in patients with thalamic and basal ganglia lesions. In the case of thalamic aphasia, the likely explanation is an acute deafferentation (loss of thalamic input) of overlying perisylvian language cortices. Acutely this resembles a mixed aphasia and can be quite severe. The specific thalamic nucleus involved appears to include the motor relay nucleus (ie, the ventral lateral nucleus). Aphasia with basal ganglia lesions is typically nonfluent, and there is continued debate as to the origin of the problem—that is, whether this is truly a basal ganglia disorder or is instead due to involvement of the overlying cortices.

- Patients with classic Broca aphasia have impaired fluency, repetition, and severe phonemic paraphasias.
- In patients with Broca aphasia, the lesion is typically in the language-dominant (typically left) frontal operculum (a motor association cortex), also known as the Broca area or as Brodmann areas 44 and 45.
- Classic Wernicke aphasia results from a lesion in the language-dominant posterior superior temporal gyrus. Wernicke aphasia is characterized by impaired comprehension, impaired repetition, and agrammatic, semantic, and phonemic paraphasias.
- Alexia without agraphia was initially described as a disconnection syndrome in a patient with a lesion damaging the left occipital lobe (causing a right homonymous hemianopia and thus allowing no direct connection within the left hemisphere between visual and comprehension regions) and corpus callosum (thus disconnecting the right visual cortex from the left hemisphere comprehension area).

Apraxia

Apraxia has been used often to describe the inability to perform certain tasks when no other explanation was obvious (eg, sensory or motor loss of function).

Ideomotor Apraxia

Ideomotor apraxia refers to disordered motor programming resulting in the inability to perform a skilled movement. The inability is not proportional to weakness, sensory loss, ataxia, or other more basic type of movement disturbance.

Ideomotor apraxia can result from lesions of the motor association cortex (supplementary motor area; medial

Brodmann area 6) and parietal lobe (Brodmann areas 5 and 7, monosynaptically connected to the motor association cortex). A left supplementary motor area infarction from anterior cerebral artery ischemia causes more severe impairment of the contralateral limbs, so that the apraxic deficit is more severe when tasks are carried out with the right hand than with the left hand, but even left-hand performance is impaired.

Degenerative causes include corticobasal ganglionic degeneration and its mimics; magnetic resonance imaging shows profound parietal atrophy. Because degenerative diseases are almost never strictly unilateral, ideomotor apraxia can result from a degenerative lesion on either side of the brain but typically is more severe when the degenerative atrophy is more pronounced in the left hemisphere.

Limb Kinetic Apraxia

Limb kinetic apraxia refers to loss of fine-movement dexterity, typically within the context of hemiparesis. It often occurs with corticospinal tract lesions.

Ideational Apraxia

Ideational apraxia is a semantic paraphasia for movement—that is, substitution of 1 form of movement for another. For example, if asked to pantomime the use of a screwdriver, the patient pantomimes the use of a hammer instead.

Other (Task-Specific) Apraxia

Task-specific apraxias may occur with various diseases, most commonly degenerative diseases. Dressing apraxia, constructional apraxia, and agraphia are examples. Gait apraxia is not a true apraxia, but simply a form of magnetic gait that is thought to be characteristic of normal-pressure hydrocephalus. It resembles the shuffling gait of parkinsonism (but patients lack other parkinsonian features) and is thought to reflect compression of, or damage to, frontal white matter. A similar form of gait disorder may develop in patients with extensive frontal white matter disease for other reasons.

- *Apraxia* has been used often to describe the inability to perform certain tasks when no other explanation was obvious.
- Ideomotor apraxia can result from lesions of the motor association cortex (supplementary motor area; medial Brodmann area 6) and parietal lobe (Brodmann areas 5 and 7, monosynaptically connected to the motor association cortex).

Agnosia

Agnosia is the inability to recognize objects, people, sounds, or smells despite intact sensation. Older literature distinguishes between apperceptive and associative agnosia, at least for visually based agnosia, but the apperceptive form is not really an agnostic disturbance, as discussed below.

Visual Agnosia

Visual cortices include the primary visual cortex (Brodmann area 17, striate cortex, and calcarine cortex) and modality-specific visual association cortices, including the dorsal occipitoparietal and ventral occipitotemporal streams (Figure 23.2).

Occipitotemporal Stream (the "What" Pathway)

Damage to the occipitotemporal stream (the "what" pathway) of the cortical visual network leads to true agnostic disturbances in which stimuli are perceived but not fully understood. Left occipitotemporal infarctions cause alexia, an inability to read a correctly perceived word. Right occipitotemporal infarctions impair the ability to distinguish familiar faces, a condition termed prosopagnosia. It is contested whether unilateral right lesions are sufficient, and it has been shown that patients with prosopagnosia due to stroke typically have bilateral occipitotemporal damage. By far, however, a more common cause is neurodegenerative disease, such as the right temporal variant of semantic variant frontotemporal dementia. Affected patients typically have asymmetrically greater atrophy of the right anterior temporal lobe than the left, but some degree of atrophy is present bilaterally and likely extends posteriorly into the salient visual association areas (anatomical localization can only be estimated in degenerative cases because of the noncircumscribed nature of the offending lesions).

Occipitoparietal Stream (the "Where" Pathway)

Bilateral superior parietal lobe damage causes asimultanagnosia, which is the inability to compute the simultaneity of a complex visual scene in space and time or to effectively scan the environment. Balint syndrome consists of asimultanagnosia with the additional elements of optic ataxia (impaired visually guided reaching) and ocular apraxia (the inability to voluntarily fixate gaze on a visual target), although the optic ataxia and ocular apraxia are the consequence of asimultanagnosia. Asimultanagnosia is an apperceptive agnosia—that is, it is more of a problem with perception than with comprehending what is perceived. Patients gaze at a visual scene and have difficulty finding targets. They have lost the ability to integrate the many parts of a scene into a coherent whole and cannot search normally for the target of interest, so that they appear functionally blind. However, when they do encounter what they are seeking, they can see it and comprehend it.

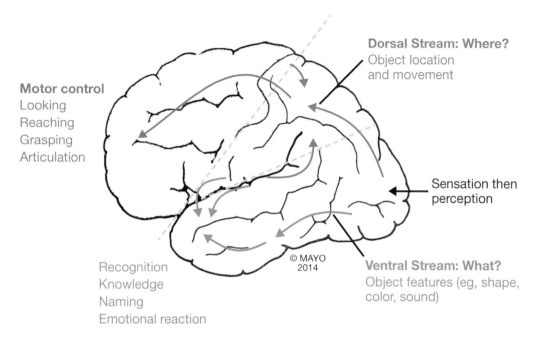

Motor control
Looking
Reaching
Grasping
Articulation

Dorsal Stream: Where?
Object location
and movement

Sensation then
perception

Recognition
Knowledge
Naming
Emotional reaction

© MAYO
2014

Ventral Stream: What?
Object features (eg, shape,
color, sound)

Figure 23.2 Parallel Processing of Sensory Information in the Dorsal and Ventral Streams.
(Used with permission of Mayo Foundation for Medical Education and Research.)

Anton Syndrome

Patients with Anton syndrome deny that they are blind. Those with complete loss of primary visual cortices retain thalamic input to the visual association cortex from the pulvinar; some patients may falsely perceive and thus report that they retain vision when they can show no such evidence for visual function. In contrast, patients with "blindsight" appear to have also lost cortical vision yet retain some evidence of function, presumably mediated by the extrafoveal-pulvino-extrastriate cortex pathway.

Auditory Agnosia

Verbal Auditory Agnosia (Wernicke Aphasia, "Pure Word Deafness")

Wernicke aphasia was the first agnostic type of disorder described. Whether it should be classified as an aphasia or as an agnosia is a matter of semantics, but it is almost universally regarded as an aphasia despite its agnostic qualities.

Nonverbal Auditory Agnosia (Amusia)

Amusia refers to difficulty comprehending music. An example is a patient who was a middle-aged professional musician with a right basal ganglia regional hemorrhage. Motor function returned to nearly normal, but his ability to comprehend music remained so impaired that he became disabled. The lesion interrupted the white matter in the right temporal stem and presumably disconnected input to his right auditory cortex and auditory association cortex.

Aprosodia

Patients with lesions in the right hemisphere and patients with parkinsonism (subcortical aprosodia) may exhibit reduced prosody of their speech.

Somatosensory Agnosia

The ventrolateral somatosensory association cortex includes the inferior parietal lobule, the parietal operculum, and possibly the posterior insula. Lesions in this area result in true tactile agnosia (analogous to a disorder in the visual "what" pathway), a subtle disturbance that is typically unilateral (affecting the contralateral hand). Patients can describe a felt object's basic qualities, such as length, weight, material composition, and texture, yet they may not precisely identify the specific object and usually make an error that describes a similar object (eg, a pen for a screwdriver). If people normally can identify more than 90% of felt objects, patients with tactile agnosia may recognize only 75% (so the deficit is indeed subtle and typically nondisabling).

The dorsomedial somatosensory association cortex includes the medial aspects of Brodmann areas 5 and 7 (medial parietal lobe), and damage to this region produces a tactile deficit that is analogous to asimultanagnosia, or a disorder in the visual "where" pathway. Patients with damage to this area generally also have damage to more anterior parts of the hemisphere, specifically the supplementary motor area, and so patients with ideomotor apraxia have somatosensory problems and cannot localize where they have been touched on the affected limb. This is less of an agnostic disorder than a perceptual disorder.

Astereognosis is sometimes classified as an agnosia. That some consider this an agnosia at all is a reflection of how poorly the somatosensory system is understood in clinical neurology. Patients with primary somatosensory cortical damage (or ventral posterolateral thalamic damage) lose elemental somesthetic function, including, importantly, proprioception and 2-point discrimination and even the sense of touch itself. It is therefore no surprise that within this tactually blinded context patients cannot discern shapes and objects. This is not an agnosia but a severe perceptual deficit.

- Bilateral or right occipitotemporal lesions may result in prosopagnosia (inability to recognize faces).
- Bilateral superior parietal lobe damage causes asimultanagnosia, which is the inability to compute the simultaneity of a complex visual scene in space and time or to effectively scan the environment.
- Balint syndrome consists of asimultanagnosia with the additional elements of optic ataxia (impaired visually guided reaching) and ocular apraxia (the inability to voluntarily fixate gaze on a visual target), although the optic ataxia and ocular apraxia are the consequence of asimultanagnosia.
- Anton syndrome (denial of blindness with confabulation) results from bilateral occipital lesion.

Hemineglect

The ascending consciousness pathway includes autorhythmic neurons in the brainstem: 1) the mesencephalic reticular formation with projection to the nucleus reticularis of the thalamus, which serves a gating function for all thalamocortical projections; and 2) a right hemisphere–dominant thalamocortical projection that includes, most importantly, the parietal heteromodal region (including both inferior and superior parietal cortices). Damage to right parietal cortices, in particular, essentially extinguishes consciousness of the contralateral space and is reflected by a widely encompassing spatial perceptual and constructional disorder most prominently manifested by left hemispatial neglect. In severe (typically acute) cases, patients do not orient to stimuli in the left hemispace. Many patients (probably most patients) also have left hemiplegia (typically resulting from a large right middle cerebral artery territory infarction); yet when asked, they deny it. Some, when shown their plegic left arm, deny that it is theirs, and when asked to move it, they will instead move the right and say that it was the left (typically they are not argumentative, but they simply give short responses).

Patients with milder cases have evidence of extinction of left-sided stimuli with double simultaneous stimulation that may be detectable in all sensory modalities (showing that this is not a modal disorder but rather a supramodal one). Interestingly, hemineglect often improves even if initially severe. Patients who have large right hemisphere infarctions and acutely severe neglect syndromes may have little evidence of neglect after a year, but assessment of tactile object recognition may show residual impairment even in the normal ipsilateral hand as a chronic manifestation of impaired global cortical arousal.

- Damage to right parietal cortices, in particular, essentially extinguishes consciousness of the contralateral space and is reflected by a widely encompassing spatial perceptual and constructional disorder most prominently manifested by left hemispatial neglect.

Inferior Parietal Lobe Signs

Gerstmann Syndrome

The inferior parietal lobe comprises Brodmann areas 39 and 40; grossly, it is represented by the angular gyrus. This is a heteromodal association area, and, as previously noted, it is unique to humans, although it retains some somesthetic function (reflecting our primate ancestry) that is practically of little consequence. In this heteromodal region, deficits resulting from damage tend to be conceptually complex and not limited to a particular sensory modality. Also, there are laterality differences: Right parietal lesions tend to be associated with neglect, and nonneglect parietal syndromes generally imply left hemisphere lesions.

After left inferior parietal damage, the following constitute the angular gyrus syndrome: alexia, agraphia, anomia with or without additional elements of aphasia, acalculia, constructional apraxia (Figure 23.3), right-left confusion, and finger anomia. The last 4 elements (acalculia, constructional apraxia, right-left confusion, and finger anomia) constitute Gerstmann syndrome, an older carryover term of little heuristic value. Language and spatial deficits are the most prominent aspects of left inferior parietal damage, reflecting the language-dominant hemisphere and the posterior (spatial perception) cortices. However, there is 1 additionally interesting element—acalculia. Quantity, a feature shared by all our senses, is subserved by the multimodal inferior parietal cortex. Lesions of this region disrupt arithmetic skills and our ability to accurately judge magnitude.

- Gerstmann syndrome is characterized by acalculia, constructional apraxia, right-left confusion, and finger anomia and is due to a lesion of the left inferior parietal lobe (angular gyrus).

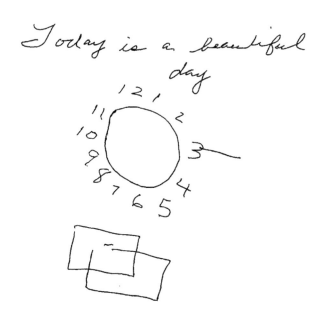

Figure 23.3 Constructional Apraxia.
The patient was asked to draw a clock with hands indicating the time "11:10" and to copy a drawn cube.

Frontal Lobe Dysfunction

The frontal lobes are the largest of the cerebral hemispheres and do not constitute a unitary structure, yet common parlance refers to frontal lobe signs. In fact, the frontal lobes contain 1) the primary motor cortex (damage results in contralateral spastic hemiparesis); 2) motor association areas, including the supplementary motor area (left-sided damage results in ideomotor apraxia), the Broca area (nonfluent aphasia), and the frontal eye fields (monosynaptically connected to the parietal visual association cortices that map space and so control voluntary eye movements); 3) the dorsolateral prefrontal cortices (important for working memory, behavioral inhibition, and probably metacognition); and 4) ventromedial and orbitofrontal cortices (reward-based behavior).

In addition, a more primitive structure, the anterior cingulate gyrus (which may or may not be considered a true part of the frontal lobe) is anatomically associated with this region, so that syndromes resulting from frontal damage may also reflect damage to this structure (resulting in akinetic mutism). Also, the frontal lobes are interconnected with the basal ganglia and other subcortical structures, so that it may be more appropriate to refer to frontostriatal signs (eg, bradykinesia) individually rather than to lump them in a general category of frontal lobe signs.

Three brain regions or systems are central in reward and punishment: the hypothalamus, the mesolimbic dopaminergic system (comprising the ventral tegmental area [VTA] and the nucleus accumbens in the ventral striatum),

and the orbitofrontal cortex (linked by the medial forebrain bundle). VTA dopaminergic reward neurons are most strongly activated by rewarding events that are better than expected. VTA neurons also contain opiate receptors that lead to dopaminergic transmission of VTA neurons to the ventral striatum. Further, some orbitofrontal and striatal neurons show greater activity for the more highly rewarding of 2 outcomes before the outcome has occurred. The more rewarding the envisioned reward, the greater the neuronal activation.

The basolateral amygdala forms associations between sensory cues and rewarding or aversive stimuli. It acts as a fear center but does not encode the rewarding or aversive properties of the stimulus itself. The basolateral amygdala is interconnected with sensory cortices and the hippocampus, allowing it to detect emotionally salient aspects of a stimulus and so influence perception and memory encoding of the stimulus.

The interplay of appetitive and aversive signals defines a most rewarding (or least punishing) goal, and a plan for action to attain it must ensue. The activity of anterior cingulate neurons, in the earliest anatomical stage of action planning and movement, is influenced by reward signals. Immediately preceding a change in response to a diminished reward, neurons in the anterior cingulate fire, marking the first step that results in the altered behavior in response to the reduced reward.

Akinetic Mutism

Lesions of the anterior cingulate disrupt the first step in the network of motivated behavior. Input from reward centers are lost as are ascending signals to the motor association and other upstream areas. Consequently, patients are in an extreme amotivational state characterized by little or no speech or movement. Butterfly gliomas crossing the anterior corpus callosum as well as anterior cerebral artery territory infarctions can cause this syndrome. Patients who have glioma and are treated with dexamethasone (to reduce the associated cerebral edema) may have a rapid recovery. When questioned about their experience in the akinetic mutism state, they respond that they felt nothing, they did not feel imprisoned, and they simply lacked spontaneous thought.

Acquired Sociopathy

Lesions of the orbitofrontal cortex, as in the historical case of Phineas Gage, produce disarmingly subtle but disabling problems with social behavior. Interpersonal interactions are vital for the creation of societies and so for survival. Socially relevant behavior, including cooperation, the decision to enact justice-related punishment, and the expectation of its delivery, activate orbitofrontal and ventral striatal regions (in functional imaging studies). In a developing relationship between 2 people who are learning the degree to which they can trust one another, changes in the reward center and associated brain region activity occur in an interpersonally synchronized fashion. When patients have orbitofrontal cortex lesions, appreciation of these social relationships is impaired as is the ability to alter their behavior according to the pattern of expected or observed rewards and outcomes; these impairments have led to business failures among the previously successful. This is one of the defining characteristics of the frontal lobe syndrome.

Perseveration

On the basis of the relative reward value of any given action, people adjust their behavior accordingly. Lesions that impair this ability include those involving the reward centers directly or other initial steps in the action pathway. Lesions can also occur at a later cognitive step mediated by the dorsolateral prefrontal cortices. These heteromodal regions receive ascending input about the state of the body (eg, hunger) and other motivational drives from reward centers, as well as information from posterior sensory areas, particularly heteromodal parietal cortices. They integrate this information ("How am I feeling and what do I want?" and "What is the state of the world around me?") to formulate a strategic plan of action. Patients with damage in this area have trouble changing actions and instead tend to continue in the same way even if it is not advantageous.

Cognitive Disorder

The frontal lobes are important for working memory that, simply defined, is the ability to hold multiple bits of information in the mind's eye while working on it (Table 23.2). Reciting a string of digits backward, performing mental arithmetic, or trying to recall a person's phone number while still speaking with the person are simple examples. The frontal lobes, in conjunction with their subcortical connections, are also important for psychomotor speed. Timed tasks, such as saying as many words as possible beginning with the letter *c* or naming as many kinds of animals as possible in 1 minute, are examples. Problem solving (which typically involves shifting mental states—ie, not perseverating on an unsuccessful strategy) is another frontally mediated cognitive operation. All these activities are impaired by damage to frontal heteromodal cortices.

Disinhibition

In disinhibition, which is possibly related to spasticity, the involuntary reflexive display of emotion results from frontal damage. This can manifest as pathologic crying (or, less often, laughing), anger outbursts, expression of profanity, or other socially inappropriate (but provoked) behavior.

This is not quite the same as acquired sociopathy, which is not reflexive.

Metacognition

Metacognition refers to the ability to think about thought itself. Patients with frontal lobe damage may have trouble imagining how another person feels in a given situation, a function called theory of mind. They may also lack insight into their deficiencies, a problem called anosognosia, which is particularly frequent in patients with degenerative dementia due to Alzheimer disease and frontotemporal dementia. Denial of hemiparesis in patients with right hemisphere infarctions causing hemineglect is also considered anosognosia, but it may have a different basis (eg, unawareness of left space).

- Three brain regions or systems are central in reward and punishment: the hypothalamus, the mesolimbic dopaminergic system (comprising the VTA and the nucleus accumbens in the ventral striatum), and the orbitofrontal cortex (linked by the medial forebrain bundle).
- The basolateral amygdala detects emotionally salient aspects of a stimulus and so influences perception and memory encoding a stimulus.
- The activity of anterior cingulate neurons, in the earliest anatomical stage of action planning and movement, is influenced by reward signals.
- Lesions of the anterior cingulate disrupt the first step in the network of motivated behavior.
- Lesions of the orbitofrontal cortex, as in the historical case of Phineas Gage, produce disarmingly subtle but disabling problems with social behavior.

Amnesia

Memory loss, as an isolated finding, should be regarded as a focal neurologic sign. It results most frequently from degenerative brain disease, particularly Alzheimer disease, but even when it is isolated it reflects focal brain dysfunction.

Strictly speaking, memory is any lasting change in function caused by prior experience. Memory is a reflection of neuronal plasticity, and, in this sense, all parts of the brain are plastic. The usual meaning of *memory loss* is the inability to retrieve information, which is also called explicit or declarative memory (Table 23.2). Procedural (or implicit) memory reflects the development of a skill, or familiarity with a test paradigm. For example, learning the format of a test is procedural memory, but knowing the actual answers is declarative memory. *Working memory* refers to a frontal lobe function in which people hold things in their mind's eye while they use the rest of their brain to work on the task. Reciting a string of numbers

Table 23.2 • Comparison of Memory Systems

Type of Memory	Function	Anatomy
Working memory	Maintains information for a short period after transient exposure to a stimulus to guide behavior	Prefrontal cortex
Declarative memory		
Episodic	Learning and retrieving personal events and facts	Medial temporal lobe Medial thalamus, mammillary bodies, basal forebrain cholinergic system
Semantic	General fund of knowledge	Heteromodal association cortex (particularly left lateral and anterior temporal areas)
Priming	Experience of a stimulus influences later processing of the same or related stimulus	Occipital, temporal, parietal, and frontal cortices
Emotional memory	Associative learning of a link between a perceptual stimulus and its emotional significance	Amygdala
Procedural (implicit) memory	Motor skill learning	Striatum, cerebellum

Adapted from Benarroch EE, Daube JR, Flemming KD, Westmoreland BF. Mayo Clinic medical neurosciences: organized by neurologic systems and levels. 5th ed. Rochester (MN): Mayo Clinic Scientific Press and Florence (KY): Informa Healthcare USA; c2008. Chapter 16, Part B, The supratentorial level: telencephalon; p. 701–63. Used with permission of Mayo Foundation for Medical Education and Research.

backward, performing mental arithmetic, and multitasking are examples of working memory.

When a person first tries to learn something, the initial experience must be encoded. The paralimbic cortices are a cytoarchitecturally defined ring of allocortical structures that include the hippocampus, parts of the cingulate gyrus, and the periamygdaloid cortex with connections to the hypothalamus (the anchoring limbic structure that defines these as paralimbic) and are thought to be involved in early memory formation, including encoding. Within this series of structures a circuit called the Papez circuit, which may or may not be important for encoding has been defined anatomically. The Papez circuit is the hippocampus, fornix, hypothalamus (mamillary bodies), mamillothalamic tract, anterior nucleus of the thalamus, cingulate gyrus, and a return to the hippocampus. Although the role of the Papez circuit is unclear, the forniceal projections to the septal formation and hypothalamus provide the hippocampus with connections to powerful reward centers, and, conceivably, this is the specific contribution to learning and memory. It is easier to remember something that is salient (ie, rewarding or punishing) than something of no consequence.

Confabulation refers to an amnestic patient's attempt to recall what may have happened, when the patient actually does not remember. Patients may appear to be lying, but they may truly believe what they are saying. Sometimes equated with Korsakoff syndrome, confabulation does occur in other contexts, including Alzheimer disease.

Three anatomical locations should be considered in amnestic patients: the hippocampus and medial temporal lobe, the dorsomedial nucleus of the thalamus, and the hypothalamic and septal region.

The medial temporal lobe structures are among the brain regions that are most sensitive to metabolic insults, including ischemia, hypoxia, hypoglycemia, toxic exposure, trauma, epilepsy, and neurodegeneration. The single most common cause is Alzheimer disease, which outnumbers all other causes of amnesia in all locations combined.

The dorsomedial nucleus of the thalamus is another anatomical structure that may be involved in amnesia when affected bilaterally. The vascular supply of the thalamus is primarily derived from the posterior circulation (thalamic perforators at the tip of the basilar artery or proximal posterior cerebral arteries), particularly the medial thalamus. A basilar artery embolus, therefore, can simultaneously affect both sides of the thalamus. In brain mapping studies of patients with thalamic amnesia, the dorsomedial nucleus of the thalamus is involved most often, possibly because of connections with the hippocampus; the anterior nucleus is not involved, despite its presence in the Papez circuit. A typical presentation is that of "top of the basilar" syndrome with initial coma, followed by delirium that gradually clears to a more circumscribed and permanent amnestic state.

The hypothalamic and septal region near the area of the fornix is also a location where amnesia may result. Uncommonly, patients with suprasellar tumors (most often craniopharyngiomas) may present with memory loss that may develop gradually or abruptly, presumably from compression of the septal nuclei and hypothalamus and the termination of the fornix in these structures. Another cause is Wernicke-Korsakoff syndrome that results from thiamine deficiency; patients typically present with coma or delirium in an acute neurologic emergency. Patients have oculomotor disturbances with diplopia and nystagmus, ataxia, peripheral neuropathy (dry beriberi), and congestive heart failure (wet beriberi). If they survive Wernicke encephalopathy, they eventually improve but have Korsakoff psychosis, which is not a psychosis at all but is a dense amnestic syndrome with prominent confabulation. Patients have damage to periaqueductal gray structures from the brainstem up to those surrounding the third ventricle, prominently including the hypothalamic mammillary bodies.

Questions and Answers

Questions

Multiple Choice (choose the best answer)

I.1. Which of the following statements about cerebrovascular anatomy is most correct?
   a. The lenticulostriate branches of the middle cerebral artery typically arise from both M2 segments
   b. The recurrent artery of Heubner supplies the anterior portion of the ventromedial nucleus of the thalamus
   c. Although cerebrovascular anatomy may vary considerably, bilateral A1 and P1 segments are always present
   d. The vertebral arteries arise from the subclavian arteries bilaterally
   e. Superficial cerebral veins include the superior anastomotic vein of Trolard, the inferior anastomotic vein of Labbé, and the great cerebral vein of Galen

I.2. An 18-year-old man presents with pain in the right side of the neck, veering to the right, and numbness on the right side of the face and in the left arm and leg that came on acutely with lifting heavy weights. His examination shows right hemiataxia, right miosis and ptosis, poor palatal elevation on the right, and decreased sensation to pinprick of the right side of the face and the left arm and leg. To which of the following structures does the lesion best localize?
   a. Right lateral medulla
   b. Left lateral medulla
   c. Right cerebellum
   d. Left midbrain
   e. Central pons

I.3. You order magnetic resonance angiography of the head and neck for a patient with pain in the left side of the neck, a tendency to veer to the left, and numbness on the left side of the face and right arm and leg that came on after a car accident. On examination, you had noted left hemiataxia, left miosis and ptosis, poor left palatal elevation, and decreased sensation to pinprick of the left side of the face and the right arm and leg. Which artery is most likely to show possible dissection?
   a. Right posterior inferior cerebellar artery
   b. Right vertebral artery
   c. Left posterior inferior cerebellar artery
   d. Left vertebral artery
   e. Basilar artery

I.4. Which of the following is the first major branch off of the internal carotid artery?
   a. Anterior choroidal artery
   b. Posterior choroidal artery
   c. Ophthalmic artery
   d. Posterior communicating artery
   e. Anterior communicating artery

I.5. Which of the following structures are supplied by the posterior spinal arteries?
   a. Spinothalamic tracts
   b. Dorsal column-medial lemniscal pathways
   c. Spinoreticular tracts
   d. Rubrospinal tracts
   e. Tectospinal tracts

I.6. Which of the following best approximates the volume of cerebrospinal fluid in an average adult at any single point in time?
   a. 50 mL
   b. 35 mL
   c. 150 mL
   d. 500 mL
   e. 725 mL

I.7. Which of the following best reflects a typical, normal cerebrospinal fluid opening pressure in a healthy adult?
   a. -20 mm H_2O
   b. 10 mm H_2O
   c. 150 mm H_2O
   d. 450 mm H_2O
   e. 700 mm H_2O

I.8. The falx cerebri is composed of which of the following tissues?
   a. Dura mater
   b. Arachnoid
   c. Pia mater
   d. Cartilage
   e. Periosteum

I.9. In a patient with a known Chiari I malformation, burning pain develops in both shoulders. On examination, strength is normal in the limbs, but the sensation to pinprick is reduced in a capelike distribution around the shoulders extending to the upper part of the arms. To what structure does the lesion best localize?
   a. Bilateral dorsal columns
   b. Right lateral funiculus
   c. Central spinal cord
   d. Bilateral ventral funiculus
   e. Bilateral ventral horns

I.10. An anterior spinal artery stroke might result in which of the following symptoms and signs?
   a. Reduced proprioception and vibration bilaterally below the level of the lesion
   b. Decreased pain and temperature ipsilaterally and upper motor neuron weakness contralaterally below the level of the lesion
   c. Paraparesis or quadriparesis with reduced pain and temperature sensation below the level of the lesion
   d. Reduced pain and temperature in the limbs with sacral sparing
   e. Loss of pinprick sensation in the left side of the face and right upper and lower limbs

I.11. A 65-year-old man presents with a left footdrop. On examination, the left anterior tibialis, extensor hallucis longus, and posterior tibialis muscles are weak. The strength of the quadriceps, gastrocnemius, and gluteus maximus muscles is normal. Stretch reflexes of the quadriceps and ankle muscle are normal. To which structure does the lesion best localize?
a. Peroneal nerve
b. L4 spinal root
c. L5 spinal root
d. Sciatic nerve
e. Thoracic spinal cord

I.12. A 47-year-old woman presents with paresthesias in the medial aspect of the right hand. On examination, you find moderate weakness of the right opponens pollicis and adductor pollicis muscles. Stretch reflexes of the biceps, triceps, and brachioradialis muscles are normal. To which structure does the lesion best localize?
a. C8 spinal root
b. Middle trunk
c. Lateral cord
d. Anterior interosseous nerve
e. Ulnar nerve

I.13. A 72-year-old man with diabetes presents with subacute left thigh pain and weakness. On examination, you note moderate weakness of the left quadriceps muscles and hip adductors. The stretch reflexes of the quadriceps muscle are reduced, but the ankle jerks are preserved. To which structure does the lesion best localize?
a. S1 spinal root
b. Lumbar plexus
c. Femoral nerve
d. Obturator nerve
e. Sciatic nerve

I.14. A 15-year-old boy presents for evaluation of right shoulder pain. On examination, you find that his right scapula moves posteriorly when he leans forward against the wall with both hands. To which structure does the lesion best localize?
a. Left precentral gyrus
b. Long thoracic nerve
c. Spinal accessory nerve
d. Dorsal scapular nerve
e. Suprascapular nerve

I.15. Which of the following is the primary postsynaptic receptor at the neuromuscular junction?
a. Nicotinic acetylcholine receptor
b. γ-Aminobutyric acid receptor
c. Muscarinic acetylcholine receptor
d. Glutamate receptor
e. Glycine receptor

I.16. Which of the following statements about sensory systems is most correct?
a. All sensory modalities relay through the thalamus except the olfactory system
b. Most pathways do not maintain topographic representations of receptive fields
c. There are no parallel pathways of sensory integration through the ventral and dorsal streams
d. All sensory systems contain at least 3 precortical synapses
e. All sensory systems are mediated via extraparenchymal sensory ganglia

I.17. Which of the following modalities is primarily carried by the dorsal column-medial lemniscal system?
a. Pain and temperature from the face
b. Bulbar joint position sense
c. Light touch from the face
d. Pain and temperature from the body
e. Vibration and joint position sense from the body

I.18. Which of the following nerve fiber types are the primary carriers of nociception?
a. A delta and C
b. Type IIa
c. A beta
d. Type IIb
e. A alpha

I.19. The affective component of pain is relayed primarily to which of the following areas of the brain?
a. Ventral posterolateral nucleus of the thalamus and the primary sensory cortex
b. Ventral posteromedial nucleus of the thalamus and the posterior cingulate gyrus
c. Anterior nucleus of the thalamus and the prefrontal cortex
d. Pulvinar of the thalamus and the insular cortex
e. Mediodorsal nucleus of the thalamus and the anterior cingulate gyrus

I.20. Mutations affecting which of the following channels may cause hereditary erythromelalgia?
a. $Na_v1.7$ channel
b. P/Q-type calcium channel
c. TRPV1 channel
d. $Na_v1.9$ channel
e. $K_v\alpha11$ channel

I.21. The trigeminothalamic tract travels in which of the following portions of the pons and midbrain?
a. Medial
b. Ventral
c. Lateral
d. Central (near the fourth ventricle and cerebral aqueduct)
e. Dorsal

I.22. In which of the following functions does the superior olive participate?
a. Comparing actual with intended movement
b. Sound localization
c. Visual relay to the superior colliculus
d. Coordination of motor programming
e. Vestibulo-ocular reflex efferent pathway

I.23. The dorsal stream for sensory processing codes for which of the following types of information?
a. "Who" (identification of faces)
b. "What" (identification of an object)
c. "When" (temporal sequencing)
d. "Where" (where in time and space an object is)
e. "Why" (purpose or intent of action)

I.24. A 68-year-old woman presents with difficulty lifting her right shoulder, hoarseness of the voice, and intermittent episodes of syncope. The face, palate, and tongue have normal strength. There are no abnormal sensory findings. To which of the following structures does this process best localize?
a. Pons
b. Medial medulla
c. Jugular foramen
d. Retropharyngeal space
e. Foramen magnum

I.25. The nucleus solitarius is involved in which of the following functions?
a. Motor innervation of muscles of the pharynx and larynx
b. Receiving information about taste
c. Unconscious proprioception of the jaw
d. Relay nuclei in the auditory pathway
e. Vestibulospinal reflex

I.26. A 55-year-old man presents with acute weakness of the right arm and leg and left tongue weakness. To which of the following structures does the lesion best localize?
a. Left lateral cerebral cortex

b. Bilateral ventral pons
c. Right lateral pons
d. Left ventral medulla
e. Right lateral medulla

I.27. The mandibular portion of the trigeminal nerve exits the skull through which of the following structures?
a. Jugular foramen
b. Foramen ovale
c. Internal auditory canal
d. Hypoglossal canal
e. Foramen lacerum

I.28. An 82-year-old woman presents with sensory symptoms of the right side of the face and left side of the body, dysarthria, and dysphagia. Diffusion-weighted magnetic resonance imaging shows an acute right lateral medullary infarction. Impairment of which of the following structures is likely responsible for these symptoms?
a. Hypoglossal nucleus
b. Nucleus solitarius
c. Nucleus ambiguus
d. Raphe nucleus
e. Inferior olivary nucleus

I.29. Which of the following functions is mediated by the trigeminal nerve?
a. Innervation of the stapedius muscle
b. Carrying pain and temperature, but not touch, sensation of the face
c. Innervation of muscles of facial expression
d. Carrying unconscious proprioception sensation of the jaw to the motor nucleus of cranial nerve V
e. Carrying gustatory sensation to the spinal trigeminal nucleus

I.30. A 39-year-old man presents with subacute simultaneous left abducens and facial palsies. To which of the following locations does the lesion best localize?
a. Dorello canal
b. Internal auditory canal
c. Facial colliculus
d. Cavernous sinus
e. Area postrema

I.31. The sphenopalatine ganglion is the postganglionic parasympathetic ganglion for which of the following cranial nerves?
a. III
b. VII
c. IX
d. X
e. XI

I.32. A 29-year-old woman presents with acute bilateral visual loss associated with somnolence and diplopia. Which of the following clinical syndromes does this represent?
a. Locked-in syndrome
b. Wallenberg syndrome
c. Foville syndrome
d. Nothnagel syndrome
e. Top-of-the-basilar syndrome

I.33. A 75-year-old man with diabetes and hypertension presents with an acute right pupil-sparing third nerve palsy. Which of the following is the most likely cause?
a. Ischemia of the third nerve bundle
b. Posterior communicating artery aneurysm
c. Pituitary macroadenoma and apoplexy
d. Basilar artery aneurysm
e. Ischemic infarction of the right medial midbrain

I.34. A 21-year-old man presents with right eye pain, pulsatile tinnitus, and double vision. Examination shows a right abducens nerve palsy, proptosis, and reduced sensation to pinprick on the right side of the forehead. To which of the following structures does the lesion best localize?
a. Right jugular foramen

b. Right pons
c. Right cavernous sinus
d. Right Dorello canal along the petrous ridge
e. Right middle cerebral fossa

I.35. Turning the head to the right results in which of the following responses?
a. Increased frequency of action potentials in the right vestibular nerve
b. Increased frequency of action potentials in the left vestibular nerve
c. Decreased frequency of action potentials in the right vestibular nerve
d. Decreased frequency of action potentials in the left vestibular nerve
e. No change in action potential frequency in any cranial nerve

I.36. A 41-year-old woman with a history of smoking and hypertension presents with an acute third nerve palsy affecting the pupil and a severe headache. Computed tomography of the head is negative, but cerebrospinal fluid analysis is suggestive of subarachnoid hemorrhage. What is the most likely localization of the responsible lesion?
a. Posterior communicating artery
b. Anterior choroidal artery
c. Carotid-cavernous segment
d. Vertebral artery
e. Artery of Percheron

I.37. A 37-year-old man presents with galactorrhea after taking haloperidol for visual hallucinations. Interruption of which of the following pituitary-hypothalamic hormones is likely responsible?
a. Oxytocin
b. Somatostatin
c. Follicle-stimulating hormone
d. Prolactin
e. Antidiuretic hormone

I.38. A 25-year-old man sustains a severe traumatic brain injury after a snowmobile accident. While he is in the neurology intensive care unit, his serum sodium level and urine output increase. Which of the following is the most likely mechanism?
a. Syndrome of inappropriate antidiuretic hormone
b. Pituitary stalk disruption resulting in diabetes insipidus
c. Dehydration
d. Pharmacy error in intravenous fluid concentrations
e. Cerebral salt wasting

I.39. The paraventricular nucleus of the hypothalamus participates in which of the following functions?
a. Feeding and energy metabolism
b. Osmoregulation
c. Circadian rhythm
d. Ovulation
e. Stress response and autonomic control

I.40. Which of the following structures can serve as a thalamic target for deep brain stimulation in a patient with tremor?
a. Pulvinar
b. Anterior nucleus
c. Lateral geniculate body
d. Ventrolateral nucleus
e. Mediodorsal nucleus

I.41. Which of the following promotes synchronized 3-Hz rhythmic burst firing in thalamocortical circuits?
a. γ-Aminobutyric acid (GABA) A receptor–mediated inhibition within the reticular thalamic nucleus
b. Activation of GABA B receptors in thalamocortical neurons
c. Activation of cholinergic receptors in the reticular thalamic nucleus
d. Blockade of T-channels in thalamocortical neurons
e. Blockade of glutamatergic receptors in the reticular thalamic nucleus

I.42. The ventroposterolateral nucleus of the thalamus participates in which of the following functions?
a. Limbic relay
b. Lemniscal relay
c. Executive function and behavior
d. Visual processing
e. Auditory processing

I.43. The head of the caudate is an important structure in which of the following circuits?
a. Motor programming
b. Behavioral processing
c. Sensory-motor transition
d. Autonomic processing
e. Language decoding

I.44. The pedunculopontine nucleus is most closely tied to which of the following functions?
a. Locomotor pattern generation
b. Pain and temperature sensation of the face and supratentorial meninges
c. General visceral afferent input to the hypothalamus
d. Vestibular relay
e. Electrolyte monitoring and homeostasis

I.45. Which of the following structures serves as the main output for basal ganglia circuits?
a. Striatum
b. Substantia nigra pars compacta and globus pallidus externa
c. Substantia nigra pars reticulata and globus pallidus interna
d. Fornix
e. Substantia nigra pars compacta and subthalamic nucleus

I.46. Which of the following processes defines the activity of the globus pallidus internus?
a. Phasic excitatory glutamatergic output facilitated by the striatum
b. Tonic inhibitory GABAergic output facilitated by the subthalamic nucleus
c. Phasic inhibitory GABAergic output facilitated by the striatum
d. Silent at rest, tonically inhibited by the striatum
e. Silent at rest, phasically activated by the subthalamic nucleus

I.47. A 50-year-old man is evaluated for abrupt onset of violent involuntary right-arm movements that started 12 hours ago. Magnetic resonance imaging shows an acute infarction in the left subthalamic nucleus. Which of the following is the most likely consequence of the lesion?
a. Decreased glutamatergic activation of the right globus pallidus
b. Decreased glutamatergic activation of the left globus pallidus
c. Increased GABAergic inhibition of the right striatum
d. Decreased GABAergic inhibition of the right striatum
e. Increased GABAergic inhibition of the left thalamus

I.48. A 45-year-old man with hypertension has a hemorrhage affecting the left dentate nucleus. Which of the following will be the most likely consequence of the lesion?
a. Impaired excitation of the left ventral intermedius (ventral lateral, VL) nucleus thalamus
b. Impaired excitation of the right ventral intermedius (VL)
c. Impaired inhibition of the left inferior olivary nucleus
d. Impaired excitation of the left inferior olivary nucleus
e. Impaired inhibition of the right ventral intermedius (VL)

I.49. Which of the following statements regarding the insular cortex is most correct?
a. The primary gustatory cortex is located in the posterior insula
b. It receives visceral nociceptive input via sympathetic afferents
c. It receives mechanical visceral input via sympathetic afferents
d. It does not receive visceral afferent input via the thalamus
e. It receives gustatory afferent input via the medial geniculate body

I.50. Which of the following statements regarding preganglionic sympathetic neurons is most correct?
a. Cell bodies are located in the ventral column of the spinal cord

b. They receive the majority of afferent input from neocortex
c. They release norepinephrine which acts on postganglionic neurons
d. They directly innervate the adrenal medulla
e. They release epinephrine to mediate hidrosis

I.51. A 32-year-old man with a history of traumatic brain injury presents with short-term memory loss, hyperphagia, hypersexuality, and docility. Damage to which of the following structures is most likely responsible for this syndrome?
a. Prefrontal cortex bilaterally
b. Habenular nucleus
c. Bilateral temporal lobes, including amygdala and hippocampus
d. Bilateral dorsomedial thalamus
e. Occipital cortex resulting in frequent seizures

I.52. Input to the hippocampus comes primarily from which of the following structures?
a. Entorhinal cortex
b. Posterior cingulate gyrus
c. Olfactory cortex
d. Mammillothalamic tract
e. Fornix

I.53. Which of the following statements best describes the function of the amygdala?
a. Primary input to the hippocampus
b. Does not participate in associative learning leading to classically conditioned responses
c. Critical for social recognition and behavior
d. Unilateral lesions result in profound anterograde amnesia
e. Primary regulator of sleep-wake cycles

I.54. Which of the following cortical structures has 3 layers?
a. Primary motor cortex
b. Visual association cortex
c. Prefrontal heteromodal cortex
d. Hippocampus
e. Heschl gyrus

I.55. Injury to which of the following cerebral cortical structures results in behavioral disinhibition?
a. Anterior cingulate gyrus
b. Posterior cingulate gyrus
c. Dorsolateral prefrontal cortex
d. Orbitofrontal cortex
e. Paramedian prefrontal cortex

I.56. A 76-year-old woman has slowly progressive cognitive decline presenting initially with an amnestic syndrome. On examination she has poor naming ability and comprehension. Fluency is preserved, as is repetition. Which of the following classic aphasia syndromes do these findings most closely resemble?
a. Transcortical sensory aphasia
b. Transcortical motor aphasia
c. Broca aphasia
d. Wernicke aphasia
e. Global aphasia

I.57. A 57-year-old man presents with difficulty identifying familiar faces, such as family members. However, when they speak, he then can identify them by voice. A lesion resulting in this syndrome would typically localize to which of the following structures?
a. Prefrontal cortex
b. Nondominant occipitotemporal lobe
c. Nondominant occipitoparietal lobe
d. Occipital cortex
e. Dominant occipitoparietal lobe

I.58. Which of the following terms best describes the inability to assimilate a complex visual scene in space and time?
a. Alexia without agraphia
b. Prosopagnosia
c. Anosognosia

d. Gerstmann syndrome

e. Asimultanagnosia

I.59. Amnesia may result from a lesion of which of the following structures?

    a. Right temporal neocortex

    b. Left fornix

    c. Bilateral mamillary bodies

    d. Surgical resection of the dentate nuclei of the left hippocampus

    e. Bilateral prefrontal cortices

I.60. Which of the following structures serves as the primary output of the hippocampus?

    a. Dentate gyrus

    b. Subiculum

    c. Cingulate gyrus

    d. Fornix

    e. Habenula

I.61. A lesion of the anterior cingulate gyrus may result in which of the following syndromes?

    a. Akinetic mutism

    b. Anosognosia

    c. Prosopagnosia

    d. Balint syndrome

    e. Anton syndrome

Answers

I.1. Answer d.

Brazis PW, Masdeu JC, Biller J. Localization in clinical neurology. 6th ed. Philadelphia (PA): Wolters Kluwer Health/ Lippincott Williams & Wilkins; c2011. 657 p.

I.2. Answer a.

Brazis PW, Masdeu JC, Biller J. Localization in clinical neurology. 6th ed. Philadelphia (PA): Wolters Kluwer Health/ Lippincott Williams & Wilkins; c2011. 657 p.

I.3. Answer d.

Brazis PW, Masdeu JC, Biller J. Localization in clinical neurology. 6th ed. Philadelphia (PA): Wolters Kluwer Health/ Lippincott Williams & Wilkins; c2011. 657 p.

I.4. Answer c.

Osborn AG. Diagnostic cerebral angiography. 2nd ed. Philadelphia (PA): Lippincott-Raven; c1999. 462 p.

I.5. Answer b.

Brazis PW, Masdeu JC, Biller J. Localization in clinical neurology. 6th ed. Philadelphia (PA): Wolters Kluwer Health/ Lippincott Williams & Wilkins; c2011. 657 p.

I.6. Answer c.

Benarroch EE, Daube JR, Flemming KD, Westmoreland BF. Mayo Clinic medical neurosciences: organized by neurologic systems and levels. 5th ed. Rochester (MN): Mayo Clinic Scientific Press and Florence (KY): Informa Healthcare USA; c2008. 808 p.

I.7. Answer c.

Benarroch EE, Daube JR, Flemming KD, Westmoreland BF. Mayo Clinic medical neurosciences: organized by neurologic systems and levels. 5th ed. Rochester (MN): Mayo Clinic Scientific Press and Florence (KY): Informa Healthcare USA; c2008. 808 p.

I.8. Answer a.

Benarroch EE, Daube JR, Flemming KD, Westmoreland BF. Mayo Clinic medical neurosciences: organized by neurologic systems and levels. 5th ed. Rochester (MN): Mayo Clinic Scientific Press and Florence (KY): Informa Healthcare USA; c2008. 808 p.

I.9. Answer c.

Brazis PW, Masdeu JC, Biller J. Localization in clinical neurology. 6th ed. Philadelphia (PA): Wolters Kluwer Health/ Lippincott Williams & Wilkins; c2011. 657 p.

I.10. Answer c.

Haines DE, editor. Fundamental neuroscience for basic and clinical applications. 4th ed. Philadelphia (PA): Elsevier/ Saunders; c2013. 492 p.

I.11. Answer c.

Haines DE, editor. Fundamental neuroscience for basic and clinical applications. 4th ed. Philadelphia (PA): Elsevier/ Saunders; c2013. 492 p.

I.12. Answer a.

Brazis PW, Masdeu JC, Biller J. Localization in clinical neurology. 6th ed. Philadelphia (PA): Wolters Kluwer Health/ Lippincott Williams & Wilkins; c2011. 657 p.

I.13. Answer b.

Brazis PW, Masdeu JC, Biller J. Localization in clinical neurology. 6th ed. Philadelphia (PA): Wolters Kluwer Health/ Lippincott Williams & Wilkins; c2011. 657 p.

I.14. Answer b.

Brazis PW, Masdeu JC, Biller J. Localization in clinical neurology. 6th ed. Philadelphia (PA): Wolters Kluwer Health/ Lippincott Williams & Wilkins; c2011. 657 p.

I.15. Answer a.

Benarroch EE, Daube JR, Flemming KD, Westmoreland BF. Mayo Clinic medical neurosciences: organized by neurologic systems and levels. 5th ed. Rochester (MN): Mayo Clinic Scientific Press and Florence (KY): Informa Healthcare USA; c2008. 808 p.

I.16. Answer a.

Benarroch EE. Basic neurosciences with clinical applications. Philadelphia (PA): Butterworth Heinemann/Elsevier; c2006. 1087 p.

I.17. Answer e.

Benarroch EE, Daube JR, Flemming KD, Westmoreland BF. Mayo Clinic medical neurosciences: organized by neurologic systems and levels. 5th ed. Rochester (MN): Mayo Clinic Scientific Press and Florence (KY): Informa Healthcare USA; c2008. 808 p.

I.18. Answer a.

Benarroch EE. Basic neurosciences with clinical applications. Philadelphia (PA): Butterworth Heinemann/Elsevier; c2006. 1087 p.

I.19. Answer e.

Benarroch EE. Basic neurosciences with clinical applications. Philadelphia (PA): Butterworth Heinemann/Elsevier; c2006. 1087 p.

I.20. Answer a.

Benarroch EE. Basic neurosciences with clinical applications. Philadelphia (PA): Butterworth Heinemann/Elsevier; c2006. 1087 p.

I.21. Answer c.

Benarroch EE, Daube JR, Flemming KD, Westmoreland BF. Mayo Clinic medical neurosciences: organized by neurologic systems and levels. 5th ed. Rochester (MN): Mayo Clinic Scientific Press and Florence (KY): Informa Healthcare USA; c2008. 808 p.

I.22. Answer b.

Haines DE, editor. Fundamental neuroscience for basic and clinical applications. 4th ed. Philadelphia (PA): Elsevier/ Saunders; c2013. 492 p.

I.23. Answer d.

Benarroch EE. Basic neurosciences with clinical applications. Philadelphia (PA): Butterworth Heinemann/Elsevier; c2006. 1087 p.

I.24. Answer c.

Brazis PW, Masdeu JC, Biller J. Localization in clinical neurology. 6th ed. Philadelphia (PA): Wolters Kluwer Health/ Lippincott Williams & Wilkins; c2011. 657 p.

I.25. Answer b.

Benarroch EE, Daube JR, Flemming KD, Westmoreland BF. Mayo Clinic medical neurosciences: organized by neurologic systems and levels. 5th ed. Rochester (MN): Mayo Clinic Scientific Press and Florence (KY): Informa Healthcare USA; c2008. 808 p.

I.26. Answer d.

Brazis PW, Masdeu JC, Biller J. Localization in clinical neurology. 6th ed. Philadelphia (PA): Wolters Kluwer Health/Lippincott Williams & Wilkins; c2011. 657 p.

I.27. Answer b.

Benarroch EE, Daube JR, Flemming KD, Westmoreland BF. Mayo Clinic medical neurosciences: organized by neurologic systems and levels. 5th ed. Rochester (MN): Mayo Clinic Scientific Press and Florence (KY): Informa Healthcare USA; c2008. 808 p.

I.28. Answer c.

Benarroch EE, Daube JR, Flemming KD, Westmoreland BF. Mayo Clinic medical neurosciences: organized by neurologic systems and levels. 5th ed. Rochester (MN): Mayo Clinic Scientific Press and Florence (KY): Informa Healthcare USA; c2008. 808 p.

I.29. Answer d.

Haines DE, editor. Fundamental neuroscience for basic and clinical applications. 4th ed. Philadelphia (PA): Elsevier/Saunders; c2013. 492 p.

I.30. Answer c.

Benarroch EE, Daube JR, Flemming KD, Westmoreland BF. Mayo Clinic medical neurosciences: organized by neurologic systems and levels. 5th ed. Rochester (MN): Mayo Clinic Scientific Press and Florence (KY): Informa Healthcare USA; c2008. 808 p.

I.31. Answer b.

Benarroch EE, Daube JR, Flemming KD, Westmoreland BF. Mayo Clinic medical neurosciences: organized by neurologic systems and levels. 5th ed. Rochester (MN): Mayo Clinic Scientific Press and Florence (KY): Informa Healthcare USA; c2008. 808 p.

I.32. Answer e.

Brazis PW, Masdeu JC, Biller J. Localization in clinical neurology. 6th ed. Philadelphia (PA): Wolters Kluwer Health/Lippincott Williams & Wilkins; c2011. 657 p.

I.33. Answer a.

Benarroch EE, Daube JR, Flemming KD, Westmoreland BF. Mayo Clinic medical neurosciences: organized by neurologic systems and levels. 5th ed. Rochester (MN): Mayo Clinic Scientific Press and Florence (KY): Informa Healthcare USA; c2008. 808 p.

I.34. Answer c.

Haines DE, editor. Fundamental neuroscience for basic and clinical applications. 4th ed. Philadelphia (PA): Elsevier/Saunders; c2013. 492 p.

I.35. Answer a.

Benarroch EE. Basic neurosciences with clinical applications. Philadelphia (PA): Butterworth Heinemann/Elsevier; c2006. 1087 p.

I.36. Answer a.

Osborn AG. Diagnostic cerebral angiography. 2nd ed. Philadelphia (PA): Lippincott-Raven; c1999. 462 p.

I.37. Answer d.

Benarroch EE. Basic neurosciences with clinical applications. Philadelphia (PA): Butterworth Heinemann/Elsevier; c2006. 1087 p.

I.38. Answer b.

Benarroch EE, Daube JR, Flemming KD, Westmoreland BF. Mayo Clinic medical neurosciences: organized by neurologic systems and levels. 5th ed. Rochester (MN): Mayo

Clinic Scientific Press and Florence (KY): Informa Healthcare USA; c2008. 808 p.

I.39. Answer e.

Benarroch EE. Basic neurosciences with clinical applications. Philadelphia (PA): Butterworth Heinemann/Elsevier; c2006. 1087 p.

I.40. Answer d.

Benarroch EE. Basic neurosciences with clinical applications. Philadelphia (PA): Butterworth Heinemann/Elsevier; c2006. 1087 p.

I.41. Answer b.

Benarroch EE. Basic neurosciences with clinical applications. Philadelphia (PA): Butterworth Heinemann/Elsevier; c2006. 1087 p.

I.42. Answer b.

Benarroch EE. Basic neurosciences with clinical applications. Philadelphia (PA): Butterworth Heinemann/Elsevier; c2006. 1087 p.

I.43. Answer b.

Benarroch EE. Basic neurosciences with clinical applications. Philadelphia (PA): Butterworth Heinemann/Elsevier; c2006. 1087 p.

I.44. Answer a.

Benarroch EE. Basic neurosciences with clinical applications. Philadelphia (PA): Butterworth Heinemann/Elsevier; c2006. 1087 p.

I.45. Answer c.

Benarroch EE, Daube JR, Flemming KD, Westmoreland BF. Mayo Clinic medical neurosciences: organized by neurologic systems and levels. 5th ed. Rochester (MN): Mayo Clinic Scientific Press and Florence (KY): Informa Healthcare USA; c2008. 808 p.

I.46. Answer b.

Benarroch EE, Daube JR, Flemming KD, Westmoreland BF. Mayo Clinic medical neurosciences: organized by neurologic systems and levels. 5th ed. Rochester (MN): Mayo Clinic Scientific Press and Florence (KY): Informa Healthcare USA; c2008. 808 p.

I.47. Answer b.

Benarroch EE. Basic neurosciences with clinical applications. Philadelphia (PA): Butterworth Heinemann/Elsevier; c2006. 1087 p.

I.48. Answer b.

Benarroch EE. Basic neurosciences with clinical applications. Philadelphia (PA): Butterworth Heinemann/Elsevier; c2006. 1087 p.

I.49. Answer b.

Benarroch EE. Basic neurosciences with clinical applications. Philadelphia (PA): Butterworth Heinemann/Elsevier; c2006. 1087 p.

I.50. Answer d.

Benarroch EE, Daube JR, Flemming KD, Westmoreland BF. Mayo Clinic medical neurosciences: organized by neurologic systems and levels. 5th ed. Rochester (MN): Mayo Clinic Scientific Press and Florence (KY): Informa Healthcare USA; c2008. 808 p.

I.51. Answer c.

Brazis PW, Masdeu JC, Biller J. Localization in clinical neurology. 6th ed. Philadelphia (PA): Wolters Kluwer Health/Lippincott Williams & Wilkins; c2011. 657 p.

I.52. Answer a.

Benarroch EE. Basic neurosciences with clinical applications. Philadelphia (PA): Butterworth Heinemann/Elsevier; c2006. 1087 p.

I.53. Answer c.

Benarroch EE. Basic neurosciences with clinical applications. Philadelphia (PA): Butterworth Heinemann/Elsevier; c2006. 1087 p.

I.54. Answer d.

Haines DE, editor. Fundamental neuroscience for basic and clinical applications. 4th ed. Philadelphia (PA): Elsevier/Saunders; c2013. 492 p.

I.55. Answer d.

Brazis PW, Masdeu JC, Biller J. Localization in clinical neurology. 6th ed. Philadelphia (PA): Wolters Kluwer Health/Lippincott Williams & Wilkins; c2011. 657 p.

I.56. Answer a.

Brazis PW, Masdeu JC, Biller J. Localization in clinical neurology. 6th ed. Philadelphia (PA): Wolters Kluwer Health/Lippincott Williams & Wilkins; c2011. 657 p.

I.57. Answer b.

Benarroch EE. Basic neurosciences with clinical applications. Philadelphia (PA): Butterworth Heinemann/Elsevier; c2006. 1087 p.

I.58. Answer e.

Brazis PW, Masdeu JC, Biller J. Localization in clinical neurology. 6th ed. Philadelphia (PA): Wolters Kluwer Health/Lippincott Williams & Wilkins; c2011. 657 p.

I.59. Answer c.

Haines DE, editor. Fundamental neuroscience for basic and clinical applications. 4th ed. Philadelphia (PA): Elsevier/Saunders; c2013. 492 p.

I.60. Answer b.

Haines DE, editor. Fundamental neuroscience for basic and clinical applications. 4th ed. Philadelphia (PA): Elsevier/Saunders; c2013. 492 p.

I.61. Answer a.

Brazis PW, Masdeu JC, Biller J. Localization in clinical neurology. 6th ed. Philadelphia (PA): Wolters Kluwer Health/Lippincott Williams & Wilkins; c2011. 657 p.

SUGGESTED READING

Benarroch EE. Basic neurosciences with clinical applications. Philadelphia (PA): Butterworth Heinemann/Elsevier; c2006. 1087 p.

Benarroch EE. Circumventricular organs: receptive and homeostatic functions and clinical implications. Neurology. 2011 Sep 20;77(12):1198–204.

Benarroch EE. Neural control of feeding behavior: Overview and clinical correlations. Neurology. 2010 May 18;74(20):1643–50.

Benarroch EE. Paraventricular nucleus, stress response, and cardiovascular disease. Clin Auton Res. 2005 Aug;15(4):254–63.

Benarroch EE, Daube JR, Flemming KD, Westmoreland BF. Mayo Clinic medical neurosciences: organized by neurologic systems and levels. 5th ed. Rochester (MN): Mayo Clinic Scientific Press and Florence (KY): Informa Healthcare USA; c2008. 808 p.

Benarroch EE, Westmoreland BF, Daube JR, Reagan TJ, Sandok BA. Medical neurosciences: an approach to anatomy, pathology, and physiology by systems and levels. 4th ed. Philadelphia (PA): Lippincott Williams & Wilkins; c1999. 631 p.

Brazis PW, Masdeu JC, Biller J. Localization in clinical neurology. 6th ed. Philadelphia (PA): Wolters Kluwer Health/Lippincott Williams & Wilkins; c2011. 657 p.

Carpenter MB. Core text of neuroanatomy. 4th ed. Baltimore (MD): Lippincott Williams & Wilkins; c1991. 481 p.

Caselli RJ, Tariot PN. Alzheimer's disease and its variants: a diagnostic and therapeutic guide. Oxford (UK): Oxford University Press; c2010. 252 p.

Dyck PJ, Thomas PK, editors. Peripheral neuropathy. 4th ed. Philadelphia (PA): Elsevier Saunders; c2005.

Eggers SDZ, Zee DS, editors. Vertigo and imbalance: clinical neurophysiology of the vestibular system. Amsterdam (NETHERLANDS): Elsevier Health Sciences; c2010. 575 p. (Daube JR, Mauguiere F, editors. Handbook of clinical neurophysiology; vol. 9).

Engel AG, Franzini-Armstrong C, editors. Myology. 3rd ed. New York (NY): McGraw-Hill Medical Publishing Division; c2004. 1960 p.

Feinberg TE, Farah MJ, editors. Behavioral neurology and neuropsychology. 2nd ed. New York (NY): McGraw-Hill; c2003. 910 p.

Haines DE, editor. Fundamental neuroscience. 2nd ed. New York (NY): Churchill Livingstone; c2002. 582 p.

Haines DE, editor. Fundamental neuroscience for basic and clinical applications. 4th ed. Philadelphia (PA): Elsevier/Saunders; c2013. 492 p.

Heilman KM, Valenstein E, editors. Clinical neuropsychology. 5th ed. Oxford (UK): Oxford University Press; c2011. 690 p.

Hubel DH, Wiesel TN. Brain mechanisms of vision. Sci Am. 1979 Sep;241(3):150–62.

Hubel DH, Wiesel TN. Ferrier lecture. Functional architecture of macaque monkey visual cortex. Proc R Soc Lond B Biol Sci. 1977 Jul 28;198(1130):1–59.

Jones DT, Vemuri P, Murphy MC, Gunter JL, Senjem ML, Machulda MM, et al. Non-stationarity in the "resting brain's" modular architecture. PLoS One. 2012;7(6): e39731. Epub 2012 Jun 28.

Kandel ER, Schwartz JH, Jessell TM, editors. Principles of neural science. 4th ed. New York (NY): McGraw-Hill, Health Professions Division; c2000. Chapters 25-29, Review of entire visual system. p. 492–589.

Kline LB, Foroozan R, Bajandas FJ (deceased). Neuro-ophthalmology: review manual. 7th ed. Thorofare (NJ): SLACK; c2013. 288 p.

Kolb H. How the retina works. Am Scientist. 2003 Jan-Feb;91(1):28–35.

Kolb H, Nelson R, Fernandez E, Jones B, editors. Webvision: the organization of the retina and visual system. Webvision; c2014. Available from: http://www.webvision.med.utah.edu.

Low PA, Benarroch EE, editors. Clinical autonomic disorders. 3rd ed. Philadelphia (PA): Wolters Kluwer Health/Lippincott Williams & Wilkins; c2008. 780 p.

Mesulam M-M, editor. Principles of behavioral and cognitive neurology. 2nd ed. Oxford (UK): Oxford University Press; c2000. 540 p.

Moore JK. The human brainstem auditory system. In: Jackler RK, Brackmann DE, editors. Neurotology. 2nd ed. Philadelphia (PA): Mosby; c2005. p. 45–51.

Myssiorek D. Recurrent laryngeal nerve paralysis: anatomy and etiology. Otolaryngol Clin North Am. 2004 Feb;37(1):25–44.

Osborn AG. Diagnostic cerebral angiography. 2nd ed. Philadelphia (PA): Lippincott-Raven; c1999. 462 p.

Parent A. Carpenters' human neuroanatomy. 9th ed. Baltimore (MD): Lippincott Williams & Wilkins; c1996. 1011 p.

Rizzo M, Eslinger PJ, editors. Principles and practice of behavioral neurology and neuropsychology. Philadelphia (PA): W.B. Saunders; c2004. 1168 p.

Section II

Cellular
Neuroscience
Eduardo E. Benarroch, MD,
editor

24 Cellular Signaling

NATHAN P. STAFF, MD, PHD

Overview

Cell communication in the nervous system is finely tuned to respond rapidly to external stimuli, learn from those stimuli, and produce more effective responses in the future. The physical basis for this cell communication is the manipulation of ion gradients via ion pumps and channels, chemical neurotransmission, and synaptic plasticity, all of which are discussed in this chapter.

Neuronal Excitability

The majority of cell communication that occurs in the nervous system relies on maintenance of a transmembrane electrochemical potential, which at rest is approximately −70 mV. This transmembrane potential is primarily developed by the action of the sodium-potassium-adenosine triphosphatase transport that shuttles 3 sodium ions out of the cell while bringing 2 potassium ions into the cell. Four main ions have electrochemical gradients across the plasma membrane and contribute substantially to neuronal excitability, and each ion acts independently to achieve equilibrium, according to the Nernst equation. These ions (and their approximate equilibrium potentials) are sodium (0 mV), potassium (−75 mV), calcium (+20 mV), and chloride (−90 mV). Thus, when a selective ion channel (eg, sodium) is opened under resting conditions (−70 mV), the transmembrane potential rapidly moves toward the equilibrium potential of that channel (eg, +20 mV).

Ion channels are transmembrane proteins that have a selectivity pore for specific ions. Most ion channels are not constitutively open and are thus gated by an external mechanism, which in most cases is from either a change in transmembrane voltage (voltage-gated ion channels) or binding of a chemical neurotransmitter or second messenger cascade (ligand-gated ion channels). Additionally, once the external force opens a given ion channel, it likely has a mechanism to transition into an inactivated state shortly thereafter. The classic voltage-gated ion channel is the fast-activating, fast-inactivating voltage-gated sodium channel. When the transmembrane potential becomes more positive (depolarization) from the resting potential, the voltage-gated sodium channel is more likely to be in the open or activated state. This leads to more depolarization via sodium flow through the channel toward its equilibrium potential. As the membrane becomes more depolarized, a second independent process takes place within the voltage-gated ion channel wherein a portion of the channel gains access to a binding site within the ion pore that effectively plugs the pore, thus inactivating the channel.

The voltage-gated sodium channel is the key determinant of the nerve action potential, which is an all-or-none phenomenon that occurs within the axon and propagates along the axon to its target. The depolarizing phase of the action potential is driven by the voltage-gated sodium channel (Figure 24.1). As the membrane potential becomes depolarized, delayed activation of voltage-gated potassium channels helps the potential become more negative (hyperpolarization), moving it toward the potassium equilibrium potential (−75 mV).

The speed of action potential propagation along an axon is determined by several factors: axonal diameter (larger is faster), temperature (warmer is faster), and myelination. In the peripheral nervous system, there are both myelinated and small unmyelinated axons. Large myelinated axons have conduction velocities of about 60 m/s, whereas small

---

Abbreviations: AMPA, α-amino-3-hydroxy-5-methyl-4-isoxazolepropionic acid; GABA, γ-aminobutyric acid; NMDA, N-methyl-D-aspartate; SNAP-25, synaptosomal-associated protein 25

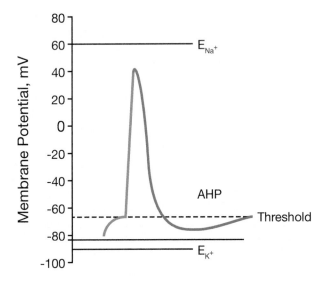

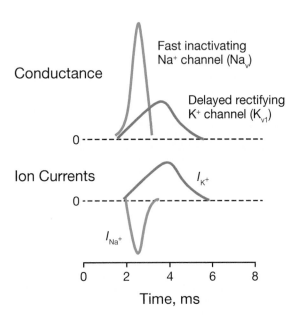

Figure 24.1 Ionic Basis of the Action Potential in Axons. Action potentials occur as a result of opening and closing of specific voltage-gated ion channels. The depolarizing upstroke of the action potential is mediated by a voltage-gated sodium (Na^+) channel that has a fast activation, allowing the membrane potential to approach the equilibrium potential (E) for sodium (E_{Na^+}). The voltage-gated sodium channel has fast inactivation (Na_v). The repolarization is then mediated by a voltage-gated potassium (K^+) channel (delayed rectifying potassium channel; K_{v1}) that brings the membrane potential toward the equilibrium potential for potassium (E_{K^+}). AHP indicates afterhyperpolarization; I, current.

unmyelinated axons have conduction velocities of approximately 2 m/s. Myelination leads to a much faster conduction velocity due to saltatory conduction than can be achieved by increasing axonal diameter. Myelination (by either Schwann cells in the peripheral nervous system or oligodendrocytes in the central nervous system) forms an insulating wrap along a segment of axon (internode); between regions of myelination, there is a small region (the node of Ranvier) that does not contain myelin and is highly enriched for the voltage-gated sodium and potassium channels that underlie the action potential (see Figure 25.1 in Chapter 25). In saltatory conduction, the action potentials effectively skip along the nodes, quickly propagating to their intended target.

Many varieties of voltage-gated ion channels are distributed along neuronal axons, somata, and dendrites in a cell-specific manner. Because each voltage-gated ion channel has a unique pattern of activation and inactivation, and depending on a channel's placement within a given neuron (which may have one of many different morphologies), there exists a bewildering array of neuronal phenotypes that are specialized for their given tasks. There are 10 types of voltage-gated sodium channels (Na_v1-9 and Na_vx), many of which are blocked by the pufferfish toxin (ie, tetrodotoxin) or local anesthetics (eg, lidocaine). Potassium channels come in many varieties, some of which are voltage gated, calcium activated (typically activating after extensive neuronal firing), or second messenger gated. Voltage-gated calcium channels are distributed throughout the nervous system. Some types are involved in the burst firing of action potentials, in pacemaker properties, and in the presynaptic terminal (P/Q type) where they are critical for chemical neurotransmission.

Chemical Neurotransmission

Cell communication in the central nervous system (and neuromuscular junction) occurs primarily at synaptic terminals and is mediated by chemical neurotransmission. As the action potential enters the presynaptic terminal, voltage-gated calcium channels (P/Q type) are activated, allowing calcium ions to enter the neuron. In the majority of neurons, entry of calcium ions leads to a cascade of events that causes a neurotransmitter-filled synaptic vesicle to fuse with the plasma membrane, thus releasing its neurotransmitter into the region between the presynaptic and postsynaptic neuron (ie, the synaptic cleft). The neurotransmitter then diffuses across the synaptic cleft and binds to postsynaptic receptors. These postsynaptic receptors are often ligand-gated ion channels, which then open and either depolarize (excitatory effect) or hyperpolarize (inhibitory effect) the postsynaptic neuron. Mechanisms exist to remove the neurotransmitter from the synaptic cleft by either hydrolyzing the neurotransmitter in the cleft (ie, acetylcholinesterase) or pumping the neurotransmitter into either the presynaptic terminal or the glia, which then completes the cycle of chemical neurotransmission in neuronal communication.

The presynaptic terminal is a complex and highly regulated structure within the neuron. Synaptic vesicles are filled with the neurotransmitter and then eventually are docked along the plasma membrane by a series of specialized synaptic proteins. Toxins target several synaptic proteins. Botulinum toxin targets synaptobrevin, synaptosomal-associated protein 25 (SNAP-25), and syntaxin in the neuromuscular and autonomic presynaptic terminals, whereas tetanus toxins target synaptobrevin in the central inhibitory presynaptic terminals.

Key Peripheral Nervous System Neurotransmitter System: Neuromuscular Junction

Alpha motor neurons in the anterior horn of the spinal cord innervate skeletal muscle and use acetylcholine as their neurotransmitter. The presynaptic terminal releases acetylcholine as described above (Figure 24.2). Acetylcholine diffuses across the synaptic cleft and binds to nicotinic acetylcholine receptors, which then open a nonselective cation channel that depolarizes the muscle membrane. The depolarizing wave across the muscle membrane enters T tubules and activates a voltage-gated calcium channel that causes calcium influx and muscle contraction via the interaction of troponin, tropomyosin, actin, and myosin. Acetylcholinesterase (inhibited by pyridostigmine) resides in the synaptic cleft and hydrolyzes acetylcholine to inactivate it.

Various myasthenic syndromes help illustrate the function of the neuromuscular junction. In autoimmune myasthenia gravis, autoantibodies may target either the acetylcholine receptor or a closely associated muscle-specific kinase. In Lambert-Eaton myasthenic syndrome, autoantibodies target the presynaptic P/Q voltage-gated calcium channel, thus hampering adequate presynaptic calcium levels for exocytosis. Many forms of congenital myasthenic syndromes are caused by mutations in various components of the neuromuscular junction, including the acetylcholine receptor, acetylcholinesterase, and choline acetyltransferase (protein that pumps acetylcholine into synaptic vesicles).

Key Central Nervous System Neurotransmitter Systems: Glutamate and [γ]-Aminobutyric Acid

Postsynaptic receptors for neurotransmitters are often categorized as excitatory (causing depolarization), inhibitory

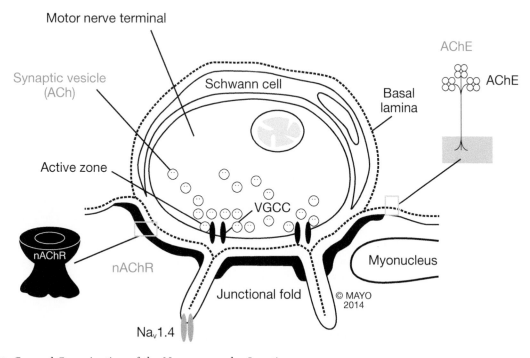

Figure 24.2 *General Organization of the Neuromuscular Junction.*
The neuromuscular junction comprises the presynaptic motor nerve terminal, the postsynaptic myocyte structures, and an enveloping Schwann cell. In the presynaptic terminal, synaptic vesicles are filled with acetylcholine (ACh) and prepared by exocytosis, which is dependent on activation of closely aligned voltage-gated calcium channels (VGCCs). Postsynaptically, the myocyte has ultrastructural organization that increases the surface area via junctional folds that are studded with nicotinic acetylcholine receptors (nAChRs). Acetylcholinesterase (AChE) fills the synaptic cleft and rapidly degrades ACh within the cleft, ensuring a rapid, nonsustained response. $Na_v1.4$ indicates voltage-gated sodium channel 1.4.

(Used with permission of Mayo Foundation for Medical Education and Research.)

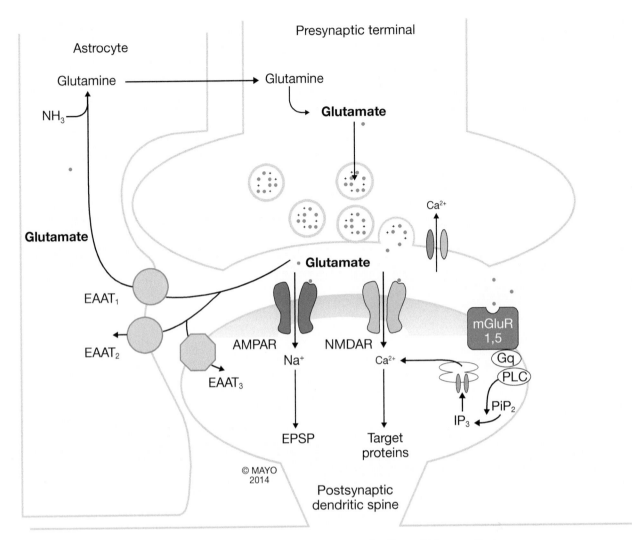

Figure 24.3 *General Organization of the Glutamatergic Synapse in the Central Nervous System.*
The central nervous system glutamatergic synapses comprise a presynaptic glutamatergic axonal nerve terminal, a postsynaptic dendritic spine, and an enveloping astrocytic process. Glutamate is formed from glutamine and packaged into synaptic vesicles that are released via exocytosis in a calcium-dependent fashion. The postsynaptic dendritic spine contains 3 main glutamate receptors, the α-amino-3-hydroxy-5-methyl-4-isoxazolepropionic acid receptor (AMPAR), the N-methyl-D-aspartate receptor (NMDAR), and the metabotropic glutamate receptor (mGluR). When fully activated, the postsynaptic spine depolarizes and has increased intracellular calcium, a signal involved in synaptic plasticity. Glutamate is taken up by excitatory amino acid transporters (EAATs) to ensure efficient neurotransmission and prevent excitotoxicity. Ca^{2+} indicates calcium ion; EPSP, excitatory postsynaptic potential; Gq, Gq protein; IP, inositol phosphate; Na^+, sodium ion; NH_3, ammonia; PiP, phosphatidylinositol phosphate; PLC, phospholipase C.
(Used with permission of Mayo Foundation for Medical Education and Research.)

(causing hyperpolarization), or neuromodulatory (causing slow changes in potentials or provoking second messenger cascades). The most ubiquitous excitatory neurotransmitter is glutamate (produced by metabolism of glutamic acid), which is mediated through α-amino-3-hydroxy-5-methyl-4-isoxazolepropionic acid (AMPA) and N-methyl-D-aspartate (NMDA) receptors (Figure 24.3). The AMPA receptor is a ligand-gated ion channel that binds glutamate and opens a sodium-predominant cation channel whose

equilibrium potential is near 0 mV. This is the main receptor responsible for fast excitatory neurotransmission in the brain. The NMDA-type glutamate receptor has properties that implicate it as a major mediator of neuronal plasticity (and presumably learning and memory). The NMDA receptor requires glutamate binding for activation and concomitant depolarization to achieve its full effect. This binding is necessary because, at normal resting membrane potential, there is a magnesium ion in the pore that

Table 24.1 • Neurotransmitters in the Central Nervous System

Neurotransmitter	Receptors	Receptor Type	Anatomical Cell Body Distribution	Anatomical Receptor Distribution	Key Points	Clinically Relevant Pharmacology or Toxicology[a]
Glutamate	AMPA	Excitatory	Ubiquitous CNS	Ubiquitous CNS	Primary mediator of fast excitatory neurotransmission	
	NMDA	Excitatory	Ubiquitous CNS	Ubiquitous CNS	Critical for synaptic plasticity	Memantine (−) Autoimmune NMDAR encephalitis
	Metabotropic	Neuromodulatory	Ubiquitous CNS	Ubiquitous CNS		
GABA	$GABA_A$	Inhibitory (fast kinetics)	Ubiquitous CNS	Ubiquitous CNS	Primary mediator of fast inhibitory neurotransmission	Benzodiazepines (+) Barbiturates (+) Volatile anesthetics (+) Ethanol (+)
	$GABA_B$	Inhibitory (slow kinetics)	Ubiquitous CNS	Ubiquitous CNS		Baclofen (+)
Glycine	Glycine	Inhibitory	Brain stem and spinal cord	Brain stem and spinal cord		Strychnine (−)
Acetylcholine	Nicotinic	Excitatory	Spinal motor neuron, spinal sympathetic neurons CNS (basal forebrain, mesopontine tegmentum)	Neuromuscular junction, autonomic ganglia Ubiquitous CNS		Pyridostigmine and donepezil (increase ACh via reduced degradation) Succinylcholine (−) Vecuronium (−)
	Muscarinic	Excitatory (M_1) Inhibitory (M_2)	Autonomic ganglia CNS (basal forebrain, mesopontine tegmentum)	Parasympathetic targets Ubiquitous CNS	Excess causes much of cholinergic toxidrome	Pyridostigmine and donepezil (increase ACh via reduced degradation) Pilocarpine (+) Atropine (−) Scopolamine (−)
Dopamine	D_1 type (D_1 and D_5) D_2 type (D_2, D_3, D_4)	Neuromodulatory (excitatory) Neuromodulatory (inhibitory)	SNc VTA	Caudate and putamen (SNc) nucleus accumbens, amygdala, hippocampus, prefrontal cortex (VTA)	Deficient in Parkinson disease; Important role in reward system	Levodopa (+) Dopamine agonists (eg, pramipexole) (+) Antipsychotics (eg, quetiapine) (−)

(continued)

Table 24.1 • Continued

Neurotransmitter	Receptors	Receptor Type	Anatomical Cell Body Distribution	Anatomical Receptor Distribution	Key Points	Clinically Relevant Pharmacology or Toxicology[a]
Serotonin	5-HT$_1$	Neuromodulatory (inhibitory)	Raphe nuclei	Ubiquitous	Mood regulation (SSRI effect); sleep-wake cycle	Buspirone (+) Triptans (+) Trazodone (−)
	5-HT$_2$	Neuromodulatory (excitatory)				
	5-HT$_3$	Excitatory				Ondansetron (−)
Histamine	H$_1$	Neuromodulatory (excitatory)	Tuberomammillary nucleus of hypothalamus	Ubiquitous	Important in states of arousal; sleep-wake cycle	Sedating antihistamines Amitriptyline (−)
	H$_2$	Neuromodulatory (excitatory)				
	H$_3$	Neuromodulatory (inhibitory)				
Norepinephrine	α$_1$	Neuromodulatory (excitatory)	Locus ceruleus; lateral tegmental system	Ubiquitous	Important in states of arousal; sleep-wake cycle	Norepinephrine reuptake blocked by amphetamine/cocaine Prazosin (−) Amitriptyline (−)
	α$_2$	Neuromodulatory (inhibitory)				Clonidine (+) Mirtazapine (−)
	β	Neuromodulatory (variable)				Propranolol (−)

Abbreviations: ACh, acetylcholine; AMPA, α-amino-3-hydroxy-5-methyl-4-isoxazolepropionic acid; CNS, central nervous system; GABA, γ-aminobutyric acid; 5-HT, 5-hydroxytryptamine receptor 1; 5-HT$_2$, 5-hydroxytryptamine receptor 2; 5-HT$_3$, 5-hydroxytryptamine receptor 3; NMDA, N-methyl-D-aspartate; NMDAR, N-methyl-D-aspartate receptor; SNc, sustantia nigra pars compacta; SSRI, selective serotonin reuptake inhibitor; VTA, ventral tegmental area.

[a] Minus sign indicates inhibitory at this receptor; plus sign, excitatory at this receptor.

is released on depolarization and results in calcium influx into the postsynaptic terminal. This local influx of calcium can lead to synapse-specific changes in the postsynaptic neuron that are considered to be the cellular basis for learning and memory.

γ-Aminobutyric acid (GABA) is the main mediator of inhibitory neurotransmission in the brain. It is produced by decarboxylation of L-glutamate by glutamic acid decarboxylase; antibodies against this enzyme are associated with stiff person syndrome. There are 2 main types of GABA receptors: type A (GABA$_A$) and type B (GABA$_B$). GABA$_A$ receptors mediate fast inhibitory neurotransmission by means of a ligand-gated chloride channel mechanism and are the target of benzodiazepines, barbiturates, and ethanol. GABA$_B$ receptors mediate inhibitory neurotransmission but have slower kinetics because they work by means of a second messenger cascade that activates a potassium channel.

The vast neuromodulatory neurotransmitter system is distributed throughout the central nervous system, and the key points are listed in Table 24.1.

- The voltage-gated sodium channel is the key determinant of the nerve action potential, which is an all-or-none phenomenon that occurs within the axon and propagates along the axon to its target.
- The speed of action potential propagation along an axon is determined by several factors: axonal diameter (larger is faster), temperature (warmer is faster), and myelination.
- Postsynaptic receptors are often ligand-gated ion channels, which open and either depolarize (excitatory effect) or hyperpolarize (inhibitory effect) the postsynaptic neuron.
- Botulinum toxin targets synaptobrevin, SNAP-25, and syntaxin in the neuromuscular and autonomic presynaptic terminals, whereas tetanus toxins target synaptobrevin in the central inhibitory presynaptic terminals.
- Alpha motor neurons in the anterior horn of the spinal cord innervate skeletal muscle and use acetylcholine as their neurotransmitter.
- The most ubiquitous excitatory neurotransmitter is glutamate (produced by metabolism of glutamic acid), which is mediated through AMPA and NMDA receptors.
- GABA is the main mediator of inhibitory neurotransmission in the brain.

25 Cellular Processes

NATHAN P. STAFF, MD, PHD

Introduction

Although cells in the nervous system contain all the cellular machinery that exists in other cells throughout the body, nervous system cells have many specialized functions that present unique challenges in the maintenance of cell functionality and homeostasis. The unique morphology of neurons demands elaborate cytoarchitecture, energy production, and cellular processing machinery that are unparalleled in other parts of the body. In this chapter, a broad overview of cellular processes related to cytoskeleton, axonal transport, protein processing, and energy metabolism within the nervous system are discussed. Foreshadowing subsequent chapters, many diseases of the nervous system are due to breakdowns of the intricate processes that are outlined in this chapter.

Cellular Structure

The plasma membrane of neurons is formed by a lipid bilayer that forms a barrier between the internal and external cellular environment. Within this lipid bilayer are many proteins that provide cell-cell signaling (eg, ligand-gated ion channels, neural cell adhesion molecules) or anchor the membrane to internal (cytoskeletal) or external (extracellular matrix) proteins.

Within neurons, the cytoskeleton is composed of several components and plays an important role as a dynamic scaffold (Figure 25.1). Microtubules are 25-nm-diameter polymers of α- and β-tubulin that span the lengths of axons and dendrites and serve as the tracks for axonal transport. Microtubules are dynamic and have polarity, with a plus end and a minus end, which determine the directionality of axonal transport proteins. Neurofilaments (10-nm diameter) are intermediate filaments that provide static structure for axonal processes. Microfilaments (7-nm diameter) are polymers made up of actin. Microfilaments are located primarily just beneath the plasma membrane where they form a dense matrix that anchors integral membrane proteins via linker proteins, such as spectrin-ankryn or dystrophin. This interaction between microfilaments, linker proteins, and integral proteins keeps membrane integral proteins in their proper location within the cell (eg, voltage-gated sodium channels at the node of Ranvier, N-methyl-D-aspartate receptors at the postsynaptic terminal, and active zones for synaptic vesicle release at the presynaptic terminal). Microfilaments are also very dynamic and are involved in protein trafficking and morphologic changes in neurons (eg, growth cones and dendritic spines).

While the cytoskeleton provides the architecture of the neuron, axonal transport is needed to shuttle cellular cargo to and from the prime manufacturing center in the cell body. Anterograde (away from the cell body) transport is accomplished by the kinesin family of proteins. In an adenosine triphosphate (ATP)–dependent fashion, kinesin proteins (and their bound cargoes) progress along the microtubules (toward the plus end) at a rate of 200 to 400 mm/d (ie, fast transport). When kinesin molecules are carrying larger cargo, such as mitochondria or neurofilaments, they advance in a stop-and-start fashion at a slower rate of 1 to 10 mm/d (ie, slow transport). Retrograde (toward the cell body) transport is performed by the dynein-dynactin complex, which is able to move toward the minus end of microtubules at a rate of 150 to 300 mm/d.

Abbreviations: acetyl CoA, acetyl coenzyme A; ER, endoplasmic reticulum; mRNA, messenger RNA; SNAP, soluble N-ethylmaleimide–sensitive factor attachment protein; SNARE, soluble N-ethylmaleimide–sensitive factor attachment protein receptors; TCA, tricarboxylic acid

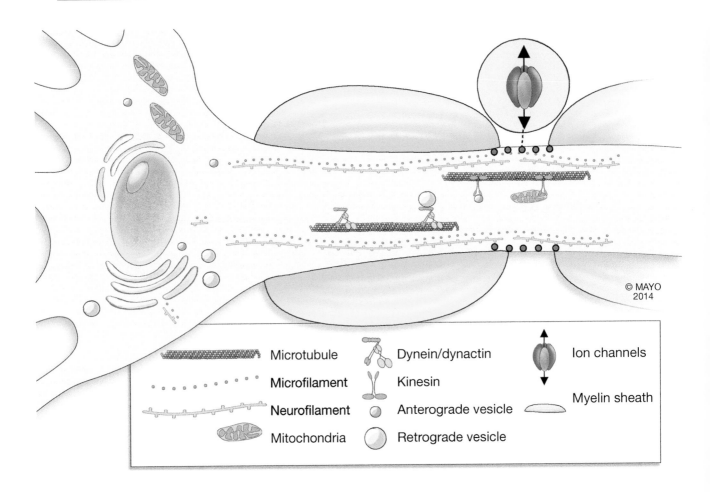

Figure 25.1 Cytoskeletal Components.
Node of Ranvier illustrates cytoskeleton, protein localization, and axonal transport.
(Used with permission of Mayo Foundation for Medical Education and Research.)

Abnormalities in axonal transport are linked to neurologic disease via genetic etiologies (kinesin mutations causing Charcot-Marie-Tooth disease type 2A1 or hereditary spastic paraparesis type 10) or toxic effects (vincristine or taxane toxicity to microtubules causing peripheral neuropathy). It is further hypothesized that axonal transport dysfunction plays a key role in many neurodegenerative diseases.

Protein Processing

The central dogma dictates that DNA within the nucleus encodes for RNA, which is then spliced into messenger RNA (mRNA). The mRNA transcript is then translated into polypeptides via transfer RNA in the ribosomes. If proteins are bound for membrane vesicles within the cell, they pass via the ribosome-studded rough endoplasmic reticulum and Golgi apparatus where they are then shuttled away from the cell body by the axonal transport process

described above (Figure 25.2). There is often extensive posttranslational modification to proteins involving glycosylation (adding sugars to the proteins) or phosphorylation (adding phosphate groups) that affects protein stability, function, and localization within a cell.

Membranous vesicles continuously bud off and fuse with other membranes throughout the cell. For example, vesicles bud off from the endoplasmic reticulum and fuse with the Golgi network, where they eventually bud off and fuse either with an endosome or the plasma membrane. Also, within the plasma membrane, vesicles that are endocytosed are either recycled or destined for degradation via lysosomes. In either instance, regions of membrane destined to become vesicles are coated with a protein (eg, clathrin), which initiates the budding process. Specific posttranslational modifications to integral membrane proteins within the vesicle target the vesicle for its final destination. One example is that lysosomal proteins are tagged with a mannose 6-phosphate within the Golgi network. Additionally, integral membrane proteins known as

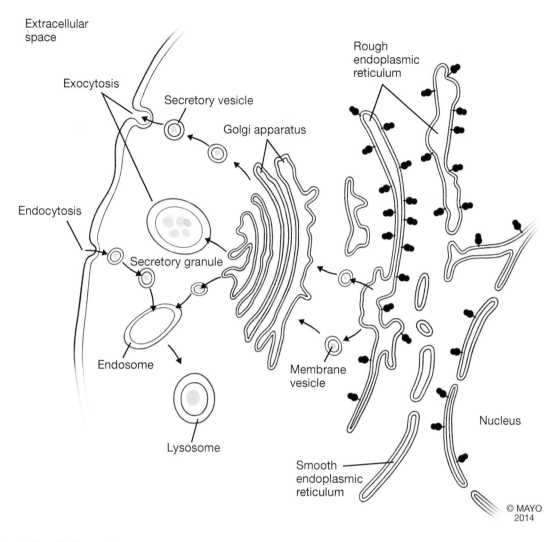

Figure 25.2 *Protein Processing.*
Shown are protein and vesicular trafficking from rough endoplasmic reticulum, the Golgi apparatus, plasma membrane, endosome, lysosome, and the ubiquitin-proteasome system.
(Adapted from Benarroch EE. Basic neurosciences with clinical applications. Philadelphia [PA]: Butterworth Heinemann/Elsevier; c2006. Chapter 3, Protein processing, membrane organization, and cytoskeleton; p. 45–68. Used by permission of Mayo Foundation for Medical Education and Research.)

SNAREs (soluble *N*-ethylmaleimide–sensitive factor attachment protein [SNAP] receptors) are important for vesicles fusing with their targets. The vesicle contains vesicle SNAREs and the target membrane contains complementary target SNAREs that interact and are critical for the vesicle fusion process (also important in neurotransmitter release; see Chapter 24, "Cellular Signaling").

Proteins are eventually degraded within a cell; this degradation may be a programmed process or a response to a given stimulus. Proteins are degraded primarily by 2 processes: endosomal and lysosomal destruction or ubiquitination and proteasome removal. Endosomes are vesicular organelles that are made up of vesicles from the endoplasmic reticulum (ER)–Golgi complex and endocytosed vesicles. Endosomes contain proteins that pump protons into the endosome and thus acidify the environment. As endosomes become more acidic and incorporate more degradative enzymes from the ER-Golgi complex, they become lysosomes. Lysosomes contain acid hydrolases that activate only at acidic levels and serve to hydrolyze proteins within the lysosome. In the cytosol, proteins are primarily degraded via the ubiquitin-proteasome system. As a result of programmed degradation or misfolding or as a stress response, targeted proteins are tagged with ubiquitin (a small protein). Once tagged by ubiquitin, the 26S proteasome binds to the ubiquitinated protein, releases the ubiquitin for reuse, and breaks down the accompanying protein. Many examples of abnormal protein processing

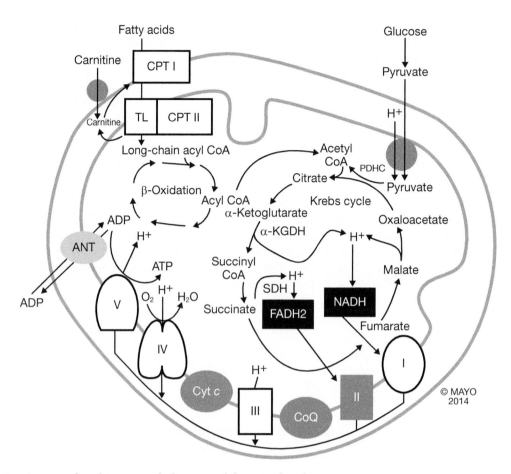

Figure 25.3 *Key Structural and Functional Elements of the Mitochondria.*
Acetyl coenzyme A (CoA) derived from pyruvate transport or β-oxidation of fatty acids enters the Krebs cycle. The production of nicotinamide adenine dinucleotide (NADH) and flavine adenine dinucleotide (FADH2) then supplies electrons to the electron transport chain, producing most cellular adenosine triphosphate (ATP) (from adenosine diphosphate [ADP]). ANT indicates adenine nucleotide translocator; CoQ, coenzyme Q; CPT (I, II), carnitine palmitoyl transferase; Cyt c, cytochrome c; α-KGDH, α-ketoglutarate dehydrogenase; PDHC, pyruvate dehydrogenase complex; SDH, succinate dehydrogenase; TL, carnitine-acylcarnitine translocase.
(Adapted from Benarroch EE. Basic neurosciences with clinical applications. Philadelphia [PA]: Butterworth Heinemann/Elsevier; c2006. Chapter 26, Energy metabolism in the nervous system; p. 953–81. Used by permission of Mayo Foundation for Medical Education and Research.)

are associated with neurologic diseases. Lysosomal storage diseases (Volume 2, Chapter 74, "Lysosomal Storage Disorders") are a broad array of primarily pediatric disorders caused by dysfunctional lysosomal function. Many neurodegenerative diseases (eg, frontotemporal dementia, Lewy body disease) are associated with intracellular inclusions that frequently are tagged with ubiquitin.

Energy Metabolism

As in all tissues, the nervous system requires energy metabolism for proper functioning. The brain, while only 2% of body weight, consumes 20% of energy in the body. Phosphate bonds (eg, ATP) are used as energy fuel to

facilitate the many enzymatic reactions within the cell and are produced primarily through the processes of glycolysis, lipid metabolism, the tricarboxylic acid (TCA) cycle (Krebs cycle), and ultimately oxidative phosphorylation in the electron transport chain.

The main energy manufacturer in cells is the mitochondria (Figure 25.3). Thought to be a remnant of a prokaryotic symbiosis with a primitive eukaryote, the mitochondria have their own DNA encoding 37 proteins (most mitochondrial proteins are encoded in nuclear DNA). Within the mitochondria, the main fuel for the TCA cycle is acetyl coenzyme A (acetyl CoA), which is produced primarily from 2 substrates. In the brain, most acetyl CoA is produced when pyruvate dehydrogenase transforms pyruvate (a cytosolic glycolysis end product).

Of note, pyruvate dehydrogenase requires thiamine pyrophosphate as a cofactor (see Volume 2, Chapter 78, "Neurologic Complications of Nutritional Disorders"). Elsewhere in the body, especially in muscle, fatty acid oxidation provides considerable amounts of acetyl CoA. Long-chain fatty acids have a specific transport mechanism into the mitochondria that depends on L-carnitine and carnitine palmitoyltransferases I and II, defects of which are associated with neurologic disease. Alterations in several other steps in fatty acid oxidation cause neurologic and systemic disease and are discussed further in Volume 2, Chapter 73, "Neurometabolic Disorders Associated With Disturbances of Small Molecule Metabolism." Acetyl CoA then feeds the TCA cycle and results in production of nicotinamide adenine dinucleotide after reduction (NADH) and flavin adenine dinucleotide, hydroquinone form (FADH2). These molecules serve as electron donors in the electron transport chain, which help produce a hydrogen gradient along the internal mitochondrial membrane and the outer mitochondrial membrane. The hydrogen gradient is then exploited via ATP synthase, wherein most of the ATP in the body is produced via oxidative phosphorylation.

Blood glucose is the substrate for most of the energy for oxidative metabolism in the brain, and it enters the brain via the facilitative glucose transporters 1 (astrocytes and endothelial cells) and 3 (neurons). Astrocytes store glucose in the form of glycogen and provide an energy reserve for the brain in times of hypoglycemia. If there is severe hypoglycemia, the brain is also able to use either mannose (which can enter glycolytic pathway) or ketone bodies (transformed into acetyl CoA) as energy sources.

- Anterograde (away from the cell body) transport is accomplished by the kinesin family of proteins, which is able to move toward the plus end of microtubules at a rate of 200 to 400 mm/d.
- Retrograde (toward the cell body) transport is performed by the dynein-dynactin complex, which is able to move toward the minus end of microtubules at a rate of 150 to 300 mm/d.
- Proteins are degraded primarily by 2 processes: endosomal and lysosomal destruction or ubiquitination and proteasome removal.
- As a result of programmed degradation or misfolding or as a stress response, targeted proteins are tagged with ubiquitin (a small protein).
- The mitochondria have their own DNA encoding 37 proteins.
- Long-chain fatty acids have a specific transport mechanism into the mitochondria that is dependent on L-carnitine and carnitine palmitoyltransferases I and II, defects of which are associated with neurologic disease.

26 Cellular Injury and Death

BRIAN S. KATZ, MD; EDUARDO E. BENARROCH, MD

Introduction

Cell death is a result of several complex interconnected mechanisms simultaneously occurring in the cell's organelles, namely, necrosis, apoptosis, and autophagy. While different morphologically and biochemically, these processes are not mutually exclusive and commonly coexist in cell loss in vascular, inflammatory, and degenerative conditions.

Mechanisms of Cell Death

The 3 pathways of cellular injury and death are 1) external forced cell death or necrosis; 2) programmed nuclear cell death, including apoptosis; and 3) autophagic cell death (Table 26.1). These processes may affect neurons, glial cells, endothelial cells, and ependymal cells. The cell death pathways differ in their triggering factors, temporal profile, biochemical mechanisms, and morphologic markers.

While necrosis and apoptosis appear very different biochemically and histologically, they are not mutually exclusive processes. In general, acute injury leading to severe adenosine triphosphate (ATP) depletion (such as ischemia or status epilepticus) triggers necrosis, whereas slower processes, such as neurodegeneration, may lead primarily to apoptosis, which requires some residual ATP levels. Both pathways critically involve the mitochondria (Figure 26.1).

Eventually all the cellular injury and death pathways coalesce to form the "final common pathway" of cell death. Because of the multiple triggers of multiple interconnecting pathways, no single specific element has been identified to prevent cellular injury and death. This may explain the difficulty involved in creating "neuron-protective" agents for acute and chronic neurologic diseases.

Necrosis

Necrosis is a process of cell injury attributable to abrupt and severe loss of energy. Examples include cerebral ischemia and severe head trauma. Impaired mitochondrial function results in ATP depletion leading to failure of ion pumps (such as the sodium-potassium–adenosine triphosphatase pump), leading to cell swelling and neuronal depolarization (Figure 26.2). Impaired astrocytic reuptake of glutamate leads to an increase in synaptic levels of glutamate, and activation of N-methyl-D-aspartate (NMDA) receptors leads to glutamate-triggered excitotoxicity mediated by an increase in intracellular calcium. Calcium-triggered cascades result in production of nitric oxide, calpain-induced destruction of the cytoskeleton, and DNA damage. Mitochondrial respiratory chain dysfunction also leads to production of superoxide, triggering oxidative stress that damages cell membranes and DNA. Cells undergoing necrosis show evidence of mitochondrial swelling and extensive vacuolization of the cytoplasm, and the chromatin becomes coarse with loss of nuclear staining (karyolysis). The cell swelling eventually results in lysis, and this then triggers a secondary inflammatory response.

Apoptosis

Apoptosis is a form of programmed cell death that occurs normally in development but also occurs under certain abnormal conditions and results in early cell death. Triggering stimuli may be intrinsic, such as oxidative stress, or extrinsic, such as the inflammatory cytokine tumor necrosis factor. The final effectors are caspases, which are

---

Abbreviations: AMPA, α-amino-3-hydroxy-5-methyl-4-isoxazolepropionic acid; ATP, adenosine triphosphate; NMDA, N-methyl-D-aspartate

Table 26.1 • Microscopic and Histologic Appearance of Cell Death Pathways

Pathway	Necrosis	Apoptosis	Autophagy
Cell membrane permeability	Increased membrane permeability or disruption (characteristic) leads to inflammation (see apoptosis triggers)	Preserved until late Cells and organelles shrink; cell membrane invaginates (blebs)	Normal
Cell or organelle swelling	Yes	No	No
Nucleus	Swelling	Chromatin condensation (as a result of nuclear cytokine triggers or direct nuclear toxins) Nuclear breakdown	No change
ATP levels	Depleted early	Preserved until very late	...
PARP activity	Increased	Decreased	...
Triggers	Acute energy failure (hypoxemia, ischemia, acute exposure to toxins, status epilepticus)	Inflammation (necrosis, TNF-α) DNA damage (nuclear, mitochondrial, or both) Oxidative stress Endoplasmic reticulum stress response	Accumulation of misfolded proteins or damaged organelles Imbalance of homeostasis of proteins
Mechanisms	Excitotoxicity (glutamate) Cellular or organelle membrane leakage Calcium-triggered cascades (phospholipases, endonucleases, cathepsin, NOS)	Death receptor activation Mitochondria produce and release proapoptotic signals Caspases or nuclease activation	Macroautophagy Microautophagy or chaperone-mediated autophagy

Abbreviations: ATP, adenosine triphosphate; NOS, nitric oxide synthase; PARP, poly adenosine diphosphate ribose polymerase; TNF-α, tumor necrosis factor α.

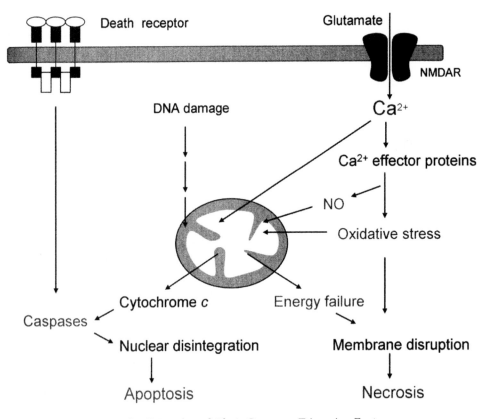

Figure 26.1 *The 2 Main Mechanisms of Cell Death and Their Common Triggering Factors.*
The mitochondria are involved in both necrosis and apoptosis. Whether the cell dies of necrosis depends on the adenosine triphosphate concentration, which is determined in part by the intensity and temporal profile of the insult. Ca²⁺ indicates calcium; NMDAR, N-methyl-D-aspartate receptor; NO, nitric oxide.
(Adapted from Benarroch EE. Basic neurosciences with clinical applications. Philadelphia [PA]: Butterworth Heinemann/Elsevier; c2006. Chapter 28, Mechanisms of neuronal injury and death; p. 1017–43. Used with permission of Mayo Foundation for Medical Education and Research.)

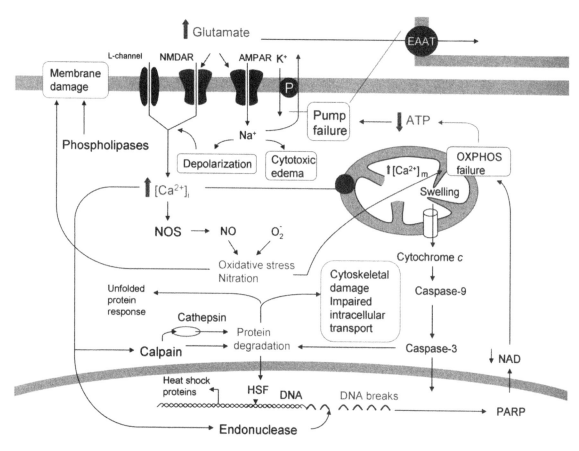

Figure 26.2 Excitotoxic Cascade.

Activation of glutamate α-amino-3-hydroxy-5-methyl-4-isoxazolepropionic acid receptors (AMPAR) and N-methyl-D-aspartate receptors (NMDAR) leads to sodium (Na⁺) influx and cell swelling, cell depolarization, and massive influx of calcium (Ca²⁺) via voltage-gated and N-methyl-D-aspartate channels. Ca²⁺ activates potentially damaging cascades, including phospholipases, calpain, cathepsin, nitric oxide synthase (NOS), and endonucleases. This results in generation of free radicals, including nitric oxide (NO) and the superoxide radical (O₂⁻), leading to oxidative stress and protein nitration, membrane damage, impairment of oxidative phosphorylation (OXPHOS), and therefore adenosine triphosphate (ATP) production and pump failure, impaired cytoskeletal and transport function, and DNA breaks. Markers of cell stress include activation of heat shock factor (HSF) and poly adenosine diphosphate ribose polymerase (PARP). PARP consumes nicotinamide adenine dinucleotide (NAD), and this contributes to OXPHOS failure. Accumulation of intramitochondrial Ca²⁺ leads to mitochondrial swelling, which further impairs energy metabolism and triggers opening of a permeability transition pore and release of cytochrome c, triggering apoptosis. EAAT indicates excitatory amino acid transporter; K⁺, potassium; P, sodium-potassium–adenosine triphosphatase pump.

(Adapted from Benarroch EE. Basic neurosciences with clinical applications. Philadelphia [PA]: Butterworth Heinemann/Elsevier; c2006. Chapter 28, Mechanisms of neuronal injury and death; p. 1017–43. Used with permission of Mayo Foundation for Medical Education and Research.)

proteases that damage DNA. For example, oxidative stress, excessive calcium loading, or accumulation of unfolded proteins (as typically occurs in neurodegenerative disorders) triggers the intrinsic mitochondrial pathway of apoptosis that involves the formation of a mitochondrial pore and the release of cytochrome *c* and other mediators that activate caspases, leading to DNA fragmentation. Caspases also cleave cytoskeletal proteins and lamins that result in cell dysfunction and death. Cells undergoing apoptosis shrink. The nucleus shrinks, and the chromatin condenses (pyknosis) and collapses into patches. The cell breaks into dense spheres called apoptotic bodies. The DNA fragments and marginates along the inner aspect of the nuclear envelope. Phagocytosis of apoptotic bodies occurs by neighboring cells. There is no inflammation.

Autophagy

Autophagy refers to lysosomal-mediated degradation of intracellular contents. It occurs in chaperone-mediated autophagy, microautophagy, and macroautophagy. Chaperone-mediated autophagy is initiated by heat-shock proteins that recognize accumulated unfolded proteins (such as Aβ amyloid or α-synuclein) that have escaped normal degradation by the ubiquitin-proteasome system. The proteins are degraded by autophagy, and impairment of this process leads to accumulation of abnormal inclusions, such as Lewy bodies. Autophagic removal of mitochondria (mitophagy) is important for mitochondrial quality control, because poor-quality mitochondria may increase intracellular oxidative stress and generate apoptotic signals.

- The 3 pathways of cellular injury and death are 1) external forced cell death or necrosis; 2) programmed nuclear cell death, including apoptosis; and 3) autophagic cell death.

- Eventually all the cellular injury and death pathways coalesce to form the "final common pathway" of cell death.
- Necrosis is a process of cell injury attributable to abrupt and severe loss of energy (eg, cerebral ischemia).
- Apoptosis is a form of programmed cell death that occurs normally in development but also occurs under certain abnormal conditions and results in early cell death.
- *Autophagy* refers to lysosomal-mediated degradation of intracellular contents.

Clinical Correlation

Ischemic Stroke

After vessel occlusion and deprivation of oxygen to the brain, a series of events occur in the ischemic cascade.

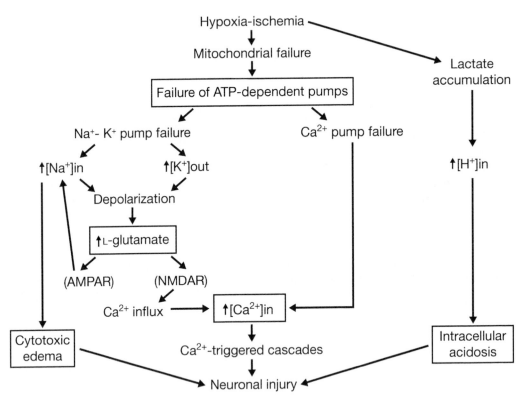

Figure 26.3 *Cerebral Blood Flow and Cerebral Oxygen and Glucose Consumption.*
The cascade of events leads to ischemic neuronal injury. The initial mechanism is mitochondrial failure, adenosine triphosphate (ATP) depletion, and pump failure. This leads to neuronal depolarization due to an increase of extracellular potassium (K^+), a decrease in uptake of L-glutamate, and an increase in intracellular sodium (Na^+) and calcium (Ca^{2+}). Calcium-triggered cascades, including phospholipases, proteases, and nucleases, together with intracellular acidosis (from accumulation of lactate), lead to production of oxygen free radicals, disruption of the cytoskeleton, and neuronal death. AMPAR indicates α-amino-3-hydroxy-5-methyl-4-isoxazolepropionic acid receptor; H^+, hydrogen; NMDAR, N-methyl-D-aspartate receptor.
(Adapted from Benarroch EE, Daube JR, Flemming KD, Westmoreland BF. Mayo Clinic medical neurosciences: organized by neurologic systems and levels. 5th ed. Rochester [MN]: Mayo Clinic Scientific Press and Florence [KY]: Informa Healthcare USA; c2008. Chapter 12, The vascular system; p. 447–88. Used with permission of Mayo Foundation for Medical Education and Research.)

Table 26.2 • Self-aggregating Misfolded Proteins

Normally Expressed Protein	Abnormally Processed Protein	Pathology	Example of Disease
Amyloid precursor protein	Aβ42	Neuritic plaque	Alzheimer disease
Cellular prion protein (PrP^c)	Scrapie prion protein (PrP^{Sc})	Florid plaque	Creutzfeldt-Jakob disease
Tau	Hyperphosphorylated tau (paired helical filaments)	Neurofibrillary changes	Alzheimer disease
Tau	Hyperphosphorylated tau (single filament)	Rounded inclusion or balloon neurons	Pick disease
α-Synuclein	α-Synuclein	Lewy body	Lewy body disease
α-Synuclein	α-Synuclein	Glial cytoplasmic inclusion	Multiple systems atrophy
Superoxide dismutase 1	Superoxide dismutase 1	Inclusion body	Amyotrophic lateral sclerosis

Cerebral blood flow and cerebral oxygen and glucose consumption decrease at the center of the ischemic area (Figure 26.3). Local autoregulatory mechanisms become impaired. Anaerobic glycolysis is initiated as oxygen and glucose levels decrease. The tissue lactate level increases, and thus, pH decreases, resulting in intracellular acidosis. Substrate depletion leads to failure of mitochondrial function and inefficient ATP generation, with resultant leakage of potassium from cells and intracellular accumulation of sodium, chloride, and calcium. Transmembrane potential diminishes and cellular water increases. The energy loss also results in increased release of excitatory neurotransmitters such as glutamate. Subsequently, there is activation of NMDA and α-amino-3-hydroxy-5-methyl-4-isoxazolepropionic acid (AMPA) receptors, resulting in increased permeability to sodium and further cellular swelling and lysis. Calcium enters the postsynaptic neuron, and calcium-induced release of excitatory neurotransmitters heightens further necrosis. The intracellular calcium can activate phospholipases, proteases, and endonucleases and generate oxygen free radicals and nitric oxide. Ultimately, these events lead to cell destruction.

Paraneoplastic Disease

Paraneoplastic disease is caused by autoreactive antibodies against neuronal antigens from tumor cells. These antigens are recognized as foreign and create an autoantibody response and cytotoxic T cells. Autoantibodies invade neurons and disrupt critical cell proteins, leading to apoptotic cell death.

Neurodegenerative Disease

Neurodegenerative diseases have variable clinical and pathologic manifestations, with some underlying similarities: They occur late in life; there is selective neuronal loss with synaptic alteration; and they are characterized by abnormal deposits of misfolded proteins (Table 26.2). While much of the pathophysiology of these disorders is not completely understood, mechanisms triggering the misfolding include genetic mutations or environmental damage.

- Neurodegenerative diseases are associated with selective neuronal loss and characterized by abnormal deposits of misfolded proteins (Table 26.2).

Questions and Answers

Questions

Multiple Choice (choose the best answer)

II.1. Which of the following statements regarding neuronal trans-membrane potentials is most correct?
  a. In most cases, the neuronal resting membrane potential is approximately +70 mV
  b. Maintenance of the resting membrane potential is primarily done via passive membrane ion transport
  c. The depolarizing phase of the action potential is mediated primarily by voltage-gated sodium channels that have a fast activation
  d. The speed of action potential propagation is entirely independent of axonal diameter
  e. The equilibrium potential of potassium is highly positive (around +75 mV) and therefore does not contribute meaningfully to the resting membrane potential

II.2. Which of the following statements regarding neurotransmission is most correct?
  a. γ-Aminobutyric acid (GABA) is the primary inhibitory neurotransmitter in the central nervous system
  b. GABA A receptors have slower kinetics because they work by means of a second messenger cascade that activates a potassium channel
  c. Glycine receptors are widely distributed in the central nervous system and have a primarily excitatory effect
  d. The AMPA (α-amino-3-hydroxy-5-methyl-4-isoxazole propionic acid) glutamate receptor is primarily responsible for central nervous system neuronal plasticity
  e. The D2-type dopamine receptor system is the primary excitatory receptor population in the ventral tegmental area

II.3. Which of the following is the primary neurotransmitter synthesized by spinal alpha motoneurons?
  a. Dopamine
  b. Serotonin
  c. Norepinephrine
  d. Acetylcholine
  e. Glutamate

II.4. Which of the following statements regarding axonal transport is most correct?
  a. Anterograde axonal transport is accomplished along neurofilaments (10-nm diameter intermediate filaments)
  b. Retrograde axonal transport is capable of rates up to 15 to 30 mm/d
  c. Microfilaments (7-nm diameter) provide the primary static structure for axonal processes
  d. Microtubules are static structures and as a result have no contribution to the directionality of axonal transport

  e. Retrograde axonal transport is performed by the dynein-dynactin complex

II.5. Which of the following statements regarding neuronal oxidative metabolism in the brain is most correct?
  a. Ketones are the primary neuronal energy source in the setting of normoglycemia
  b. Glycogen stored in astrocytes can serve as a neuronal energy reserve in the setting of hypoglycemia
  c. Neurons are unable to utilize mannose in times of oxidative stress
  d. Pyruvate dehydrogenase does not require a thiamine cofactor to transform pyruvate into acetyl coenzyme A
  e. Neurons are unique in that they do not metabolize substrates via the tricarboxylic acid cycle

II.6. Which of the following statements regarding neuronal protein processing is most correct?
  a. Mitochondria are the primary intracellular site of protein processing and degradation
  b. Endosomal alkalinization results in the formation of lysosomes
  c. Clathrin proteins are intimately involved in vesicle budding
  d. Mitochondrial proteins are tagged with a mannose 6-phosphate within the Golgi network
  e. The ubiquitin-proteasome system is the primary process of protein degradation within lysosomes

II.7. Misfolding of which of the following proteins typically occurs in patients with multiple systems atrophy?
  a. Superoxide dismutase 1
  b. α-Synuclein
  c. Tau
  d. Cellular prion protein (PrPc)
  e. Amyloid precursor protein

II.8. Which of the following statements regarding mechanisms of neuronal death is most correct?
  a. Cell membrane permeability decreases during autophagy
  b. Apoptosis is marked by prominent swelling of mitochondria, nuclei, and lysosomes
  c. Early adenosine triphosphate depletion is a characteristic feature of necrosis
  d. Accumulation of misfolded proteins or damaged organelles is a common apoptotic trigger
  e. Poly (adenosine diphosphate-ribose) polymerase (PARP) activity is decreased in the setting of cellular necrosis

II.9. Accumulation of which of the following abnormally processed proteins is responsible for the pathologic observation of neuritic plaques in patients with Alzheimer disease?
  a. Scrapie prion protein (PrPSc)
  b. Hyperphosphorylated tau
  c. α-Synuclein
  d. Superoxide dismutase
  e. Aβ42

II.10. Which of the following statements regarding neurotransmitter receptor mechanisms is most correct?
   a. D_5 dopamine receptors have an excitatory neuromodulatory function
   b. $5-HT_1$ serotonin receptors have an excitatory neuromodulatory function
   c. M_1 muscarinic receptors are primarily inhibitory
   d. Glycine receptors have a combination of excitatory and inhibitory functions
   e. AMPA (α-amino-3-hydroxy-5-methyl-4-isoxazole propionic acid) glutamate receptors are exclusively inhibitory

Answers

II.1. Answer c.
   Kandel ER, Schwartz JH, Jessell TM, Siegelbaum SA, Hudspeth AJ. Principles of neural science. 5th ed. New York (NY): McGraw-Hill Medical; c2013. 1709 p.

II.2. Answer a.
   Benarroch EE. Basic neurosciences with clinical applications. Philadelphia (PA): Butterworth Heinemann/Elsevier; c2006. 1087 p.

II.3. Answer d.
   Benarroch EE, Daube JR, Flemming KD, Westmoreland BF. Mayo Clinic medical neurosciences: organized by neurologic systems and levels. 5th ed. Rochester (MN): Mayo Clinic Scientific Press and Florence (KY): Informa Healthcare USA; c2008. 808 p.

II.4. Answer e.
   Benarroch EE. Basic neurosciences with clinical applications. Philadelphia (PA): Butterworth Heinemann/Elsevier; c2006. 1087 p.

II.5. Answer b.
   Kandel ER, Schwartz JH, Jessell TM, Siegelbaum SA, Hudspeth AJ. Principles of neural science. 5th ed. New York (NY): McGraw-Hill Medical; c2013. 1709 p.

II.6. Answer c.
   Benarroch EE. Basic neurosciences with clinical applications. Philadelphia (PA): Butterworth Heinemann/Elsevier; c2006. 1087 p.

II.7. Answer b.
   Benarroch EE. Basic neurosciences with clinical applications. Philadelphia (PA): Butterworth Heinemann/Elsevier; c2006. 1087 p.

II.8. Answer c.
   Kandel ER, Schwartz JH, Jessell TM, Siegelbaum SA, Hudspeth AJ. Principles of neural science. 5th ed. New York (NY): McGraw-Hill Medical; c2013. 1709 p.

II.9. Answer e.
   Benarroch EE. Basic neurosciences with clinical applications. Philadelphia (PA): Butterworth Heinemann/Elsevier; c2006. 1087 p.

II.10. Answer a.
   Kandel ER, Schwartz JH, Jessell TM, Siegelbaum SA, Hudspeth AJ. Principles of neural science. 5th ed. New York (NY): McGraw-Hill Medical; c2013. 1709 p.

SUGGESTED READING

Benarroch EE. Basic neurosciences with clinical applications. Philadelphia (PA): Butterworth Heinemann/Elsevier; c2006. 1087 p.

Benarroch EE, Daube JR, Flemming KD, Westmoreland BF. Mayo Clinic medical neurosciences: organized by neurologic systems and levels. 5th ed. Rochester (MN): Mayo Clinic Scientific Press and Florence (KY): Informa Healthcare USA; c2008. 808 p.

Bredesen DE. Key note lecture: toward a mechanistic taxonomy for cell death programs. Stroke. 2007 Feb;38(2 Suppl):652–60.

Johri A, Beal MF. Mitochondrial dysfunction in neurodegenerative diseases. J Pharmacol Exp Ther. 2012 Sep;342(3):619–30. Epub 2012 Jun 13.

Kandel ER, Schwartz JH, Jessell TM, Siegelbaum SA, Hudspeth AJ. Principles of neural science. 5th ed. New York (NY): McGraw-Hill Medical; c2013. 1709 p.

Neuropharmacology
Jeffrey W. Britton, MD, *editor*

Section
III

27 Neuropharmacology

AMY Z. CREPEAU, MD; JEFFREY W. BRITTON, MD

Introduction

Medications used in the treatment of nervous system disorders typically modulate neurotransmitter function or action potential propagation to result in alterations in neurologic function. This chapter begins with a discussion of principles of pharmacokinetics. Targets for drug action and a basis for understanding how medications exert their action are also discussed. Finally, disease-specific treatments are detailed.

Principles of Pharmacokinetics

Pharmacokinetic principles of neurologic medications are important to understand for the purposes of medication prescribing and ordering (Figure 27.1). Multiple routes of administration—intravenous, sublingual, intramuscular, subcutaneous, rectal, oral, and transdermal—are available for neurologic therapeutic agents. Oral administration is affected by gastric pH, gastric contents, gastric emptying time, transmembrane transport mechanisms, and gastrointestinal tract motility. These factors can be altered by medication coadministration, medical conditions, and age.

The bioavailability of a drug, once absorbed, or the drug's distribution is affected by body fat percentage, which varies with age, and protein binding. The volume of distribution is the ratio of total amount of drug in the body to drug blood plasma concentration and reflects how the drug will be distributed throughout the body per dose,

based on a number of parameters. The expected serum concentration (C_o) after the administration of a specific dose (D) is calculated using the volume of distribution (V_d): $C_o = D/V_d$. Understanding the volume of distribution is important in order to predict duration of drug effect for certain drugs. A common example is comparing the duration of effect of lorazepam and diazepam. Diazepam has a large volume of distribution compared with that of lorazepam. As a result, a bioequivalent dose of diazepam has a shorter duration of anticonvulsant action than lorazepam as it is effectively diluted by its wide distribution after administration.

Factors affecting volume of distribution include body mass, body fat percentage, solubility, and protein binding. Serum proteins that bind drugs include albumin, lipoprotein, glycoprotein, and α-, β-, and γ-globulins. Protein binding is impacted by factors intrinsic to the drug and by serum protein concentration. The latter is affected by age, concurrent illnesses, and other medications taken by the patient (Box 27.1). A decrease in protein binding results in an increased concentration of free drug. Neurologic drugs in which serum protein binding plays an important clinical role include phenytoin, valproic acid, and carbamazepine. Use of serum-free concentrations in monitoring therapy is important with use of these drugs in patients in whom serum protein binding is affected.

Hepatic metabolism of neurologic therapeutics is primarily through the cytochrome P-450 and uridine-glucuronyl transferase enzyme systems. The activity of these systems is influenced by age, genetic factors, and

---

Abbreviations: ACh, acetylcholine; AED, antiepileptic drug; AMPA, α-amino-3-hydroxy-5-methyl-4-isoxazolepropionic acid; cAMP, cyclic adenosine monophosphate; CNS, central nervous system; COMT, catechol O-methyltransferase; DHE, dihydroergotamine; dopa, 3,4-dihydroxyphenylalanine; GABA, γ-aminobutyric acid; 5-HIAA, 5-hydroxyindolacetic acid; 5-HT$_{1B}$, 5-hydroxytryptamine receptor 1B; 5-HT$_{1D}$, 5-hydroxytryptamine (serotonin) receptor 1D; MAO, monoamine oxidase; MAO-A, monoamine oxidase type A; MAO-B, monoamine oxidase type B; NMDA, N-methyl-D-aspartate; PD, Parkinson disease; REM, rapid eye movement; SERT, serotonin transporter; SNRI, selective noradrenergic reuptake inhibitors; SSRI, selective serotonin reuptake inhibitor; T$_H$1, type 1 helper T cell; T$_H$2, type 2 helper T cell; VMAT, vesicular monoamine transporter

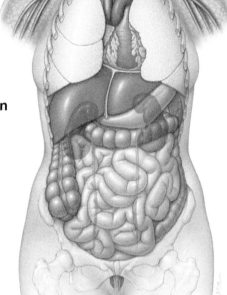

Routes of Administration
Intravenous (30-60 s)
Sublingual (3-5 min)
Intramuscular (10-20 min)
Subcutaneous (15-30 min)
Oral (30-90 min)
Transdermal (variable)

Blood-Brain Barrier
Lipophilic molecules
Tight junctions
Transport proteins

Volume of Distribution
Body fat percentage
Protein binding

Metabolism/Excretion
Hepatic metabolism
  CYP systems
  UGT systems
Renal elimination
  Glomerular filtration

Gastric Absorption
Gastric pH
Gastric contents
Gastric emptying time
GI motility

© MAYO
2012

Figure 27.1 *Principles of Pharmacokinetics.*
CYP indicates cytochrome P-450; GI, gastrointestinal; UGT, uridine-glucuronyl transferase.
(Used with permission of Mayo Foundation for Medical Education and Research.)

Box 27.1 • Causes for a Decrease in Serum Protein Binding

Catabolism
Malnutrition
Liver disease
Renal disease
Advanced age
Infancy
Concurrent administration of other highly
  protein-bound medications

other medications. Renal excretion is heavily influenced by age and renal disease.

Medications that act on the central nervous system (CNS) have the additional challenge of needing to cross the blood-brain barrier. Lipid-soluble molecules are able to cross the blood-brain barrier relatively easily, while water-soluble molecules are often unable to cross the barrier or require the assistance of transport channels. The integrity of the blood-brain barrier is maintained by tight junctions between endothelial cells in the capillaries, choroid plexus, and the meninges. These tight junctions limit the passage of compounds in either direction, particularly for large and water-soluble molecules.

- Pharmacokinetic principles of neurologic medications are important to understand for the purposes of medication prescribing and ordering.
- Lipid-soluble molecules are able to cross the blood-brain barrier relatively easily, while water-soluble molecules are often unable to cross the barrier or require the assistance of transport channels.

Major Neurologic Targets

The functions of the neurologic system depend on signaling across synapses and axonal propagation, which allow communication between different brain regions in neural networks. Synaptic and axonal propagation mechanisms provide the target for many neurologic therapeutic agents.

Ion Channels

Electrical signals in the nervous system are propagated by alterations in the resting membrane potential, which is determined by the relative balance of the fluxes of sodium (Na^+), potassium (K^+), chloride (Cl^-), and calcium (Ca^{2+}) across the membrane. At rest, the neurons and their processes show a predominance of Na^+, Ca^{2+}, and Cl^- concentrations in the extracellular space, and a higher concentration of K^+ in the intracellular space, resulting in a resting membrane potential of -70 mV, reflecting relative negativity in the intracellular region. Increases in Na^+ and Ca^{2+} conductance lead to reductions in the magnitude of negative potential intracellularly, increasing the intracellular potential, until the threshold is reached (the threshold is typically -40 to -55 mV). When the transmembrane potential supersedes the threshold, this triggers the opening of fast-inactivating voltage-gated Na^+ channels, leading to rapid membrane depolarization and transient overshoot (transient intracellular positivity). These same voltage-gated channels rapidly inactivate, leading to a reduction in transmembrane potential. In addition, at the threshold, slow-inactivating K^+ channels are also opened, leading to K^+ efflux. Increasing K^+ conductance eventually leads to membrane hyperpolarization, decreasing excitability, and eventually restores the membrane to resting membrane potential. Opening Ca^{2+} channels also leads to cellular depolarization and excitation. Medications that block voltage-gated Na^+ or Ca^{2+} channels or activate voltage-gated K^+ channels decrease neuronal excitability.

γ-Aminobutyric Acid

γ-Aminobutyric acid (GABA) plays an important role in neuronal inhibition. Ionotropic $GABA_A$ receptors reside in synapses, providing quick-acting phasic inhibition, whereas metabotropic $GABA_B$ receptors are localized in extrasynaptic regions, giving rise to tonic inhibition.

In the presynaptic neuron, glutamate, an excitatory neurotransmitter, is converted to GABA by glutamic acid decarboxylase. This reaction is dependent on pyridoxine (vitamin B_6). GABA is then stored in presynaptic vesicles. When GABA is released and binds to postsynaptic $GABA_A$ receptors, Cl^- flows into the postsynaptic neuron, resulting in hyperpolarization and neuronal inhibition. $GABA_B$ receptor activation, in contrast, leads to efflux of intracellular K^+, resulting in neuronal hyperpolarization, and thus, inhibition. GABA is taken back up into the presynaptic neuron by GABA transporter and broken down by the enzyme GABA transaminase. GABAergic mechanisms are important in the mechanisms of action of many antiepileptic drugs (AEDs).

Glutamate

Glutamate is the primary excitatory neurotransmitter in the CNS. It is an amino acid, which does not cross the blood-brain barrier but is synthesized within the CNS from glucose from α-ketoglutarate in the tricarboxylic acid cycle (Krebs cycle). After glutamate is released into the synapse, it is taken up into glial cells by excitatory amino acid transporters and converted into glutamine by glutamine synthetase. Glutamine is converted back to glutamate by glutaminase. The bidirectional conversion between glutamate and glutamine allows for rapid neurotransmission.

Glutamate acts on a number of ionotropic and metabotropic glutamatergic receptors. The functional classes of the ionotropic subtypes are the *N*-methyl-D-aspartate (NMDA), α-amino-3-hydroxy-5-methyl-4-isoxazolepropionic acid (AMPA), and kainate receptors. When glutamate binds to one of these receptors, the channel opens, allowing Ca^{2+} and Na^+ influx to the postsynaptic terminal, resulting in depolarization. At membrane potentials more negative than -50 mV, magnesium ions (Mg^{2+}) in the extracellular space block NMDA receptor channels, preventing influx of cations. Activation of NMDA receptors requires concurrent binding of glutamate and glycine. Glutamatergic pathways are important in the mechanisms of seizures and long-term potentiation underlying memory formation.

The metabotropic glutamate receptors activate a G-protein–coupled reaction, which either leads to release of postsynaptic Ca^{2+} vesicle stores, leading to apoptosis, or inhibition of cyclic adenosine monophosphate (cAMP) formation, leading to inhibition of neurotransmitter release and a decrease in neuronal excitability.

Monoamines

The monoamines norepinephrine, epinephrine, and dopamine are neurotransmitters which are synthesized from tyrosine through a shared pathway. Tyrosine hydroxylation of tyrosine to levodopa is the rate-limiting step in monoamine synthesis. Levodopa in turn is converted by 3,4-dihydroxyphenylalanine (dopa) decarboxylase to dopamine. Dopamine then undergoes hydroxylation to norepinephrine, which undergoes methylation to epinephrine. The rate-limiting step in monoaminergic synthesis is the hydroxylation of tyrosine to levodopa.

Five dopamine receptor subtypes are further categorized into 2 main dopamine receptor families, the D1-like families (D1 and D5), which lead to increased cAMP activity, and D2-like families (D2, D3, and D4), which lead to reduction in cAMP activity. D1 and D2 are located primarily in the corpus striatum and frontal lobes, and D3 and D4 in the frontal cortex, hippocampus, amygdala, and nucleus accumbens. D1 and D2 play a crucial role in modulating motor activity in the basal ganglia. D2 agonists lead to presynaptic inhibition of neurotransmitter release and decreased neuronal excitation. Dopamine agonists are used in the treatment of Parkinson disease (PD). Conversely, dopamine antagonists are used in the treatment of schizophrenia, which may lead to parkinsonism and tardive dyskinesia.

Norepinephrine is synthesized in preganglionic neurons and stored in vesicles with the assistance of vesicular monoamine transporter (VMAT) proteins. Inhibition of norepinephrine production or its ability to bind with α- and β-adrenergic receptors results in decreased activity in the sympathetic nervous system, an effect which is commonly exploited in the treatment of hypertension, cardiac disease, and urinary retention. Adrenergic receptor antagonists and α_2-receptor presynaptic agonists such as prazosin, which lead to reduced presynaptic norepinephrine release, may cause orthostatic hypotension–related presyncope and dizziness, which may necessitate a neurology consultation. Conversely, agonists of α-receptors, such as modafinil, lead to increases in blood pressure and are used in the management of neurogenic orthostatic hypotension, such as in multiple system atrophy (Shy-Drager syndrome).

Serotonin

Serotonin is synthesized from the amino acid tryptophan. Serotonergic neurons are located in the dorsal raphe nuclei in the midbrain, which project to the cerebral cortex, medulla, spinal cord, and forebrain structures. Serotonin is stored in vesicles for eventual release with the assistance of VMATs. After release, serotonin reuptake is modulated by the serotonin transporter (SERT). SERT blockage allows for prolonged serotonergic activity. Serotonin is broken down to 5-hydroxyindolacetic acid (5-HIAA) by monoamine oxidase (MAO), and in the pineal gland, it is converted to melatonin.

Medications to enhance serotonin activity through inhibition of serotonin uptake (selective serotonin reuptake inhibitors or SSRIs) are widely used in the treatment of depression. Serotonin receptor agonists are used in the treatment of migraine. Drugs that inhibit norepinephrine and serotonin reuptake (selective noradrenergic reuptake inhibitors or SNRIs) are also used in the treatment of depression.

Acetylcholine

Acetylcholine (ACh) is widely distributed in the CNS and has many roles related to memory, attention, induction of rapid eye movement (REM) sleep, regulation of behavior, and muscle excitation and in the functioning of the autonomic nervous system.

ACh is synthesized by the binding of acetyl coenzyme A and choline by choline acetyltransferase. It is subsequently broken down to acetate by acetylcholinesterase intrasynaptically. There are 2 main types of ACh receptors: nicotinic and muscarinic.

Nicotinic ACh receptors are located at neuromuscular junctions, adrenal medulla, and CNS and in the preganglionic synapses in the autonomic nervous system. Activation of these ionotropic receptors results in influx of Na$^+$ and Ca^{2+}, depolarizing the postsynaptic target.

Muscarinic ACh receptors are located in the postganglionic synapses of the parasympathetic autonomic nervous system, peripheral tissue, and CNS. Many medications, such as tricyclic antidepressants, have antagonistic effects on muscarinic ACh receptors which lead to reduced parasympathetic activity resulting in symptoms such as urinary retention, xerostomia, constipation, and erectile dysfunction.

Deactivation of ACh activity occurs through degradation of ACh by acetylcholinesterase. Inhibitors of acetylcholinesterase are used to enhance ACh activity in the treatment of neurologic diseases such as Alzheimer disease, which is associated with reductions in ACh due to degeneration of cholinergic neurons in the basal forebrain, and myasthenia gravis, which is due to antibody blockage of postsynaptic nicotinic ACh receptors.

- Ionotropic GABA$_A$ receptors reside in synapses, providing quick-acting phasic inhibition, whereas metabotropic GABA$_B$ receptors are localized in extrasynaptic regions, giving rise to tonic inhibition.
- The monoamines norepinephrine, epinephrine, and dopamine are neurotransmitters which are synthesized from tyrosine through a shared pathway.
- Five dopamine receptor subtypes are further categorized into 2 main dopamine receptor families, the D1-like families (comprising D1 and D5), which lead to increased cAMP activity, and D2-like families (D2, D3, and D4), which lead to reduction in cAMP activity.
- Dopamine agonists are used in the treatment of Parkinson disease. Conversely, dopamine antagonists are used in the treatment of schizophrenia, which may lead to parkinsonism and tardive dyskinesia.

- Serotonin receptor agonists are used in the treatment of migraine. Drugs that inhibit norepinephrine and serotonin reuptake (selective noradrenergic reuptake inhibitors or SNRIs) are also used in the treatment of depression.
- Inhibitors of acetylcholinesterase are used to enhance ACh activity in the treatment of neurologic diseases such as Alzheimer disease, which is associated with reductions in ACh due to degeneration of cholinergic neurons in the basal forebrain, and myasthenia gravis, which is due to antibody blockage of postsynaptic nicotinic ACh receptors.

Disease-Specific Medications

Epilepsy

AEDs function generally through decreasing neuronal excitation or increasing neuronal inhibition. Some AEDs have a single mechanism of action, while others are known to have more than one. In some AEDs, the anticonvulsant mechanism remains unclear.

Selection of an AED takes into account a number of factors in addition to its mechanism of action. Seizure type is often the first consideration (Table 27.1). Pharmacokinetics also need to be considered carefully, particularly in patients on multiple medications and with concurrent medical ailments, such as liver and renal disease, because AEDs have a relatively narrow therapeutic range, and these factors can affect serum concentrations. Finally, the potential adverse effects of particular medications may be especially important in the management of certain patients. Considering these 3 factors, the complete list of AED options can usually be pruned to a few preferences for an individual patient (Table 27.2).

Parkinson Disease

The symptoms and signs of PD are related to loss of dopaminergic activity due to loss of dopaminergic neurons in the substantia nigra. The primary goal of current PD treatment is to increase dopaminergic activity in the CNS. This is accomplished pharmacologically by drugs that increase production or decrease degradation of dopamine or through stimulation of dopamine receptors by synthetic dopamine agonists. Levodopa, a precursor of dopamine, which unlike dopamine can cross the blood-brain barrier, is considered the gold standard of PD treatment.

Some pharmacokinetic factors are important to keep in mind with use of levodopa. Levodopa is converted to dopamine by dopa decarboxylase in dopaminergic neurons. To prevent peripheral conversion of levodopa to dopamine by peripheral dopa decarboxylase, which would markedly decrease the amount of levodopa available for transport across the blood-brain barrier and lead to elevated systemic dopamine levels resulting in nausea and other adverse

Table 27.1 • Antiepileptic Drug Selection by Seizure Type

Seizure Type	Drug
Focal epilepsy	Phenytoin
	Carbamazepine
	Oxcarbazepine
	Lamotrigine
	Valproic acid
	Levetiracetam
	Lacosamide
	Gabapentin
	Pregabalin
	Tiagabine
	Vigabatrin
	Topiramate
	Zonisamide
	Felbamate
	Ezogabine
	Perampanel
Primarily generalized tonic clonic	Valproic acid
	Felbamate
	Lamotrigine
	Levetiracetam
	Topiramate
	Zonisamide
Generalized atonic or tonic	Lamotrigine
	Rufinamide
	Topiramate
	Clobazam
	Felbamate
	Valproic acid
Absence	Ethosuximide
	Valproic acid
	Lamotrigine
Myoclonic	Levetiracetam
	Valproic acid
	Zonisamide
Infantile spasms	Adrenocorticotropic hormone
	Vigabatrin
	Topiramate
	Clonazepam
	Valproic acid
	Corticosteroids

Table 27.2 • Commonly Used Antiepileptic Drugs

Drug	Mechanism of Action	Half-life, h	Metabolism/Excretion	Major Adverse Effects
Phenytoin	Blocks sodium channels	14–22	Hepatic	Long-term use: gingival hyperplasia, peripheral neuropathy
Carbamazepine or oxcarbazepine	Inhibits rapid firing of sodium channels	12–17	Hepatic	Hyponatremia, dizziness
Lamotrigine	Blocks voltage-dependent sodium channels, inhibits glutamate release	12–70	Hepatic	Stevens-Johnson syndrome, insomnia
Lacosamide	Inhibits slow firing of sodium channels	13	Hepatic	Dizziness, imbalance, prolonged PR interval
Rufinamide	Modulates voltage-dependent sodium channels	6–10	Hepatic	Nausea, shortened QT interval
Zonisamide	Blocks voltage-dependent sodium channels, T-type calcium channels, weak carbonic anhydrase inhibitor	63–105	Hepatic or renal	Somnolence, mental slowing, nephrolithiasis
Phenobarbital	Increases duration of $GABA_A$ receptor opening	48–168	Hepatic	Sedation, mental slowing
Valproic acid	Enhances GABA activity	9–16	Hepatic	Weight gain, sedation, tremor, pancreatitis, hepatotoxicity
Clobazam	Increases frequency of $GABA_A$ receptor opening	36–42	Hepatic	Sedation, tolerance
Vigabatrin	Irreversibly binds to GABA transaminase	7–7.5	Renal	Drowsiness, loss of peripheral vision
Tiagabine	Inhibits GABA transporter-1	7–9	Hepatic or renal	Dizziness, emotional lability
Topiramate	Inhibits AMPA receptors, weak carbonic anhydrase inhibitor	21	Renal or hepatic	Cognitive blunting, paresthesias, decreased appetite, nephrolithiasis
Felbamate	Blocks NMDA receptors, voltage-dependent calcium channels	13–23	Hepatic	Insomnia, decreased appetite, aplastic anemia, hepatic failure
Perampanel	AMPA receptor antagonist	66–90	Hepatic	Dizziness, somnolence, headache
Ethosuximide	Blocks T-type calcium channels	40–60[a]	Hepatic	Nausea, abdominal upset
Gabapentin	Inhibits opening of voltage-dependent calcium channels, enhances GABA	5–7	Renal	Sedation, dizziness, ataxia
Pregabalin	Inhibits opening of voltage-dependent calcium channels, enhances GABA	6.3	Renal	Sedation, dizziness, weight gain
Ezogabine	Potassium channel opener	7–11	Hepatic	Urinary retention
Levetiracetam	Binds to SV2A transport protein	6–8	Renal	Irritability, emotional lability

Abbreviations: AMPA, α-amino-3-hydroxy-5-methyl-4-isoxazolepropionic acid; GABA, γ-aminobutyric acid; NMDA, N-methyl-d-aspartate; SV2A, synaptic vesicle glycoprotein 2A.
[a] Duration is for adults.

effects, levodopa is usually coadministered with carbidopa or a benserazide, both dopa decarboxylase inhibitors. Also, levodopa has amino acid properties and is transported to the blood from the gut via amino acid transporters in the mucosa. As a result, coadministration of levodopa with a protein meal can interfere with levodopa absorption.

Levodopa leads to indiscriminant increases in dopamine levels. Therefore, its dopaminergic effects are nonselective, leading to agonism of all CNS and peripheral dopaminergic receptor subtypes. This leads to adverse effects of nausea, orthostatic hypotension, and hallucinosis. Because levodopa leads to increased dopamine production, the serum half-life of levodopa is generally unimportant in selecting dose intervals early in the course of PD. As the disease progresses and the number of dopaminergic neurons declines, the duration of effect of every levodopa dose often shortens considerably, and the frequency of administration increases.

Dopamine agonists do not require conversion to dopamine but bind directly to dopamine receptors. While more selective than levodopa in terms of affected dopaminergic receptor subtypes, dopamine agonists still can lead to orthostatism and hallucinosis because of activation of dopaminergic receptors.

Monoamine oxidase type B (MAO-B) inhibitors block degradation of dopamine, increasing the half-life of dopamine. These are distinct from monoamine oxidase type A (MAO-A) inhibitors used in the treatment of depression. Catechol O-methyltransferase (COMT) inhibitors prevent degradation of levodopa, increasing its duration of action.

Anticholinergic medications are also used in PD primarily as a preferential treatment for tremor. Amantadine, an antiviral medication, was serendipitously found to be effective in decreasing tremor and dyskinesias in PD.

The primary mechanism of action is the enhancement of dopamine release from presynaptic terminals, but it is postulated that amantadine has a neuroprotective effect by way of acting as an NMDA receptor antagonist (Table 27.3).

Migraine

Treatment of migraine headaches is divided into acute and preventive strategies. A number of medication classes have been used in migraine prevention. These include AEDs (valproic acid, topiramate); antidepressants (nortriptyline, amitriptyline); β-blockers (propranolol); calcium channel antagonists (verapamil); and neurotoxins (onabotulinumtoxinA). These classes have various mechanisms, and the exact method by which they prevent migraines is not completely understood.

Triptans are selective agonists of 5-hydroxytryptamine receptor 1B (5-HT$_{1B}$) and 5-hydroxytryptamine (serotonin) receptor 1D (5-HT$_{1D}$) used in the acute treatment of migraine. The postulated mechanisms of action of the triptans are intracranial vasoconstriction (5-HT$_{1B}$), inhibition of peripheral pain signal transmission and neuropeptide release (5-HT$_{1D}$), and presynaptic dorsal horn stimulation (5-HT$_{1D}$), inhibiting central pain transmission. There is a risk of serotonin toxicity if triptans are taken in conjunction with SSRIs, and they are contraindicated in patients with a history of unstable coronary artery disease, stroke, and uncontrolled hypertension.

Ergot alkaloids are less specific serotonin receptor agonists that can also be used in the acute treatment of migraine. Intravenous dihydroergotamine (DHE) is indicated for status migrainosus and can be effective in migraines that have failed to respond to other acute

Table 27.3 • Treatment of Parkinson Disease

Drug	Major Adverse Effects
Levodopa	Nausea, hypotension, dyskinesias
Dopamine agonists	
Bromocriptine	Nausea, orthostatic hypotension, vasospasm
Pramipexole	Nausea, orthostatic hypotension, hallucinations, compulsive behaviors
Ropinirole	Nausea, orthostatic hypotension, hallucinations, compulsive behaviors, sudden sleep attacks
Apomorphine	Hypotension, somnolence
Monoamine oxidase type B inhibitors	
Selegiline	Insomnia, dizziness, nausea, hallucinations, chorea, potential for serotonin syndrome
Rasagiline	Insomnia, anorexia, nausea, hallucinations, chorea, potential for serotonin syndrome
Catechol O-methyltransferase inhibitors	
Entacapone	Diarrhea, orange discoloration of bodily fluids
Tolcapone	Hepatic failure
Anticholinergics	
Trihexyphenidyl	Dizziness, anxiety, disrupted sleep, delirium, constipation, dry mouth
Benztropine	Dizziness, anxiety, delirium, constipation, dry mouth
Dopamine release enhancer	
Amantadine	Mood changes, nausea, dizziness

Table 27.4 • Migraine-Specific Acute Treatment

Medication	T_{max}, h	Half-life, h	Route of Administration
Triptans			
Sumatriptan	2–2.5 (oral), 1–1.75 (intranasal), 0.2 (subcutaneous)	3	Oral, intranasal, subcutaneous
Rizatriptan	1–2.5	2–3	Oral
Eletriptan	2	4	Oral
Zolmitriptan	1	3	Oral, intranasal
Almotriptan	1–3	3–4	Oral
Frovatriptan	2–4	26	Oral
Naratriptan	2–3	6	Oral
Ergots			
Dihydroergotamine	(0.2	9–10	Intravenous, intranasal

treatments, including triptans. Intravenous DHE is given every 6 to 8 hours, until the migraine has abated. The drug is associated with severe nausea, and pretreatment with an antiemetic is required. It should not be administered within 24 hours of triptan use because of concerns about vasoconstriction. As a class, ergots interact with multiple receptor types, resulting in multiple potential adverse effects. The primary adverse effects are nausea and vasoconstriction, and thus, ergots are contraindicated in patients with vascular disease, hypertension, and pregnancy (Table 27.4).

Multiple Sclerosis

Medications used in multiple sclerosis are distinct from those used in other neurologic diseases because they do not exert their action through alterations of neural transmission but rather act to alter immune function in the nervous system. Injectable disease-modifying therapies promote an anti-inflammatory state by decreasing type 1 helper T cell (T_H1) (proinflammatory) activity and increasing type 2 helper T cell (T_H2) (anti-inflammatory) activity. Natalizumab and fingolimod have different mechanisms of limiting lymphocyte entry into the CNS. Teriflunomide inhibits pyrimidine synthesis, inhibiting rapidly dividing cells. All the medications currently in use struggle to balance immunosuppression and immunomodulation, with adverse effects associated with these alterations (Table 27.5).

Common symptoms in multiple sclerosis require additional symptomatic treatment. Spasticity is treated with muscle relaxants, including baclofen, tizanidine, and diazepam. Trigeminal neuralgia commonly occurs in multiple sclerosis and is typically treated with carbamazepine,

Table 27.5 • Treatment of Multiple Sclerosis

Drug	Mechanism of Action	Route of Administration	Dosing Frequency	Major Adverse Effects
Glatiramer acetate	Promotes suppressor cells of T_H2	Subcutaneous	Daily	Injection site reaction, chest pain, palpitations, flushing
Interferon beta-1a	Promotes shift of T_H1 to T_H2	Intramuscular or subcutaneous	Weekly or 3 times per week	Flulike symptoms, leukopenia, elevated LFTs
Interferon beta-1b	Antiviral/anti-inflammatory action	Subcutaneous	Every other day	Flulike symptoms, elevated LFTs
Mitoxantrone	Antineoplastic action	Intravenous	Every 3 mo	Congestive heart failure, leukemia
Natalizumab	Prevents entry of T cells into the CNS	Intravenous	Every 4 wk	Increased risk of progressive multifocal leukoencephalopathy
Fingolimod	Modulates sphingosine-1-phosphate receptors, sequestering lymphocytes in lymph nodes	Oral	Daily	Headache, fatigue, herpesvirus infection, bradycardia
Teriflunomide	Pyrimidine synthesis inhibitor	Oral	Daily	Hepatotoxicity, peripheral neuropathy

Abbreviations: CNS, central nervous system; LFT, liver function test; T_H1, type 1 helper T cell; T_H2, type 2 helper T cell.

Table 27.6 • Alzheimer Disease

Drug	Mechanism of Action	Major Adverse Effects
Donepezil	Cholinesterase inhibitor	Nausea, anorexia, bradycardia, vivid dreams
Galantamine	Cholinesterase inhibitor	Nausea, anorexia, abdominal discomfort
Rivastigmine	Cholinesterase inhibitor	Nausea, vomiting
Memantine	NMDA receptor antagonist	Confusion, dizziness, insomnia, agitation

Abbreviation: NMDA, *N*-methyl-D-aspartate.

gabapentin, or pregabalin. Fatigue may be treated with amantadine or modafinil or with paroxetine or sertraline when depression is a factor. Bladder spasticity can be treated with oxybutynin or bethanechol.

Dementia

Dementia, both as a group of diseases and as individual neurodegenerative diseases, lacks definitive treatment. Medications approved for use in dementia aim either to improve memory and attention or to protect neurons from excitotoxicity (Table 27.6).

Cholinesterase inhibitors are available in both oral and transdermal forms for use in Alzheimer disease, which is associated with degeneration of cholinergic neurons in the basal forebrain. Rivastigmine is available as a transdermal patch, which has been shown to increase compliance. The slow release from a transdermal patch allows for steady dosing of the medication and has been associated with fewer adverse effects, particularly abdominal upset.

Behavioral adverse effects in dementia often require symptomatic treatment. Antipsychotic medications can be used to treat agitation or hallucinations, although caution needs to be taken in patients with Lewy body dementia because of the drugs' antagonistic effects on dopamine receptors. Clozapine has minimal dopamine receptor binding, decreasing the risk of extrapyramidal adverse effects, but it carries a risk of agranulocytosis and seizures. The use of antipsychotic medications in elderly patients

with dementia has been associated with increased mortality, with greater risk when using first-generation, as opposed to second- and third-generation antipsychotics.

- Levodopa has amino acid properties and is transported to the blood from the gut via amino acid transporters in the mucosa. As a result, coadministration of levodopa with a protein meal can interfere with levodopa absorption.
- Levodopa causes indiscriminant increases in dopamine levels. Therefore, its dopaminergic effects are nonselective, leading to agonism of all CNS and peripheral dopaminergic receptor subtypes. This leads to adverse effects of nausea, orthostatic hypotension, and hallucinosis.
- Triptans are selective agonists of 5-hydroxytryptamine receptor 1B (5-HT$_{1B}$) and 5-hydroxytryptamine (serotonin) receptor 1D (5-HT$_{1D}$) used in the acute treatment of migraine. The postulated mechanisms of action of the triptans are intracranial vasoconstriction (5-HT$_{1B}$), inhibition of peripheral pain signal transmission and neuropeptide release (5-HT$_{1D}$), and presynaptic dorsal horn stimulation (5-HT$_{1D}$), inhibiting central pain transmission.
- Antipsychotic medications can be used to treat agitation or hallucinations, although caution needs to be taken in patients with Lewy body dementia because of the drugs' antagonistic effects on dopamine receptors.

Questions and Answers

Questions

Multiple Choice (choose the best answer)

III.1. Which of the following antiepileptic medications has the shortest half-life?
a. Perampanel
b. Clobazam
c. Phenobarbital
d. Zonisamide
e. Pregabalin

III.2. You have recently diagnosed intermittent migraine headache without aura in a 25-year-old woman. Her headaches are occurring multiple times each week, and you have discussed starting preventive therapy with topiramate. The patient should be aware of which of the following groups of potential adverse effects?
a. Insomnia, decreased appetite, aplastic anemia, hepatic failure
b. Drowsiness, loss of peripheral vision
c. Cognitive slowing, paresthesias, decreased appetite, nephrolithiasis
d. Weight gain, sedation, tremor, pancreatitis, hepatotoxicity
e. Dizziness, imbalance, prolonged PR interval

III.3. You are seeing a 72-year-old man with slowly progressive asymmetric resting tremor and imbalance. Your diagnosis is idiopathic Parkinson disease. Which of the following medications is least likely to be associated with nausea?
a. Selegiline
b. Apomorphine
c. Levodopa
d. Pramipexole
e. Ropinirole

III.4. A 22-year-old man presents with infrequent intermittent pulsatile headaches associated with nausea and vomiting, often preceded by a transient visual scotoma. You diagnose intermittent migraine with aura. Which of the following abortive medications has the longest half-life?

a. Sumatriptan
b. Naratriptan
c. Zolmitriptan
d. Frovatriptan
e. Rizatriptan

III.5. A 33-year-old woman with relapsing-remitting multiple sclerosis has continued to experience frequent clinical and radiographic relapses. On further questioning, you learn that she has not been compliant with her current disease-modifying agent because of severe aichmophobia (fear of needles). Which of the following medications would be the most reasonable alternative in this setting?
a. Mitoxantrone
b. Interferon beta-1b
c. Natalizumab
d. Glatiramer acetate
e. Fingolimod

III.6. The family of an 82-year-old woman brings her in for evaluation of slowly progressive cognitive decline. You diagnose likely Alzheimer dementia. Which of the following medications acts primarily as an NMDA (*N*-methyl-ᴅ-aspartate)-receptor antagonist?
a. Rivastigmine
b. Memantine
c. Galantamine
d. Tacrine
e. Donepezil

III.7. A 61-year-old woman with long-standing migraine headache without aura presents with increasing headache frequency. She has a history notable for severe depression, nephrolithiasis, and unexplained syncope currently being evaluated by her cardiologist. Which of the following medications would you recommend for headache prevention?
a. Propranolol
b. Verapamil
c. Topiramate
d. Amitriptyline
e. OnabotulinumtoxinA

Answers

III.1. Answer e.
White HS, Rho JM. Mechanisms of action of antiepileptic drugs. Professional Communications: West Islip (NY); c2010.

III.2. Answer c.
White HS, Rho JM. Mechanisms of action of antiepileptic drugs. Professional Communications: West Islip (NY); c2010.

III.3. Answer a.
Minagar A, Benarroch EE, Koller WC. Basic pharmaceutical principles and the blood-brain barrier. In: Noseworthy JH, editor. Neurological therapeutics: principles and practice. 2nd ed. Abingdon (UK): Informa Healthcare and Boca Raton (FL): Taylor & Francis; c2006. p. 3–24.

III.4. Answer d.
Minagar A, Benarroch EE, Koller WC. Basic pharmaceutical principles and the blood-brain barrier. In: Noseworthy JH, editor. Neurological therapeutics: principles and practice. 2nd ed. Abingdon (UK): Informa Healthcare and Boca Raton (FL): Taylor & Francis; c2006. p. 3–24.

III.5. Answer e.
Freedman MS. Present and emerging therapies for multiple sclerosis. Continuum (Minneap Minn). 2013 Aug;19(4 Multiple Sclerosis):968–91.

III.6. Answer b.
Minagar A, Benarroch EE, Koller WC. Basic pharmaceutical principles and the blood-brain barrier. In: Noseworthy JH, editor. Neurological therapeutics: principles and practice. 2nd ed. Abingdon (UK): Informa Healthcare and Boca Raton (FL): Taylor & Francis; c2006. p. 3–24.

III.7. Answer e.
Minagar A, Benarroch EE, Koller WC. Basic pharmaceutical principles and the blood-brain barrier. In: Noseworthy JH, editor. Neurological therapeutics: principles and practice. 2nd ed. Abingdon (UK): Informa Healthcare and Boca Raton (FL): Taylor & Francis; c2006. p. 3–24.

SUGGESTED READING

Freedman MS. Present and emerging therapies for multiple sclerosis. Continuum (Minneap Minn). 2013 Aug;19(4 Multiple Sclerosis):968–91.

Minagar A, Benarroch EE, Koller WC. Basic pharmaceutical principles and the blood-brain barrier. In: Noseworthy JH, editor. Neurological therapeutics: principles and practice. 2nd ed. Abingdon (UK): Informa Healthcare and Boca Raton (FL): Taylor & Francis; c2006. p. 3–24.

White HS, Rho JM. Mechanisms of action of antiepileptic drugs. Professional Communications: West Islip (NY); c2010.

Section IV

Sleep Pathophysiology

Pablo R. Castillo, MD, *editor*

28 Sleep Pathophysiology

MICHAEL F. PRESTI, MD, PHD

Introduction

Sleep is a natural, reversible, and periodic behavioral state characterized by perceptual inattention and decreased responsiveness to external stimuli. The processes governing sleep, sleep-wake transitions, and maintenance of wakefulness are mediated via complex physiologic mechanisms, the primary neurobiological substrates of which include the neocortex, basal forebrain, thalamus, hypothalamus, pontine tegmentum, and brainstem monoaminergic nuclei. Moreover, the integrity of brainstem autonomic respiratory control networks becomes critical in the maintenance of ventilation during sleep. Pathologic insults to these systems may result in a broad constellation of clinical deficits. This chapter reviews the normal stages of sleep, age-related changes in sleep composition, physiologic mechanisms mediating the generation and maintenance of sleep and wakeful states, and homeostatic and circadian control of sleep. Common clinical manifestations associated with derangement of these physiologic processes are discussed in Volume 2, Section XIV, "Sleep Disorders."

Sleep Architecture

Overview

Sleep is a dynamic process that comprises 2 distinct states: rapid eye movement (REM) sleep and non–rapid eye movement (NREM) sleep (Table 28.1). The latter is further classified into 3 separate stages, N1, N2, and N3, which are roughly associated with a depth-of-sleep continuum characterized by progressively decreasing muscle tone, responsiveness to the environment, cerebral blood flow, heart rate, blood pressure, and minute ventilation.

Whereas NREM sleep represents progressively deepening levels of physiologic relaxation, REM sleep can be conceptualized as a state of internal arousal, with an activated brain in a paralyzed body. Dreaming is the most characteristic phenomenon of REM sleep, and skeletal muscle atonia during REM sleep (which involves all but the diaphragm, extraocular, and middle ear ossicular musculature) likely developed as an adaptive protective mechanism; indeed, loss of such atonia during REM sleep (a condition often associated with neurodegenerative disease) may result in serious physical injury. Other physiologic characteristics associated with REM sleep include a desynchronized electroencephalogram (EEG) resembling that of wakefulness, increased cerebral blood flow, cardiorespiratory abnormalities, poikilothermia, and penile erection or clitoral engorgement.

A normal night of adult sleep typically consists of between 4 and 6 cycles of NREM and REM states, each lasting approximately 90 minutes, with a shift in state predominance from NREM to REM sleep over the course of the night. In a healthy young adult, the normal percentages of stage N1, N2, N3, and REM sleep are approximately 5%, 50%, 20%, and 25%, respectively. Although the functional distinctions among sleep states and stages remain largely unclear, each is associated with a specific and well-defined electrophysiologic profile.

NREM Sleep

NREM sleep is characterized by the EEG presence of several named waveforms, including V waves, K complexes, sleep spindles, and high-voltage slow waves. These

Abbreviations: DMH, dorsomedial nucleus of the hypothalamus; EEG, electroencephalogram, electroencephalographic; eVLPO, extended ventrolateral preoptic nucleus; I$_t$, transient Ca^{2+} current; MnPN, median preoptic nucleus; NREM, non–rapid eye movement; NRPO, nucleus reticularis pontis oralis; REM, rapid eye movement; SCN, suprachiasmatic nucleus; VLPO, ventrolateral preoptic nucleus

Table 28.1 • Characteristics of Sleep Stages

Sleep Stage	Signature EEG	Eye Movement	Muscle Tone
NREM			
N1	4–7 Hz (theta) V waves	Slow, roving horizontal movements	Decreases
N2	Low amplitude; mixed frequencies K complex Sleep spindle	Usually absent; slow eye movements may persist	Decreases more than N1
N3	0.5–2.0 Hz; synchronized	Usually absent	Decreased more than N2
REM	Asynchronous, low amplitude, mixed frequency EEG; sawtooth waves	Rapid eye movements	Minimal or absent

Abbreviations: EEG, electroencephalogram; NREM, non–rapid eye movement; REM, rapid eye movement.

waveforms represent highly coordinated reciprocal interactions between widespread intracortical and thalamocortical networks and are thus commonly referred to as synchronous patterns.

Sleep is typically ushered in via stage N1 sleep, which is characterized on EEG by a shift in the posterior dominant alpha rhythm (8–13 Hz) to low-amplitude, mixed-frequency, predominantly theta activity (4–7 Hz); development of sharply contoured vertex waves (V waves) with a duration of less than 0.5 second and maximal expression over the central head regions; and emergence of slow roving horizontal eye movements. Muscle tone is variable but generally decreases with the onset of stage N1 sleep relative to wakefulness.

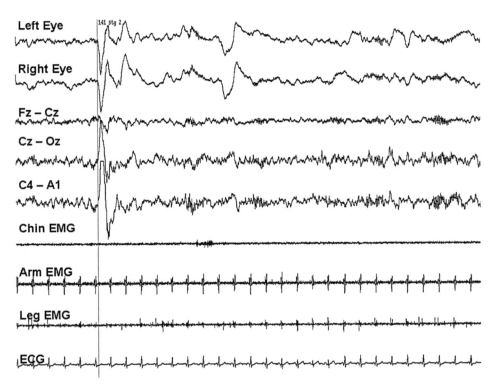

Figure 28.1 Stage N2 Sleep.

Note the K complex on the left of the tracing and several sleep spindles on the right (30-second epoch). Left eye and right eye leads are applied to left and right outer canthi and referenced to frontopolar midline electrode. Fz—Cz references frontal midline to central midline electrode; Cz—Oz, central midline to occipital midline electrode; C4—A1, right parasagittal to left ear electrode; chin electromyogram (EMG), EMG lead on chin muscles; arm EMG, upper extremity EMG; leg EMG, anterior tibialis EMG; ECG, electrocardiogram.

(Adapted from Young TJ, Tippmann-Peikert M. Neurology of sleep disorders. In: Mowzoon N, Flemming KD, editors. Neurology board review: an illustrated study guide. Rochester [MN]: Mayo Clinic Scientific Press and Florence [KY]: Informa Healthcare USA; c2007. p. 719–52. Used with permission of Mayo Foundation for Medical Education and Research.)

Stage N2 sleep is defined by 2 EEG phenomena, namely, K complexes and sleep spindles (Figure 28.1). K complexes are defined as waveforms with a well-delineated negative sharp wave immediately followed by a positive component with a duration of 0.5 second or longer, usually maximal when recorded over frontal derivations. Sleep spindles are defined as a train of distinct waves with a frequency of 11 to 16 Hz (most commonly 12–14 Hz) and a duration of 0.5 second or longer, usually maximal in amplitude in central head derivations. These 2 waveforms often occur sequentially, with a sleep spindle closely following a K complex. The arousal threshold is higher in stage N2 than N1, and the same stimuli that produce arousal from N1 sleep often result in an evoked K complex but no awakening in stage N2 sleep. In addition to such stimulus-evoked K complexes, these waveforms are also generated spontaneously with a periodicity of approximately 30 seconds. Such intermittent partial arousals may have evolved as a protective mechanism for sleep under hazardous conditions. Muscle tone is typically lower in stage N2 sleep than during wake or N1 but higher than in stage N3 or REM sleep.

Stage N3 sleep, often referred to as slow-wave sleep, is characterized by the presence of high-amplitude synchronized EEG activity with a frequency of 0.5 to 2.0 Hz (Figure 28.2). These waveforms are of maximal amplitude over the frontal derivations. Such slow-wave sleep is considered to be the deepest stage of sleep, associated with the highest arousal threshold and very low resting muscle tone. N3 sleep is considered to be a restorative and reparative state and plays an important role in numerous physiologic processes, including cognition (eg, declarative memory consolidation); endocrine function (eg, growth hormone and prolactin expression); and neuroimmunologic signaling (eg, interleukin 1 and tumor necrosis factor α expression).

REM Sleep

In contrast to the many named waveforms associated with the synchronous patterns of NREM sleep, REM sleep is characterized by asynchronous, low-amplitude, mixed-frequency EEG activity resembling that of wakefulness (hence the term *paradoxical sleep*) (Figure 28.3). Other defining features of REM sleep are the presence of rapid eye movements (ie, conjugate, irregular, sharply peaked eye movements with an initial deflection usually less than 500 milliseconds) on an electro-oculogram and skeletal muscle atonia. Sawtooth waves are the only named waveform characteristic of REM sleep and are defined as a train

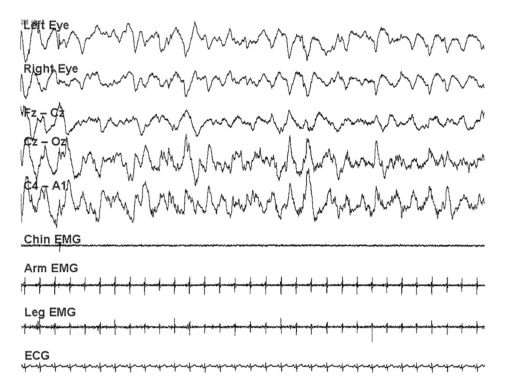

Figure 28.2 Slow-Wave Sleep.
High-amplitude delta waves predominate. The montage is the same as in Figure 28.1, with a 30-second epoch. Note the ECG artifact in arm and leg EMG channels.
(Adapted from Young TJ, Tippmann-Peikert M. Neurology of sleep disorders. In: Mowzoon N, Flemming KD, editors. Neurology board review: an illustrated study guide. Rochester [MN]: Mayo Clinic Scientific Press and Florence [KY]: Informa Healthcare USA; c2007. p. 719–52. Used with permission of Mayo Foundation for Medical Education and Research.)

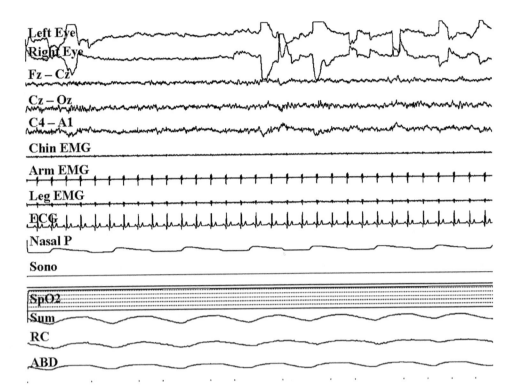

Figure 28.3 Rapid Eye Movement Sleep.
Low-voltage, mixed-frequency pattern. Note rapid eye movements in the eye channels. Normal muscle atonia is evident in the chin, arm, and leg EMG channels (30-second epoch). The montage is the same as in Figure 28.1, with additional leads ABD, abdominal respiratory band; Nasal P, nasal airflow; RC, rib cage respiratory band; Sono, snore microphone; SpO₂, oxygen saturation; Sum, sum of the rib cage and abdominal respiratory bands.
(Adapted from Young TJ, Tippmann-Peikert M. Neurology of sleep disorders. In: Mowzoon N, Flemming KD, editors. Neurology board review: an illustrated study guide. Rochester [MN]: Mayo Clinic Scientific Press and Florence [KY]: Informa Healthcare USA; c2007. p. 719–52. Used with permission of Mayo Foundation for Medical Education and Research.)

of sharply contoured or triangular, often serrated 2- to 6-Hz waves of maximal amplitude over the central head regions. REM becomes more predominant in the second half of the night, which explains the much higher likelihood of recalling a dream when woken in the morning by one's alarm clock than when woken at midnight by one's pager. The functions of REM sleep remain unclear but probably include consolidation of procedural and spatial memory.

- Sleep is a dynamic process that comprises 2 distinct states: rapid eye movement (REM) and non–rapid eye movement (NREM) sleep.
- NREM sleep is classified into 3 separate stages, N1, N2, and N3.
- NREM sleep represents progressively deepening levels of physiologic relaxation.
- REM sleep can be conceptualized as a state of internal arousal, with an activated brain in a paralyzed body.
- A normal night of adult sleep typically consists of between 4 and 6 cycles of NREM and REM states, each lasting approximately 90 minutes.

Age-Related Alterations in Sleep

Both NREM and REM sleep states are normally present throughout a human lifetime, but their expression shifts over time. In neonates, NREM and REM sleep are referred to as quiet and active sleep, respectively. In the first few months of life, active sleep comprises approximately half of total sleep time, and over the first decade of life, the proportion of REM sleep declines while the latency to the first REM period of sleep increases. Similarly, total daily sleep time and slow-wave sleep time decrease with age.

All named sleep-related waveforms are generally present by about 6 months of age. As parents of teenagers know, the timing of sleep (or sleep phase) also varies with age, such that young children and the elderly generally get to sleep and wake from sleep earlier than middle-aged adults (ie, advanced sleep phase pattern), whereas normal sleep onset and wake times are normally later in adolescents (ie, delayed sleep phase pattern).

- In the first few months of life, active sleep comprises approximately half of total sleep time.

- Total daily sleep time and slow-wave sleep time decrease with age.
- All named sleep-related waveforms are generally present by about 6 months of age.

Neurophysiologic Control of Sleep and Wakefulness

Overview

Expression of distinct conscious states depends on the coordinated activity of diffuse sleep- or wake-promoting neuronal networks involving the neocortex, basal forebrain, thalamus, hypothalamus, pontine tegmentum, and brainstem monoaminergic nuclei. The activity profiles of important regulatory nuclei during wakefulness, REM sleep, and NREM sleep states are summarized in Table 28.2. These systems can be most easily understood using the engineering concept of the flip-flop switch, in which distinct state transitions occur as a function of reciprocal inhibition between 2 control nodes. In this context, brainstem and posterior hypothalamic arousal systems can be viewed as engaging in a tug-of-war with anterior hypothalamic somnogenic systems, where the relative strength of these opposing forces oscillates as a function of circadian and homeostatic influences. Moreover, a second flip-flop switch involving circuits within the pontine tegmentum, periaqueductal gray, and anterior hypothalamus can be invoked to explain transitions between NREM and REM sleep states.

State-Dependent Thalamic Activity

The activity across these neurobiological switches results in differential patterns of thalamic firing and thalamocortical synchronization, which account for the fundamental EEG distinctions of wakefulness, REM, and NREM states. Specifically, these thalamocortical circuits exhibit a state of tonic activation and desynchrony during wakefulness and

REM sleep and a state of rhythmic, synchronized activity during NREM sleep. These 2 modes of thalamocortical activity are mediated on the cellular level by specialized membrane properties involving a voltage-sensitive calcium current, known as the transient Ca^{2+} current, I_t. This I_t is inactive during periods of thalamic activation (membrane potential less negative than -65 mV) associated with REM sleep and wakeful states, and under such circumstances, a depolarizing input results in standard single-spike firing. During periods of relative cellular inhibition (membrane potential more negative than -65 mV) associated with NREM sleep states, however, the I_t becomes active, and under such circumstances, excitatory thalamic input evokes slow Ca^{2+}-mediated depolarization, which culminates in a burst of 3 to 8 action potentials followed by inactivation of I_t and restoration of a hyperpolarized state. Thus, the transient Ca^{2+} current, I_t, enables thalamocortical neurons to generate a tonic firing pattern when stimulated from a relatively depolarized state or a burst-pause firing pattern when stimulated from a relatively hyperpolarized state. The resting membrane potentials governing these thalamic firing patterns, the reactivity of cortical neurons to such thalamic activity, and the temporal stability of such activated states depend on the influence of diverse arousal systems.

Wake-Promoting Systems

The arousal networks promoting wakefulness can be divided into ascending and stabilizing systems. Ascending systems include cholinergic nuclei of the midbrain and pontine tegmentum, as well as monoaminergic brainstem and hypothalamic neurons. The wakefulness stabilizing system consists of the hypocretinergic (or orexinergic) neurons of the perifornical and posterolateral hypothalamus.

Cholinergic ascending arousal networks involve the pedunculopontine and laterodorsal tegmental nuclei. These nuclei exert an excitatory influence on thalamocortical relay neurons and help establish the relatively depolarized cellular environment discussed above, in which I_t currents are inactivated and thalamocortical neurons demonstrate tonic single-spike firing in response to afferent input. Such activity facilitates transmission of sensory information to the cortex, a key feature of wakefulness.

The monoaminergic ascending arousal system involves noradrenergic neurons of the locus coeruleus, serotonergic neurons of the midbrain dorsal raphe, dopaminergic neurons of the ventral periaqueductal gray, and histaminergic neurons of the hypothalamic tuberomammillary nucleus. This system innervates several targets, including the cerebral cortex, wake-stabilizing systems of the posterolateral and perifornical hypothalamus, and sleep-promoting centers of the anterior hypothalamus and basal forebrain. In the cortex, these monoaminergic influences render pyramidal neurons more responsive to thalamic relays, facilitating behavioral reaction to environmental stimuli, which

---

Table 28.2 • Neurotransmitter Systems in Sleep and Wakefulness

Affected Neurons	Wake	NREM Sleep	REM Sleep
Cholinergic	Active	Silent	Active
Noradrenergic	Active	Partially active	Silent
Serotonergic	Active	Partially active	Silent
Hypocretinergic	Active	Silent	Silent

Abbreviations: NREM, non–rapid eye movement; REM, rapid eye movement.

Adapted from Silber MH, Krahn LE, Morgenthaler TI. Sleep medicine in clinical practice. 2nd ed. New York (NY): Informa Healthcare; c2010. Chapter 1, Physiological basis of sleep; p. 3–24. Used with permission of Mayo Foundation for Medical Education and Research.

is necessary for adaptive wakefulness. Monoaminergic innervation of the posterolateral hypothalamus activates the hypocretin system, which provides both excitatory feedback to these monoaminergic nuclei and inhibitory feedback to sleep-promoting centers of the preoptic area (ie, ventrolateral preoptic nucleus [VLPO] and median preoptic nucleus [MnPN]). Finally, these monoaminergic nuclei comprise 1 arm of the flip-flop switch between sleep- and wake-promoting centers, with direct inhibitory influences over the NREM sleep-generating neurons of the VLPO and MnPN (see Sleep-Promoting Systems, below).

The stabilizing arousal system comprises a small group of neurons in the posterolateral and perifornical region of the hypothalamus. These neurons express the peptide neurotransmitter hypocretin (also known as orexin) and project widely throughout the brain to targets in the neocortex, limbic system, diencephalon, and brainstem cholinergic and monoaminergic ascending arousal systems. The potential role of the posterolateral hypothalamus in the maintenance of wakefulness was first proposed in the early 20th century by von Economo (Wiener Klin Wochenschr. 1917 May 10;30:581–5), who reported that postmortem examination of patients with encephalitis lethargica consistently demonstrated inflammatory lesions in this area of the brain. Of note, von Economo (Wiener Klin Wochenschr. 1917 May 10;30:581–5) was also the first to postulate the role of the anterior hypothalamus in induction and maintenance of sleep, noting that encephalitic patients with severe insomnia had lesions involving the preoptic area. More recently, studies in narcoleptic animal models and patients with narcolepsy have confirmed the role of the hypocretin or orexin nuclei of the posterolateral hypothalamus in enhancing alertness and stabilizing the waking state. Depletion of these neurons results in persistent hypersomnolence and intrusion of elements of REM sleep into wakefulness (see the text on narcolepsy in Volume 2, Chapter 86, "Hypersomnias and Sleep-Related Movement Disorders"). This system stabilizes wakefulness via excitatory influences on the ascending cholinergic and monoaminergic arousal systems and inhibitory influences on the sleep-promoting centers of the preoptic area (ie, VLPO and MnPN). The hypocretin or orexin arousal system is activated largely via glutamatergic input from the dorsomedial nucleus of the hypothalamus (DMH), which in turn is regulated by circadian inputs from the suprachiasmatic nucleus (SCN) and ventral subparaventricular zone. Conversely, both the VLPO and MnPN (sleep-promoting centers, see Sleep-Promoting Systems, below) provide reciprocal inhibitory innervation of the posterolateral hypothalamus, thereby inhibiting the hypocretin arousal system during sleep.

Sleep-Promoting Systems

The 2 most important brain regions involved in the generation and maintenance of sleep are the anterior hypothalamus (and adjacent basal forebrain) and the pontine tegmentum. Specifically, the preoptic nuclei of the anterior hypothalamus, including the VLPO and the MnPN, are involved in the mediation of NREM sleep, whereas pontine tegmental nuclei, including the subcoeruleus region of the lateral nucleus reticularis pontis oralis (NRPO), mediate REM sleep. State transitions between wake, NREM sleep, and REM sleep are regulated by 2 flip-flop switches.

The concept of a biological flip-flop switch regulating distinct states of arousal was introduced in preceding paragraphs, where the monoaminergic ascending arousal system was described as the stimulatory pole of the wake-NREM switch. Conversely, the preoptic area nuclei (as well as the substantia innominata and diagonal band nucleus of the basal forebrain) can be considered the somnogenic pole of this switch, as their widespread GABAergic and galaninergic projections inhibit the monoaminergic, cholinergic, and hypocretinergic arousal nuclei. While the VLPO discharges at high rates throughout NREM periods, the MnPN is most active early in NREM sleep, especially after a period of prolonged wakefulness, suggesting that MnPN activity induces NREM sleep, which is then sustained via VLPO activity.

A second important flip-flop switch regulates state transitions between REM and NREM sleep. The poles of this switch include REM-on cells of the subcoeruleus region in the lateral NRPO and REM-off cells of other parts of the lateral pontine tegmentum and ventrolateral periaqueductal gray. These poles are mutually inhibitory via dense reciprocal GABAergic innervation. However, the REM-on cells have additional outputs, including cholinergic innervation of the thalamus and glutamatergic innervation of the basal forebrain and nucleus magnocellularis. The thalamic and basal forebrain projections establish a wakelike state of thalamic gating and a desynchronized EEG, whereas the medullary projections to the nucleus magnocellularis are involved in mediating skeletal muscle atonia during REM sleep. Activity between the 2 poles of the REM switch is largely influenced by input from the extended VLPO (eVLPO) to REM-off cells. Specifically, these REM-off cells are periodically inhibited via GABAergic input from the eVLPO during NREM sleep, resulting in disinhibition of the subcoeruleus region and transition to REM sleep. Finally, REM periods are terminated when excitatory inputs to the REM-off neurons from the posterolateral hypothalamus, locus coeruleus, and midbrain raphe are sufficient to overcome inhibitory influences of the REM-on cells.

- Arousal networks promoting wakefulness can be divided into ascending and stabilizing systems. Ascending systems include cholinergic nuclei of the midbrain and pontine tegmentum, as well as monoaminergic brainstem and hypothalamic neurons.

The wakefulness stabilizing system consists of the hypocretinergic or orexinergic neurons of the perifornical and posterolateral hypothalamus.

- The 2 most important brain regions involved in the generation and maintenance of sleep are the anterior hypothalamus (and adjacent basal forebrain) and the pontine tegmentum.
- The preoptic nuclei of the anterior hypothalamus, including the VLPO and the MnPN, are involved in the mediation of NREM sleep.
- Pontine tegmental nuclei, including the subcoeruleus region of the lateral NRPO, mediate REM sleep.

Homeostatic and Circadian Influences on Sleep

There are 3 basic influences on sleep and wake patterns, namely, homeostatic, circadian, and allostatic forces (Table 28.3). Homeostatic and circadian influences wax and wane in a relatively predictable manner throughout the day in accordance with one's recent sleep history (eg, sleep deprived vs well rested) and endogenous rhythms trained to periodic environmental stimuli (eg, sunlight vs darkness). These forces normally influence the activity of the regulatory neural systems discussed in the preceding section to produce the characteristic diurnal human sleep-wake cycle. Allostatic forces represent less predictable environmental conditions that require urgent modification to sleep-wake cycles (eg, in response to a predator encounter or mating opportunity). Such allostatic forces involve more complex, less well-delineated biological mechanisms beyond the scope of this chapter.

The primary function of the homeostatic force, termed *process S*, is to maintain an equilibrium between wake and sleep times. Process S can be viewed as sleep debt, which progressively increases with time spent awake and decreases with time asleep. This sleep debt is tallied independently for slow-wave sleep (stage N3) and REM sleep,

and selective deprivation of either of these states results in rebound of that state when sleep restrictions are removed. Recent evidence suggests that adenosine, which accumulates extracellularly as a result of astrocytic cellular metabolism, may be a primary substrate through which the homeostatic force is expressed. Adenosine may exert a depolarizing or hyperpolarizing influence on target cell membranes, depending on the receptor subtypes to which it binds. It is postulated that adenosine exerts its sleep-promoting influence via both inhibitory A1 receptors expressed in arousal-related nuclei (ie, locus coeruleus, tuberomammillary, and perifornical hypothalamic nuclei) as well as A2a excitatory receptors expressed in meningeal cells adjacent to the preoptic area (which subsequently activate VLPO and MnPN neurons). This mechanism explains why coffee, which contains caffeine, an adenosine antagonist, may help stave off process S to maintain wakefulness.

The second major influence on periodic sleep-wake transitions comes from the circadian system. In humans, circadian rhythms are driven primarily through activity of the SCN of the hypothalamus, often referred to as the biological clock. Accordingly, neurons in this structure express an array of clock genes, which function as transcription factors regulating the temporal expression of other genes controlling periodic functions, such as sleep, feeding, locomotion, and immunologic and hormonal activity. The SCN is both intrinsically rhythmic and sensitive to external entraining stimuli. These entraining environmental stimuli are termed *zeitgebers*, among which light is by far the most salient. Light exerts this entraining influence even in blind (but not enucleated) individuals through intrinsically photosensitive retinal ganglion cells that express the photopigment melanopsin. Although the SCN itself has no notable direct connections to the sleep- and wake-promoting neural systems discussed herein, it provides dense innervation of the ventral subventricular zone nucleus, which in turn innervates the DMH. Finally, the DMH exerts a GABAergic inhibitory influence over the sleep-promoting neurons of the VLPO and MnPN, as well as a glutamatergic excitatory influence over the wake-promoting neurons in the posterolateral hypothalamus. This connectivity pattern suggests that the main function of the circadian system is to promote wakefulness during the active period, which explains why lesions of the SCN, subparaventricular zone, or DMH, as well as experimental disruption of clock genes, reduce total wake time.

- There are 3 basic influences on sleep and wake patterns, namely, homeostatic, circadian, and allostatic forces.
- The primary function of the homeostatic force, termed *process S*, is to maintain an equilibrium between wake and sleep times.

Table 28.3 • Influences on Sleep and Wake Patterns

Influence	Definition	Example
Homeostatic	Maintain equilibrium between wake and sleep times	Sleep debt accumulates if one stays up late studying
Circadian	Influence of light on activity; functions to promote wakefulness during the active period	Higher alertness during light or daytime hours
Allostatic forces	Unpredictable environmental influences	Being woken by a predator coming into one's home

Questions and Answers

Questions

Multiple Choice (choose the best answer)

IV.1. Which of the following characteristics is typical of rapid-eye-movement (REM) sleep?
a. K complexes
b. Sawtooth waves
c. 4- to 7-Hz background
d. Sleep spindles
e. V waves

IV.2. Which of the following statements regarding neurotransmitter systems controlling sleep and wakefulness is most correct?
a. Hypocretinergic neurons are active during nonREM sleep
b. Noradrenergic neurons are active during REM sleep
c. Cholinergic neurons are silent in the waking state
d. Serotonergic neurons are active in the waking state
e. The only silent neurons during nonREM sleep are noradrenergic and serotonergic neurons

IV.3. Which of the following statements regarding influences on sleep and wake patterns is most correct?
a. Exposure to light is a typical allostatic force
b. Process S is the primary function of allostatic forces
c. The main function of the circadian system is to promote wakefulness during the inactive period
d. Homeostatic forces function independently of sleep debt
e. The suprachiasmatic nucleus of the hypothalamus is the primary driver of the circadian rhythm

IV.4. Which of the following pairs of structures is most important in the generation and maintenance of sleep?
a. The anterior hypothalamus and pontine tegmentum
b. The ventrolateral preoptic nucleus and anterior hypothalamus
c. The nucleus reticularis pontis oralis and pontine tegmentum
d. The median preoptic nucleus and dorsomedial nucleus of the hypothalamus
e. The suprachiasmatic nucleus and dorsomedial nucleus of the hypothalamus

IV.5. The subcoeruleus region of the lateral nucleus reticularis pontis oralis is primarily associated with the mediation of which of the following stages of sleep?
a. Drowsiness
b. N1
c. N2
d. N3
e. REM

Answers

IV.1. Answer b.
Iber C, Ancoli-Israel S, Chesson AL Jr, Quan SF. The AASM manual for the scoring of sleep and associated events: rules, terminology and technical specifications. Westchester (IL): American Academy of Sleep Medicine; c2007. 59 p.

IV.2. Answer d.
Silber MH, Krahn LE, Morgenthaler TI. Sleep medicine in clinical practice. 2nd ed. New York (NY): Informa Healthcare; c2010. 332 p.

IV.3. Answer e.
Silber MH, Krahn LE, Morgenthaler TI. Sleep medicine in clinical practice. 2nd ed. New York (NY): Informa Healthcare; c2010. 332 p.

IV.4. Answer a.
Kryger MH, Roth T, Dement WC, editors. Principles and practice of sleep medicine. 5th ed. Philadelphia (PA): Saunders/Elsevier; c2011. 1723 p.

IV.5. Answer e.
Kryger MH, Roth T, Dement WC, editors. Principles and practice of sleep medicine. 5th ed. Philadelphia (PA): Saunders/Elsevier; c2011. 1723 p.

SUGGESTED READING

Iber C, Ancoli-Israel S, Chesson AL Jr, Quan SF. The AASM manual for the scoring of sleep and associated events: rules, terminology and technical specifications. Westchester (IL): American Academy of Sleep Medicine; c2007. 59 p.

Kryger MH, Roth T, Dement WC, editors. Principles and practice of sleep medicine. 5th ed. Philadelphia (PA): Saunders/Elsevier; c2011. 1723 p.

Saper CB, Fuller PM, Pedersen NP, Lu J, Scammell TE. Sleep state switching. Neuron. 2010 Dec 22;68(6):1023–42.

Silber MH, Krahn LE, Morgenthaler TI. Sleep medicine in clinical practice. 2nd ed. New York (NY): Informa Healthcare; c2010. 332 p.

Neurogenetics

Ralitza H. Gavrilova, MD,

editor

29 Patterns of Inheritance in Neurogenetic Disease

RALITZA H. GAVRILOVA, MD; VIRGINIA V. MICHELS, MD

Introduction

The human genome consists of approximately 25,000 genes that are encoded within the nuclear DNA and embedded in the chromosome. Mitochondria are the only cytoplasmic organelles that have their own DNA.

Nuclear gene and mitochondrial inheritance are discussed in this chapter. Basic genetic terms are defined in Box 29.1.

Nuclear Gene Disorders

Overview

Nuclear gene disorders follow the patterns of inheritance originally described by Gregor Mendel. They often are referred to as *single-gene disorders* because 1 or more alleles of only 1 locus are the major determinants of phenotype. *Mendelian patterns* are autosomal dominant (AD), autosomal recessive (AR), X-linked, and Y-linked (rare).

Box 29.1 • **Basic Genetic Terms**

Allele—A copy of a gene. Each nuclear gene consists of 2 copies (ie, alleles), 1 maternal and 1 paternal.

Allelic heterogeneity—There may be many mutations at a given gene locus.

Expressivity—The degree or severity to which a disease phenotype is expressed among individuals with the same mutation. Many autosomal dominant conditions show variable expressivity, even within the same family. For example, within 1 family, persons who have neurofibromatosis type 1 may have any number of neurofibromas, from a few to hundreds.

Heterozygous—Nonidentical alleles for a gene.

Homozygous—Identical alleles for a gene.

Locus heterogeneity—The same phenotype may be caused by mutations in different genes at different loci. For example, Charcot-Marie-Tooth disease can be caused by mutations in the *PMP22* or *MPZ* gene.

Penetrance—The percentage of persons carrying a particular genotype who express the associated trait or phenotype. When penetrance is reduced, a person who is heterozygous for a disease-causing allele shows no signs of the disorder. The penetrance of some genes is age dependent. For example, the penetrance of Huntington disease is nearly 50% by 45 years and 100% by 75 years.

Phenotypic heterogeneity—Different mutations in the same gene may cause different phenotypes or conditions. For example, *LMNA* gene mutations have been associated with Emery-Dreifuss muscular dystrophy, dilated cardiomyopathy, and Charcot-Marie-Tooth disease.

Pleiotropy—A single gene mutation is responsible for several signs and symptoms from various systems. For example, neurofibromatosis type 1 can cause neurofibromas, skeletal abnormalities, learning difficulties, café au lait macules, and involvement in many other organ systems.

Abbreviations: AD, autosomal dominant; AR, autosomal recessive; mtDNA, mitochondrial DNA

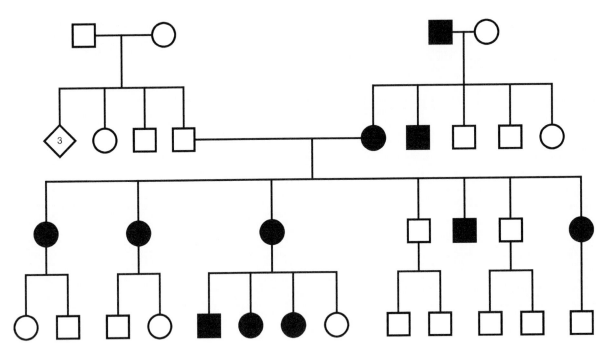

Figure 29.1 Pattern of Inheritance for Autosomal Dominant Disorders.
Square indicates male; circle, female; diamond, sex not designated for that number of children; shading, affected.

In contrast, in *polygenic inheritance*, several different genes intersect to produce a phenotype; when environmental factors are also involved, the term *multifactorial* is used.

AD Disorders

An *AD disorder* is one in which the mutant allele, located on an autosome, is expressed in the heterozygote (ie, the mutant allele is dominant to the wild-type allele). The pedigree pattern of transmission is vertical, with successive generations affected. Both males and females are affected and can transmit the disease. The hallmark is male-to-male transmission, which excludes X-linked inheritance (Figure 29.1). However, new mutations can occur, so that the antecedent family history may be negative.

Infrequently, an apparently unaffected parent has gonadal mosaicism for the mutant allele, and 1 or more offspring may have full penetrance (ie, expresses the disease). Since persons with an AD condition are heterozygous, with 1 mutant and 1 normal allele, for each child of an affected parent, the risk of inheriting the disease-causing mutation is 50%, or 1 in 2.

AR Disorders

An *AR disorder* is due to 2 mutant alleles and no normal allele at a given locus. Persons with an AR disorder can be homozygous for the same mutation or compound heterozygous for 2 different mutations. The parents are typically carriers for 1 of these mutations and are unaffected because

they have 1 normal allele that compensates for the mutant allele. The transmission of an AR disease typically is horizontal or confined to 1 sibship, the children of the carrier parents (Figure 29.2). Occasionally, the parents are consanguineous, which increases the risk of homozygosity and the risk of rare diseases in such families. Males and females are equally likely to be affected. The term *pseudodominant* refers to successive generations of affected individuals with an AR disease, which can occur by chance, especially for common disorders. However, pseudodominant is particularly common in inbred populations. The risk for each child of carrier parents to receive 2 mutant alleles and become affected is 0.5 × 0.5, or 1 in 4 (25%). Incomplete penetrance and variable expressivity also can occur in AR diseases.

X-Linked Disorders

Inheritance of *X-linked disorders* is distinct from autosomal patterns of inheritance. The X and Y chromosomes encode genes that are responsible for sex determination, among other traits, and therefore are distributed unequally to males and females. As a result, diseases caused by genes on the X chromosome have a sex predilection and a characteristic pattern of inheritance. Because the Y chromosome has very few genes, mostly related to fertility, a single-gene pattern of inheritance is rare and is not discussed further in this chapter. However, it is important to know that Y inheritance is characterized by male-to-male transmission.

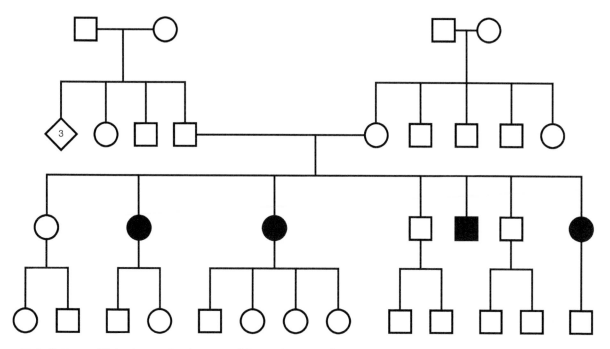

Figure 29.2 Pattern of Inheritance for Autosomal Recessive Disorders.
Square indicates male; circle, female; diamond, sex not designated for that number of children; shading, affected.

X-linked dominant inheritance patterns can be distinguished from X-linked recessive inheritance patterns on the basis of the phenotype in heterozygous females. If the disorder is consistently expressed in heterozygous females, the inheritance pattern is X-linked dominant (eg, Rett syndrome). X-linked recessive conditions are expressed in hemizygous males (these conditions are sometimes lethal in the embryo or fetus and therefore are not observed clinically) and variably expressed in heterozygous females. This is explained by random inactivation of 1 of the 2 X chromosomes in the female embryo, which occurs soon after fertilization. The pattern of X chromosome inactivation in a female determines the presence and degree of severity of symptoms. Usually heterozygous females for an X-linked recessive condition are affected more mildly than their male relatives. An example of X-linked recessive inheritance is Fabry disease, in which males uniformly exhibit symptoms, whereas females rarely show signs of disease and generally present with a milder phenotype. Clinically, this distinction between X-linked dominant and X-linked recessive conditions can be a continuum.

The pedigree pattern for X-linked disorders is vertical, affecting multiple generations, but there is no male-to-male transmission (Figure 29.3). Because a heterozygous female has 1 mutant and 1 normal X chromosome, the risk for each son and daughter to inherit the mutation is 1 in 2, or 50%. Because an affected male transmits an X chromosome to all his daughters and to none of his sons, the risk for each daughter to inherit the mutant gene is 100% and the risk for each son is 0%. New mutations in mothers of

boys with X-linked recessive diseases, such as Duchenne muscular dystrophy, are not uncommon.

DNA Repeat Disorders

In a group of hereditary conditions, the mutation is characterized by an unstable nucleotide repeat expansion. The repeating unit within the affected gene may consist of 3 or more nucleotides (CAG, CCGT, etc). Normal alleles have a stable, low number of repeat units. This low number may vary among individuals. When the repeats expand beyond a certain size (mutate), the expanded allele becomes unstable and may expand further in successive meioses (gamete cell divisions). Expanded mutant alleles are associated with increased severity or earlier onset of disease in successive generations, a phenomenon called *anticipation*. With some diseases, the stability of the expanded allele varies, depending on whether the allele is maternally or paternally inherited. Repeat expansion diseases can be inherited in any of the mendelian patterns of inheritance, but anticipation is characteristic of only the ones inherited in an AD fashion (Table 29.1).

Alleles with abnormal repeat numbers that do not cause disease but are unstable and capable of expanding into the disease-causing range in subsequent generations are known as *premutations*. However, some premutation carriers may have symptoms. For example, premutation carriers of the fragile X gene (*FMR1*) are susceptible to tremor/ataxia syndrome, a neurologic condition of adult onset, in contrast to the classic childhood developmental disorder, fragile X intellectual disability syndrome.

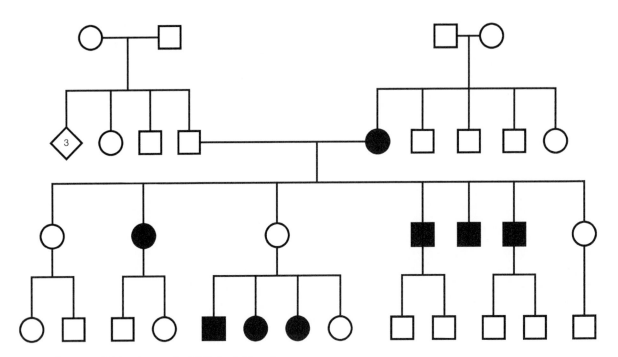

Figure 29.3 *Pattern of Inheritance for X-Linked Disorders.*
Square indicates male; circle, female; diamond, sex not designated for that number of children; shading, affected.

Multifactorial Inheritance

The concept of *multifactorial inheritance* is a formal construct in medical genetics. Of the multiple different genes that may influence a disease or trait, some may be more important than others. In the era of genome-wide association studies and microarrays that detect copy number variants, it is important to realize that variations in the genome influence development of not only classic multifactorial conditions, such as some birth defects, diabetes mellitus, atherosclerosis, and hypertension, but also expression and penetrance of single-gene disorders.

Genomic Imprinting

Genomic imprinting is a normal process of controlling gene expression by alterations in chromatin but not in the DNA sequence. Imprinting is equivalent to silencing the

Table 29.1 • Neurologic Disorders Associated With Unstable Repeat Expansions[a]

Feature	Huntington Chorea (Huntington Disease)	Fragile X-Associated Tremor/Ataxia Syndrome	Friedreich Ataxia	Myotonic Dystrophy Type 1	Myotonic Dystrophy Type 2	Spinobulbar Muscular Atrophy	DRPLA
Inheritance	AD	X-linked dominant	AR	AD	AD	X-linked recessive	AD
Gene	*HD*	*FMR1*	*FXN*	*DMPK*	*CNBP* (*ZNF9*)	*AR* (androgen receptor)	*ATN1* (atrophin)
Repeat location in the gene	5′ untranslated region	Exon 1	Intron 1	Noncoding 3′ untranslated region	Intron 1	Exon 1	Coding region
Repeat	CAG	CGG	GAA	CTG	CCTG	CAG	CAG
Repeat size, No. of repeats							
Normal	10–26	<55	5–33	5–34	11–26	≤34	6–35
Premutation	27–35	55–200	34–65	35–49	27–74	0	36–47
Disease-causing	≥40; 36–39 (reduced penetrance)	>200	≥66	>50	>75	>35	≥48

Abbreviations: AD, autosomal dominant; AR, autosomal recessive; DRPLA, dentatorubral-pallidoluysian atrophy.

[a] These and other repeat disorders, including *C9orf72*-associated frontotemporal dementia and spinocerebellar ataxias, are discussed in other chapters.

expression of a gene. Genomic imprinting occurs before fertilization in the germline of 1 parent (that allele is not expressed in the offspring) and not in the other parent (that allele is expressed in the offspring). Imprinting occurs at only a limited number of chromosome regions. In contrast, nonimprinted genes are expressed from both paternal and maternal alleles in each cell.

The process of imprinting includes the covalent methylation of cytosine to form 5-methylcytosine and the modification of histones. The imprinted state generally persists into adulthood (except in some disease states), so that only the maternal or only the paternal copy of the gene is expressed. The imprint is reversible in the gamete, so that a paternally derived allele is converted in the female germline into a maternal imprint. Imprinting is important in mendelian disorders and in chromosomal abnormalities. Imprinting disorders may become evident when *uniparental disomy* occurs—that is, when both copies of a chromosome or a chromosomal region are received from the same parent. Disorders of imprinting are discussed in Chapter 30, "Chromosomal Syndromes."

Mutations sometimes result in aberrant imprinting or silencing of a gene. Such abnormal silencing occurs in fragile X syndrome and results in a lack of the FMR protein.

- An *AD disorder* is one in which the mutant allele, located on an autosome, is expressed in the heterozygote. The pedigree pattern of transmission is vertical, with successive generations affected.
- The transmission of an AR disease typically is horizontal or confined to 1 sibship, the children of the carrier parents.
- The pattern of X chromosome inactivation in a female determines the presence and degree of severity of symptoms.
- The pedigree pattern for X-linked disorders is vertical, affecting multiple generations, but there is no male-to-male transmission.
- Expanded mutant alleles are associated with increased severity or earlier onset of disease in successive generations, a phenomenon called *anticipation*.

Mitochodrial Inheritance

Mitochondrial inheritance differs from nuclear gene inheritance, reflecting the unique characteristics of mitochondrial biology and its genome. Mitochondrial DNA (mtDNA) is a double-stranded circular molecule that contains 37 genes. It encodes 13 protein respiratory chain subunits and 24 RNAs (2 ribosomal RNAs and 22 transfer RNAs) that are required within the mitochondria for translation of the protein-coding units. It has a high mutation rate compared with that of nuclear DNA. Each mitochondrion contains approximately 5 copies of mtDNA. Most cells contain thousands of mtDNA molecules.

Mitochondrial inheritance has the following unique features: maternal inheritance, mitotic segregation, homoplasmy, heteroplasmy, and threshold effect.

Transmission of mitochondrial diseases is through *maternal inheritance*. All mitochondria in the zygote are derived from the ovum. Therefore, a mother carrying an mtDNA mutation may pass it on to her male and female children, but only her daughters may transmit it to their offspring.

Mitotic segregation is unique to mitochondrial inheritance. The random redistribution of mitochondria during cell division can alter the proportion of mutant mtDNAs received by daughter cells.

Homoplasmy refers to the presence of all normal or all mutant mtDNA. If a female is homoplasmic for an mtDNA mutation, such as in Leber hereditary optic neuropathy, all her children will inherit the mutation. *Heteroplasmy* refers to cells that harbor both normal (wild-type) and mutant mtDNA. A minimal number of mutant mtDNAs must be present before oxidative dysfunction occurs and clinical signs become apparent, a phenomenon known as *threshold effect*.

These unique features of mitochondrial inheritance underlie the age-related and tissue-related variability of clinical features in mtDNA-related diseases. Thus, the risk of disease for offspring varies from 0% to 100%. Children of mothers with heteroplasmic mitochondrial mutations receive only a subset of their mother's mtDNA. Therefore, the risk and severity of mitochondrial disease in children of mothers with mtDNA mutation depends on the fraction of mutant mitochondria in their mother and in their tissues and on the random chance of inheriting mutant mitochondria. An exception to maternal inheritance occurs when the mother is heteroplasmic for an mtDNA deletion, because deletions are generally not transmitted from mothers to their children. A possible explanation is that mtDNA containing deletions may disrupt an important mitochondrial function and be removed by natural selection.

It is important to note that mitochondria are semiautonomous, because their replication structure and function depend on nuclear-encoded genes. Therefore, mitochondrial diseases can also be due to nuclear gene mutations and, therefore, inherited in mendelian patterns. The most common mendelian pattern of inheritance in mitochondrial disorders is AR.

- Mitochondrial inheritance has the following unique features: maternal inheritance, mitotic segregation, homoplasmy, heteroplasmy, and threshold effect.

30 Chromosomal Syndromes[a]

RALITZA H. GAVRILOVA, MD; VIRGINIA V. MICHELS, MD

Introduction

The chromosomal syndromes are due to numerical, structural, or functional abnormalities of chromosomes. These include numerary changes of chromosomes in some or all cells, structural rearrangements, deletions or duplications of parts of chromosomes, and, in some cases, changes in small segments of the chromosomes as in fragile X syndrome.

The most common chromosomal syndromes are discussed in this chapter. Inherited diseases that are not related to chromosomal abnormalities are discussed in other chapters in the context of their corresponding pathophysiologic category (eg, inherited peripheral neuropathies are discussed in Volume 2, Chapter 40, "Peripheral Nerve Disorders").

Numerary Chromosomal Abnormalities

Down Syndrome

Overview and Epidemiology

Down syndrome is the result of 3 copies of chromosome 21 and the increased expression of critical genes on this chromosome. The incidence of trisomy 21 is approximately 1 in 800 births in the general population; the incidence increases with advancing maternal age.

Clinical Characteristics

Down syndrome is characterized by mild to moderate intellectual impairment (average IQ, 50–60), distinctive facial features (flat facial profile, upslanted palpebral fissures, and small mandible), infantile hypotonia, heart defects, childhood leukemia, and early-onset Alzheimer disease (Box 30.1).

Physical abnormalities that may be present in Down syndrome include heart defects (40% of patients), particularly atrioventricular septal defect, and gastrointestinal tract abnormalities, such as duodenal stenosis or atresia, imperforate anus, and Hirschsprung disease. Hypothyroidism and conductive hearing loss (90% of patients) are common and may develop over time. Transient myeloproliferative reaction may occur in the neonatal period. On average, children with Down syndrome tend to be relatively short compared with other family members; shortness and inactivity, or an

---

Box 30.1 • Common Features in Down Syndrome

Mild to moderate intellectual impairment

Distinctive facies

Short stature

Associated abnormalities

  Heart defects (40%)

  Gastrointestinal tract defects: duodenal stenosis, Hirschsprung disease, imperforate anus

  Hypothyroidism

  Conductive hearing loss

  Rare associations: celiac disease, moyamoya disease, leukemia

  Increased risk of early-onset Alzheimer disease

---

[a] Portions of the sections on Prader-Willi and fragile X syndrome previously published in Cassidy SB, Schwartz S, Miller JL, Driscoll DJ. Prader-Willi syndrome. Genet Med. 2012 Jan;14(1):10-26 and Jacquemont S, Hagerman RJ, Hagerman PJ, Leehey MA. Fragile-X syndrome and fragile X-associated tremor/ataxia syndrome: two faces of *FMR1*. Lancet. 2007 Jan;6(1):45-55, respectively. Used with permission

Abbreviations: CGH, comparative genomic hybridization; FISH, fluorescence in situ hybridization; FMRP, fragile X mental retardation protein; FXTAS, fragile X–associated tremor/ataxia syndrome; MRI, magnetic resonance imaging; mRNA, messenger RNA

unwillingness to control dietary intake, may lead to being overweight. Children with Down syndrome have an increased risk of odontoid hypoplasia that may cause impingement of the cervical spinal cord.

Associated Diseases

A subset of these children are at increased risk for leukemia (acute myelogenous leukemia or acute lymphoblastic leukemia), but this risk is less than 1%. Children with Down syndrome have a slightly higher frequency of cataracts, esotropia, and astigmatism and an increased risk of celiac disease and moyamoya disease.

The increased risk of early-onset Alzheimer disease is possibly due to the triplication of the amyloid-β precursor protein gene (*APP*). Senile plaques and neurofibrillary tangles are present in the brain of all adults with Down syndrome older than 40 years.

Diagnosis and Management

Down syndrome is diagnosed by clinical features and chromosomal analysis. The diagnosis can be made by chromosomal analysis on peripheral blood or by chromosomal microarray. Prenatally, it may be diagnosed by chromosomal analysis of amniocytes or chorionic villi. Most patients with Down syndrome (95%) have 3 free copies of chromosome 21 (47,XX,+21 karyotype or 47,XY,+21 karyotype). In 5% of patients, Down syndrome results from chromosomal translocation of acrocentric chromosomes, with chromosome 21 most commonly translocated to chromosome 14.

Imaging of the brain of Down syndrome patients shows a smaller brain volume, and the size of the hippocampus and cerebellum are particularly affected.

Management is symptomatic. Recommendations in childhood include screening for refractive errors and conductive hearing loss, dietary management to prevent obesity, and flexion and extension radiography of the neck at 3 years of age to screen for atlantoaxial instability. Memantine, a noncompetitive *N*-methyl-D-aspartic acid receptor antagonist, has been proposed to improve cognition in adults with Down syndrome.

Klinefelter Syndrome

Overview and Epidemiology

Klinefelter syndrome is the most common sex chromosome abnormality, with an incidence of 1 in 700 male live births. Nondisjunction of the sex chromosomes during meiosis results in an extra copy of the X chromosome in males (47,XXY karyotype).

Clinical Features

In childhood, the diagnosis can be suspected in boys presenting with clumsiness or mild learning difficulties, particularly in relation to verbal skills. Mean cognitive ability is in the normal range, but overall verbal IQ is 10 to 20 points less than that of unaffected siblings and controls. Language difficulties with articulation, word processing, and retrieval, in addition to general delayed expressive language skills are common (70%-80% of patients). Approximately 50% to 75% of boys demonstrate reading comprehension and spelling difficulties, and some have problems with arithmetic skills. Some studies have shown deficits in executive function and attention. School-aged boys display maturational delays that affect gross and fine (poor writing) motor skills. They have mild impairment of coordination, speed, and strength, giving the impression of clumsiness.

Adults with Klinefelter syndrome tend to be slightly taller than average, with long lower limbs. Approximately 30% of adult males with Klinefelter syndrome have moderately severe gynecomastia, and almost all are infertile and have small testes. Occasional males are fertile, especially if the condition is mosaic (the presence of ≥2 cell lines with different genotypes in 1 individual, such as a 47,XXY cell line and a 46,XY cell line). Adults have an increased incidence of leg ulcers, osteoporosis, and carcinoma of the breast.

Diagnosis and Treatment

Klinefelter syndrome is diagnosed with chromosomal analysis of a peripheral blood sample or with chromosomal microarray. Prenatally, it may be diagnosed with chromosomal analysis of amniocytes or chorionic villi. Functional neuroimaging has suggested reduced leftward functional asymmetry in the temporal-parietal brain regions that may relate to the characteristic language difficulties and reading disabilities of patients with Klinefelter syndrome.

Treatment with testosterone from puberty onward is beneficial for the development of secondary sexual characteristics and long-term prevention of osteoporosis. In vitro fertilization techniques that use aspirated sperm precursors have been used to achieve fertility in some cases.

- Down syndrome is the result of 3 copies of chromosome 21 and the increased expression of critical genes on this chromosome.
- Klinefelter syndrome is the most common sex chromosome abnormality. Nondisjunction of the sex chromosomes during meiosis results in an extra copy of the X chromosome in males (47,XXY karyotype).

Microdeletion Syndromes

Overview

Microdeletion refers to the loss of a small piece of chromosome that is not seen readily through a microscope by routine chromosomal analysis (ie, by karyotype). Common microdeletion syndromes are compared in Table 30.1.

Table 30.1 • Common Microdeletion Syndromes

Syndrome	Chromosome	Gene	Clinical Features
DiGeorge syndrome (velocardiofacial syndrome)	22q11.2	*TBX1*	Characteristic facies Cardiac anomalies (tetralogy of Fallot, ventricular septal defect) Developmental delay Immunodeficiency
Williams syndrome (Williams-Beuren syndrome)	7q11.23	Elastin	Mild intellectual impairment Unusual behavior (hypersocial and hyperverbal) Motor symptoms

Microdeletions can be detected by high-resolution chromosomal banding, by molecular chromosomal analysis with fluorescence in situ hybridization (FISH), or by comparative genomic hybridization (CGH) microarray. FISH uses fluorescent probes for detecting and localizing the presence or absence of specific DNA sequences on chromosomes. A DNA microarray is a collection of submicroscopic DNA sequences attached to a solid surface. Each specific sequence is known as a *probe* (or an *oligo*). These probes can be a short section of a gene or another DNA element that is used to hybridize a complementary DNA sample (called the *target*). Probe-target hybridization is quantified by detection of fluorophore-, silver-, or chemiluminescence-labeled targets to determine the relative abundance of nucleic acid sequences in the target.

Chromosome 22q11.2 Deletion Syndrome

Overview and Epidemiology

Chromosome 22q11.2 deletion syndrome is also referred to as velocardiofacial syndrome or DiGeorge syndrome. Its prevalence is estimated to be around 1 in 5,000 people. Its frequency is relatively high because the 22q region is flanked by low copy number repeats, which predispose to mispairing of sister chromatids during meiosis, resulting in unequal crossing over and, subsequently, a deletion. This mechanism underlies the occurrence of new cases. Medical advancements have allowed the survival of mildly affected patients to reproductive age.

Pathophysiology

The *TBX1* gene located within the deleted interval is important for cardiac development. The *COMT* (catechol *O*-methyltransferase) gene has been previously implicated in psychiatric diseases because of its role in dopamine metabolism and its expression in the prefrontal cortex. Therefore, haploinsufficiency of the *COMT* gene may contribute to the psychiatric and behavioral abnormalities in patients with chromosome 22q11.2 deletion syndrome.

Several imaging studies have been performed to investigate the cause of developmental abnormalities in patients with chromosome 22q11.2 deletion syndrome, but a specific explanation has not been found. Microcephaly is seen in 10% of patients. Reduced gray matter in the frontal lobes, cingulate gyrus, and cerebellum may correlate with executive dysfunction, poor attention, and a tendency for schizophrenia to develop. A small cerebellar vermis has been linked to the social awkwardness of patients with 22q11.2 deletion because the cerebellar vermis has been implicated in social drive. Functional magnetic resonance imaging (MRI) has raised the possibility of aberrant neural connections in the parietal and occipital lobes, possibly explaining visuospatial processing difficulties in patients.

Clinical Features

Clinical features vary widely, even within families, but the variable combination of characteristic facial features, cardiac anomalies (most commonly tetralogy of Fallot or ventricular septal defect), palatal defect, developmental delay, and immunodeficiency should raise the possibility of chromosome 22q11.2 deletion syndrome.

The main neurologic feature of chromosome 22q11.2 deletion syndrome is cognitive and speech delay. Most patients (70%-90%) have an IQ that ranges from normal to moderately disabled. However, two-thirds of patients have nonverbal learning disability (important for educational interventions) with a higher verbal IQ. The areas of deficit include visuospatial memory, abstract reasoning, and mathematics. Speech delay is another important developmental aspect of patients with chromosome 22q11.2 deletion syndrome. Receptive skills are nearly normal, but expressive language is delayed and typically develops around 30 months of age. Motor skills are less severely affected. The mean age at walking is 18 months.

Psychiatric and behavioral abnormalities are well correlated to the chromosome 22q11.2 deletion syndrome. Mainly characterized in children, behavioral abnormalities include generalized anxiety, phobias, obsessive-compulsive disorder, attention-deficit/hyperactivity disorder, impulsivity, poor social interaction, and autism spectrum disorder. Psychiatric conditions, such as schizophrenia, schizoaffective disorder, and bipolar disease are described in up to 10% to 30% of adult patients.

Affected children have several common facial features, including hooded eyelids, narrow palpebral fissures, a nose with a rectangular shape and a bulbous nasal tip, a small chin, and posteriorly rotated ears with folded helices. The palate is affected in the majority of patients (69%), causing feeding and speech difficulties. Velopharyngeal weakness, the most common difficulty, leads to an inability to close the nasopharynx when swallowing or speaking. Babies may have nasal regurgitation, and older children have hypernasal speech. Palatal clefts are seen in up to 27% of patients, but cleft lip is uncommon. Some patients with cardiac defects also have shortness of breath, contributing to feeding difficulties.

Patients also have a modest T-cell (CD3$^+$) immunodeficiency as a result of thymic hypoplasia, resulting in frequent upper respiratory infections. They may be more prone to various autoimmune diseases (eg, juvenile idiopathic arthritis, celiac disease, and hematologic autoimmunity). Less common features that may also affect the quality of life include hypocalcemia; hearing loss; renal anomalies; ophthalmologic defects in 75% of patients (characteristic Schwalbe line defect called posterior embryotoxon, refractive errors, and tortuous retinal vessels); psychiatric disorders; vertebral abnormalities (C2-C3 fusion, hemivertebrae, and butterfly vertebrae); and gastrointestinal tract issues (intestinal malrotation, imperforate anus, esophageal atresia in infancy, constipation, and gastroesophageal reflux).

Diagnosis and Treatment

Level II prenatal ultrasonography at 16 weeks' gestation may show compatible clinical signs, including conotruncal cardiac anomaly, polyhydramnios (16% of patients), cleft palate (11%), or polydactyly (6%), which are particularly suggestive of the diagnosis in the presence of a positive family history. Prenatal diagnosis can be made with FISH or CGH microarray by means of chorionic villus sampling at 12 weeks' gestation or amniocentesis at 16 weeks.

A multidisciplinary approach to management is essential. Most patients are identified at birth because of the presence of a cardiac anomaly. In newborns, management should target screening for hypocalcemia, intestinal malrotation, and severe immunodeficiency. During infancy, feeding difficulties may become evident. In early childhood, attention is given to developmental and speech abnormalities. Behavioral abnormalities may become evident in school-aged children, and psychiatric disease may develop in teenagers or adults.

In most cases the deletion is submicroscopic and not visible on routine karyotyping. Therefore, the diagnosis is made by using FISH or CGH microarray. Fewer than 5% of patients with clinical symptoms of the chromosome 22q11.2 deletion syndrome have normal results on routine chromosomal analysis and negative FISH testing. These cases might be due to *TBX1* gene mutation.

Because the syndrome is a result of haploinsufficiency (1 missing copy of the critical chromosome region), the deletion is inherited like an autosomal dominant disorder.

Each child of an affected parent has a 1 in 2 (50%) chance of inheriting the deletion. Males and females are equally affected.

Williams Syndrome

Overview and Epidemiology

Williams syndrome (also called Williams-Beuren syndrome) is a multisystem disorder caused by a microdeletion of 26 to 28 genes, including the elastin (*ELN*) gene on chromosome 7q11.23. Transmission is in an autosomal dominant manner. Most cases represent de novo occurrence. Prevalence is estimated to be around 1 in 7,500 people.

Clinical Features

Neurologic features of Williams syndrome include mild intellectual impairment, unusual behavior, and motor symptoms. The cognitive profile is characterized by weakness in visuospatial construction. Patients with Williams syndrome have relative strength in language and nonverbal reasoning. However, they have difficulty with the pragmatics of language, such as maintaining a conversation.

Behaviorally, patients with Williams syndrome have been described as empathetic, hyperverbal, hypersociable, and socially disinhibited. Attention-deficit/hyperactivity disorder (67% of patients) and anxiety are other common psychiatric issues.

Patients with Williams syndrome may also have poor motor skills, including low muscle tone or cerebellar signs such as intention tremor, dysmetria, and gait imbalance. Adults are described as having an unusual, stiff gait. Sensorineural hearing loss and hypersensitivity to sound are also common.

Systemic manifestations include supravalvular aortic stenosis (also pulmonary or renal artery stenosis) and connective tissue abnormalities (inguinal hernias, soft skin, bladder and bowel diverticula, and lax joints due to the *ELN* gene deletion). Children with Williams syndrome have distinctive facial features, including periorbital fullness, strabismus, stellate iris pattern, flat nasal bridge, a long and smooth philtrum, a pointed chin, and a wide mouth with fullness of the lower cheeks. In infancy, they may have hypercalcemia or feeding difficulties. Other endocrine abnormalities include hypercalciuria, hypothyroidism, and early puberty.

Diagnosis and Management

Diagnosis may be confirmed with FISH or CGH microarray. MRI has shown a decrease in grey matter, most pronounced in the parietal lobe. Functional MRI studies have suggested impaired regulation of the amygdala by the orbitofrontal cortex, which may contribute to impaired social judgment.

Children with Williams syndrome require developmental intervention programs to address developmental disabilities. Behavioral counseling and psychotropic medication are used to manage behavioral problems, including attention-deficit/hyperactivity disorder and anxiety. Surgery may be required for supravalvular aortic stenosis, mitral valve insufficiency, or renal artery stenosis. Children with Williams syndrome should not be given multivitamins containing vitamin D and calcium because of an increased risk of hypercalcemia, hypercalciuria, and nephrocalcinosis. Adults should be monitored for glucose tolerance, mitral valve prolapse, aortic insufficiency, arterial stenoses, hypertension, and cataracts.

- *Microdeletion* refers to the loss of a small piece of chromosome that is not seen readily through a microscope by routine chromosomal analysis (ie, by karyotype).
- The main neurologic feature of chromosome 22q11.2 deletion syndrome is cognitive and speech delay.
- Psychiatric and behavioral abnormalities are well correlated to the chromosome 22q11.2 deletion syndrome.
- Neurologic features of Williams syndrome include mild intellectual impairment, unusual behavior, and motor symptoms.
- Behaviorally, patients with Williams syndrome have been described as empathetic, hyperverbal, hypersociable, and socially disinhibited.
- Children with Williams syndrome should not be given multivitamins containing vitamin D and calcium because of an increased risk of hypercalcemia, hypercalciuria, and nephrocalcinosis.

Genomic Imprinting Disorders

Overview

Genomic imprinting disorders are compared in Table 30.2.

Prader-Willi Syndrome

Overview and Epidemiology

Prader-Willi syndrome results from loss of expression of the normally paternally expressed genes on chromosome 15q11.2. The lack of paternal expression results in total absence of expression, because normally the maternal copy of these genes is programmed by epigenetic factors to be silenced. This lack of expression occurs by 1 of 3 main mechanisms: deletion of the paternal chromosome 15q11.2 region (65%-75% of patients); maternal uniparental disomy (20%-30%); or imprinting control center defects (1%-3%).

Imprinting defects due to deletion or uniparental disomy are usually sporadic, and the risk to siblings is less than 1%. However, parental chromosomal translocation and mutation in the imprinting control center may be associated with an increased recurrence risk of up to 50% for siblings. Prader-Willi syndrome has an estimated prevalence of 1 in 20,000 people.

Clinical Features

Prader-Willi syndrome is characterized by low birth weight, infantile hypotonia with poor suck, weight gain due to hyperphagia beginning at 1 to 6 years of age, and gradual development of morbid obesity at around 8 years.

Patients have characteristic facial features (narrow bifrontal diameter, almond-shaped palpebral fissures, esotropia, thin upper lip, and downturned corners of the mouth); a distinctive behavioral phenotype (temper tantrums, stubbornness, and manipulative and obsessive-compulsive behavior); and mild intellectual impairment (mean IQ, 60–70). Motor milestones and language development are delayed, and articulation difficulties are common. Hypogonadism is present in both males and females and manifests as genital hypoplasia, incomplete pubertal development, cryptorchidism in males, and infertility in

Table 30.2 • Genomic Imprinting Disorders

Syndrome	Genetics	Clinical Features	Other
Prader-Willi	Chromosome 15q11.2	Infantile hypotonia Hyperphagia with weight gain and obesity Behavioral abnormalities Short stature	Diagnose with DNA methylation testing Management: weight control, hormone assessment, and hormone replacement therapy
Angelman	Chromosome 15q11.2	Intellectual and language disability Seizure Happy, sociable, inappropriate laughter	Diagnose with molecular genetic testing EEG: rhythmic activity
Fragile X	X-linked recessive *FMR1* mutation	Intellectual impairment Characteristic facies Autistic behavior and gaze avoidance	Premutation can lead to neurodegenerative disorder in men older than 50 y (tremor, ataxia, parkinsonism)
Rett	X-linked dominant *MECP2* mutation	Typically girls present by age 6-18 mo Developmental regression or delay with spoken words Nonspecific hand rubbing or hand-mouth movements	Supportive management

Abbreviation: EEG, electroencephalogram.

the majority. Short stature is common and is related to growth hormone insufficiency. Other features include an increased incidence of sleep disturbance and non–insulin-dependent diabetes mellitus (mean age at onset, 20 years) in obese patients.

Diagnosis and Management

The diagnosis of Prader-Willi syndrome is confirmed by DNA-based methylation testing to detect abnormal parent-specific imprinting within the Prader-Willi critical region on chromosome 15. This testing determines whether the region is maternally inherited only (ie, the paternally contributed region is absent) or whether the paternal copy also is silent; testing detects more than 99% of affected patients. Neuroimaging studies have shown ventriculomegaly, decreased parietal-occipital lobe volume, sylvian fissure polymicrogyria, and incomplete insular closure in some cases, but the implication of these findings is unknown.

Management is symptomatic. In infancy, steps that may be helpful include the use of special nipples or gavage feeding to ensure adequate nutrition and the use of physical therapy to improve muscle strength. Hormonal and surgical treatments may be considered for hypogonadism and cryptorchidism.

In children with Prader-Willi syndrome, strict supervision of daily food intake to provide energy requirements while limiting weight gain is critical. Growth hormone replacement therapy to normalize height, decrease fat mass, and increase mobility has been recommended. Although reports of sudden death during sleep initially were attributed to growth hormone therapy, this therapy now seems unrelated to the increased risk for persons with Prader-Willi syndrome. Evaluation and treatment of sleep disturbance is important. Patients should be monitored for scoliosis and treated appropriately. Selective serotonin reuptake inhibitors are helpful to treat behavioral problems. Replacement of sex hormones at puberty produces adequate secondary sexual characteristics. Recommendations for adults include weight control to avoid development of diabetes mellitus and calcium supplementation to avoid osteoporosis.

- Prader-Willi syndrome is characterized by low birth weight, infantile hypotonia with poor suck, weight gain due to hyperphagia beginning at 1–6 years of age, and gradual development of morbid obesity at around 8 years.
- In children with Prader-Willi syndrome, strict supervision of daily food intake to provide energy requirements while limiting weight gain is critical.

Angelman Syndrome

Overview and Epidemiology

Angelman syndrome is a neurodevelopmental disorder caused by loss of the normally expressed maternal copy of the imprinted 15q11.2 chromosome region. There are 4 main genetic mechanisms: 1) interstitial deletion of the maternal chromosome 15q11-q13 (70%-75% of patients); 2) paternal uniparental disomy, usually of the entire chromosome (2%-3%); 3) imprinting center defect (3%-5%); and 4) ubiquitin protein ligase (*UBE3A*) gene mutation (20% of sporadic cases and 75% of familial cases). The *UBE3A* gene is expressed from only the maternal allele in the brain (hippocampus, Purkinje cells) but has biallelic expression elsewhere. Angelman syndrome has a prevalence of 1 in 12,000 to 20,000 people.

Clinical Characteristics

Angelman syndrome is characterized by severe intellectual disability, marked impairment of language acquisition, ataxia, a seizure disorder with a characteristic electroencephalogram, subtle distinctive facial features (wide smiling mouth, prominent chin, and deep-set eyes), and a happy sociable disposition. Most children present with delays in milestones and slowing of head growth during the first year of life. The behavior is unique, with paroxysms of inappropriate laughter, a happy demeanor, a love of water, hyperactivity, and sleep disturbance. Most patients do not develop speech, but higher receptive and nonverbal communication skills allow understanding of simple commands and expression of likes and dislikes. Independent walking begins at a mean age of 4 years. The gait is slow, stiff, and ataxic, and the arms are raised and held flexed at the wrists and elbows. Muscle tone is abnormal with truncal hypotonia and hypertonicity of the limbs. Many patients have cortical myoclonus and jerky movements. In 80% of patients, epilepsy starts at 1 to 5 years of age. Various seizures are observed in childhood and may be difficult to control. Atypical absence and myoclonic seizures frequently occur in adults. Patients with Angelman syndrome require constant supervision but acquire basic life skills. If patients lack some of these features or have milder impairments, recognition of the disease is based on diagnostic testing.

Diagnosis and Management

Molecular genetic testing (methylation analysis and *UBE3A* sequencing) identifies alterations in approximately 90% of patients. The other 10% who have classic features of Angelman syndrome have an unidentified genetic mechanism.

Siblings of an affected person have a risk that depends on the genetic mechanism leading to the loss of *UBE3A* function: the risk varies from typically less than 1% with a deletion or uniparental disomy to as high as 50% with an imprinting center defect or a mutation of *UBE3A*.

The electroencephalogram is characteristic with 1) persistent rhythmic activity (4–6/s); 2) runs of triphasic activity (2–3/s) that is maximal over the frontal regions and is mixed with spikes and sharp waves; and 3) posterior spikes mixed with waves (3–4/s) provoked by eye closure.

Management is symptomatic and targets the specific cognitive profile and behavioral features of Angelman syndrome. Carbamazepine, vigabatrin, and tiagabine should be avoided because they may exacerbate seizures. Sedatives may be used for nighttime wakefulness. Annual evaluations for scoliosis and ophthalmologic screening for strabismus or refractory errors are recommended. Evaluation of older children for obesity associated with an excessive appetite is necessary.

- Angelman syndrome is characterized by severe intellectual disability, marked impairment of language acquisition, ataxia, a seizure disorder with a characteristic electroencephalogram, subtle distinctive facial features (wide smiling mouth, prominent chin, and deep-set eyes), and a happy sociable disposition.

Fragile X Syndrome

Overview and Epidemiology

Fragile X syndrome is the most common inherited cause of intellectual disability and the most common single-gene cause of autism. The estimated prevalence is 20 in 100,000 males. This disorder was named for the cytogenetically visible region on the X chromosome that was apparent by karyotype after culture in folate-deficient media. However, molecular analysis is more sensitive and specific and is now used for diagnosis.

Fragile X syndrome is inherited in an X-linked recessive fashion. All mothers of persons who have an *FMR1* full mutation are carriers of an *FMR1* mutation. Female premutation carriers are at increased risk for fragile X–associated tremor/ataxia syndrome (FXTAS) and premature ovarian failure; those with a full mutation may have signs of fragile X syndrome. All are at increased risk for having offspring with FXTAS or, because the repeat size can expand when transmitted, fragile X syndrome. (*Anticipation* is defined and discussed in Chapter 29, "Patterns of Inheritance in Neurogenetic Disease.") Males with a premutation are at increased risk for FXTAS. Males with FXTAS will transmit their *FMR1* premutation expansion to none of their sons and to all their daughters, who also will be premutation carriers because the repeat size does not expand when transmitted through males.

Clinical Features

Classic clinical features in a male include intellectual impairment, a characteristically long face with prominent ears, autistic behavior, postpubertal macro-orchidism, connective tissue abnormalities (mitral valve prolapse or aortic dilatation), and seizures (20% of patients). About 30% of boys with fragile X syndrome meet the criteria for autism. Strong gaze avoidance, even when the patient is seeking interaction, is a hallmark of fragile X syndrome. In addition, tactile defensiveness and tantrum behavior with excessive auditory or visual stimuli suggest sensory processing problems. Epilepsy resolves during childhood in most people with fragile X syndrome.

Because fragile X syndrome is an X-linked disorder, the production of fragile X mental retardation protein (FMRP) by the normal allele generally results in a less severe phenotype in girls and women. Half of female carriers also have cognitive, behavioral, facial, or connective tissue signs and symptoms. IQ is generally in the borderline to low-normal range (75–90) in affected females. Shyness and social anxiety are common.

Fragile X syndrome is caused by an expanded trinucleotide CGG repeat of the *FMR1* gene 5′ region. The normal range of less than 55 CGG repeat sequences is stably transmitted. Full mutation alleles (>200 repeats) are associated with abnormal gene methylation and turning off of the gene, resulting in absent FMRP. FMRP is a messenger RNA (mRNA)-binding protein that regulates synaptic proteins. Absence of FMRP results in abnormal synaptic connections.

Premutation (55–200 CGG repeats) carriers have a specific set of signs and symptoms that are clearly distinguishable from those of patients with full-mutation fragile X syndrome. The signs and symptoms seem to correspond to an excess of mRNA.

Premutation leads to a progressive neurodegenerative disorder, FXTAS, in males older than 50 years (40%), but FXTAS is rare in females (8%). The clinical signs and symptoms include intention tremor, cerebellar ataxia, parkinsonism, peripheral neuropathy, psychiatric disorders, cognitive dysfunction, and hearing loss (see Volume 2, Chapter 26, "Cerebellar Disorders and Ataxias").

Diagnosis and Management

MRI features of FXTAS include T2-signal abnormalities in the periventricular and subcortical white matter. Increased T2-signal intensities of the middle cerebellar peduncles are a distinctive feature of FXTAS. Global brain atrophy is most evident in the frontal and parietal regions and in the pons and cerebellum.

The principal neuropathologic characteristic of FXTAS is ubiquitin-positive inclusions located in the nuclei of neurons and astrocytes. The inclusions contain *FMR1* mRNA, which implies a toxic gain-of-function effect.

No known pharmacologic treatment specifically overcomes the fragile X defect. Some children with fragile X syndrome, like children with other forms of developmental delays or learning disabilities, may benefit from medication designed to overcome attention-deficit/hyperactivity disorder or other disorders.

- Fragile X syndrome is the most common inherited cause of intellectual disability and the most common single-gene cause of autism.

- Fragile X syndrome is caused by an expanded trinucleotide CGG repeat of the *FMR1* gene 5′ region.
- Premutation leads to a progressive neurodegenerative disorder, FXTAS, in males older than 50 years (40%), but FXTAS is rare in females (8%).

Rett Syndrome

Overview and Epidemiology

Rett syndrome occurs with a frequency of approximately 1 in 10,000 females. It is an X-linked dominant disorder that formerly had been considered lethal in hemizygous males. However, it is now known that both males and females can be affected and that there is a wide range of variability in the clinical condition.

Rett syndrome is caused by mutations in the methyl-CpG-binding protein 2 gene (*MECP2*) located on chromosome Xq28. The methyl-CpG-binding protein 2 binds to methylated CpG dinucleotides within the human genome, which results in regulation of gene expression. Deficiency of the protein results in dysfunction of GABAergic neurons, which contribute to the neuropsychiatric features of Rett syndrome. Patients with Rett syndrome are reported to have reduced dendritic complexity of cortical neurons of the motor, association, and limbic cortices.

Most mutations are sporadic, but some mothers may be asymptomatic carriers or gonadal mosaics. Males typically have severe infantile encephalopathy due to absence of functional methyl-CpG-binding protein 2. Affected females are heterozygous for a mutation; severity depends in part on the degree of skewed X inactivation. The risk for the offspring of an affected mother to inherit the *MECP2* mutation is 50%. Affected males transmit the mutation to all their daughters.

Clinical Features

Classically, affected girls are often considered to have developed normally for the first 6 to 18 months of life, and then their development slows and arrests. A period of regression and social withdrawal follows; this period may persist for months. Loss of purposeful hand use and loss of spoken language are important features. The presence of nonspecific hand rubbing or hand-mouth movements and of truncal instability or ataxia may also suggest a diagnosis of Rett syndrome.

After the period of regression, social contact returns and progress can be made in the learning of limited skills.

However, girls affected by the classic form of Rett syndrome often remain profoundly mentally handicapped and many have progressive physical problems, such as scoliosis and spasticity. Many affected girls also have behavioral and emotional problems, including anxiety, depressed mood, and self-injurious behavior. Autistic behaviors may be present. If they had any speech capabilities before the period of regression, affected girls sometimes continue to utter a word or phrase; occasionally, this is in an appropriate context. However, there is virtually no useful speech.

Dystonia may occur, and more than 50% of patients have seizures. Growth is characterized by an early deceleration of head growth and the subsequent deceleration in the linear growth, leading to short stature in later childhood. Some patients have episodes of hyperventilation followed by central apnea, but the reason for these episodes is not known. Rett syndrome is not associated with specific dysmorphic features.

Now it is known that this classic description is too limited. Some patients may have preserved speech or remain ambulatory. Some males and females have only mild and nonspecific autism, pervasive development delay, or intellectual disability.

Diagnosis and Management

Currently there is no curative therapy for Rett syndrome. Certain aspects of the disorder may be controlled by medications, such as risperidone for treating agitation. Chloral hydrate, hydroxyzine, and diphenhydramine also are sometimes helpful. Melatonin may improve sleep disturbances. Treatment is provided as necessary for seizures, constipation, gastroesophageal reflux, scoliosis, prolonged QT interval, and spasticity.

Prognosis

Survival is shortened for patients with Rett syndrome. Causes of death may be related to aspiration during a seizure or to QT interval electrocardiographic changes. Autonomic abnormalities associated with Rett syndrome reduce heart rate variability. These autonomic changes also may account for the abnormal breathing pattern of many Rett syndrome patients. The nature of the autonomic dysfunction in Rett syndrome is not well understood.

- The presence of nonspecific hand rubbing or hand-mouth movements and of truncal instability or ataxia may suggest a diagnosis of Rett syndrome.

Questions and Answers

Questions

Multiple Choice (choose the best answer)

V.1. A 41-year-old patient with trisomy 21 is brought to the clinic by his mother for evaluation of progressive cognitive decline. In addition to your discussion with them of the higher risk of Alzheimer disease in patients with this condition, he also is at increased risk and should undergo additional surveillance for which of the following conditions?
a. Conductive hearing loss
b. Osteoporosis
c. Melanoma
d. Pulmonary fibrosis
e. Retinitis pigmentosa

V.2. Which of the following statements regarding genomic imprinting disorders is most accurate?
a. Results of DNA methylation studies are typically normal in patients with Prader-Willi syndrome
b. Mutations in *UBE3A*, whose brain expression is entirely derived from the maternal allele, can result in fragile X syndrome
c. Patients with Angelman syndrome need strict dietary supervision given the risk of hyperphagia and morbid obesity
d. Uniparental disomy is a potential mechanism of some imprinting disorders
e. Because these disorders are by definition sporadic, genetic counseling is unnecessary

V.3. Which of the following disorders is associated with a trinucleotide repeat expansion?
a. Type 2 myotonic dystrophy
b. Miyoshi myopathy (dysferlinopathy)
c. Hereditary neuropathy with liability to pressure palsies (HNPP)
d. Primary torsion dystonia (DYT1)
e. Friedreich ataxia

V.4. You are asked to evaluate a 41-year-old man for generalized seizures. On examination, you note short stature, bilateral hearing loss, and mild symmetric proximal muscle weakness. Which of the following statements regarding this category of inherited disorders is most accurate?
a. A high degree of homoplasmy may limit the sensitivity of tissue-based genetic testing
b. These disorders are usually passed via maternal inheritance
c. Mitotic segregation does not affect mutation expression in downstream cell lines
d. Mendelian patterns of inheritance for these disorders is impossible given autonomy of the mitochondrial genome
e. The mitochondrial genome has a lower basal mutation rate than the nuclear genome

V.5. Which of the following statements regarding patterns of inheritance is most correct?
a. If both parents are heterozygous for the same autosomal dominant mutation in a gene, their offspring have a 100% chance of inheriting the disorder
b. If a patient has no family history of a given mendelian disorder, then it is impossible for the patient to carry a disease-causing mutation
c. Each offspring of 2 carriers of a recessive disorder has a 25% chance of inheriting the disorder
d. X-linked disorders are typically passed from fathers to sons
e. Daughters of fathers with mitochondrial genome mutations are obligate carriers of the disorder

V.6. A neonate is diagnosed with velocardiofacial syndrome. Which of the following statements regarding this disorder is most accurate?
a. Clinically significant psychiatric disease occurs rarely in these patients
b. Most mutations consist of a 22q11.2 duplication
c. Microcephaly occurs in more than 50% of patients
d. Some degree of cognitive impairment is present in most patients
e. The disorder is uniformly fatal in infancy or childhood

Answers

V.1. Answer a.

Vance JM, Tekin D, Baloh RH, Barbouth DS, Estabrooks Hahn S, Fogel BL, et al. Neurogenetics. Contin. Lifelong Learn Neurol. 2011 Apr;17(2):233–427.

V.2. Answer d.

Vance JM, Tekin D, Baloh RH, Barbouth DS, Estabrooks Hahn S, Fogel BL, et al. Neurogenetics. Contin. Lifelong Learn Neurol. 2011 Apr;17(2):233–427.

V.3. Answer e.

Vance JM, Tekin D, Baloh RH, Barbouth DS, Estabrooks Hahn S, Fogel BL, et al. Neurogenetics. Contin. Lifelong Learn Neurol. 2011 Apr;17(2):233–427.

V.4. Answer b.

Vance JM, Tekin D, Baloh RH, Barbouth DS, Estabrooks Hahn S, Fogel BL, et al. Neurogenetics. Contin. Lifelong Learn Neurol. 2011 Apr;17(2):233–427.

V.5. Answer c.

Vance JM, Tekin D, Baloh RH, Barbouth DS, Estabrooks Hahn S, Fogel BL, et al. Neurogenetics. Contin. Lifelong Learn Neurol. 2011 Apr;17(2):233–427.

V.6. Answer d.

Vance JM, Tekin D, Baloh RH, Barbouth DS, Estabrooks Hahn S, Fogel BL, et al. Neurogenetics. Contin. Lifelong Learn Neurol. 2011 Apr;17(2):233–427.

SUGGESTED READING

Vance JM, Tekin D, Baloh RH, Barbouth DS, Estabrooks Hahn S, Fogel BL, et al. Neurogenetics. Contin. Lifelong Learn Neurol. 2011 Apr;17(2):233–427.

Neurodiagnostics
Ruple S. Laughlin, MD,
editor

Electroencephalography[a]

DAVID B. BURKHOLDER, MD; JEFFREY W. BRITTON, MD

Electroencephalography (EEG) is a useful procedure for diagnosis, evaluation, and prognosis of cerebral diseases and related conditions. EEG is particularly helpful for evaluation of transient neurologic disorders, altered states of consciousness, and encephalopathies.

Basics of EEG: Technical Factors

EEG electrodes are placed according to the International 10–20 System, which uses the inion and nasion and the ear or mastoid regions as landmarks to facilitate uniform placement. Typical electrode placement and nomenclature are summarized in Figure 31.1.

Each oscillation on the displayed EEG represents the potential difference between the electrode of interest for that channel (G1) and a reference electrode (G2). A differential amplifier amplifies the potential difference between G1 and G2 and displays this difference on the EEG. By convention, if G1 is of lower potential ("voltage") than G2, the display is an upward deflection, and vice versa. Comparison of neighboring derivations can help localize the regional source of detected potentials on the EEG (Figure 31.2).

The multiple derivations acquired in an EEG recording are displayed in an anatomical format known as a montage. Bipolar montages are composed of derivations in which G1 and G2 represent neighboring electrodes. Localized abnormalities on bipolar montages typically show phase reversal involving the electrode derivations where the potential is maximal (Figure 31.2A). Referential montages are composed of derivations in which G1 consists of a particular head region of interest and G2 represents a single electrode selected as a reference for all

derivations. In contrast to bipolar montages, localization using referential montages is based on determining the electrode in which the potential shows highest amplitude (Figure 31.2B).

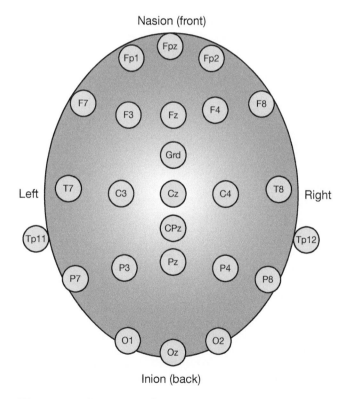

Figure 31.1 International 10-20 System.
C indicates central; F, frontal; Fp, frontopolar; Grd, ground; O, occipital; P, parietal; T, temporal; Tp, reference (ear or mastoid). F7 and F8 are considered the anterior temporal regions, and P7 and P8 are considered the posterior temporal regions.

---

[a] The electrode designations used in the illustrations are explained in the legend for Figure 31.1.

Abbreviations: CA, conceptional age; EEG, electroencephalography; REM, rapid eye movement; RTTD, rhythmic temporal theta of drowsiness

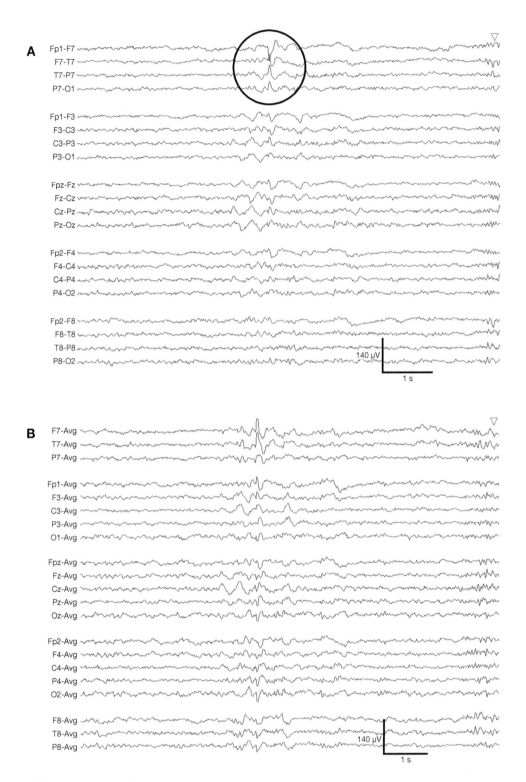

Figure 31.2 *Left Frontotemporal Spike.*
A, Bipolar montage. Phase reversal is present in circled area. B, Average (Avg) referential montage. Localization is determined by identifying the derivation and channel in which the spike amplitude is highest, which in this case are F7 and T7.

EEG activity is categorized in terms related to specific frequency bands: alpha (8.5–13 Hz), beta (>13 Hz), theta (4–7 Hz), and delta (0.5–4 Hz). Any frequency may be either normal or abnormal depending on the context of the recording, such as patient wake-sleep status, age, and administered medications. Other factors to consider when analyzing EEG recordings are waveform shape, distribution, and localization; overall background symmetry; amplitude; and reactivity.

- The multiple derivations acquired in an EEG recording are displayed in an anatomical format known as a montage.
- EEG activity is categorized in terms related to specific frequency bands: alpha (8.5–13 Hz), beta (>13 Hz), theta (4–7 Hz), and delta (0.5–4 Hz).

The Normal EEG

The appearance of the normal EEG depends on the patient's age and state of wakefulness.

Adult Awake EEG

The adult awake EEG is characterized by a posterior dominant (alpha) rhythm with normal frequency ranging from 8.5 to 13 Hz that attenuates with eye opening. The alpha rhythm may not be conspicuous in 10% to 20% of adults, particularly in the elderly. The remainder of the awake EEG background is typically composed of low-amplitude theta, beta, and delta components. Additional features of the normal awake EEG include a sharply contoured surface negative mu rhythm of 7 to 12 Hz present over the central head regions, either unilaterally or bisynchronously; this rhythm attenuates with movement of the contralateral hand. Eye blink artifact consisting of a high-amplitude triangular deflection over the frontopolar head regions is a hallmark of the awake EEG. Sail-shaped surface positive lambda waves are seen over the posterior head regions when the patient looks at images with sharp repeating contrasts.

Adult Sleep EEG

Sleep is composed of 2 main stages: non–rapid-eye movement (REM) and REM sleep. Non-REM sleep is further broken down into 3 substages: N1, N2, and N3. These stages have characteristic EEG features (Figure 31.3).

Drowsiness, or N1 sleep, makes up 5% of total sleep time. The EEG hallmarks of N1 sleep include slow horizontal eye movements, slowing and attenuation of alpha, decreases in myogenic artifact, and, in some cases, enhancement of frontocentral beta. Positive occipital sharp transients of sleep, which are surface positive, sharply contoured waveforms present over the occipital head regions, can be seen in N1 sleep, and persist into N2 sleep. They may be mistaken for epileptiform sharp waves.

The features of N2 sleep include V waves, sleep spindles, and K complexes. V waves consist of 200- to 500-millisecond high-amplitude, surface negative depolarizations localized to the central midline (Cz) head region. Sleep spindles consist of bisynchronous 1- to 2-second oscillations of 10 to 16 Hz maximal over the frontocentral head regions. K complexes are high-amplitude 500- to 1,000-millisecond depolarizations that are maximal in amplitude over the frontal head regions. Positive occipital sharp transients of sleep persist into N2 sleep. Benign variants most commonly occur in N1 and N2 sleep. Epileptogenic abnormalities are most common in N2 sleep.

N3 sleep is characterized by the presence of diffuse, frontally predominant delta waveforms making up 20% or more of the EEG epoch under review. Many parasomnias occur out of N3 sleep, including sleep walking, night terrors, bed wetting, and confusional arousals.

REM sleep is characterized by marked attenuation of myogenic activity and the presence of rapid multidirectional conjugate saccadic eye movements. The EEG background is typically composed of low-voltage activity in the 7- to 8-Hz range over the posterior head region. Sawtooth waves may be present over the central midline head regions. Clinical conditions involving REM sleep include narcolepsy and REM sleep behavior disorder. REM sleep is rarely recorded during the routine EEG. EEG changes in sleep are further discussed in Volume 2, Chapter 83, "Polysomnography and Other Sleep Testing."

Premature Infant, Full-term Neonate, and Pediatric Awake and Sleep EEG

Premature Infant

The EEG goes through several changes from conceptional age (CA) 27 weeks through full term. The EEG from 27 to 29 weeks shows a discontinuous pattern known as *tracé discontinue*. This evolves to a *tracé alternant* pattern, which shows shorter interburst intervals, between 34 and 36 weeks CA. A delta brush pattern consisting of delta waves with superimposed fast activity most prominent over the central, occipital, and temporal regions is also characteristic; these waves typically resolve by 42 weeks CA.

Between 32 and 34 weeks CA, infrequent multifocal sharp transients can be seen in normal patients. By 40 weeks CA, these multifocal sharp transients begin to resolve considerably, although they may persist in normal infants to a slight degree.

By 34 to 37 weeks CA, features of REM sleep begin to appear. Sleep in the premature infant (and full-term neonate) is separated into active and quiet sleep. Quiet sleep is analogous to non-REM sleep, and active sleep is analogous to REM sleep.

Full-term Neonate Through 3 Months

The awake record in the full-term neonate is characterized by irregular theta and delta activity known as *activité moyenne*. At full term, quiet sleep continues to show a

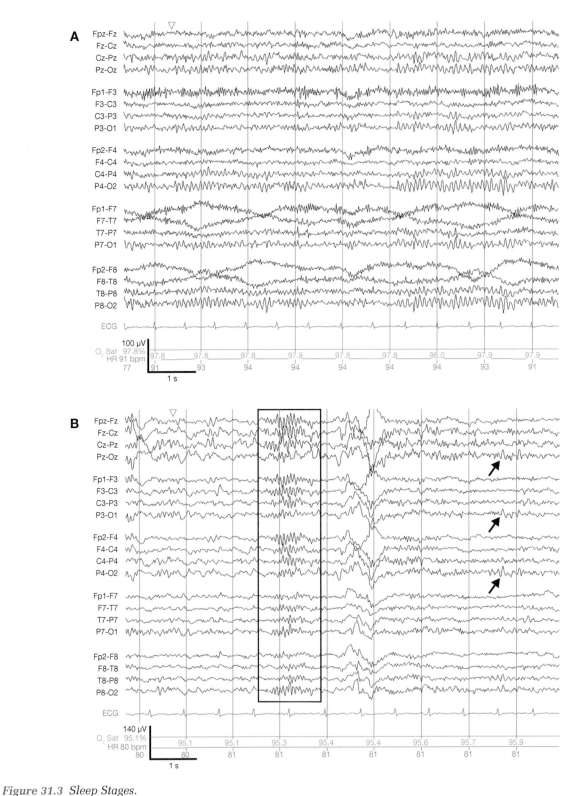

Figure 31.3 *Sleep Stages.*

A, N1 sleep, or drowsiness. Note slow eye movements at F7 and F8. B, N2 sleep. Sleep spindles (box). A few positive occipital sharp transients of sleep are present at Pz-Oz at the end of the sample (arrows). V waves, an additional feature of N2 sleep, are not depicted in this sample. C, N3 sleep, characterized by continuous diffuse anterior predominant slow waves that compose more than 20% of the electroencephalographic epoch. D, Rapid-eye movement (REM) sleep, marked by saccadic multidirectional eye movement artifact involving F7 and F8, absence of myogenic artifact, and a low-voltage background. Central midline sawtooth waves, an additional feature of REM, are not depicted in this example. bpm indicates beats per minute; ECG, electrocardiogram; HR, heart rate; O₂ Sat, oxygen saturation.

(continued on next page)

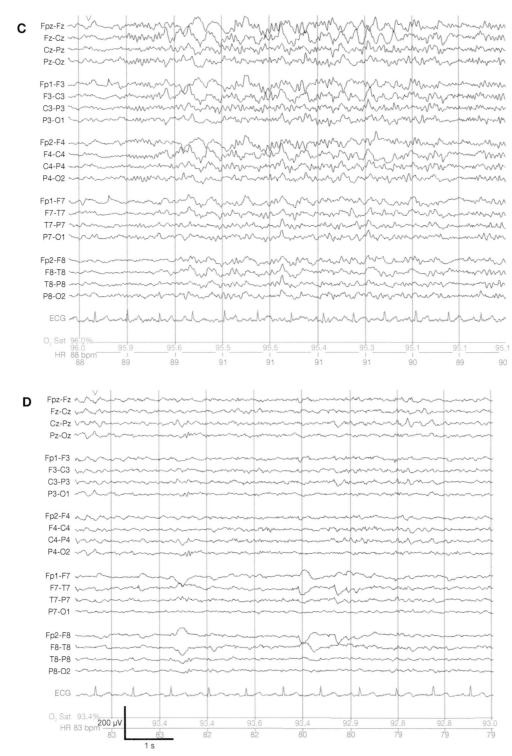

Figure 31.3 Continued.

tracé alternant pattern. Sleep spindles begin to emerge, which are prolonged and asynchronous in this age group. The posterior dominant rhythm should consist of 3- to 4-Hz activity; this can be brought out by passive eye closure. There may be organized central rhythmic activity in the range of 5 to 6 Hz that does not attenuate with eye opening; this is a precursor of the mu rhythm. The background otherwise consists of irregular and low-amplitude delta activity. Delta brushes and multifocal sharp transients should resolve in this interval.

Age 4 Months to 2 Years

The posterior dominant rhythm becomes better organized in the range of 5 to 6 Hz during infancy, which gradually increases to 6 to 8 Hz by age 2 years. A photic driving response may also be seen. During sleep, sleep spindles gradually become synchronous and shorter in duration and should be synchronous by 2 years of age. V waves and K complexes are now also seen.

Age 2 to 5 Years

The posterior dominant rhythm should reach a range of 6 to 8 Hz, although there can still be variation down to 5 Hz until 3 years of age. There is also a decrease in prominence of theta and delta frequencies during this time. During wakefulness, transient posterior wave forms, known as posterior slow waves of youth, are present. During sleep, high-voltage posterior predominant O waves may be seen as part of the normal record.

Age 6 to 16 Years

The posterior dominant rhythm should reflect that of an adult pattern, ranging between 9 and 12 Hz. Despite an adult-appearing posterior rhythm, the frontal, central, and temporal regions often still show relatively prominent theta components, which are normal in childhood.

- The adult awake EEG is characterized by a posterior dominant (alpha) rhythm with normal frequency ranging from 8.5 to 13 Hz that attenuates with eye opening.
- The features of N2 sleep include V waves, sleep spindles, and K complexes.
- REM sleep is characterized by marked attenuation of myogenic activity and the presence of rapid multidirectional conjugate saccadic eye movements.

Benign Variants in EEG

There are several nonspecific benign variants in the normal EEG that can resemble epileptiform abnormalities, leading to misdiagnosis (Box 31.1). Some of these variants are shown in Figure 31.4.

Box 31.1 • Benign Variants on Normal Electroencephalograms

Wicket waves
Rhythmic temporal theta of drowsiness
Benign small sharp spikes
6-Hz spike-and-wave pattern
14 & 6 positive spike bursts
Subclinical rhythmic epileptiform discharges of adults

Wicket Waves

Wicket waves are seen in N1 sleep and begin to resolve in N2 sleep. They may occur singly or in 1- to 2-second trains with a frequency of 6 to 11 Hz and phase reverse over the midtemporal regions (Figure 31.4A). When in trains, they often have a crescendo-decrescendo, piranha-teeth appearance. They may be bilateral or unilateral in distribution.

Rhythmic Temporal Theta of Drowsiness

Rhythmic temporal theta of drowsiness (RTTD) is also sometimes known as the *psychomotor variant*. RTTD is composed of rhythmic theta-range bursts present over the midtemporal regions (Figure 31.4B). RTTD may be unilateral or bisynchronous and may last several seconds. The feature that most distinguishes RTTD from a true epileptogenic discharge is that RTTD has a monomorphic appearance that does not evolve in frequency or spread anatomically over time. The theta waveforms may have a notched appearance.

Benign Small Sharp Spikes

Benign small sharp spikes are low-voltage, short-duration spikes seen predominantly in N1 and N2 sleep (Figure 31.4C). They may be unilateral or bilateral in distribution. They are typically most prominent over the temporal derivations. They may have an associated low-amplitude aftercoming slow wave.

6-Hz Spike-and-Wave Pattern

This variant has also been called *phantom spike and wave* because the spike is often less apparent than the slow-wave component and sometimes may be hidden altogether. It is characterized by bursts of bisynchronous 5- to 7-Hz spike-and-wave activity lasting 1 to 2 seconds and is most common in N1 sleep.

Other examples of benign variants include 14 & 6 positive spike bursts and subclinical rhythmic epileptiform discharges of adults.

Artifacts

Artifacts are common in EEG and can lead to misdiagnosis if not recognized. Examples are shown in Figure 31.5. Electrode artifacts result from excessive impedance between the electrode surface and scalp and can lead to "pops" that can be confused with epileptiform spikes and to rhythmic activity that can be confused with focal seizures (Figure 31.5A). Eye movements cause alterations in the frontotemporal regions. Nystagmus, horizontal eye movements of drowsiness, and unilateral artifact in patients with one eye can all be mistaken for focal

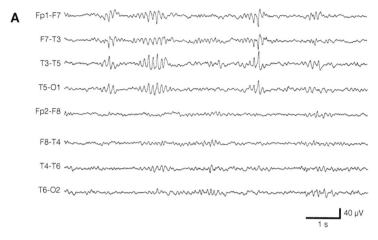

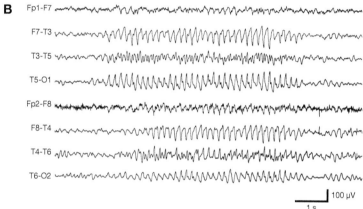

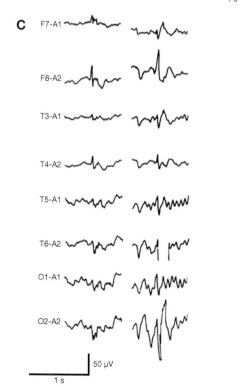

Figure 31.4 *Benign Electroencephalographic Variants.*
A, Wicket waves in left temporal region. B, Rhythmic temporal theta of drowsiness. C, Benign small, sharp spikes.

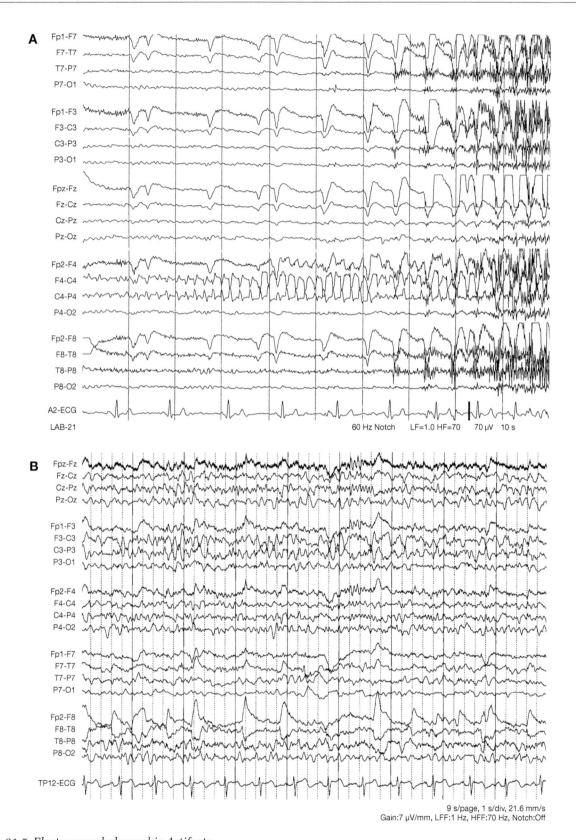

Figure 31.5 *Electroencephalographic Artifacts.*
A, Electrode artifact at C4 mimicking seizure discharge. B, Artifact due to nystagmus (F8) resembling periodic lateralized epileptiform discharges. C, Pulse artifact at Fp1 mimicking focal delta. D, Breach rhythm involving C3 after craniotomy. ECG indicates electrocardiogram; HF, high frequency; HFF, high-frequency filter; LF, low frequency; LFF, low-frequency filter.

(continued on next page)

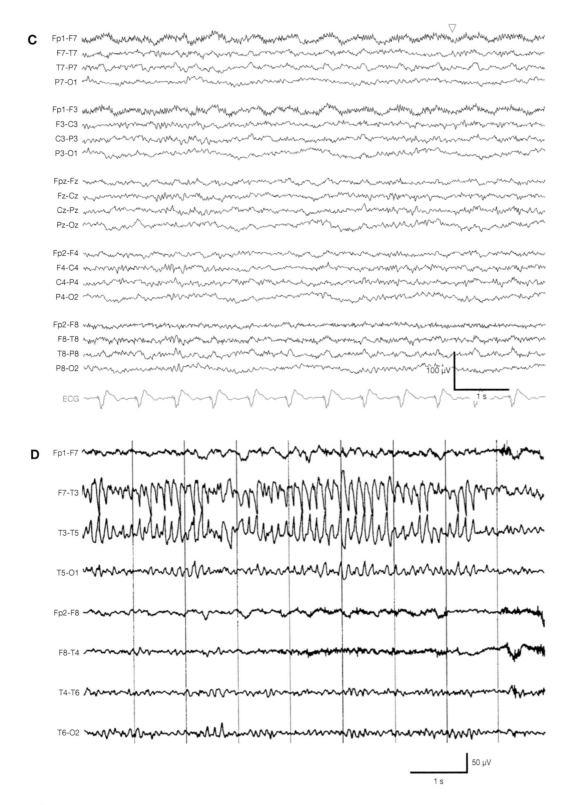

Figure 31.5 Continued.

frontotemporal dysrhythmias (Figure 31.5B). Electrocardiography commonly causes periodic spikelike alterations, predominantly in the temporal regions, which can cause confusion with epileptiform abnormalities. Pulse artifact is composed of rounded 1-Hz activity, which can be confused with focal delta (Figure 31.5C). After craniotomy, the EEG may show an excess of focal slow wave and sharply contoured activity known as a breach rhythm over the affected region, which can be confused with focal delta and spikes and sharp waves (Figure 31.5D).

EEG in the Epilepsies

Epileptiform Discharges

There are 3 main types of epileptiform discharges: spikes, sharp waves, and spike-and-wave discharges. Spikes have a steep ascent and descent and are brief, with a duration of less than 70 milliseconds (Figure 31.6A, C, and D). Sharp waves, in contrast, are longer in duration, lasting between 70 and 200 milliseconds (Figure 31.6B). Spike-and-wave discharges consist of a spike followed by an aftercoming slow wave. All of the discharges may occur singly or in trains, and any may be present in either focal or generalized epilepsy.

Focal Epilepsies

Interictal Activity in the Focal Epilepsies

Epileptiform discharges in the focal epilepsies typically correlate with the area of seizure onset. For example, frontotemporal or anterior temporal sharp waves typically suggest seizure onset in the temporal region. Certain zones of seizure onset are more difficult to appreciate on the scalp EEG than others. For instance, spikes and sharp waves may not always be evident in the frontal, parietal, or occipital lobes because of the anatomy of these structures relative to the scalp surface. Not all interictal abnormalities in focal epilepsy are sharply contoured: temporal intermittent rhythmic delta activity, for example, which consists of rounded, rhythmic monomorphic delta over one or both temporal regions, suggests seizure onset in the temporal lobe.

Ictal EEG Patterns in the Focal Epilepsies

Temporal lobe seizures typically begin with rhythmic theta or delta activity arising from the temporal region. The discharge usually increases in frequency to the high theta or alpha range and spreads to neighboring derivations and the central midline region. The discharge then slows to the delta frequency range in the terminal phase of the seizure and then stops. After the seizure, focal postictal delta

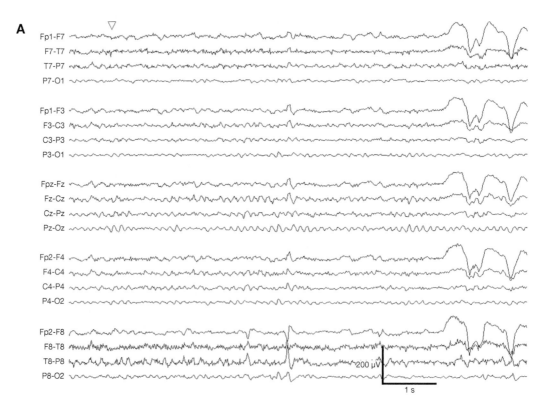

Figure 31.6 Epileptiform Discharges.
A, Right anterior temporal spikes at F8. B, Left frontopolar sharp wave localized to Fp1. ECG indicates electrocardiogram.
C, Left central spikes localized to C3. D, Left occipital spikes.

(continued on next page)

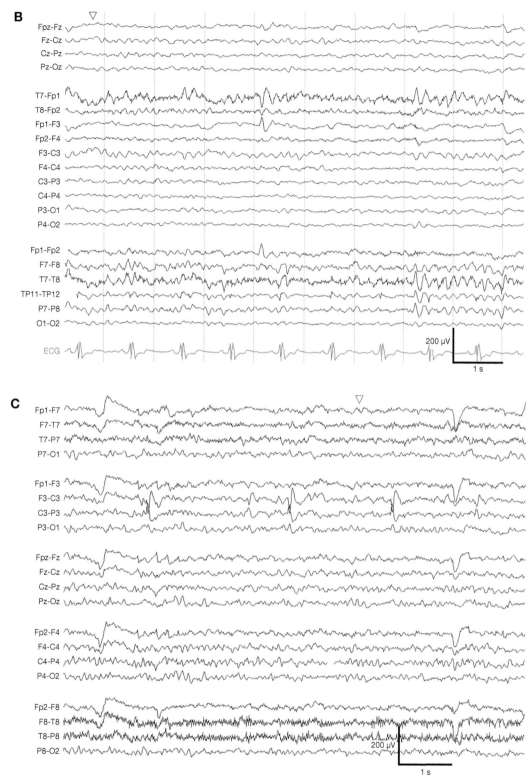

Figure 31.6 Continued on next page

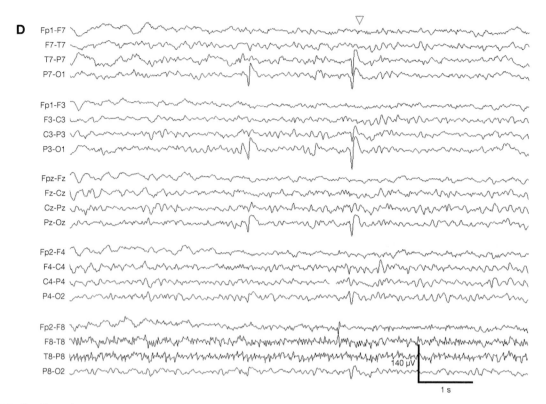

Figure 31.6 Continued

slowing may be seen, maximal over the area of seizure onset (Figure 31.7). Ictal discharges in the extratemporal focal epilepsies may show discharges overlying the lobe of onset, but in many cases the onset may be obscure. Sometimes, the clearest early discharge may actually be in an area of propagation (and not the area of onset) because of neural networks involved in rapid seizure spread.

Generalized Epilepsies

Interictal Activity in the Generalized Epilepsies

The interictal patterns seen in the generalized epilepsies include generalized spike and wave, generalized paroxysmal fast activity, and hypsarrhythmia. The 3 main spike-and-wave discharge subtypes are 3-Hz spike and wave, slow spike and wave, and atypical spike and wave. Differentiation among these generalized spike-and-wave types may help with diagnosis. The 3-Hz spike-and-wave discharges are classically seen in absence epilepsy (Figure 31.8). In practice, the frequency often begins at 4 Hz, remains at 3 Hz during the majority of the discharge, and terminates at 2 Hz. Slow spike-and-wave discharges occur at a frequency of 1 to 2.5 Hz. This pattern is typically seen in Lennox-Gastaut syndrome and is often associated with considerable developmental abnormalities and intellectual disability. Atypical spike-and-wave patterns do not share the same regularity displayed by the 3-Hz pattern

and are higher frequency than slow spike-and-wave pattern. The frequency may be variable, and there can be a polyspike component to the discharges, in which case the pattern is termed *polyspike and wave*. The latter is typically seen in idiopathic generalized epilepsies, such as juvenile myoclonic epilepsy. Generalized paroxysmal fast activity is often seen in patients with severe symptomatic generalized epilepsy and in those with tonic and atonic seizures. Hypsarrhythmia is characteristic of infantile spasms.

Ictal EEG Patterns in the Generalized Epilepsies

Generalized tonic-clonic seizures usually begin with a buildup of generalized high-frequency spike or spike-and-wave activity. During the tonic phase, continuous high-frequency activity and myogenic artifact often render the screen black. This activity is then interrupted by periodic silent periods during the clonic phase. After the seizure, the EEG is typically markedly suppressed (Figure 31.9).

Drop attacks, tonic, and atonic seizures are typically associated with a generalized electrodecremental response with or without a high-frequency, low-amplitude generalized fast discharge. These are usually not followed by post-ictal suppression, and recovery is more prompt than after a generalized tonic-clonic seizure.

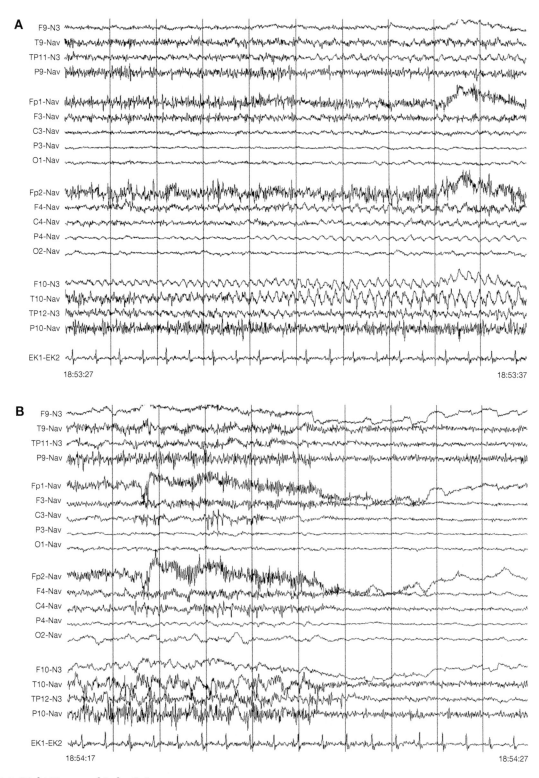

Figure 31.7 *Right Temporal Lobe Seizure.*
A, At F10 and T10. B, Seizure termination.

Infantile spasms are characterized by an interictal EEG showing a hypsarrhythmia pattern characterized by high-voltage delta and multifocal sharp complexes. The infantile spasms themselves are typically correlated in time by brief electrodecremental periods lasting seconds in duration on the EEG. These electrodecrements may also show very low-amplitude, high-frequency components (Figure 31.10).

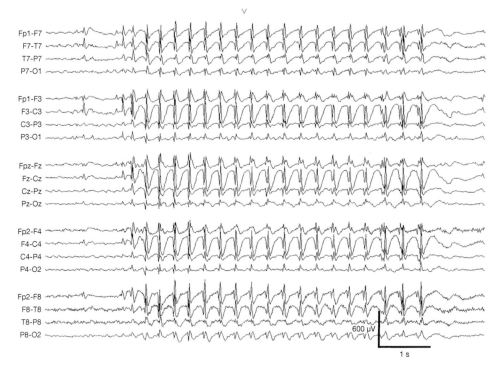

Figure 31.8 *Absence Seizure With 3-Hz Spike and Wave.*

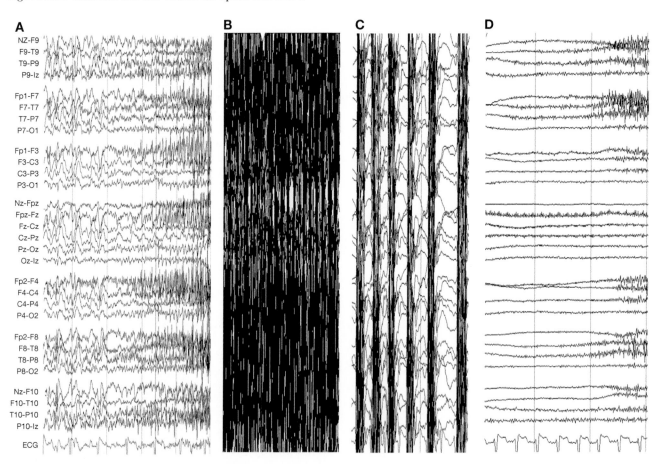

Figure 31.9 *Generalized Tonic-Clonic Seizure.*
A, Seizure onset, consisting of diffuse high-frequency discharge maximal over the anterior head regions. B, Tonic phase: interference pattern is due to continuous myogenic artifact and high-frequency seizure discharge. C, Clonic phase: repetitive bursts with intervening silent periods occurring at regular intervals correspond with clonic activity. D, Postictal phase: marked diffuse suppression of cerebral activity correlates with postictal unresponsiveness. ECG indicates electrocardiogram.

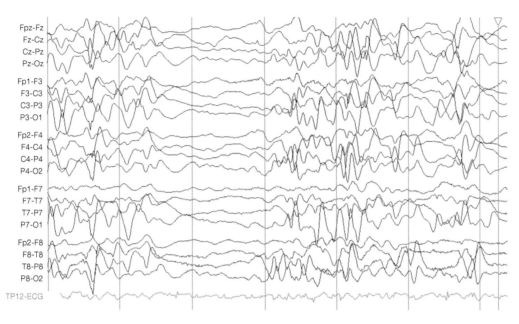

Figure 31.10 Hypsarrhythmia With Electrodecrement.
ECG indicates electrocardiogram.

Ictal EEG in Status Epilepticus

Status epilepticus is operationally defined as a convulsive seizure lasting longer than 5 minutes or as 2 or more convulsive seizures without return to baseline consciousness. Nonconvulsive status epilepticus is defined as a nonconvulsive seizure associated with changes in mental status lasting at least 30 minutes.

Convulsive status epilepticus is typically accompanied by continuous high-frequency generalized spike or spike-and-wave activity on the EEG. In cases of prolonged status epilepticus, the EEG typically evolves to show generalized periodic (usually 1 per second) epileptiform discharges as opposed to generalized spike-and-wave activity. Because the clinical correlates of status epilepticus may become more subtle over time, continuous EEG is recommended in the monitoring of affected patients.

The EEG during nonconvulsive status epilepticus may show various patterns depending on the type of status present. Generalized absence status epilepticus typically shows continuous generalized 3- to 4-Hz spike-and-wave activity. Focal nonconvulsive status epilepticus typically shows continuous rhythmic theta activity over the region involved with the seizure activity.

- There are 3 main types of epileptiform discharges: spikes, sharp waves, and spike-and-wave discharges.
- Epileptiform discharges in the focal epilepsies typically correlate with the area of seizure onset.
- The interictal patterns seen in the generalized epilepsies include generalized spike and wave, generalized paroxysmal fast activity, and hypsarrhythmia.

- The 3-Hz spike-and-wave discharges are classically seen in absence epilepsy.
- Slow spike-and-wave discharges occur at a frequency of 1 to 2.5 Hz. This pattern is typically seen in Lennox-Gastaut syndrome.
- Infantile spasms are characterized by an interictal EEG showing a hypsarrhythmia pattern characterized by high-voltage delta and multifocal sharp complexes.
- Convulsive status epilepticus is typically accompanied by continuous high-frequency generalized spike or spike-and-wave activity on the EEG.

EEG in Diffuse Disorders

Degenerative Disorders

The EEG in Alzheimer disease typically shows diffuse slowing in later stages, but it may show minimal abnormalities in early and moderate stages. In dementia with Lewy bodies, slowing may occur at an earlier stage than in Alzheimer disease. In Huntington disease, the EEG characteristically shows a markedly low voltage background. In degenerative disease in which seizures are a prominent feature (eg, neuronal lipofuscinosis), epileptiform abnormalities are common.

Encephalopathies

The EEG in encephalopathies shows slowing of the background. In moderate encephalopathies, slowing is typically in the theta range, and when severe, slowing is usually in the delta range in a generalized distribution. In addition, other characteristic waveforms may be present

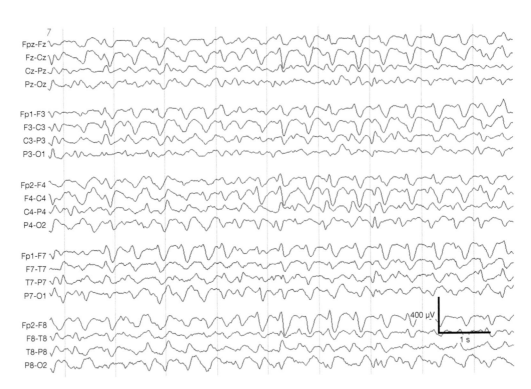

Figure 31.11 Generalized Triphasic Waves.

in severe encephalopathies. Triphasic waves are characteristic of metabolic encephalopathies, often hepatic or renal in origin, and consist of high-amplitude anterior predominant periodic waveforms (Figure 31.11). Triphasic waves characteristically show an anterior-posterior lag. In some diffuse encephalopathies, multifocal sharp waves and seizures may be present. In addition, periodic attenuation of the EEG may occur in severe encephalopathies.

Generalized periodic complexes are generalized sharp waves with a diphasic or triphasic morphologic pattern that typically discharge at a rate of 1 to 2 Hz. Periodic sharp-wave complexes may be difficult to distinguish from triphasic waves; however, unlike triphasic waves, there should not be an anterior-posterior lag. These are classically seen in patients with Creutzfeldt-Jakob disease, but they may also be seen in other conditions such as toxic and hypoxic encephalopathies.

Encephalopathies may also be associated with frontal intermittent rhythmic delta activity. This activity can be seen with toxic-metabolic encephalopathies but also with hydrocephalus, midline deep-seated tumors, and frontal lobe lesions.

- The EEG in Alzheimer disease typically shows diffuse slowing in later stages, but it may show minimal abnormalities in early and moderate stages.
- Triphasic waves are characteristic of metabolic encephalopathies, often hepatic or renal in origin, and consist of high-amplitude anterior predominant periodic waveforms.

EEG in Focal Lesions

Focal Slowing

In patients with focal lesions, focal polymorphic delta activity may be present. This consists of focal persistent, nonreactive delta activity overlying the lesion. It can be seen in the setting of cerebral infarcts, hemorrhages, tumor, and other focal abnormalities. Focal delta is typically seen in lesions that involve the underlying white matter.

Periodic Patterns in Focal Disorders: Periodic Lateralized Epileptiform Discharges

Periodic lateralized epileptiform discharges are periodic waveforms consisting of spikes, sharp waves, or slow waves that repeat at regular intervals of 0.2- to 2-Hz frequency and are typically continuous throughout the recording (Figure 31.12). They are focal or lateralized moderate- to high-amplitude sharp-wave discharges and are typically seen in the setting of focal acute to subacute cerebral lesions such as abscesses, infarcts, and intracerebral and subdural hemorrhages. They can also be seen in patients with high-grade primary brain tumors and cerebral metastases and are a classic EEG finding in herpes encephalitis.

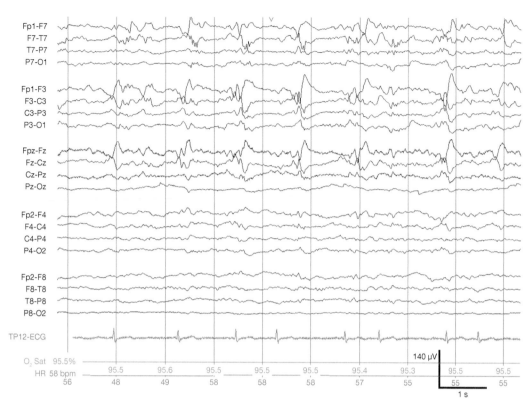

Figure 31.12 Left frontotemporal periodic lateralized epileptiform discharges in a semicomatose patient after a stroke. bpm indicates beats per minute; ECG, electrocardiogram; HR, heart rate; O₂ Sat, oxygen saturation.

Other EEG Findings in Focal Disorders

Patients with focal lesions may also show focal interictal epileptiform discharges and electrographic seizures arising from the affected brain regions. In addition, asymmetry over homologous brain regions may be seen with certain lesions. For example, focal suppression may be present over large chronic cerebral infarcts or overlying unilateral subdural hematomas, hygromas, or empyemas.

- Periodic lateralized epileptiform discharges are periodic waveforms consisting of spikes, sharp waves, or slow waves that repeat at regular intervals of 0.2- to 2-Hz frequency and are typically continuous throughout the recording.
- Periodic lateralized epileptiform discharges are focal or lateralized moderate- to high-amplitude sharp-wave discharges and are typically seen in the setting of focal acute to subacute cerebral lesions such as abscesses, infarcts, and intracerebral and subdural hemorrhages.

Coma and Brain Death

Coma

Various EEG patterns can be seen in comatose patients. It is critical to take into account a patient's medications and core body temperature before basing prognosis on any of the EEG coma patterns because these factors can affect the EEG independent of the underlying cerebral disease. In severe coma due to cortical lesions, the EEG may show generalized suppression, particularly in cases with severe intractable intracranial hypertension and in the setting of severe hypoxic ischemic encephalopathy. A characteristic feature of the EEG in comatose patients is the presence of background activity that does not show evidence of reactivity to external stimuli. Several monorhythmic coma patterns have been described in which one background frequency is predominant on the EEG tracing. These monorhythmic coma pattern types are named after the predominant frequency or waveforms present (specifically, alpha coma, theta coma, beta coma, and spindle coma patterns). These patterns are most commonly seen in severe hypoxic ischemic encephalopathies but may also be seen in posttraumatic coma. Beta coma may be seen in pharmacologic coma. The prognostic value of EEG is dependent on the underlying cause of coma; no EEG pattern has inherent prognostic meaning outside its clinical context.

Burst suppression pattern consists of intermittent bursts of polyphasic, sharply contoured or spiky activity interspersed with periods of suppression, each lasting several seconds (Figure 31.13). Burst suppression pattern can be seen in the context of anesthesia and hypothermia, in

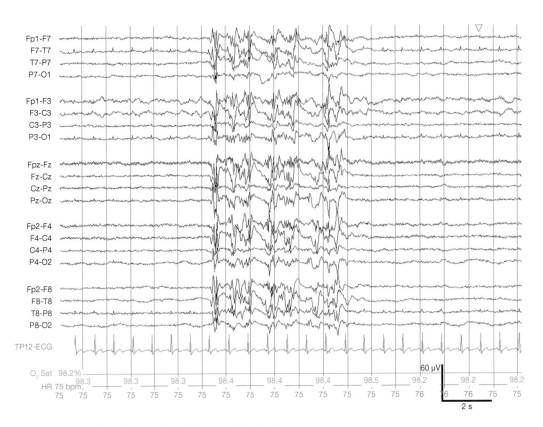

Figure 31.13 Burst Suppression Pattern in a Comatose Patient.
bpm indicates beats per minute; ECG, electrocardiogram; HR, heart rate; O₂ Sat, oxygen saturation.

which case it may be reversible. When burst suppression pattern is present in the setting of hypoxic ischemic encephalopathy, it portends a very poor prognosis.

Brain Death

Brain death is a clinical diagnosis and should be based on clinical examination and investigation, and it cannot be diagnosed with EEG in isolation. For cases in which a clinical brain death examination cannot be performed in its entirety and in which reversible causes have been effectively eliminated, EEG may be useful for establishing evidence in support for or against brain death. The EEG criteria for brain death in the adult and pediatric populations are as follows:

- At least 8 scalp electrodes must be used with at least 10 cm between any 2 electrodes. Placement and integrity must be verified by tapping.
- Impedance must not be less than 100 ohms or more than 10,000 ohms.
- The high-frequency filter must not be set below 30 Hz, and the low-frequency filter must be set at 1 Hz or lower.
- A sensitivity of 2 µV/mm must be used for at least 30 minutes of the recording.
- There should be electrocerebral silence without reactivity to stimulation throughout the recording.

- The recording must be performed by a qualified technologist.

The EEG is supportive of brain death if the above-listed criteria are met in the appropriate clinical context. If there are doubts regarding true electrocerebral silence, the study should be repeated. Although there are no strict criteria, EEG should not be repeated before 24 hours in the evaluation of brain death in children. See also Volume 2, Chapter 1, "Impaired Consciousness and Coma."

- A characteristic feature of the EEG in comatose patients is the presence of background activity that does not show evidence of reactivity to external stimuli.
- Monorhythmic coma pattern types are named after the predominant frequency or waveforms present (specifically, alpha coma, theta coma, beta coma, and spindle coma patterns).
- Monorhythmic coma patterns are most commonly seen in severe hypoxic ischemic encephalopathies but may also be seen in posttraumatic coma.
- Brain death is a clinical diagnosis and should be based on clinical examination and investigation, and it cannot be diagnosed with EEG in isolation.

Nerve Conduction Studies and Needle Electromyography

BRIAN A. CRUM, MD

Introduction

Nerve conduction studies (NCSs) and needle electromyography (EMG) should be considered extensions of the neurologic history and examination of the peripheral sensory and motor systems. NCSs assess large, myelinated sensory and motor nerve fibers. EMG assesses primarily type 1 muscle fibers. Because of the limitations of NCSs and EMG, small-fiber function (ie, small-fiber neuropathies) and, to an extent, type 2 muscle-fiber diseases (ie, steroid myopathy) cannot be excluded with these studies.

The main goal of NCSs and EMG is to obtain objective evidence of disease within the peripheral nervous system and to assist with localization of the problem. NCSs and EMG can aid in answering several clinical questions: Is the problem focal, multifocal, or diffuse? Does it involve peripheral nerve, neuromuscular junction, or muscle? For conditions affecting the nerve, one can try to assess how much of the pathophysiologic mechanism is axonal or demyelinating. The natural evolution of abnormalities found on EMG can help determine the timing of a neurologic process and assist in prognostication (eg, worsening results of needle examination over time in amyotrophic lateral sclerosis).

A valuable approach to interpret the results of EMG is to identify the pattern of abnormality. Most neuromuscular conditions demonstrate 1 of 8 clinical and electrodiagnostic patterns (Table 32.1).

• Most neuromuscular conditions demonstrate 1 of 8 clinical and electrodiagnostic patterns.

Anatomy

The main motor neuroanatomical structures that are important in NCSs and EMG include the anterior horn cell in the ventral (anterior) spinal cord, the motor root and axon traversing down the peripheral nerves, the neuromuscular junction, and the muscle fiber. In the sensory system, the dorsal root ganglion (generally located in the intervertebral foramen) and its peripheral axon arriving from a sensory receptor can be assessed with NCSs. This location of the dorsal root ganglion is an important feature to note in interpretation of NCSs because preganglionic sensory lesions (eg, radiculopathy, central nervous system process) will not show abnormalities, but postganglionic lesions (eg, plexopathy or peripheral neuropathy) will show abnormalities on sensory NCSs.

Nerve Conduction Studies

The Basics

NCSs are performed by percutaneously stimulating a peripheral nerve and then recording a response elsewhere. In motor studies the response is recorded over muscle, whereas in sensory studies the response is recorded at another point on the nerve. Various factors are measured in the resulting response, including the amplitude (size) of the response, the conduction velocity, and distal latency (time from stimulus to onset of response). Attention is also paid to change in the morphologic pattern of the resulting waveforms (Figure 32.1). Stimulation is performed with a negatively charged stimulator (cathode) applied percutaneously to the nerve being studied. Because the inside of the axon is

---

Abbreviations: CMAP, compound muscle action potential; EMG, electromyography; EPP, end plate potential; NCSs, nerve conduction studies; SNAP, sensory nerve action potential

Table 32.1 • Common Patterns of Electrodiagnostic Abnormalities

	Nerve Conduction Studies			Needle Electromyography	
Pattern	Motor	Sensory		Spontaneous Activity	Activation (Motor Unit Potential Analysis)
Motor neuron disease	Low-amplitude CMAPs Mild slowing of CV Mild prolongation of DL	Normal		Fasciculation potentials Fibrillation potentials	Reduced recruitment Large, often varying MUPs
Radiculopathy or polyradiculopathy	Low-amplitude CMAPs in distribution of affected root(s)	Normal		Fibrillation potentials (for active disorders)	Reduced recruitment Large MUPs
Plexopathy	Low-amplitude CMAPs	Low-amplitude or absent SNAPs		Fibrillation potentials Myokymic discharges (especially in radiation plexopathies)	Reduced recruitment Large MUPs
Mononeuropathy (single or multiple, as in mononeuritis multiplex)	Low-amplitude CMAPs in distribution of affected nerve(s)	Low-amplitude or absent SNAPs in distribution of affected nerve(s)		Fibrillation potentials	Reduced recruitment Large MUPs in distribution of affected nerve(s)
Axonal length-dependent sensorimotor peripheral neuropathy	Low-amplitude CMAPs Mild slowing of CV Mild prolongation of DL	Low-amplitude or absent SNAPs		Fibrillation potentials in distal muscles	Reduced recruitment Large MUPs in distal muscles
Demyelinating sensorimotor peripheral neuropathy	Pronounced slowing of conduction velocity Pronounced prolongation of distal latencies Possible temporal dispersion or conduction block Prolonged F-wave latencies	Pronounced slowing of conduction velocity Pronounced prolongation of distal latencies		May be normal or show fibrillation potentials if secondary axonal loss	Reduced recruitment MUPs may be normal
Defect of neuromuscular transmission	Normal routine motor studies Slow repetitive stimulation shows decrement CMAPs may be low amplitude in presynaptic disorders (eg, LEMS)	Normal		Typically normal May show fibrillation potentials in severe presynaptic or postsynaptic disorders	Small, varying MUPs SFEMG may be needed in mild cases
Myopathy	Typically normal In severe or distal myopathies, CMAPs may be low amplitude	Normal		May show fibrillation potentials	Small, complex MUPs

Abbreviations: CMAP, compound muscle action potential; CV, conduction velocity; DL, distal latency; LEMS, Lambert-Eaton myasthenic syndrome; MUPs, motor unit potentials; SFEMG, single-fiber electromyography; SNAPs, sensory nerve action potentials.

negatively charged, this stimulation will depolarize the axon and lead to an action potential generated at that point on the nerve. Large, myelinated axons have lower stimulation thresholds. Approximately 2 cm proximal to the cathode on the stimulator is an anode that hyperpolarizes the axon at that point on the nerve; this hyperpolarization can yield a theoretical anodal block. Thus, any component of the initiated action potential that is heading proximally may be blocked. As the stimulus intensity is increased (typically measured in milliamperes), the amplitude (size) of the resulting response increases due to excitation of more and more axons within the nerve up until a point at which further increase of stimulus intensity does not lead to

increase in the amplitude of the response. This level of stimulus intensity is called *supramaximal stimulation* and must be attained at each point of stimulation along the nerve to ensure that all axons in the nerve that are able to be stimulated have been stimulated.

In motor NCSs, the recording electrode (G1) is placed over the motor end plate of the muscle, which is typically halfway along the course of the muscle. The referential electrode (G2) is placed distally over the corresponding tendon. This arrangement allows acquisition of a compound muscle action potential (CMAP) (Figure 32.1). In sensory NCSs, the recording electrode is placed over the nerve, and the referential electrode is also placed on the

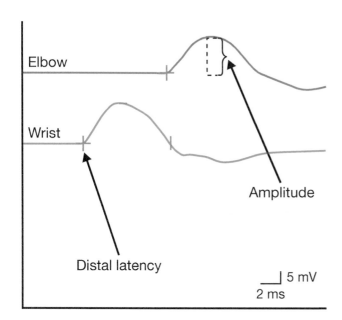

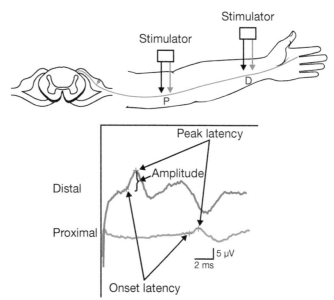

Figure 32.1 Compound muscle action potential generated by stimulation of the median nerve at 2 points; recording is over the abductor pollicis brevis. Note the similar configuration at different sites of stimulation.

(Adapted from Mowzoon N. Clinical neurophysiology. Part B: Principles of nerve conduction studies and electromyography [EMG]. In: Mowzoon N, Flemming KD, editors. Neurology board review: an illustrated study guide. Rochester [MN]: Mayo Clinic Scientific Press and Florence [KY]: Informa Healthcare USA; c2007. p. 189–223. Used with permission of Mayo Foundation for Medical Education and Research.)

Figure 32.2 Median sensory nerve action potential (antidromic) generated by stimulation of the median nerve at 2 sites and recording over the second digit. D indicates distal; P, proximal.

(Adapted from Mowzoon N. Clinical neurophysiology. Part B: Principles of nerve conduction studies and electromyography [EMG]. In: Mowzoon N, Flemming KD, editors. Neurology board review: an illustrated study guide. Rochester [MN]: Mayo Clinic Scientific Press and Florence [KY]: Informa Healthcare USA; c2007. p. 189–223. Used with permission of Mayo Foundation for Medical Education and Research.)

nerve, typically 3 to 4 cm farther away from the recording electrode. The resulting sensory nerve action potential (SNAP) often has a triphasic waveform with an initial downward (positive) deflection (Figure 32.2). Sensory NCSs can be done orthodromically (stimulating distally, recording proximally) or antidromically (stimulating proximally, recording distally). A ground electrode is used in all NCSs and EMG and is usually placed at a point between the cathode stimulus and recording (G1) electrode.

The CMAP amplitude is generally measured in millivolts. At both proximal and distal sites of stimulation, the CMAP morphologic pattern stays essentially the same without any considerable changes or decreases in amplitude. Note that, for a CMAP, the response is a measure not only of the motor axon but also of the neuromuscular junction and the muscle itself.

For sensory NCSs, because one is recording a nerve-generated potential, the amplitude is much smaller (generally on the order of microvolts). As a result, the signal-to-noise ratio is less favorable than with motor studies, and several stimuli may have to be averaged to ensure a high-quality SNAP. In normal sensory NCSs, the morphologic pattern of the waveform changes (decrease in

amplitude and prolong in duration) between proximal and distal sites because of phase cancellation of the traveling wave.

Parameters

Many different parameters are measured in NCSs. These include the amplitude, distal latency, and, at times, the conduction velocity. The amplitude of the CMAP or SNAP is the height of the response. The distal latency is the time between stimulation to the onset of the waveform when stimulating the most distal site (usually at the ankle or wrist). In motor NCSs, the distal latency is marked at the initial upward (negative) deflection of the waveform from baseline. In sensory studies, there may be an initial downward (positive) deflection and then an upward deflection. The point at which the upward deflection begins (even if there is first a downward deflection from baseline) is the point at which the onset latency is marked. Conduction velocity is calculated by measuring the distance between points of stimulation and dividing by the difference in latencies between the 2 stimulation sites.

In motor studies, the duration and area of the CMAP are also marked and may be important in certain clinical

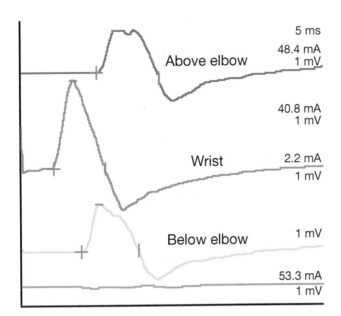

Figure 32.3 Stimulation of the ulnar nerve results in an approximately 55% drop in amplitude of the compound muscle action potential between the wrist and below-elbow stimulation sites. This finding indicates conduction block along that segment of nerve.

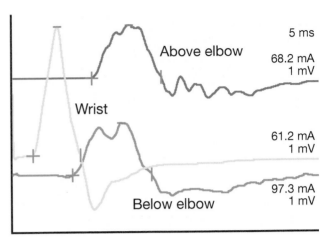

Figure 32.4 Stimulation of the ulnar nerve results in reduced amplitude (conduction block) and prolonged duration (temporal dispersion) of the compound muscle action potential waveforms between the below-elbow and wrist stimulation sites.

conditions. If there is a difference in morphologic pattern between the distal and proximal sites of stimulation, one may consider the presence of temporal dispersion or conduction block. As mentioned above, the CMAP should be almost identical with a similar amplitude and duration and overall morphologic findings along all sites of stimulation in a motor nerve. Considerable loss of amplitude or prolongation of duration at the proximal site compared with the distal site suggests conduction block or temporal dispersion, respectively. In general, a 20% decrease in CMAP amplitude is consistent with conduction block (Figure 32.3). An increase in duration of the CMAP waveform of more than 30% is consistent with temporal dispersion (Figure 32.4). Both of these findings generally indicate some degree of underlying demyelination occurring between the points of stimulation. In sensory studies, because nerve conduction amplitudes fall off as a function of distance and also increase slightly in duration simply due to distance, measurement of duration and area is not helpful.

Late Responses

The motor and sensory NCSs described above are relatively direct measures of the integrity of the more distal segments of nerves. In proximal segments of nerves, NCSs are technically limited in their ability to directly assess the nerve because of difficulty in isolated stimulation of nerves and isolated recording from nerves or muscle. Although direct measures are not reliable, indirect measures of the proximal segments of nerve are possible utilizing F waves (Figure 32.5) and the H reflex.

In elicitation of an F wave, stimulation is performed as it is routinely done for the CMAP. However, for obtaining an F wave, rotating the anode off the nerve allows the action potential generated at the point of stimulation at the distal stimulation site to travel proximally. This action potential travels exclusively up the motor axon to the anterior horn cell and causes depolarization of a small pool of anterior horn cells. These anterior horn cells, in turn, send an action potential back down the motor nerve to the muscle, where the small evoked responses can be recorded, representing the F wave. Because each stimulus will excite a different pool of anterior horn cells, the F waves elicited will vary in configuration, amplitude, and, to a lesser extent, latency. The F wave represents a signal that has traversed the entire peripheral segment of the motor nerve proximally and then back distally and therefore serves as an indirect way to assess proximal motor nerve segments (plexus and root).

Typically the F latency is measured as the time between stimuli at the distal site on the motor nerve and the appearance of the first 2 F waves. One can compare the resulting F latency to normal values or to an estimate that takes into consideration the conduction velocity of the nerve and distance of the pathway traveled to the spinal cord. If the F latency is longer than the F estimate, some proximal slowing of conduction is suggested, which is consistent with an underlying pathophysiologic mechanism of acquired demyelination.

An H reflex is another late reflex that can be measured during NCSs (Figure 32.5). It is the electrophysiologic correlate of a deep tendon reflex and is most often measured from the mixed (motor and sensory) tibial nerve. Stimulation is performed at very low levels (much less

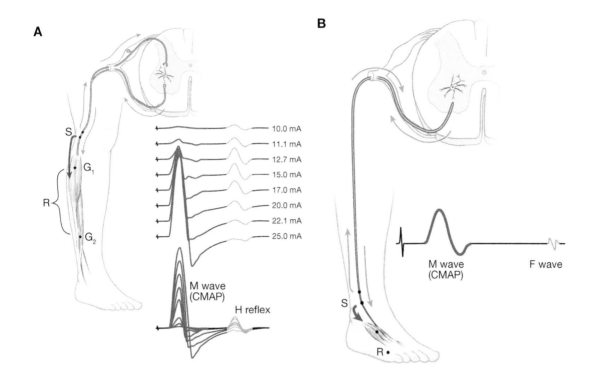

Figure 32.5 *Late Responses.*

A, The H reflex is a true monosynaptic reflex, with selective activation of Ia muscle spindle afferents (with low stimulus) and alpha motor neuron efferents supplying the gastrocnemius-soleus muscle group. B, In contrast, the F wave represents antidromic stimulation of alpha motor neuron and a small population of anterior horn cells whose action potentials then travel orthodromically to the muscle. CMAP indicates compound muscle action potential; G1, active recording electrode; G2, reference recording electrode; R, recording electrodes.

(Adapted from Jones LK Jr. Nerve conduction studies: basic concepts and patterns of abnormalities. Neurol Clin. 2012 May;30[2]:405–27. Epub 2011 Dec 28. Erratum in: Neurol Clin. 2013 Feb;31[1]:xv. Used with permission.)

than supramaximal stimulation). This causes an action potential to travel proximally up the type 1a afferent sensory fibers. Anterior horn cells are then activated by monosynaptic reflex, which leads to an action potential traveling down the motor axon and yields an evoked muscle response (monosynaptic reflex arc). The latency between the time of stimulation and onset of the H reflex can be measured and compared with normal values or compared side to side. The most common application of an H reflex is to diagnose an S1 radiculopathy.

- In motor NCSs, the recording electrode (G1) is placed over the motor end plate of the muscle (typically halfway along the course of the muscle), and the referential electrode (G2) is placed distally over the corresponding tendon—this arrangement allows acquisition of a CMAP.
- The SNAP often has a triphasic waveform with an initial downward (positive) deflection.
- Many different parameters are measured in NCSs, including amplitude, distal latency, and conduction velocity.

- A 20% decrease in CMAP amplitude is consistent with conduction block, and an increase in duration of the CMAP waveform >30% is consistent with temporal dispersion—these findings generally indicate some degree of underlying demyelination occurring between the points of stimulation.
- Indirect measures of the proximal segments of nerve are possible utilizing F waves and the H reflex.
- If the F latency is longer than the F estimate, some proximal slowing of conduction is suggested, which is consistent with an underlying pathophysiologic mechanism of acquired demyelination.

Cranial NCSs

The trigeminal blink reflex is most often performed by stimulating the supraorbital branch of the trigeminal nerve; this yields an afferent response through the V1 component of the trigeminal nerve. The efferent arc of this reflex involves the facial nucleus and facial nerve, and recording is typically performed over the nasalis muscle. When performing a blink reflex, one can identify 2 waveforms: 1) an R1 component occurs on the same side as the stimuli and 2) a later R2 component that can be recorded from both sides of the face.

The blink reflex allows assessment of the trigeminal nerve, its connections within the brainstem, and the facial nerve. In cases of a trigeminal nerve lesion, ipsilaterally the R1 and bilaterally the R2 responses may be abnormal because the afferent pathway is affected. In cases of a facial nerve lesion, the R1 and ipsilateral R2 responses may be abnormal. However, if the contralateral supraorbital nerve (normal trigeminal nerve and normal contralateral facial nerve) is stimulated, then the R1 and R2 responses on the unaffected side will be normal; however, because of connection within the brainstem to the facial nucleus on the affected side, the R2 response on the side of the facial neuropathy will be abnormal. Blink reflexes are also used to assess patients in whom polyradiculoneuropathy is suspected, and results can be abnormal in patients with acute or chronic inflammatory demyelinating polyradiculopathies.

- Blink reflexes are also used to assess patients in whom polyradiculoneuropathy is suspected, and results can be abnormal in patients with acute or chronic inflammatory demyelinating polyradiculopathies.

Repetitive NCSs

Repetitive nerve stimulation is a nerve conduction technique most commonly used to assess the neuromuscular junction in diseases such as myasthenia gravis and Lambert-Eaton myasthenic syndrome. As discussed above, when a motor nerve is stimulated and recording is done over muscle, each supramaximal stimulus should yield a CMAP identical in amplitude and morphologic pattern. Recall that the CMAP is a response recorded over muscle due to stimulation of a motor nerve and therefore reflects not only the integrity of the motor axons but also the neuromuscular junction and the muscle being recorded. In repetitive stimulation, a short train (usually 4–5) of stimuli is given with measurement of the CMAP amplitude after each stimulus.

Normally, each stimulus should yield an identical CMAP with identical amplitude. In disorders of neuromuscular transmission, the CMAP amplitude reduces, or "decrements," with each successive stimulus. After brief exercise (10 seconds) of the muscle being recorded, neuromuscular transmission improves transiently because calcium influx enables calcium-mediated exocytosis of acetylcholine vesicles. This release may repair the decrement, and one may even see an increase, or increment, in the CMAP amplitude after brief exercise (*facilitation* is another term used to describe this phenomenon). The degree of increment can help distinguish a presynaptic disorder from a postsynaptic one.

Each stimulus of the nerve elicits presynaptic release of vesicles containing acetylcholine. The acetylcholine traverses the synaptic space and binds acetylcholine receptors. This process opens sodium channels and leads to an action potential down the muscle fiber. The end plate potential (EPP) is the amplitude recorded at the muscle fiber after the release of vesicles of acetylcholine. Normally, every action potential down a nerve will result in an EPP sufficient enough to elicit an action potential through the muscle. A safety factor built into neuromuscular transmission ensures that this action potential is always elicited, even with some normal variation in the EPP. In a disorder of neuromuscular transmission, however, that safety factor is compromised, and the EPP is not sufficient to elicit an action potential down the muscle fiber, and neuromuscular transmission fails. This failure causes fatiguable weakness. Short trains of repetitive stimulation (typically 4 stimuli at 2–3 Hz) in a normal person will reduce the acetylcholine released and the EPP somewhat, but it will always be above the threshold needed (because of the safety factor). These repetitive stimuli will result in essentially identical CMAP amplitudes. In neuromuscular junction disorders, the EPP at baseline is low. Thus, by reducing the amount of acetylcholine released (which happens with repetitive stimulation), the EPP is reduced even further (sometimes below the threshold), and some action potentials will not be transferred to the muscle fiber. The result is a decrement, or reduction, of the CMAP amplitude. With a short course of exercise (typically 10 seconds), the amount of acetylcholine available for release may increase briefly. This increase will, in the short term, repair the decrement (typically within a few seconds). If repetitive stimulation is repeated a minute or 2 later, the decrement tends to return and be more severe because the stores of acetylcholine have been depleted with that brief exercise. This is postexercise exhaustion, or potentiation (Figure 32.6).

In some cases, there may be not only a repair of decrement but also an increment, or facilitation, of the CMAP amplitude compared with baseline. The degree of facilitation can sometimes be helpful for distinguishing a presynaptic disorder such as Lambert-Eaton myasthenic syndrome from a postsynaptic process such as myasthenia gravis (Figure 32.7). In cases of Lambert-Eaton myasthenic syndrome, facilitation is usually more than 200%.

Abnormal decrement is generally defined as a 10% decrease in CMAP amplitude between the first and last response in a train of 4 stimuli. The maximal relative decrement should always be greatest between the first and second responses. If there is a baseline decrement during repetitive stimulation studies, then brief exercise (10 seconds or brief rapid stimulation at 20–50 Hz if exercise is not possible) is given to look for any repair of the decrement and perhaps increment (facilitation) of the CMAP.

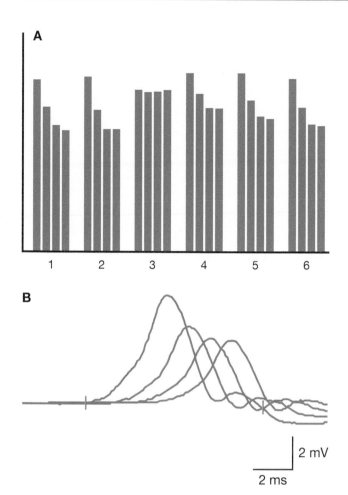

Figure 32.6 Repetitive Stimulation in Myasthenia Gravis.
A, Histogram shows decremental response with 2-Hz
repetitive stimulation with greatest decrement between first
and second responses in the train of 4 responses. Repair of
the decrement occurs with brief exercise (A, bar graph 3); B,
Individual waveforms indicating decremental response is
again observed some time after exercise (corresponding to bar
graph 6 in A).
(Adapted from Mowzoon N. Clinical neurophysiology. Part B: Principles of nerve conduction studies and electromyography [EMG]. In: Mowzoon N, Flemming KD, editors. Neurology board review: an illustrated study guide. Rochester [MN]: Mayo Clinic Scientific Press and Florence [KY]: Informa Healthcare USA; c2007. p. 189–223. Used with permission of Mayo Foundation for Medical Education and Research.)

The train of 4 stimuli is repeated every 30 to 60 seconds for 2 to 5 minutes after exercise to look for a worsening of the decrement (known as exhaustion). The possibility of a technical abnormality giving false-positive results can be lessened, by demonstrating decrement in at least 2 motor nerves before diagnosing a neuromuscular junction disorder. As mentioned above, these findings can be nonspecific and have to be taken in the context of the clinical scenario. In addition, patients who are receiving

acetylcholine esterase inhibitors such as pyridostigmine should have the medication withheld for at least 12 hours before repetitive stimulation studies.

In all NCSs, temperature must be measured. If a patient is too cold, the conduction velocities can be artificially slow, amplitudes can be artificially high, and distal latencies may be artificially prolonged. The result could be a diagnosis of peripheral neuropathy or a distal mononeuropathy (ie, median neuropathy at the wrist) simply due to a technical error. Also, cold temperature may normalize neuromuscular transmission in milder cases of myasthenia gravis, falsely normalizing the results of repetitive nerve conduction studies.

- Repetitive nerve stimulation is a nerve conduction technique most commonly used to assess the neuromuscular junction in diseases such as myasthenia gravis and Lambert-Eaton myasthenic syndrome.
- In some cases, there may be not only a repair of decrement but also an increment, or facilitation, of the CMAP amplitude compared with baseline.
- The degree of facilitation can sometimes be helpful for distinguishing a presynaptic disorder such as Lambert-Eaton myasthenic syndrome from a postsynaptic process such as myasthenia gravis.

Needle EMG

Spontaneous Activity

Needle EMG assesses electrical activity with the muscle fibers themselves. This technique is typically performed on an awake patient who can both relax a muscle and voluntarily contract it with mild force because the needle study includes analysis of electrical activity with the muscle at rest and assessment with mild levels of voluntary contraction.

Spontaneous activity is assessed with the muscle at rest. A needle is inserted through the skin into the muscle, and spontaneous activity is assessed with no movement of the needle in several areas of the muscle. Insertional activity occurs with each movement of the needle. Fibrillation potentials indicate denervation of individual muscle fibers. These are regular, rhythmic discharges of muscle fibers and can only be heard or seen with EMG. They are not visible clinically. Positive sharp waves have a pathophysiologic meaning similar to that of fibrillation potentials but have a different morphologic pattern in that they have a downward (positive) deflection rather than upward (negative) deflection. Fibrillation potentials or positive sharp waves can be seen as early as 2 weeks after injury to a nerve and almost always by 21 days. With reinnervation of muscle, fibrillation potentials may decrease or resolve. Fibrillation potentials can be found in any neurogenic

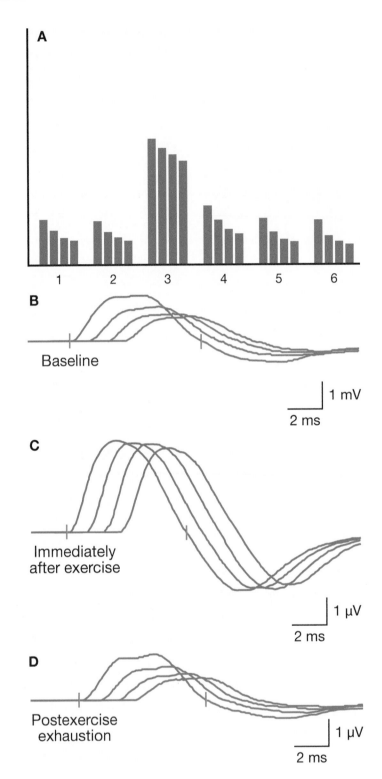

Figure 32.7 *Repetitive Stimulation in Lambert-Eaton Myasthenic Syndrome.*
A, Histogram shows facilitation of amplitudes after brief exercise (bar graph 3). B, Baseline repetitive stimulation at 2 Hz demonstrates a decremental response, as in myasthenia gravis. C, Facilitation (increment) of the amplitude of compound muscle action potential with brief exercise, as demonstrated in A, graph 3. D, This facilitation usually resolves by 60 to 120 seconds after exercise.
(Adapted from Mowzoon N. Clinical neurophysiology. Part B: Principles of nerve conduction studies and electromyography [EMG]. In: Mowzoon N, Flemming KD, editors. Neurology board review: an illustrated study guide. Rochester [MN]: Mayo Clinic Scientific Press and Florence [KY]: Informa Healthcare USA; c2007. p. 189–223. Used with permission of Mayo Foundation for Medical Education and Research.)

process. When found in muscle disorders, they correlate with the pathologic findings of muscle fiber necrosis, vacuolization, or muscle fiber splitting.

Fasciculation potentials are irregular discharges of motor units (one anterior horn cell and all the muscle fibers it innervates); as a result, they are larger than fibrillation potentials and can be seen clinically under the skin. Unlike fibrillation potentials, which are indicative of a pathologic process, fasciculations can be seen in normal persons but are also seen as part of disorders involving anterior horn cells, motor roots, or motor nerves. Fasciculations are not seen in neuromuscular junction disorders or muscle diseases.

Myotonic discharges are another spontaneous discharge characterized by waxing and waning frequency and amplitude with a typical dive-bomber sound. They are noted in various disorders affecting muscle, including several channelopathies. Myotonic discharges are not typically seen with the naked eye. Patients who have electrical myotonia may not always have clinical myotonia.

Myokymic potentials are most commonly due to radiation damage to nerves. These are regularly occurring bursts of motor units that fire spontaneously, giving rise to a marching-soldiers sound. They are not usually visible to the naked eye. They are occasionally found in demyelinating neuropathies and in mononeuropathies. When occurring in the face, they are often associated with brainstem disorders such as multiple sclerosis or glioma.

Neuromyotonic discharges are very fast spontaneous discharges of muscle fibers. These have a typical Indy-car sound. These can be associated with hyperexcitable nerve disorders such as Isaacs syndrome or Morvan syndrome.

Voluntary Activation

Voluntary motor units are assessed during muscle contraction. Several parameters are assessed, the most important of which is the motor unit potential duration. The morphologic pattern of the waveform is also analyzed for polyphasia or complexity. Recruitment of motor unit potentials is also an important component to the examination and refers to the number of motor unit potentials firing at a given force. As a muscle is contracted more forcefully, more and more motor units are recruited to supply the force needed. In a neurogenic process, a reduced number of motor units are available. Despite stronger force of contraction, fewer motor units are present to supply that force, and reduced recruitment occurs (ie, an inappropriately small number of motor unit potentials fire at inappropriately high frequencies). In myopathic disorders, because the motor units themselves are

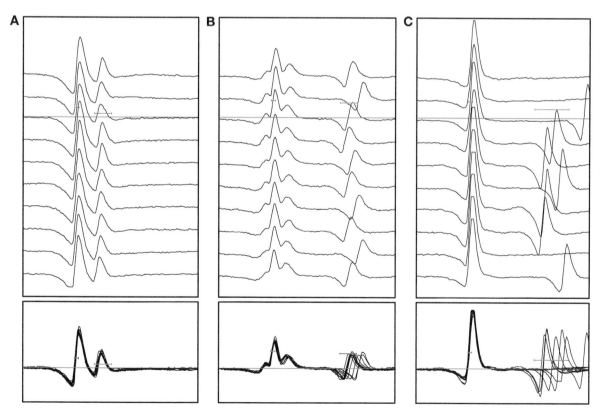

Figure 32.8 Single-Fiber Electromyographic Recordings.
A, Normal recording. B, Increased jitter with no blocking. C, Increased jitter with blocking.
(Courtesy of W. Neath Folger, MD, Mayo Clinic, Rochester, Minnesota. Used with permission.)

smaller from loss of muscle fibers, more motor units need to be recruited more quickly to supply the same level of force, and rapid recruitment occurs.

In neurogenic disorders, the typical EMG pattern includes fibrillation potentials, fasciculation potentials, and large, occasionally complex, motor units firing with reduced recruitment. In myopathic disorders, the pattern is fibrillation potentials (but not fasciculation potentials) and small, often complex, motor units firing with rapid recruitment.

An additional technique known as single-fiber EMG allows assessment of the variability in neuromuscular transmission recorded at the level of a single muscle fiber. Routine EMG, as described above, records from the 10 to 20 muscle fibers of a given motor unit that are closest to the recording needle. Single-fiber EMG is the most sensitive electrophysiologic test to assess the neuromuscular junction, and results can be abnormal in patients with normal repetitive nerve stimulation. Single-fiber EMG allows assessment of jitter, which is the variability in neuromuscular transmission at a single muscle fiber level. In some cases, there is failure of the neuromuscular transmission, which leads to blocking of muscle fiber action potentials (Figure 32.8). Abnormally prolonged jitter or blocking indicates abnormal neuromuscular transmission. As is the case with repetitive nerve stimulation, abnormal results of single-fiber EMG are nonspecific. Findings are typically abnormal in myasthenia gravis or Lambert-Eaton myasthenia syndrome, and they can also be abnormal in other disorders of the nerve or muscle in which there may be immaturity at the nerve terminal.

- Fibrillation potentials indicate denervation of individual muscle fibers.
- Fibrillation potentials or positive sharp waves can be seen as early as 2 weeks after injury to a nerve and almost always by 21 days.

- Fasciculation potentials are irregular discharges of motor units.
- In neurogenic disorders, the typical EMG pattern includes fibrillation potentials, fasciculation potentials, and large, occasionally complex, motor units firing with reduced recruitment. In myopathic disorders, the pattern is fibrillation potentials (but not fasciculation potentials) and small, often complex, motor units firing with rapid recruitment.

Evolution and Timing of EMG Abnormalities

After an initial nerve injury, immediate reduced recruitment of motor units will be seen on needle EMG given the loss of action potentials firing down the nerve. Fibrillation potentials appear in about 2 weeks, and voluntary motor unit prolongation may take 1 to 2 months to start appearing. On NCSs, conduction block can be identified by stimulating above and below the site of the injury. Acutely (within 10 days), identifying conduction block with NCS identifies *where* a lesion is but will not identify the pathophysiologic process. In a focal process that affects axons (axonotmesis), there will be wallerian degeneration, and repeat NCSs 2 to 4 weeks later will yield low-amplitude CMAPs stimulating at both proximal and distal sites. In this case, localization will not be possible, but pathophysiologic findings would be consistent with an axonal lesion. Needle EMG would show fibrillation potentials and reduced numbers of large motor units. However, with a focal demyelinating process (neurapraxia), a focal conduction block will continue to be seen when stimulating both proximal and distal to the lesion at 2 to 4 weeks. The EMG will again show reduced recruitment; however, fibrillation potentials and increased duration of motor units may be absent or very mild.

Cerebrospinal Fluid

RUPLE S. LAUGHLIN, MD

Introduction

The total volume of cerebrospinal fluid (CSF) within ventricles and subarachnoid space is about 150 mL. The absorption of CSF is directly linked to intracranial pressure. In steady states, the rate of CSF absorption equals CSF formation, where the normal resting pressure of CSF is typically between 150 and 180 mm H_2O and ranges of normal vary from 65 to 200 mm H_2O (5–15 mm Hg). The major cause of error in measurement of CSF pressure is failure to position the patient properly (correct is lateral decubitus, where the right atrium pressure then can serve as the reference 0). This chapter focuses on the utility of spinal fluid evaluation and on the aspects of CSF evaluation that are useful clinically. The anatomy and physiologic aspects of the ventricles and spinal fluid are discussed in Volume 1, Chapter 2, "Meninges and Ventricles."

- The normal resting pressure of CSF is typically between 150 and 180 mm H_2O.

Clinical Examination of the CSF

Lumbar Puncture

The most common method used to obtain and analyze CSF is lumbar puncture (LP). LP should be performed only after careful review of the indications and contraindications because it is an invasive procedure; fortunately, however, the frequency of serious complications is low. For example, LP is clearly indicated if meningitis is suspected and in some cases when subarachnoid hemorrhage is suspected. For other, less precise clinical circumstances (eg, fluctuating encephalopathy), alternative causes (eg, drugs, metabolic compromise) should first be excluded.

The most serious outcome of LP to be considered is aggravating a potential herniation syndrome. A comprehensive neurologic examination needs to be performed to exclude signs of increased cranial pressure due to a mass lesion (eg, papilledema).

A post-LP headache is the most common complication of LP. This occurs in 15% to 25% of patients and has a very characteristic postural component (onset when upright and improvement or resolution when supine). If it occurs, it usually does so 24 to 48 hours after LP. In most cases (85%), supportive management in the form of fluids, simple analgesics such as caffeine, and rest is all that is needed. In a small percentage of cases, more aggressive measures such as intravenous caffeine or autologous epidural blood patch may be required. Studies have supported that the modifiable factor most influencing the development of a post-LP headache is needle gauge (the larger the needle, the larger the dural puncture); no studies show any relationship with the volume of fluid removed or a benefit of supine rest after LP.

CSF Composition

CSF should be clear and colorless. In most instances, 4 main CSF variables are examined: glucose level (relative to serum glucose), quantity and type of red and white blood cells, CSF protein level, and the opening CSF pressure.

Abnormalities in one or more of these variables may provide clues to the underlying process and thus narrow the differential diagnosis and work-up. In cases of suspected bacterial meningitis, lifesaving antibiotic treatment should always be initiated immediately, even if there is a delay to LP.

Abbreviations: CSF, cerebrospinal fluid; Ig, immunoglobulin; LP, lumbar puncture

Table 33.1 • Patterns of Cerebrospinal Fluid Abnormalities in Infection Disorders of the Central Nervous System

Pattern	Protein, mg/dL	Glucose, % of Serum Glucose	WBC, cells/mm³	Cell Type
Normal	15–45	>40%	<5	Lymphocytes
Bacterial	>100	<40%	>500	PMNs
Viral	<120	>40%	10–500	Lymphocytes
Granulomatous	>50	<40%	10–1,000	Lymphocytes

Abbreviations: PMNs, polymorphonuclear leukocytes; WBC, white blood cells.

Patterns of CSF abnormalities are often helpful for distinguishing various infections from one another and from other central nervous system inflammatory or neoplastic disorders (Table 33.1).

CSF Glucose

The CSF glucose value should be no less than 40% of the serum level, and an absolute CSF glucose level less than 40 mg/dL is suspicious for an infectious or other inflammatory process (Table 33.1). The CSF glucose value is difficult to interpret in patients with diabetes because of wide swings in serum levels and the latency for equilibration at high levels of serum glucose. A CSF to serum ratio of glucose less than 30% should be considered abnormal in patients with diabetes. Ideally, the serum glucose value should be measured *1 hour before* LP to account for CSF glucose equilibration; however, this schedule is at times logistically challenging to coordinate.

A low glucose value in the CSF (hypoglycorrhachia) may be indicative of central nervous system infection, inflammation, or other meningeal reactive processes. A low spinal fluid glucose value in bacterial meningitis is currently thought to mainly result from the shutdown of the glucose transporter system. Leukocyte utilization contributes to a lesser extent, but bacterial consumption does not contribute. The differential diagnosis of a low CSF glucose value is outlined in Box 33.1.

CSF Cell Count

The quality and quantity of cellular reaction in the CSF are important with regard to the causative agent. In healthy patients, the CSF should be essentially acellular (<5 cells). Acute bacterial meningitis produces a polymorphonuclear leukocyte response, usually more than 1,000 cells/mm³. Viral meningoencephalitis produces a polymorphonuclear leukocyte response early, which converts to a lymphocytic response, but the cell count uncommonly exceeds 1,000 white blood cells/mm³. Lymphocytic reactions associated with a low glucose value imply tuberculous or fungal meningitis, occasionally viral meningoencephalitis (see above) or some other noninfectious inflammatory mechanism. An eosinophilic meningeal reaction implies a parasitic or fungal infection, but it has been found in other noninfectious conditions, including hypereosinophilic syndrome, Wegener granulomatosis, Hodgkin disease, and glioblastoma invading meninges.

Blood (red blood cells) may also spill into the CSF. This finding may be iatrogenic (due to the LP itself) or pathologic (subarachnoid or intraventricular hemorrhage). Xanthochromia (yellow color) refers to the color of CSF after bleeding; it can be due to oxyhemoglobin (4–6 hours after bleeding) or bilirubin (2 days after bleeding).

CSF Protein

Because of the large gradient between serum and CSF protein concentration, the degree of CSF protein increase reflects the degree of impairment of the blood-brain barrier. Froin syndrome refers to CSF with a very high protein value and xanthochromia, resulting in spinal fluid that coagulates spontaneously. Usually, Froin syndrome is due to loculation of the CSF in portions of the subarachnoid space, where spinal fluid circulation is compromised by an inflammatory or neoplastic obstruction. The clotting of the

---

Box 33.1 • Causes of a Low Cerebrospinal Fluid Glucose Value

Infections

    Acute bacterial meningitis

    Chronic granulomatous meningitis (TB, fungal, parasitic)

    Some viral meningitides and encephalitides (rarely) (mumps, lymphocytic choriomeningitis, herpes simplex encephalitis, chronic echovirus, and CMV polyradiculopathy associated with AIDS)

Noninfectious inflammatory conditions

    Meningeal lymphomatosis or carcinomatosis

    Meningeal gliomatosis

    Sarcoidosis

    Chemical meningitis (after dermoid or craniopharyngioma leak, post-intrathecal)

    Subarachnoid hemorrhage

Abbreviations: CMV, cytomegalovirus; TB, tuberculous.

> **Box 33.2 • Causes of a Very Increased Cerebrospinal Fluid Protein Value (>500 mg/dL)**
>
> Tuberculous meningitis
> Spinal block
> Subarachnoid hemorrhage
> Inflammatory polyneuropathy
> Meningeal involvement by a malignancy

CSF is due to leakage of fibrinogen and other clotting factors from the serum. Some causes of very increased CSF protein values are listed in Box 33.2.

- The most serious outcome of LP to be considered is aggravating a potential herniation syndrome.
- Patterns of CSF abnormalities are often helpful for distinguishing various infections from one another and from other central nervous system inflammatory or neoplastic disorders.
- A low glucose value in the CSF (hypoglycorrhachia) may be indicative of central nervous system infection, inflammation, or other meningeal reactive processes.
- In healthy patients, the CSF should be essentially acellular (<5 cells).
- Xanthochromia (yellow color) refers to the color of CSF after bleeding; it can be due to oxyhemoglobin (4–6 hours after bleeding) or bilirubin (2 days after bleeding).
- Froin syndrome refers to CSF with a very high protein value and xanthochromia, resulting in spinal fluid that coagulates spontaneously.
- Usually, Froin syndrome is due to loculation of the CSF in portions of the subarachnoid space, where spinal fluid circulation is compromised by an inflammatory or neoplastic obstruction.

CSF in Special Cases

Ventricular Fluid

CSF obtained directly from ventricles always has a *higher* glucose value than CSF from the lumbar sac (even when infection is present). The CSF protein value is normally *lower* in the ventricles than in the lumbar sac.

CSF in Central Nervous System Demyelinating Diseases

Another variable that can be assessed in CSF is the CSF immunoglobulin G (IgG) index:

$$\frac{\text{CSF IgG/serum IgG}}{\text{CSF albumin/serum albumin}} = \text{CSF IgG index}$$

The IgG index is increased in a large proportion of patients with multiple sclerosis and often is the earliest abnormality for multiple sclerosis in CSF.

In demyelinating diseases, opening pressure is normal, and usually the white blood cell count is less than 20 cells/dL. The protein value may be mildly increased, and the myelin basic protein value is often increased in the first 2 weeks after exacerbations (but also can be increased in acute infections, meningitis, encephalitis, or even neurosarcoidosis). Oligoclonal bands are increased in more than 90% of patients with multiple sclerosis, but they are usually normal in neuromyelitis optica and acute disseminated encephalomyelitis. Thus, it may be useful to distinguish these demyelinating disorders in addition to the clinical presentation.

CSF in Inflammatory Polyradiculopathies

The hallmark CSF finding in inflammatory polyradiculopathy (acute inflammatory demyelinating polyradiculoneuropathy, Guillain-Barré syndrome) and chronic inflammatory demyelinating polyradiculopathy is "cytoalbuminologic disassociation," which reflects an increased CSF protein value in the setting of a normal CSF white blood cell count. A small percentage of patients with this type of illness may have more than 10 white blood cells in the CSF, and in these cases it is important to exclude other conditions (eg, Lyme disease, human immunodeficiency virus). Not all patients with acute inflammatory demyelinating polyradiculoneuropathy or chronic inflammatory demyelinating polyradiculopathy have this finding; the CSF protein value can be normal in up to 10% of patients with an inflammatory demyelinating polyradiculoneuropathy.

- CSF obtained directly from ventricles always has a *higher* glucose value than CSF from the lumbar sac.
- Oligoclonal bands are increased in more than 90% of patients with multiple sclerosis, but they are usually normal in neuromyelitis optica and acute disseminated encephalomyelitis.
- The hallmark CSF finding in inflammatory polyradiculopathy (acute inflammatory demyelinating polyradiculoneuropathy, Guillain-Barré syndrome) and chronic inflammatory demyelinating polyradiculopathy is "cytoalbuminologic disassociation."

Evoked Potentials

JAMES C. WATSON, MD

Introduction

Evoked potentials provide a noninvasive, sensitive, and quantitative way to assess the functional integrity of the somatosensory, auditory, and visual pathways. The basic principle of evoked potentials is to apply a stimulus (sensory, auditory, or visual) in a controlled manner to create a volley of depolarization and repolarization. This stimulus volley ascends through the peripheral and central sensory, auditory, or visual pathways and can be recorded as the signals pass underneath recording electrodes. The generated evoked potential waveforms represent a transmitting volley of signals and not synaptic activity at a sensory nucleus or at the cortex. The role of somatosensory and brainstem auditory evoked potentials in the outpatient setting has declined in the past decades with the improved quality and availability of neuroimaging; however, their use has had a resurgence in electrophysiologic monitoring of surgical cases of the spine and posterior fossa, for which they are now a part of the standard of care.

- Evoked potentials provide a noninvasive, sensitive, and quantitative way to assess the functional integrity of the somatosensory, auditory, and visual pathways.

Somatosensory Evoked Potentials

Somatosensory evoked potentials (SSEPs) assess the functional integrity of the peripheral and central components of the proprioceptive (posterior column, medial-lemniscal) sensory pathways. SSEPs are a short-latency response recorded 30 to 50 milliseconds after nonpainful stimulation of a mixed sensorimotor nerve in the periphery (most commonly the tibial, median, or ulnar nerve). Although any body region can be stimulated (peripheral nerve or dermatomal segment of interest), the signal and waveforms generated are much lower in amplitude than with mixed nerve stimulation and often do not have well-defined normal values, relying instead on side-to-side comparison. Protocols that use painful stimuli are used to assess more slowly conducting pain (spinothalamic tract) pathways; however, these longer latency protocols are not a routine part of most outpatient and surgical monitoring programs.

The term *somatosensory* is partly a misnomer. Although the stimulation settings are intended to primarily bring A-beta somatosensory fibers to threshold and subsequently initiate an ascending signal volley, other axons within the mixed nerve being stimulated may reach threshold and contribute to this response. These contributors include retrograde transmission through activated motor axons whose contribution to the volley is limited by using a stimulus just adequate to initiate a motor twitch, but not to the supramaximal stimulation level used in motor nerve conduction studies. Additionally, given that there is a mild motor twitch with stimulation, the associated muscle contraction causes firing of gamma motor neurons associated with the muscle spindle, which contributes a very small amount to the ascending volley. As such, the ascending signal is primarily somatosensory, although not purely so.

The location of a lesion is more important for causing an SSEP abnormality than its size, its etiology, or the severity of associated neurologic deficits. For example, although a patient with an anterior cord syndrome is neurologically devastated (paraplegia and spinothalamic-tract sensory deficits) below the affected cord level, the posterior columns and therefore SSEPs are relatively preserved. Conversely, a patient with a small demyelinating plaque or B_{12} deficiency preferentially affecting the posterior

---

Abbreviations: BAER, brainstem auditory evoked response; SSEP, somatosensory evoked potential; VEP, visual evoked potential

columns may have more limited clinical findings yet have considerable SSEP abnormalities.

The use of SSEPs has expanded for spinal surgical monitoring and for prognosticating in cases of postanoxic coma. Despite the advances in neuroimaging, SSEPs are still useful in the outpatient setting to assess for functional impairment (or preservation) of the proprioceptive pathways in cases of known central nervous system structural (intrinsic or extrinsic) abnormality (spinal stenosis or tumor) and to provide objective identification and localization of abnormalities in imaging-negative myelopathies.

General Technical Considerations

SSEPs are low-amplitude responses that require several hundred averaged stimuli to cancel out the random background noise. Two tracings are recorded, and waveforms should be completely reproducible before marking. If the 2 averaged waveforms do not superimpose, the tracing should not be marked or interpreted. Artifact of 60 Hz is eliminated by using a stimulus rate that is a nonintegral multiple of 60. The effects of spasticity may be limited by using a slower stimulus frequency of 1 to 5 Hz.

Although unilateral stimulation is preferred for localization given the well-defined sensory pathways, if central responses are recordable from only a single site, no conclusions can be made as to whether an abnormality is related to a peripheral or central nervous system process. This situation most commonly occurs with unilateral tibial stimulation and can often be overcome with bilateral stimulation. If the bilateral tibial nerves are stimulated simultaneously, presuming nothing is affecting peripheral conduction asymmetrically, the stimulation should reach the conus from each side simultaneously. This approach summates the signal and increases the likelihood of generating a recordable potential. If 2 responses can be recorded over the central nervous system, then some conclusion can be made as to central conduction time and the functional integrity of central proprioceptive pathways.

Recording Sites and Waveforms

The SSEP responses are named on the basis of whether they are a negative (N) or positive (P) waveform; this designation is followed by a number that refers to the average time in milliseconds that the response occurs after the stimulus (Table 34.1). A negative waveform is defined as one in which the G1 electrode records a negative charge relative to the G2 electrode, and by convention the waveform is demonstrated with an upward deflection from baseline. A positive waveform is defined as one in which the G1 electrode is positive relative to the charge recorded at the G2 electrode, and by convention the waveform is demonstrated with a downward deflection from baseline.

Defining Abnormalities on SSEPs

By recording the ascending sensory volley at various points of the peripheral and central proprioceptive pathways (Table 34.1), the absolute latencies of the responses and conduction time between responses (interpeak latencies) can be compared with those of age-matched normals and used to localize a lesion. For example, if a median SSEP showed a normal brachial plexus/Erb's point N9 and cervical spine N13 absolute latency with a prolonged scalp N20 absolute and N13 to N20 (cervical to scalp) interpeak latency, the functionally impairing lesion could be localized between the cervical spine and contralateral somatosensory cortex.

If all of the absolute latencies of central waveforms are prolonged (indicating slowing of the signal volley reaching the central proprioceptive pathways) but the interpeak latencies are normal (indicating normal central conduction times), this finding could be explained by a peripheral nervous system disorder, a cold limb, or a very long limb in a tall patient. These 3 situations should be easily distinguishable clinically.

In combination with routine sensory nerve conduction studies, evidence of peripheral slowing can be further localized. Normal results of sensory nerve conduction studies indicate that the sensory nerve pathways are normal proximally to the level of the dorsal root ganglion. If a

Table 34.1 • Median and Tibial Somatosensory Evoked Potential Waveforms

Response	Recording Electrode Location	Potential Generator
Median		
N5	Median nerve in antecubital fossa	SNAP—indicates whether stimulus is adequate or there is peripheral slowing
N9	Erb's point	Brachial plexus volley
N13	Cervical spine (C7)	Cervical cord projections
N20	Scalp	Thalamocortical projections
Tibial		
N8	Tibial nerve in popliteal fossa	SNAP—indicates whether stimulus is adequate or there is peripheral slowing
N22	Lumbar spine (L1) overlying conus	Spinal cord dorsal horn projections
N30	Cervical spine (C7)	Cervical cord projections; often absent in normal populations
P38	Scalp	Thalamocortical projections

Abbreviation: SNAP, sensory nerve action potential.

patient with clinically significant peripheral-appearing sensory deficits (areflexia) had preserved sensory nerve conduction studies but prolonged absolute tibial SSEP central responses (N22, N30, and P38) with normal inter-peak latencies (normal central conduction time), then the sensory process could be localized to the sensory rootlet because the lesion must be between the dorsal root ganglion (normal sensory nerve conduction studies) and the conus (waveform generator for N22). This pattern is found in chronic inflammatory sensory polyradiculopathy, an isolated sensory rootlet variant of chronic inflammatory demyelinating polyradiculoneuropathy.

A limitation of SSEPs is that they can localize slowing over only a large segment (eg, between the cervical spine and scalp), which may not seem discriminating. However, when other data have shown a potential cause for a patient's symptoms (eg, cervical stenosis) but questions remain about the pertinence of that finding to the symptoms (eg, unsteadiness), the SSEP may be able to provide objective evidence of functional impairment of the proprioceptive pathway (slowing in the lumbar-to-cervical interpeak potential) that can be correlated with the ancillary testing to make more specific clinical conclusions.

SSEPs in Postanoxic Coma

SSEPs are less influenced by drugs and metabolic derangements than are electroencephalograms and have been validated to be useful for determining the prognosis for patients in postanoxic coma. When the bilateral median SSEP scalp responses are absent in the setting of preserved Erb's point (N9) and cervical spine (N13) responses, meta-analyses have shown that this finding invariably predicts a dire prognosis (death or persistent vegetative state) when the SSEP is performed at any point 1 day after the anoxic event (Figure 34.1). Meta-analyses have shown a false positive rate of only 0.7%. Notably, the converse is not true; a preserved median SSEP response has no positive predictive value for a good clinical outcome. If a postanoxic coma persists, it may be worthwhile to repeat the median SSEPs, because loss of the bilateral scalp responses (even if present on an earlier study) has the same grave prognostic value as if it was absent from the beginning.

With increasing use of induced hypothermia in patients who are comatose after cardiac arrest, there has been some question as to whether the hypothermia affects the specificity of absent median SSEP scalp responses. Most, but not all, studies have suggested that it does not have an effect on the predictive value of an absent response. However, delaying examinations (SSEP and clinical) until after rewarming is recommended (some authors suggest waiting at least 72 hours after rewarming).

- The use of SSEPs has expanded for spinal surgical monitoring and for prognosticating in cases of postanoxic coma.

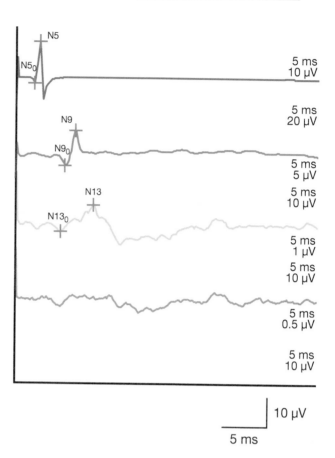

Figure 34.1 Median Somatosensory Evoked Potential.
Patient was in postanoxic coma. All responses are well-defined, except for a scalp response that is absent. In the setting of postanoxic coma, this finding is highly specific for a dire prognosis (death or persistent vegetative state).
(Adapted from Mowzoon N. Clinical neurophysiology. Part B: Principles of nerve conduction studies and electromyography [EMG]. In: Mowzoon N, Flemming KD, editors. Neurology board review: an illustrated study guide. Rochester [MN]: Mayo Clinic Scientific Press and Florence [KY]: Informa Healthcare USA; c2007. p. 189–223. Used with permission of Mayo Foundation for Medical Education and Research.)

- Despite the advances in neuroimaging, SSEPs are still useful in the outpatient setting to assess for functional impairment (or preservation) of the proprioceptive pathways in cases of known central nervous system structural (intrinsic or extrinsic) abnormality (spinal stenosis or tumor) and to provide objective identification and localization of abnormalities in imaging-negative myelopathies.
- By recording the ascending sensory volley at various points of the peripheral and central proprioceptive pathways (Table 34.1), the absolute latencies of the responses and conduction time between responses (interpeak latencies) can be compared with those of age-matched normals and used to localize a lesion.

- When the bilateral median SSEP scalp responses are absent in the setting of preserved Erb's point (N9) and cervical spine (N13) responses, meta-analyses have shown that this finding invariably predicts a dire prognosis (death or persistent vegetative state) when the SSEP is performed at any point 1 day after the anoxic event (Figure 34.1).
- With increasing use of induced hypothermia in patients who are comatose after cardiac arrest, there has been some question as to whether the hypothermia affects the specificity of absent median SSEP scalp responses.

Brainstem Auditory Evoked Potentials

Brainstem auditory evoked responses (BAERs) are also known by several other names, such as brainstem auditory evoked potentials or auditory evoked responses or potentials. BAERs are used as a functional assessment of central auditory pathways to objectively confirm brainstem dysfunction if clinical signs are equivocal or to screen for brainstem dysfunction with symptoms that are more commonly presumed to be peripheral (vertigo, dizziness, diplopia, or hearing loss). In the past, they were used to assess for functional evidence of subclinical brainstem disease as another site of nervous system involvement in the evaluation of possible multiple sclerosis; neuroimaging has now replaced this indication. They have also been used for screening or following cerebellopontine angle tumors (acoustic neuroma). However, they are primarily used today for monitoring during posterior fossa surgery.

In BAER studies, stimulation consists of auditory clicks generated by moving a diaphragm in a headphone or earplug stimulator toward (condensation) or away (rarefaction) from the eardrum. Rarefaction stimulation is more commonly used and is reported to have a slightly higher sensitivity and lower variability. However, if it is inadequate to generate well-formed waveforms, condensation or alternating rarefaction and condensation stimulation should be attempted. Some authors do not believe that rarefaction is superior to condensation, but normal values may differ between stimulation types and should be determined with each individual method. One ear is stimulated at a time while masking the other ear with white noise. Stimulation is performed at 60 to 70 dB above the hearing threshold (the sensory level). Recording electrodes are placed on the ears or mastoid processes and are referenced to Cz in the International 10–20 System for electroencephalography.

Five reproducible waveforms are elicited (Figure 34.2 and Table 34.2). Abnormalities are defined by looking at absolute and interpeak latencies to determine between which 2 waveform generators the dysfunction occurs. For example, in a severe case of acoustic neuroma, wave

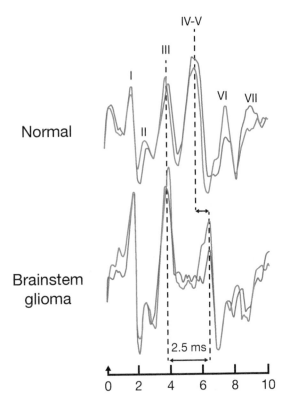

Figure 34.2 Brainstem Auditory Evoked Responses.
Top, Normal subject. Bottom, Patient with brainstem glioma. In bottom tracing, note a prolonged III-V interpeak latency (dashed lines), indicative of abnormal central auditory pathways.
(From Carter JL. Brain stem auditory evoked potentials in central disorders. In: Daube JR, Rubin DI, editors. Clinical neurophysiology. 3rd ed. New York [NY]: Oxford University Press; c2009. p. 281–93. Used with permission of Mayo Foundation for Medical Education and Research.)

I could be affected or absent without any central responses; in a milder case, wave I could be defined and normal with prolonged central waveform absolute latencies or a prolonged wave I-III interpeak latency. In a case of a demyelinating plaque in the rostral pons, waves I, II, and III may show normal absolute latencies, whereas waves IV and V have prolonged absolute latencies and the wave III-V and I-V interpeak latencies are prolonged. As with other evoked potentials, amplitudes are more variable than latencies and therefore less useful.

- BAERs are used as a functional assessment of central auditory pathways to objectively confirm brainstem dysfunction if clinical signs are equivocal or to screen for brainstem dysfunction with symptoms that are more commonly presumed to be peripheral (vertigo, dizziness, diplopia, or hearing loss).
- Five reproducible waveforms are elicited in BAERs (Figure 34.2 and Table 34.2).

Table 34.2 • Brainstem Auditory Evoked
Responses: Waveform Generators

Wave	Potential Generator
I	Cranial nerve VIII
II	Cochlear nucleus (medulla) and proximal cranial nerve VIII
III	Superior olivary nucleus (pons)
IV	Lateral lemniscus
V	Inferior colliculus (midbrain)
VI[a]	Medial geniculate body
VII[a]	Thalamocortical projections

[a] Waves VI and VII are less consistently defined than waves I through V. Routine analysis of brainstem auditory evoked responses is usually limited to wave I-V absolute and interpeak latencies.

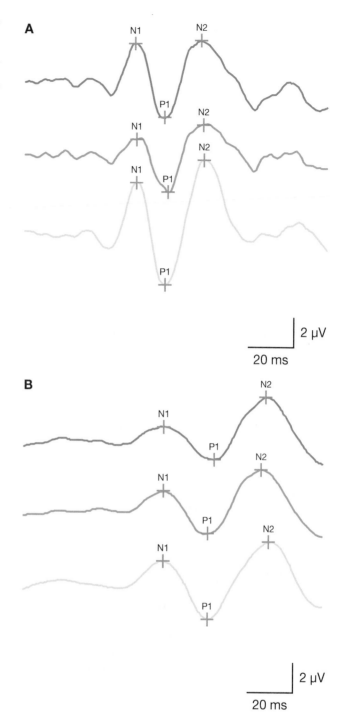

Visual Evoked Potentials

Visual evoked potentials (VEPs) are still commonly used in the work-up of suspected multiple sclerosis or neuromyelitis optica because they are sensitive to lesions of the optic nerve anterior to the optic chiasm and often remain abnormal for years after clinical resolution of symptoms of optic neuritis. Although there are stimulation techniques that allow for localization of postchiasmatic abnormalities in the visual pathways, these techniques are technically challenging, and neuroimaging has supplanted the need to perform postchiasmatic studies.

VEPs are most commonly performed with a reversing checkerboard pattern that does not change in luminance. This visual stimulation is provided to one eye at a time to ensure that the eye stays fixated on the stimulus. If VEPs fail to produce reproducible waveforms, they should be repeated with a larger check size and encouragement of the patient to visually fixate on the stimulus. If the patient is not fixating (due to volitional or cognitive impairment) or physically cannot fixate (due to esophoria, exophoria, or very poor visual acuity), then the waveforms cannot be interpreted.

Visual acuity affects VEPs only if it is severely impaired (worse than 20/200). Visual acuity should be checked before performing VEPs. During VEPs, patients should wear their glasses or contact lenses. VEPs require adequate luminance, which may be impaired if there is severe pupillary miosis (such as in patients taking opioids). Pupil dilation adversely affects visual acuity, however, and should not be performed. Males and older patients have longer normal P100 latencies than women or younger patients.

Recording electrodes are placed over Oz and referenced to Cz (in the International 10–20 System) or the ear. The VEP waveform is generated by the traveling wave of signal

Figure 34.3 Visual Evoked Potentials.
The patient had right optic neuritis due to multiple sclerosis.
A, Recording from the left eye is normal. B, Recording from the right eye shows a prolonged P1 latency.
(Adapted from Mowzoon N. Clinical neurophysiology. Part B: Principles of nerve conduction studies and electromyography [EMG]. In: Mowzoon N, Flemming KD, editors. Neurology board review: an illustrated study guide. Rochester [MN]: Mayo Clinic Scientific Press and Florence [KY]: Informa Healthcare USA; c2007. p. 189–223. Used with permission of Mayo Foundation for Medical Education and Research.)

in the geniculocalcarine projections between the lateral geniculate body and the visual cortex. It is a large, positively oriented waveform (downward deflection from baseline because the G1 electrode is positively charged relative to the G2 electrode) and occurs usually 100 milliseconds after the stimulus. This waveform is therefore referred to as the P100 waveform (Figure 34.3).

The nerve fibers innervating the nasal field of the retina pass through the optic nerve and then cross over through the optic chiasm and then back to the visual cortex on the contralateral side, and those innervating the temporal field of the retina pass through the optic nerve but remain ipsilateral as they pass posteriorly to the visual cortex. Therefore, when one eye (both the nasal and temporal retinal fields) is stimulated, the activated visual pathways include the optic nerve on the stimulated side and the bilateral visual pathways behind the optic chiasm. Performing the VEP on the opposite eye is therefore redundant in assessing postchiasmatic visual pathways, and an abnormal VEP localizes to the side of stimulation anterior to the optic chiasm. If both eyes show prolonged P100 latencies, the process causing the problem cannot be further localized. The exception is when both sides are prolonged but one side is disproportionately prolonged (>10 milliseconds) compared with the other, in which case at least part of the problem can be interpreted as occurring in the optic nerve anterior to the optic chiasm on the longer side.

No substantial visual stimulation is propagated in patients with ocular blindness, and no definable P100 waveform would be anticipated in them. In the rare case of cortical blindness, however, the visual stimulation is propagated through the visual pathways and a waveform is generated from the geniculocalcarine projections coming into the visual cortex. Because the P100 waveform is not generated from synaptic activity in the affected visual cortex, but instead represents the traveling wave coming to it, P100 responses may be preserved and normal in cortical blindness.

- Visual evoked potentials (VEPs) are still commonly used in the work-up of suspected multiple sclerosis or neuromyelitis optica because they are sensitive to lesions of the optic nerve anterior to the optic chiasm and often remain abnormal for years after clinical resolution of symptoms of optic neuritis.
- Visual acuity affects VEPs only if it is severely impaired (worse than 20/200).
- The VEP waveform is referred to as the P100 waveform.
- No substantial visual stimulation is propagated in patients with ocular blindness, and no definable P100 waveform would be anticipated in them.

Neuroimaging

DAVID F. BLACK, MD

Introduction

Neuroimaging is commonly used in the clinical setting to aid in diagnosis, prognosis, and, in certain situations, acute therapeutic decision making. Indications, pitfalls, and examples of select neuroimaging methods are reviewed in this chapter.

Magnetic Resonance Imaging

Magnetic resonance imaging (MRI) provides better contrast resolution than computed tomography (CT), and CT offers better spatial resolution than MRI. MRI findings are described by signal intensity, in contradistinction to the tissue density used in CT. Although MRI has become the workhorse of neuroimaging given its superior soft-tissue discrimination, it does have drawbacks (Box 35.1).

MRI Physics

Laying in the magnetic field (created typically by a 1.5- or 3.0-t magnet), the spins of hydrogen atoms (protons) partially align with the magnetic field of the magnet. Variation in the magnetic field strength across the patient's body creates a strength gradient such that a specific magnetic field strength maps to a specific location.

Transmission of radiofrequency (RF) energy through the patient excites the spinning protons, and they "flip." As the protons "relax" back to the low-energy configuration that aligns them with the magnetic field of the scanner, they release RF energy (at their Larmor frequency, or rate of "wobble" unique to the atom) that can be measured. The strength of this signal is measured as a function of time and converted by a Fourier transformation into a function of frequency. This 2-dimensional measurement detects the presence of protons. Protons vary in density in different tissues, and this variation provides soft-tissue contrast resolution. Rotating the calibrated magnetic gradient allows the signal to be identified in space. Images are generated using a filtered back projection technique similar to CT.

> **Box 35.1 • Advantages and Disadvantages of Magnetic Resonance Imaging**
>
> *Advantages*
>
> Better contrast resolution than CT
>
> No use of radiation
>
> Highly sensitive for acute infarct
>
> Fewer allergic reactions than CT
>
> MRA and MRV can be noncontrast
>
> *Disadvantages*
>
> Less spatial resolution than CT
>
> High cost
>
> Less availability than CT
>
> NSF with poor renal function
>
> Claustrophobia
>
> Contraindicated devices (pacer)
>
> No use of gadolinium in pregnant patients
>
> Abbreviations: CT, computed tomography; MRA, magnetic resonance angiography; MRV, magnetic resonance venography; NSF, nephrogenic systemic fibrosis.

Abbreviations: CT, computed tomography; DWI, diffusion-weighted imaging; FDG, 2-[fluorine-18] fluoro-2 deoxy-D-glucose; MRA, magnetic resonance angiography; MRI, magnetic resonance imaging; MRS, magnetic resonance spectroscopy; PET, positron emission tomography; RF, radiofrequency

T1 and T2 are time constants. T1 describes the time required for protons in a specific tissue to recover back to thermal equilibrium after RF excitation stops. This point is also when the absorbed RF energy is released into the surrounding lattice, thus allowing the spins to go from the higher to a lower energy state. T1 equals the time when 63% of the magnetization has recovered its original alignment with the scanner's main magnetic field. T1 is unique for every tissue and is a measure of how quickly a tissue can be magnetized.

T2 describes transverse relaxation. After the RF energy stops, the proton spins lose synchronization, becoming dephased. Dephasing causes the measurable signal to decay, and T2 equals the time after excitation when 63% of the signal is lost (ie, a measure of how quickly a tissue can lose its magnetization).

Standard T1 and T2 MRI Sequences

Different sequences have different time of repetition and time of echo. Time of repetition is the time between each RF pulse (time protons are allowed to align), and time of echo is the time provided for energy to be released or detected after the RF pulse stops. Box 35.2 outlines the relationships among time of repetition, time of echo, and sequence type.

T1-weighted sequences demonstrate anatomy well and are the primary sequence used for comparison of pre-gadolinium and post-gadolinium enhancement. T2-weighted sequences are useful for demonstrating inflammation, edema, and fluid, which in most cases renders pathologic processes more conspicuous. Box 35.3 summarizes the causes of hyperintensities and hypointensities on T1 and T2. See also Figures 35.1 and 35.2.

Additional MR Sequences

Fluid-attenuation inversion-recovery sequences suppress (null) bulk fluid signal (as in ventricles, cisterns, or ocular vitreous) and thus render pathologic areas more conspicuous, especially in the periventricular regions. This sequence may be used with or without gadolinium and is

---

Box 35.3 • Causes of T1 and T2 Hyperintensities and Hypointensities

T1 brightness (hyperintensity) is due to T1 shortening

Subacute blood products

Fat (myelin)

Proteinaceous material

Slow flow

Melanin

Hydrated calcium

Gadolinium

T1 darkness (hypointensity) is due to T1 prolongation

Cerebrospinal fluid

Edema

Nonhydrated calcium

Air

Most tumors

T2 brightness (hyperintensity) is due to T2 prolongation

Cerebrospinal fluid

Edema

Most tumors

T2 darkness (hypointensity) is due to T2 shortening

Bone

Hemosiderin

Ferritin

Mucinous material

Air

Box 35.2 • Relationships Among Time of Repetition, Time of Echo, and Magnetic Resonance Sequence Types

T1 = short TR, short TE (TR <500 ms, TE <20 ms)

T2 = long TR, long TE (TR >2,000 ms, TE >70 ms)

Proton density = long TR, short TE (TR >2,000-3,000 ms, TE 25-30 ms)

Gadolinium shortens T1 and T2 (T1 more than T2)

Abbreviations: TE, time of echo; TR, time of repetition.

---

particularly sensitive for acute subarachnoid blood (Figure 35.3). Because this sequence has a lower signal-to-noise ratio than T2, it is less trustworthy than T2 in the posterior fossa.

Short-tau inversion-recovery sequences are useful for highlighting fluid or edema and are most utilized for imaging of the spine, where they are more sensitive than T2 for detecting abnormal cord signal in myelopathy.

Diffusion-weighted imaging (DWI) and apparent diffusion coefficient sequences provide unique information based on the microscopic motion of water. Restricted diffusion is demonstrated when lesions are bright on DWI and dark on the apparent diffusion coefficient map. DWI demonstrates restricted diffusion immediately after a stroke, and this lasts for up to 10 to 14 days. Subacute

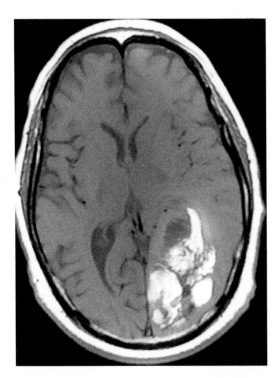

Figure 35.1 Axial T1 Magnetic Resonance Imaging.
Area of high T1 signal within this heterogenous lesion is suggestive of subacute hemorrhage. This lesion was a melanocytic neoplasm.

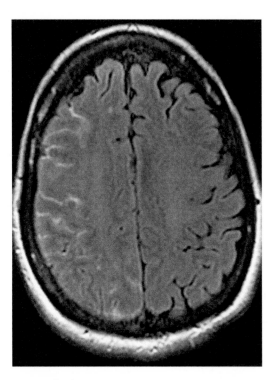

Figure35.3 Fluid-AttenuationInversion-Recovery–Sequence Axial Magnetic Resonance Imaging.
Sulcal subarachnoid blood (hyperintensity) is seen over the right hemisphere.

strokes begin to demonstrate enhancement (contingent on the degree of blood-brain barrier disruption) at about the same time DWI stops showing restriction. If a stroke clinically was suspected to have occurred 1 to 2 weeks previous to the MRI, the MRI should be performed with gadolinium because DWI may no longer be positive and the presence of enhancement aids in estimating the timing of infarction. If a lesion appears bright on the DWI and either bright or isointense to the surrounding tissue on apparent diffusion coefficient images, there is no restriction of diffusion, a result termed *T2 shine through*. DWI differentiates cytotoxic edema (infarct) from vasogenic edema, but infarcts are not the only lesions that restrict diffusion (Box 35.4). See also Volume 2,

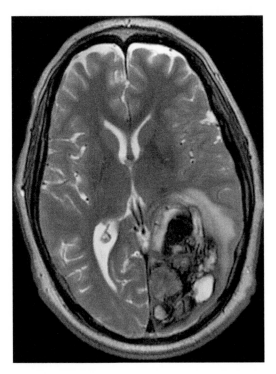

Figure 35.2 Axial T2 Magnetic Resonance Imaging.
Lesion is the same as that shown in Figure 35.1. The lesion shows mixed attenuation. Reduced T2 signal is suggestive of hemosiderin.

Box 35.4 • Lesions That Restrict Diffusion

Acute infarction

Highly cellular tumors (lymphoma, meningioma, PNETs)

Pyogenic abscesses (restrict centrally)

Cholesteatomas

Mucinous adenocarcinomas

Epidermoids

Abbreviation: PNET, primitive neuroectodermal tumor.

Chapter 10, "Ischemic Stroke: Common Causes and Diagnosis."

Perfusion-weighted imaging uses endogenous (arterial spin-labeling) or exogenous (gadolinium) sources to provide relative or absolute cerebral vascular measurements, including blood volume, blood flow, mean transit time, and time-to-peak.

Gradient-recalled echo or susceptibility-weighted imaging sequences emphasize magnetic susceptibility, a characteristic causing a "blooming" T2* hypointensity (similar to T2) that may indicate microhemorrhages, calcifications, amyloid deposition, hemorrhagic metastases, or cavernomas (Figure 35.4). See also Volume 2, Chapter 14, "Intraparenchymal Cerebral Hemorrhage." Three-dimensional constructive interference in steady-state sequence or 3-dimensional fast imaging employing steady-state acquisition are heavily T2-weighted fast sequences that are excellent for assessing small anatomical detail such as cranial nerve anatomy.

Post-gadolinium (contrast) multiplanar or 3-dimensional volume T1-weighted images are a T1 sequence obtained before and after gadolinium administration that can demonstrate abnormal enhancement, which indicates breakdown of the blood-brain barrier. In regions containing higher fat content such as the orbits or cavernous sinuses, fat-saturation techniques greatly aid the detection of enhancement. Some institutions use post-gadolinium fluid-attenuation inversion-recovery sequences, which appear especially useful for discerning meningeal processes.

MR Angiography

Typically, gadolinium (time of flight) is not used for head magnetic resonance angiography (MRA), but neck MRA is most often performed with and without bolus gadolinium. Time-of-flight imaging is direction-dependent; thus, if a vertebral artery appears absent on the time-of-flight image but present on the gadolinium bolus image, retrograde flow in this vessel is implied, most likely from a subclavian steal phenomenon. MRA data are typically reconstructed in 3 dimensions using maximum intensity projection images. These images are not trustworthy for measuring luminal diameter because this measurement varies contingent on the chosen display thresholds; thus, the source images offer the most accurate representation of true vessel caliber. MR venography can also be performed without or with a gadolinium bolus, although the latter provides a much more accurate representation of vessel patency.

Functional MRI

Functional MRI relies on the phenomenon wherein oxygen-rich hemoglobin behaves differently within a magnetic field than oxygen-poor hemoglobin. This blood oxygen level–dependent response can be measured and used as

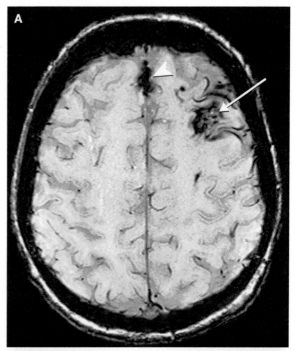

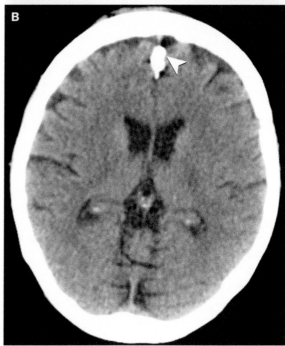

Figure 35.4 A, Susceptibility-weighted Imaging. In this patient with amyloid angiopathy, reduced signal may reflect subtle areas of hemosiderin (arrow) or calcium (arrowhead). B, Computed tomography of head. Patient is the same as that in A. Corresponding area of calcium (arrowhead) is seen.

a surrogate to image cerebral activity or function. As blood flow increases to more metabolically active areas in the brain, the ratio of oxyhemoglobin in those areas increases, resulting in a measurable difference (increase) in T2*.

MR Spectroscopy

MR spectroscopy (MRS) capitalizes on the fact that substances resonate at different frequencies in a magnetic field. MRS can identify various metabolites by their characteristic spectra. Although limited in the metabolites assessed, in certain clinical cases MRS can be useful. For example, MRS can be used to identify a lactate doublet in patients with mitochondrial cytopathies. MRS may also aid in the diagnosis of creatine deficiencies or Canavan disease in pediatric patients, and it may aid in tumor characterization.

Spine MRI

Given the distinct composition of the spine and the considerable bony component, different sequences are used in spine MRI than in head MRI. Gradient-recalled echo differentiates disk (gray) from bone (black), but it may overestimate neuroforaminal narrowing compared with conventional fast-spin echo T2. Sagittal images provide excellent coverage of the spinal canal, but axial images are the most helpful for discerning whether a process is intradural or extradural. Enhancement in primary brain tumors correlates with a higher histologic grade, but this relationship does not hold true for spine tumors. In patients who previously have had lumbar spine surgery, use of gadolinium can be useful for differentiating postoperative granulation tissue from disk material because granulation tissue enhances but disk material enhances minimally and only peripherally. The differential diagnosis of spine lesions on the basis of location is summarized in Box 35.5.

- Box 35.3 summarizes the causes of hyperintensities and hypointensities on T1 and T2 MRI.
- DWI MRI sequences demonstrate restricted diffusion immediately after an ischemic stroke, and this may last for up to 10 to 14 days.
- Gradient-recalled echo or susceptibility-weighted imaging MRI sequences emphasize magnetic susceptibility, a characteristic causing a "blooming" T2* hypointensity (similar to T2) that may indicate microhemorrhages, calcifications, amyloid deposition, hemorrhagic metastases, or cavernomas.
- Enhancement in primary brain tumors correlates with a higher histologic grade, but this relationship does not hold true for spine tumors.
- The differential diagnosis of spine lesions on the basis of location is summarized in Box 35.5.

Computed Tomography

CT uses x-ray images and filtered back projection to provide 2-dimensional and isometric voxel 3-dimensional images with better spatial resolution than MRI. Images are generated according to a tissue's density (ability to stop

---

Box 35.5 • Differential Diagnosis of Spine Lesions Based on Location

Extradural

Meningioma
Metastases (and lymphoma)
Hematoma
Abscess
Nerve sheath tumor
Disk bulge or fragment
Synovial or meningeal cyst

Intradural, extramedullary

Meningioma
Metastases (and lymphoma)
Hematoma
Abscess
Nerve sheath tumor

Intradural, intramedullary

Ependymoma (if well defined)
Astrocytoma (if ill defined)
Hemangioblastoma (enhances)
Myelitis
Infarct
Dural arteriovenous fistula (flow voids)
Metastases (and lymphoma)

---

photons) (Table 35.1). CT is the rapid and highly available test of choice for assessing for acute hemorrhage or fracture (Box 35.6) and can help estimate the age of cerebral infarction (Box 35.7).

Acute hemorrhage is hyperdense on CT. Subacute hemorrhage becomes more isodense, and chronic blood products are hypodense. Epidural hematomas do not cross suture lines unless there is an associated fracture, but they can cross the midline. This feature is more reliable diagnostically than relying on the lenticular shape that can be seen with other types of hematomas. Subdural hematomas do cross suture lines but do not cross the midline. Acute subarachnoid hemorrhage from a ruptured aneurysm typically fills the suprasellar and sylvian cisterns, but the imaging pattern is not predictive of the aneurysmal location. Pseudosubarachnoid hemorrhage occurs when marked cerebral edema causes the basal cisterns to appear relatively hyperdense, thereby mimicking the typical CT appearance of subarachnoid hemorrhage.

Acute venous sinus thromboses typically have Hounsfield units of 70 or more if measured in the first 1 to 2 days. CT attenuation correlates directly with the

Table 35.1 • Relative Densities of Tissue on Computed Tomography

Tissue	Density, Hounsfield Units
Water	0
Bone	+400–1,000
Soft tissue	40–80
Fat	−60–80
Air	−1,000
Blood	40–90 (acute = bright, chronic = dark)

hematocrit value; thus, arterial and venous density will be higher in young patients.

CT angiography and venography rely on iodinated contrast to opacify vessels. Vascular calcifications and the associated artifact often preclude accurate estimation of luminal narrowing. As with MRI, maximum intensity projection images are also not trustworthy for measuring luminal or aneurysmal diameters; the source images are most accurate.

CT perfusion is becoming more widely available and provides useful information in the acute stroke setting when the need for or helpfulness of an interventional procedure is being contemplated. CT perfusion provides maps of relative cerebral blood volume, blood flow, mean transit time, and time to peak. In acute stroke, the abnormal relative cerebral blood volume represents the infarct core, and the other parametric maps represent infarct core plus penumbra. Mismatch between the relative cerebral blood volume and relative cerebral blood flow indicates that there may be salvageable brain tissue (Figure 35.5).

Box 35.6 • Advantages and Disadvantages of Computed Tomography

Advantages

CT/CTA/CTV is widely available

Very rapid image acquisition

Claustrophobia is basically not an issue

Less expensive than MRI

Better spatial resolution than MRI

Disadvantages

Radiation

Iodine: allergy

Iodine: may impair renal function

Contrast resolution is inferior to MRI

Abbreviations: CT, computed tomography; CTA, CT angiography; CTV, CT venography; MRI, magnetic resonance imaging.

Box 35.7 • Evolution of Computed Tomography Findings in Ischemic Cerebral Infarction[a]

Hyperacute: normal or minimal blurring of gray-white junction

Acute: Indistinct gray-white junction, poorly defined hypodensity, and edema

Subacute: Hypodensity with temporal evolution toward more circumscribed focus

Chronic: Well circumscribed, low attenuation

[a] The temporal evolution of cerebral infarction on computed tomography can produce a fogging effect about 11 days after an infarct that transiently makes the previously hypodense infarct much less apparent.

- Epidural hematomas do not cross suture lines unless there is an associated fracture, but they can cross the midline. This feature is more reliable diagnostically than relying on the lenticular shape that can be seen with other types of hematomas.
- Subdural hematomas do cross suture lines and may appear acute, subacute, or chronic.
- Subarachnoid hemorrhage fills the subarachnoid space and cisterns.
- Mismatch between the relative cerebral blood volume and relative cerebral blood flow on a CT perfusion scan indicates that there may be salvageable brain tissue (Figure 35.5).

Ultrasonography

Carotid ultrasonography combines both real-time gray-scale imaging with Doppler ultrasonography. Doppler imaging relies on the shifting frequencies of returning echoes that reflect off moving objects, in this case red blood cells. Doppler ultrasonography detects the presence, direction, and velocity of blood flow, which can then be used to estimate the caliber of vessel, although tortuosity of vessels or overlying calcifications that absorb sound waves confound this measurement. Typically, ultrasonography estimations of luminal narrowing are complementary to MRA and CT angiography findings. All of these methods provide cross-sectional imaging, but with ultrasonography the quality of images is more contingent on the skill of the person acquiring the images than with CT or MRI.

Single-Photon Emission CT

Technetium Tc 99m ethyl cysteinate dimer and technetium Tc 99m hexamethylpropyleneamine oxime are radiotracers that can be used to demonstrate cerebral perfusion, which may be used to assess for brain death or seizure foci.

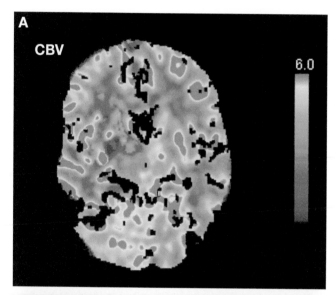

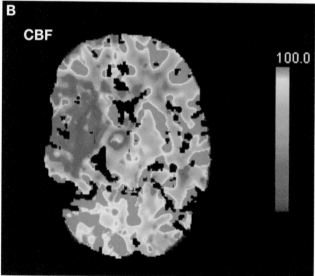

Figure 35.5 Computed Tomography Perfusion in a Patient With Acute Stroke.

A, The cerebral blood volume (CBV) is a measure of infarct core. In this patient, it appears normal without evidence of definitive infarction. B, The cerebral blood flow (CBF) is reduced in the right hemisphere. This situation, in which flow is impaired but volume remains normal, suggests a penumbra that potentially could be salvaged with reperfusion of this segment.

Acetazolamide is a selective cerebral vasodilatory agent that can be used with single-photon emission CT to assess vasodilatory reserve in patients with a fixed stenosis or when an artery may need to be sacrificed during surgery.

Positron Emission Tomography

The most commonly used positron emitter, fluorine-18, is the isotope used in the radiotracer 2-[fluorine-18] fluoro-2 deoxy-D-glucose positron emission tomography (FDG-PET). FDG is a glucose analogue that concentrates in metabolically active regions, including tumors, infections, or inflammation. Thus, full-body PET-CT can be an excellent tool for discerning metastases or the primary lesion in a paraneoplastic disorder.

Neuroimaging with PET or single-photon emission CT can be helpful for the evaluation of dementia, epilepsy, and traumatic brain injury. Because the brain primarily uses glucose for energy, FDG-PET always demonstrates relatively high cerebral uptake, which can make differentiating tumors difficult, but cerebral PET visualizes hypometabolic regions, such as those found in neurodegenerative conditions, quite well. Typical patterns of decreased metabolism suggest the clinical diagnosis, such as Alzheimer disease (temporoparietal), frontotemporal dementia (frontotemporal), or Lewy body dementia (temporoparietal and occipital).

Questions and Answers

Questions

Multiple Choice (choose the best answer)

VI.1. The electrical generators of electroencephalography (EEG) are:
- a. Action potentials
- b. Postsynaptic potentials
- c. Neurotransmitter release into the synapse
- d. Oligodendrocytes
- e. Presynaptic calcium uptake

VI.2. A 56-year-old man with a history of chronic hepatitis C is admitted to the hospital for confusion. On examination, he is encephalopathic and has asterixis. Results of an infectious evaluation, including blood cultures, chest radiography, and urinalysis, are normal. EEG is performed. What is the most likely finding?
- a. Periodic sharp waves
- b. Periodic lateralized epileptiform discharges
- c. Focal sharp waves
- d. Triphasic waves
- e. Normal results

VI.3. A 68-year-old man is evaluated for spells. EEG shows wicket waves during drowsiness. What is the significance of this finding?
- a. It is associated with temporal lobe epilepsy
- b. It is a normal variant
- c. It is the result of a space-occupying lesion
- d. It is indicative of Alzheimer dementia
- e. It is artifactual

VI.4. Which of the following best describes the relationship of diffusion restriction and enhancement after an infarction?
- a. Diffusion restriction begins immediately after an infarction and correlates with gadolinium enhancement temporally
- b. Diffusion restriction begins immediately after an infarction and lasts for several days
- c. Diffusion restriction begins immediately and begins to fade as gadolinium enhancement starts to develop
- d. Diffusion restriction begins after 2 to 3 days and starts to fade as gadolinium enhancement starts to develop
- e. Diffusion restriction does not change after an infarction

VI.5. Which of the following would not be expected to "bloom" with hypointensity on gradient recalled or susceptibility-weighted images?
- a. Calcium
- b. Microhemorrhage
- c. Amyloid
- d. Multiple sclerosis plaque
- e. Hemosiderin

VI.6. Which of the following statements is false?
- a. Epidural hematomas do not cross the midline
- b. Processes causing marked cerebral edema can mimic subarachnoid hemorrhage by causing the basal cisterns to appear relatively hyperdense
- c. Acute venous sinus thromboses typically have Hounsfield units of 70 or more
- d. Gadolinium enhancement often correlates with high-grade brain tumors, but this relationship is less reliable in spinal malignancies
- e. A small percentage of acute subarachnoid hemorrhages may be occult on computed tomography

VI.7. Which of the following is not found on electromyography in myopathic disorders?
- a. Fibrillation potentials
- b. Fasciculation potentials
- c. Small motor unit potentials
- d. Rapid recruitment of motor unit potentials
- e. Myokymic discharges

VI.8. A 32-year-old man presents with numbness and weakness in the feet and ankles. The peroneal and tibial motor conduction velocities are 22 m/s and 24 m/s, respectively. Neither temporal dispersion nor conduction block is noted. Which condition is most likely?
- a. A myopathy
- b. An axonal, likely acquired, peripheral neuropathy
- c. A demyelinating peripheral neuropathy, likely acquired
- d. A demyelinating peripheral neuropathy, likely hereditary
- e. Cool limb temperatures in a healthy patient

VI.9. A patient presents with numbness and tingling of the right fourth and fifth fingers. Mild weakness of hand intrinsic muscles is noted. All of the following electromyographic findings would fit with the diagnosis *except*:
- a. Low-amplitude ulnar compound muscle action potential (CMAP)
- b. Low-amplitude ulnar sensory nerve action potential (SNAP)
- c. A decrease in CMAP amplitude when inching the ulnar nerve across the elbow
- d. Needle electromyographic changes in abductor pollicis brevis
- e. Needle electromyographic changes in the medial flexor digitorum profundus (to the fifth digit)

VI.10. A patient is being evaluated in the electromyography laboratory for fatigue. You consider the possibility of autoimmune myasthenia gravis. What finding would help you support this diagnosis?
- a. Low-amplitude CMAPs
- b. Slowed sensory conduction velocities
- c. A decrement at rest that improves transiently after exercise
- d. A decrement of 5% at all times
- e. Large, complex, varying motor unit potentials

VI.11. The electromyographic findings in Guillain-Barré syndrome include
- a. Prolonged F-wave latencies
- b. Slowed conduction velocities
- c. Temporal dispersion or conduction block
- d. Rapid recruitment of small, complex motor unit potentials
- e. Answers a, b, and c are all correct

VI.12. A low-amplitude CMAP is least likely to be found in which of the following disorders?
- a. Peripheral neuropathy
- b. Proximal myopathy
- c. Lambert-Eaton myasthenic syndrome
- d. Amyotrophic lateral sclerosis
- e. Botulism

VI.13. Which of the following statements is most correct regarding the role of somatosensory evoked potentials (SSEPs) in the setting of anoxic coma after cardiac arrest?
- a. Preserved bilateral median N20 scalp responses are a positive prognostic indicator of an expected good clinical outcome
- b. The prognostic specificity of the median SSEP is lost with induced hypothermia in anoxic coma after cardiac arrest
- c. If the median N20 scalp response is initially present in anoxic coma, there is little use to repeating the study in a few days if the patient remains comatose
- d. SSEPs are less influenced by drugs and metabolic derangements than electroencephalography
- e. Prolonged N13 latency is the most sensitive predictor of poor outcome

VI.14. Which of the following conclusions is most correct for the reported tibial SSEP abnormality?
- a. A prolonged N22 to N30 interpeak latency indicates peripheral nerve slowing, a cold limb with slow peripheral conduction, or a long limb (tall patient)
- b. An isolated absent N30 cervical spine response in the setting of normal N22 and P38 responses is a common, normal-variant finding for tibial SSEPs
- c. Poorly defined N8, N22, N30, and P38 responses are most suggestive of diffuse disease of both the peripheral and the central proprioceptive pathways
- d. A normal N8 response, absent N22 and N30 responses, and prolonged P38 absolute latency indicate central slowing of the proprioceptive pathways in the thoracic or cervical cord
- e. Bilateral tibial nerve stimulation does not help augment N22, N30, or P38 amplitudes

VI.15. Which of the following statements is most correct regarding SSEPs?
- a. Similar to nerve conduction studies, supramaximal stimulation produces the most well-defined SSEP waveforms
- b. A faster stimulation rate is useful to overcome the effects of spasticity on SSEP recordings
- c. The tibial SSEP scalp response may be best recorded on the scalp ipsilateral to the side of stimulation
- d. An SSEP waveform represents the synaptic activity of neurons in a transmission pathway nucleus (such as the cuneate nucleus in the caudal medulla) or in the cortex
- e. Patient age and height do not affect SSEP latencies

Answers

VI.1. Answer b.

Aminoff MJ, editor. Aminoff's electrodiagnosis in clinical neurology. 6th ed. Edinburgh (UK): Elsevier/Saunders; c2012. 869 p.

VI.2. Answer d.

Aminoff MJ, editor. Aminoff's electrodiagnosis in clinical neurology. 6th ed. Edinburgh (UK): Elsevier/Saunders; c2012. 869 p.

VI.3. Answer b.

St Louis EK, Cascino GD. Patient management problem. CONTINUUM: Lifelong Learning Neurol. 2013 Jun;19(3 Epilepsy): 843–8, 849–61.

VI.4. Answer c.

Yousem DM, Grossman RI. Neuroradiology: the requisites. 3rd ed. Philadelphia (PA): Mosby/Elsevier; c2010. 619 p.

VI.5. Answer d.

Yousem DM, Grossman RI. Neuroradiology: the requisites. 3rd ed. Philadelphia (PA): Mosby/Elsevier; c2010. 619 p.

VI.6. Answer a.

Osborn AG. Osborn's brain: imaging, pathology, and anatomy. 1st ed. Salt Lake City (UT): Amirsys; c2013. 1272 p.

VI.7. Answer b.

Daube JR, Rubin DI, editors. Clinical neurophysiology. 3rd ed. New York (NY): Oxford University Press; c2009.

VI.8. Answer d.

Preston DC, Shapiro BE. Electromyography and neuromuscular disorders: clinical-electrophysiologic correlations. 3rd ed. London (UK): Elsevier/Saunders; c2013. 643 p.

VI.9. Answer d.

Preston DC, Shapiro BE. Electromyography and neuromuscular disorders: clinical-electrophysiologic correlations. 3rd ed. London (UK): Elsevier/Saunders; c2013. 643 p.

VI.10. Answer c.

Daube JR, Rubin DI, editors. Clinical neurophysiology. 3rd ed. New York (NY): Oxford University Press; c2009.

VI.11. Answer e.

Aminoff MJ, editor. Aminoff's electrodiagnosis in clinical neurology. 6th ed. Edinburgh (UK): Elsevier/Saunders; c2012. 869 p.

VI.12. Answer b.

Daube JR, Rubin DI, editors. Clinical neurophysiology. 3rd ed. New York (NY): Oxford University Press; c2009.

VI.13. Answer d.

Rossetti AO, Oddo M, Logroscino G, Kaplan PW. Prognostication after cardiac arrest and hypothermia: a prospective study. Ann Neurol. 2010 Mar;67(3):301–7.

VI.14. Answer b.

Carter JL, Stevens JC. Somatosensory evoked potentials. In: Daube JR, Rubin DI, editors. Clinical neurophysiology. 3rd ed. New York (NY): Oxford University Press; c2009. p. 257–80.

VI.15. Answer c.

Nuwer MR, Packwood JW. Somatosensory evoked potential monitoring with scalp and cervical recording. Nuwer MR, editor. Handbook of clinical neurophysiology. Vol 8. Amsterdam (Netherlands): Elsevier; c2008. p. 180–9. (Intraoperative monitoring of neural function; vol. 8).

SUGGESTED READING

Aminoff MJ, editor. Aminoff's electrodiagnosis in clinical neurology. 6th ed. Edinburgh (UK): Elsevier/Saunders; c2012. 869 p.

Barkovich AJ, Raybaud C, editors. Pediatric neuroimaging. 5th ed. Philadelphia (PA): Wolters/Kluwer Health/Lippincott Williams & Wilkins; c2012. 1125 p.

Brown PD, Davies SL, Speake T, Millar ID. Molecular mechanisms of cerebrospinal fluid production. Neuroscience. 2004; 129(4):957–70.

Carter JL. Brain stem auditory evoked potentials in central disorders. In: Daube JR, Rubin DI, editors. Clinical neurophysiology. 3rd ed. New York (NY): Oxford University Press; c2009. p. 281–93.

Carter JL. Visual evoked potentials. In: Daube JR, Rubin DI, editors. Clinical neurophysiology. 3rd ed. New York (NY): Oxford University Press; c2009. p. 311–22.

Carter JL, Stevens JC. Somatosensory evoked potentials. In: Daube JR, Rubin DI, editors. Clinical neurophysiology. 3rd ed. New York (NY): Oxford University Press; c2009. p. 257–80.

Daube JR, Rubin DI, editors. Clinical neurophysiology. 3rd ed. New York (NY): Oxford University Press; c2009.

Fishman RA. Cerebrospinal fluid in diseases of the nervous system. 2nd ed. Philadelphia (PA): Saunders; c1992. 431 p.

Latchaw RE, Kucharczyk J, Moseley ME, editors. Imaging of the nervous system: diagnostic and therapeutic applications. St. Louis (MO): Mosby; c2005.

Nuwer MR. Fundamentals of evoked potentials and common clinical applications today. Electroencephalogr Clin Neurophysiol. 1998 Feb;106(2):142–8.

Nuwer MR, Packwood JW. Somatosensory evoked potential monitoring with scalp and cervical recording. Nuwer MR, editor. Handbook of clinical neurophysiology. Vol 8. Amsterdam (Netherlands): Elsevier; c2008. p. 180–89. (Intraoperative monitoring of neural function; vol. 8).

Osborn AG. Osborn's brain: imaging, pathology, and anatomy. 1st ed. Salt Lake City (UT): Amirsys; c2013. 1272 p.

Osborn AG, Salzman KL, Barkovich AJ, editors. Diagnostic imaging: brain. 2nd ed. Salt Lake City (UT): Amirsys; c2010.

Preston DC, Shapiro BE. Electromyography and neuromuscular disorders: clinical-electrophysiologic correlations. 3rd ed. London (UK): Elsevier/Saunders; c2013. 643 p.

Rossetti AO, Oddo M, Logroscino G, Kaplan PW. Prognostication after cardiac arrest and hypothermia: a prospective study. Ann Neurol. 2010 Mar;67(3):301–7.

St Louis EK, Cascino GD. Patient management problem. CONTINUUM: Lifelong Learning Neurol. 2013 Jun; 19(3 Epilepsy): 843–8, 849–61.

Wijdicks EF, Hijdra A, Young GB, Bassetti CL, Wiebe S; Quality Standards Subcommittee of the American Academy of Neurology. Practice parameter: prediction of outcome in comatose survivors after cardiopulmonary resuscitation (an evidence-based review): report of the Quality Standards Subcommittee of the American Academy of Neurology. Neurology. 2006 Jul 25;67(2):203–10.

Yousem DM, Grossman RI. Neuroradiology: the requisites. 3rd ed. Philadelphia (PA): Mosby/Elsevier; c2010. 619 p.

Section VII

Psychiatry

Kemuel L. Philbrick, MD,

editor

36 Principles of Psychiatry and Psychology

MARY M. MACHULDA, PHD, LP

Introduction

Cognition, classic psychiatric constructs, and an approach to the evaluation of cognition and psychologic disorders are discussed in this chapter. Cognitive evaluations may include simple office-based procedures, but formal neuropsychological testing and functional imaging have aided practitioners in further understanding and treating disorders as well as understanding normal function.

Cognition

Cognition is a general term for mental processes used in processing information, such as attention, language, memory, decision making, and problem solving. *Cognitive psychology* is the specialty of psychology that examines mental processes and studies how individuals perceive, think, learn, and remember. Cognitive psychologists use scientific methods to study how individuals acquire, process, and store information. There are many practical applications of cognitive psychology research, including improving memory, increasing decision-making accuracy, and structuring educational curricula to enhance learning.

Neuropsychology is a specialty field within clinical psychology that focuses on brain functioning. A clinical neuropsychologist is a professional psychologist trained in the science of brain-behavior relationships who specializes in the application of assessment and intervention principles based on the scientific study of human behavior across the lifespan as it relates to the normal and abnormal functioning of the nervous system.

- *Cognition* is a general term for mental processes used in processing information, such as attention, language, memory, decision making, and problem solving.

Classic Psychiatric Constructs

Psychoanalytic theory is based on Freud's concept that the forces that motivate behavior are a manifestation of unconscious mental processes. The 3 parts of the mind defined in Freud's structural model of the psyche are the id, the ego, and the superego. They are functions of the mind and do not correspond to specific neuroanatomical structures. The *id* is present at birth and represents instinctive sexual and aggressive drives that cause a person to want pleasure immediately without the influence of external reality. The *ego* begins to develop at birth and controls the id as a person adapts to the outside world. It is the organized, realistic part of the personality structure. Through the ego, reality testing maintains a sense of the body and the outside world. The *superego* begins to develop at approximately 6 years of age and suppresses the unbridled urges of the id. Through the superego, the ego is shaped to function in service of morality. It serves as one's conscience and has a critical and moralizing role.

Transference refers to a patient's experience with the unconscious redirection of feelings from 1 person to another. In the context of a psychotherapeutic relationship, transference is the redirection of a patient's feelings for a

---

Abbreviations: Cho, choline; CT, computed tomography; FDG, fludeoxyglucose F 18; fMRI, functional magnetic resonance imaging; ¹H MRS, proton magnetic resonance spectroscopy; mI, *myo*-inositol; MMSE, Mini-Mental State Examination; MoCA, Montreal Cognitive Assessment; MRI, magnetic resonance imaging; NAA, *N*-acetylaspartate; PET, positron emission tomography; PRI, Perceptual Reasoning Index; PSI, Processing Speed Index; SPECT, single-photon emission computed tomography; TF-fMRI, task-free functional magnetic resonance imaging; VCI, Verbal Comprehension Index; WAIS-IV, Wechsler Adult Intelligence Scale (Fourth Edition); WMI, Working Memory Index

significant person in the patient's life (usually 1 or both parents) to the therapist. In psychoanalysis, these reactions are identified and analyzed. *Countertransference* refers to the feelings of a therapist toward the patient. Countertransference reactions can alter the therapist's judgment and be damaging. Therefore, these reactions must be identified and monitored.

Defense mechanisms (Table 36.1) are unconscious techniques of the ego that help a person cope with anxiety by blocking or diverting conflicts from conscious awareness. Mature defense mechanisms (eg, altruism, humor, sublimation, suppression) are adaptive and unlikely to have negative social consequences. Less mature defense mechanisms (eg, acting out, regression, splitting) are typically expressed in disturbed behavior and are often associated with negative social consequences. In *psychodynamic therapy*, therapists attempt to help patients learn to tolerate unpleasant emotions without resorting to maladaptive defense mechanisms

Table 36.1 • Specific Defense Mechanisms

Mechanism	Description
Acting out	Engaging in attention-getting and often socially inappropriate behavior to avoid unacceptable feelings
Altruism	Dedication to the needs of others
Denial	Ignoring or minimizing particular facts
Displacement	Transferring a feeling about one situation or person onto another situation or person
Dissociation	Trance-like detachment
Humor	Placing an emphasis on the amusing or ironic aspects of a stressor
Idealization	The attribution of exaggerated positive qualities to others
Intellectualization	The excessive use of abstract thinking
Projection	Attributing one's own unacceptable feelings to someone else
Rationalization	A false but personally acceptable explanation for one's behavior
Reaction formation	Turning an unacceptable feeling into its opposite
Regression	Returning to an earlier developmental phase
Splitting	Viewing one's self or others as all good or as all bad to avoid conflicted or ambivalent feelings
Sublimation	Redirecting unacceptable impulses into a socially approved activity
Suppression	The intentional avoidance of thinking about unwanted thoughts
Undoing	Using ritualized behavior to create an illusion of control

and to grow in self-awareness so that an individual may choose to act with conscious awareness of the intrapsychic perceptions and attitudes that shape one's behavior.

- The 3 parts of the mind defined in Freud's structural model of the psyche are the id, the ego, and the superego.
- *Transference* refers to a patient's experience with unconscious redirection of feelings from 1 person to another.
- *Countertransference* refers to the feelings of a therapist toward the patient.
- *Defense mechanisms* are unconscious techniques of the ego that help a person cope with anxiety by blocking or diverting conflicts from conscious awareness.

Mental Status Examination

A thorough evaluation of mental function is a standard part of the neurologic examination. The mental status examination is a semistructured interview during which clinicians gather information from both careful observation and direct questioning of the patient. It was developed to elicit—and to a limited extent, to quantify—the behavioral changes of individuals with organic brain dysfunction or disease.

The mental status examination provides a description of the patient's appearance, speech, actions, and thoughts during the examination. The goals are 1) to allow early detection of organically based behavioral changes when taking into account the patient's age, education, occupational history, and socioeconomic background; 2) to localize the lesion or lesions causing these changes, including the mechanism of disease, to aid in the diagnosis of neurobehavioral syndromes and disorders; 3) to determine the potential impact of cognitive dysfunction on activities of daily living; and 4) to determine whether a more comprehensive neuropsychological assessment is required. The mental status examination on a cooperative, verbally intact patient can usually be completed in 20 to 30 minutes. The key parts of the mental status examination are listed in Box 36.1.

Formal mental status tests are frequently used to evaluate the overall level of cognitive functioning. Several screening procedures or formal mental status evaluations are available for clinical use. They are brief to administer, and they provide basic information on the integrity of most cognitive functions, but they are not comprehensive and they are limited in their ability to detect subtle forms of cognitive impairment.

The most widely used general cognitive screening instrument is the Mini-Mental State Examination (MMSE). It is commonly used to screen for dementia as well as to track the course of cognitive changes in a patient over time. The MMSE provides a general summary of cognitive function but does not assess any cognitive domain in depth. It can be administered in approximately 10 minutes and includes 5 sections with a total of 30 points: Orientation (10 points), Registration (3 points), Attention and Calculation (5 points), Recall (3 points), and Language (9 points). It is currently available in 10 languages.

The Montreal Cognitive Assessment (MoCA), developed in 1996, is also a 1-page, 30-point test that can be administered in approximately 10 minutes. It includes 6 sections: Short-term Memory (5 points); Visuospatial (4 points); Executive (4 points); Attention, Concentration, and Working Memory (6 points); Language (5 points); and Orientation (6 points). The MoCA is an excellent screening measure for mild cognitive impairment and is gaining credibility over other screening tests because it offers improvements in sensitivity, uses items that evaluate frontal executive functioning, and has less susceptibility to cultural and education biases. It is currently available in 35 languages or dialects and is accessible free of charge with instructions for administration at www.mocatest.org.

• The Mini-Mental State Examination (MMSE) provides a general summary of cognitive function but does not assess any cognitive domain in depth.

Cognitive and Neuropsychological Testing

Formal neuropsychological evaluations include detailed assessment of various cognitive domains in more detail than can be covered in a mental status examination. The degree to which each of these domains is evaluated often depends on the referral question as well as on the patient's level of function. Detailed neuropsychological evaluations provide standardized assessment and quantification of cognitive functions in terms of performance compared with normative data. The evaluations allow the identification of cognitive and behavioral deficits as well as preserved areas of function. They can aid in diagnosis and treatment recommendations. A typical neuropsychological evaluation includes assessment of the following: general intellect, academic achievement, attention and concentration, learning and memory, language, visuospatial skills, sensory and motor function, and executive functions.

General Intellect

The mental abilities measured by intelligence tests include many different cognitive functions. The fourth edition of the Wechsler Adult Intelligence Scale (WAIS-IV) is the most recent version of this commonly used intelligence test. It is composed of 4 index scores: Verbal Comprehension Index (VCI), Working Memory Index (WMI), Perceptual Reasoning Index (PRI), and Processing Speed Index (PSI). Verbal IQ is derived from the VCI and WMI. Performance IQ is derived from the PRI and PSI. All 4 factors are used to create the Full Scale IQ.

Academic Achievement

These instruments focus on academic skills, such as reading, spelling, writing, language, and mathematical skills as they are acquired from elementary school through high school. For children and adolescents, these tests are typically used in conjunction with intelligence and other cognitive measures to determine the presence or absence of a learning disability and to assess deterioration of school performance. For adults, they are used to complement measures of intellectual and cognitive function and to assess baseline level of functioning.

Attention and Concentration

The ability to focus and maintain attention is a prerequisite skill for valid and reliable higher-order cognitive functions. Neuropsychological evaluations include tests of both simple forms of attention (eg, attention span) and complex forms of attention, such as the ability to divide attention, ignore distractions, and process information at a certain speed. *Working memory* refers to the ability to hold, actively process, manipulate, and transform information in short-term memory; therefore, it shares features with both complex attention and immediate memory.

Learning and Memory

Episodic memory consists of 3 steps: encoding, storage, and retrieval. *Encoding* refers to the ability to learn new information. *Storage* or consolidation is measured by free recall or retention after a delay or distractor interval. Recognition formats are used to distinguish retrieval from consolidation-based memory deficits. *Retrieval* is assessed by noting the difference between the amount of material recalled without cues or prompts and the amount identified on the recognition task. Neuropsychological evaluations often include assessment of both verbal memory and nonverbal memory. Occasionally, memory deficits may be detected with only 1 form of material. Word lists and stories are commonly used to evaluate verbal memory, and geometric designs or shapes are commonly used to evaluate nonverbal memory.

Language

Language assessment includes assessment of auditory comprehension (single words, sentences, spoken narratives); reading (word recognition, comprehension); speech and language production (intelligibility, prosody, naming, fluency, repetition); and written expression (generating automatized sequences, copying, writing to dictation, writing self-formulated material). See also Volume 2, Chapter 29, "A Review of Focal Cortical Syndromes."

Visuospatial Skills

Visuospatial skills encompass a range of cognitive functions that include the ability to analyze and understand information in space in 2 and 3 dimensions. These skills include processes such as mental imagery and navigation, distance and depth perception, and visuospatial reasoning and problem solving. Most neuropsychological evaluations include assessment of visuoperceptual, visuospatial, and visuoconstructional abilities.

Sensory and Motor Function

Auditory perception is evaluated for acuity and perception of organized sounds and rhythms. Tactile assessment is usually limited to the hands and may include assessment of tactile inattention, finger agnosia, graphesthesia, and stereognosis. Assessment of motor function includes fine motor speed, dexterity, and grip strength.

Executive Functions

Executive functions encompass the cognitive abilities necessary for complex goal-directed behavior and the ability to effectively respond to a range of environmental changes and demands. Executive functions have 4 components: 1) volition, 2) planning and decision making, 3) purposive action, and 4) effective performance. Many conceptualizations of executive function also include self-monitoring and self-awareness because these are necessary for behavioral flexibility and appropriateness. Psychometric assessment of executive function includes abilities such as mental flexibility, inhibition of responses, planning, organization, and abstract reasoning.

- *Working memory* refers to the ability to hold, actively process, manipulate, and transform information in short-term memory; therefore, it shares features with both complex attention and immediate memory.
- *Episodic memory* consists of 3 steps: encoding, storage, and retrieval.

Neuroimaging in Cognitive and Psychiatric Disorders

Structural Neuroimaging

Structural neuroimaging is useful for identifying potential structural causes of cognitive or psychiatric changes. Indications include acute changes in mental status, dementia of unknown origin, new-onset psychosis, sudden personality changes or changes in psychiatric symptoms in patients with an established psychiatric diagnosis, catatonia, or serious psychiatric illness that does not respond to front-line therapies. Computed tomography (CT) is the imaging technique of choice for agitated or uncooperative patients, for patients with claustrophobia, or for patients with other contraindications to magnetic resonance imaging (MRI). Compared with CT, MRI offers superior spatial and soft-tissue contrast, which can aid in the differential diagnosis of dementias, such as Alzheimer disease, frontotemporal lobar degeneration, and vascular dementia.

Functional Neuroimaging

Single-Photon Emission CT and Positron Emission Tomography

Single-photon emission CT (SPECT) is a functional neuroimaging technique that uses radioisotope tracers to assess brain perfusion. It is less expensive and easier to use than positron emission tomography (PET) and therefore is more widely available. It may be used clinically to support a diagnosis of Alzheimer disease and vascular dementia.

PET uses positron emitters to label glucose, amino acids, neurotransmitter precursors, and other molecules (particularly high-affinity ligands) to measure receptor densities. PET has higher sensitivity and greater spatial resolution than SPECT and can be used to assess regional brain function and blood flow. The Centers for Medicare and Medicaid Services has approved fludeoxyglucose F 18 (FDG) PET imaging as a routine examination tool for detection and differential diagnosis of Alzheimer disease, specifically to differentiate Alzheimer disease from frontotemporal lobar degeneration. FDG PET can also be used to detect early changes in glucose uptake before the onset of clinical symptoms in patients at risk of Alzheimer disease because of either family history or genetic susceptibility.

Currently, SPECT and PET are not used to diagnose primary psychiatric disorders. However, both techniques are used in research studies to examine abnormalities in blood flow, glucose uptake, and major neurotransmitter systems in conditions such as schizophrenia, obsessive compulsive disorder, and mood disorders.

Proton Magnetic Resonance Spectroscopy

Proton magnetic resonance spectroscopy (^{1}H MRS) is a noninvasive imaging technique that allows for assessment of specific brain metabolites. It is unique among imaging techniques because it allows simultaneous measurement of several different metabolites during a single measurement period. Each metabolite is sensitive to a different aspect of in vivo pathologic processes at the molecular or cellular level. Common metabolites measured include *N*-acetylaspartate (NAA), which is a marker of neuronal density; *myo*-inositol (mI), which is a marker of glial activity; and choline (Cho), which is thought to reflect the level of membrane turnover. It can also provide information about lithium and fluorinated psychopharmacologic agents. ^{1}H MRS is used in research to examine psychiatric conditions such as schizophrenia, panic disorder, obsessive compulsive disorder, autism spectrum disorders, major depression, and bipolar disorder.

Functional MRI

Functional MRI (fMRI) is a noninvasive imaging technique that is sensitive to blood flow changes that occur in response to motor, sensory, and cognitive processing. Results from functional scans are superimposed onto structural scans acquired during the same scanning session to identify neuroanatomical areas associated with activation. Psychiatric applications include understanding brain changes associated with conditions such as schizophrenia, obsessive compulsive disorder, addiction, and depression.

Resting-state fMRI, also referred to as task-free fMRI (TF-fMRI), is a type of fMRI performed without a predetermined experimental condition. It is emerging as a powerful tool for investigating the intrinsic network organization of both normal and pathologic states of the brain. Unlike activation studies that use fMRI, this technique does not require any active participation by the patient. TF-fMRI is shedding light on aberrations in intrinsic connectivity in psychiatric conditions such as depression, anxiety, attention-deficit/hyperactivity disorder, and schizophrenia.

- ^{1}H MRS is used in research to examine psychiatric conditions such as schizophrenia, panic disorder, obsessive compulsive disorder, autism spectrum disorders, major depression, and bipolar disorder.

37 Psychological Development Through the Life Cycle

MARIA I. LAPID, MD; MARK W. OLSEN, MD

Introduction

Human development from conception to death can be viewed from a number of perspectives, including biologic, cognitive, emotional, social, and moral. This chapter reviews major features of various facets of development from infancy through toddlerhood, preschool, school-aged, preadolescence, adolescence, the transition into early adulthood, adulthood, and late adulthood (Table 37.1). It includes consideration of developmental tasks and challenges as well as the importance of the environmental influence of family, peers, school, and the broader social milieu. Psychological aspects and specific stages in the elderly are also described.

Development From Infancy to Adulthood

Infancy (Birth to 1 Year)

Birth signals a major developmental milestone with an exponential increase in the range and intensity of stimuli with which the newborn is well prepared to interact. Within the first 1 or 2 weeks of life, the infant orients to the human face and voice and soon can imitate facial expressions. Overall tasks for the first year of life are to develop and maintain attachments, establish motor control, and initiate self-regulation. In Piaget's stages, the first 2 years of life comprise the *sensorimotor stage* as the infant learns by reacting to sensory inputs with motor responses (eg, turning toward the mother's nipple when the infant's cheek is touched). The infant progresses through 6 substages, by assimilation and accommodation, to achieve a sense of *object permanence.*

Freud called the first year the *oral stage*, implying that the mouth is the primary source of gratification. In Erikson's epigenetic model, this is the stage of *basic trust versus mistrust*. Through their interactions with consistent, reliable, and predictable caregivers, infants develop both a trustworthy, secure attachment and a basic hope for positive outcomes in future challenges.

Clinically, autistic spectrum disorders, with markedly impaired social reciprocity, communication deficits, and related symptoms, tend to become apparent in the first year of life.

Toddlerhood (1–2.5 Years)

During toddlerhood, progression of motor and communication skills continues at a rapid pace. Children run, jump, climb stairs, throw balls, and speak in simple sentences. Developmental tasks for toddlers include striking the proper balance between attachment and exploration, moving toward autonomy while internalizing parental values, and further refining symbolic play and communication. Toilet training may be a parental priority, and Freud termed this period the *anal stage*. As children assert their growing sense of independence, displays of emotion can be intense. This is Erikson's stage of *autonomy versus shame and doubt*. Children may chafe at parental rules, but their growing social awareness leads to an appreciation of how they might be perceived by others. Children who successfully resolve this crisis will emerge with will, the ability to make assertive choices while exercising due restraint. Mahler called the period from 15 to 24 months the time of *rapprochement*, when children become more aware of their limitations and recognize the continued importance of primary caregivers. Eventually, by 30 months, through *emotional object constancy*, children can retain a positive internal image of their primary caregivers. Toddlers observe and imitate the behaviors of others, including peers. They enjoy pretending, and they move from parallel to interactive play.

Table 37.1 • Overview of Life Stages

Age	Freud's Stage	Erikson's Stage	Characteristics
Infancy (birth to 1 y)	Oral[a]	Basic trust vs mistrust	• Maintain attachment (reliable, predictable caregivers help develop secure attachment, hope) • Establish motor control • Initiate self-regulation
Toddlerhood (1–2.5 y)	Anal[b]	Autonomy vs shame and doubt	• Motor and communication skills develop • Balance between attachment and exploration (move toward autonomy) • Internalize parental values • Toilet training • Observe and imitate others
Preschooler (2.5–6 y)	Phallic[c]	Initiative vs guilt	• Advancing motor and communication skills • Interpersonal relationships • Magical thinking moves toward logical and realistic thinking • Realize own sex • Self-regulate, follow rules
School–aged (6–11 y)	Latency[d]	Industry vs inferiority	• Competency (strive to master academic and social realms) • Understand complex rules and procedures • Understand concepts of conservation, reversibility, numeration, classification
Preadolescence (11–13 y)	. . .	. . .	• Dependence vs independence tension • Peer relationships gain ascendance • Emotional lability • Increased ability to reason and think abstractly
Early and middle adolescence (13–17 y)	Genital[e]	Identity vs role confusion	• Individual identity • Independence • Intimate relationships • Abstract thinking • Being accepted and considered attractive by peers is vitally important
Late adolescence (17–20 y)	. . .	Intimacy vs isolation	• Finding purpose and meaning • Self-identity
Adulthood	. . .	Generativity vs stagnation	• Growth in capacity for mature love • Career development • Productivity in home and family

[a] From birth to 18 months, according to Freud.
[b] From 18 months to 3 years, according to Freud.
[c] From 3 to 6 years, according to Freud.
[d] From 6 years to puberty, according to Freud.
[e] From puberty to adulthood, according to Freud.

Reactive attachment disorder may result from abusive or neglectful parenting that causes serious disruptions in separation-individuation, basic trust, and autonomy.

Preschool (2.5–6 Years)

"Play is the child's work" certainly pertains to preschool-aged children. Through play and other activities, they put their rapidly advancing communication, cognitive, and motor skills to work developing interpersonal relationships outside the family and begin to move from an egocentric and magical view of the world to one that is more logical and realistic. From the Freudian standpoint, this is the *phallic-oedipal stage*. Children become aware of their own sex and become interested in other people's bodies. They tend to enact culturally based gender roles in their play and other interactions.

Erikson considered this the time of *initiative versus guilt*. Preschoolers become better at self-regulation but also more competitive and imaginative. Their morality, termed *preconventional* by Kohlberg, is strongly influenced by parental monitoring, limit setting, and praise. Preschoolers tend to be rigid rule followers but primarily to avoid censure by the powerful people who make the rules. An authoritative parenting style, as opposed to a permissive style or an authoritarian style, tends to facilitate a process by which preschoolers navigate the challenge of *initiative versus guilt* and emerge with a firm sense of purpose. Preschoolers generally adapt very well to structured play and learning settings and are often eager to move on to their formal school years.

Psychiatric disorders that could emerge in preschool-aged children include separation anxiety, oppositional defiant disorder, and attention-deficit/hyperactivity disorder.

School-aged (6–11 Years)

Competency is the overall theme for school-aged children as they strive to achieve mastery in the academic and social realms. Motor and communication skills are well developed. Freud called this time the *latency stage*, when libido is suppressed in the interest of directing energy into school, same-sex relationships, clubs, sports, and other activities with complex rules and procedures. School-aged children, according to Piaget, are in the *concrete operational* stage. They can perform mental operations, such as logic, to better understand their world. They can grasp important concepts like conservation, seriation, classification, reversibility, and numeration. There is a decline in egocentrism (decentration) that allows better appreciation of subjectivity and objectivity.

The developmental challenge for school-aged children in the Eriksonian system is *industry versus inferiority*. Children begin the long effort to master the cognitive and social skills that will ultimately equip them for adult roles. In the process, they compare themselves with peers and may find themselves wanting academically, athletically, or socially. Parents and teachers play a vital role. By intervening in what Vygotsky called the *zone of proximal development* (ie, the gap between actual and potential skill acquisition), sensitive and patient adults can provide the cognitive scaffolding needed for the child to progress. The social network expands to include teachers, coaches, and peers' parents. Even family relationships take on a more public dimension as families interact at sports and other recreational activities. The media, too, exert a stronger—and not always positive—socializing influence. Morally, there is still a strong, rule-based sense of right and wrong. School-aged children can be quick to point out inconsistencies in adult behavior. By the time children transition into adolescence, most have established a reasonable sense of competency and can apply skills and knowledge to succeed in developmentally appropriate tasks.

Psychiatric conditions that may emerge during the school-aged period are conduct disorder, learning disorders, social and school phobia, and other anxiety disorders.

Preadolescence (11–13 Years)

By the time most children reach preadolescence, puberty is well under way, ushering in new physical potentials and a new sense of self as individuated from, yet still related to, the family. There is a reenactment of the tension between dependence and independence. Group-oriented peer relationships gain ascendance and may manifest in styles of dress, music, and other modes of expression. Emotions may become more labile and negative affects more common. For parents, this can be a challenging time as they adjust to the increasing need for independence even though their preteen may lack the wisdom to consistently make good choices. This is the onset of Piaget's stage of *formal operations*.

Preadolescents begin to develop the capacity to think abstractly and to use hypothetical and deductive reasoning to solve higher-order problems. They may start to challenge social norms but were considered by Kohlberg to generally have conventional morality. They tend to stress the value of shared rules in sustaining good social relationships and maintaining social order.

Preadolescence is also a time when social media can exert profound influence. Difficult to monitor, instantly accessible, and seemingly irresistible, social media can enhance a sense of connectivity, but they can also have potentially devastating effects, such as cyberbullying.

Other psychiatric conditions that may emerge in preadolescence are mood disorders and substance use disorders.

Early and Middle Adolescence (13–17 Years)

In adolescence, the developmental tasks are to establish an individual identity, achieve or at least progress toward independence, and form intimate relationships. Cognitively, adolescents continue to develop their capacity for abstract thought and ability to think about thinking (*metacognition*). They start to solidify their sense of who they are and what they want to become while strengthening affective self-regulation. From a moral standpoint, adolescents who use their capacity for thinking abstractly and challenging the status quo move into Kohlberg's *postconventional* level of morality. They may think about moral issues in terms of individual rights, the social contract, and universal principles.

Freud termed adolescence the *genital stage* to indicate a return of libidinal energy to that domain. Peer relationships typically take on a sexual dimension as the adolescent begins the process that for many will lead to the formation of a new family. Erikson saw the developmental task of adolescence as *identity versus role confusion*. On a basic level, adolescents may need to become familiar with their transformed bodies and minds after puberty has run its course. More broadly, though, they have to form a revised social identity. Being accepted and considered attractive by peers is vitally important. There is evidence that early maturing females and late maturing males may receive more negative evaluations by peers and adults. Adolescent groups can be intolerant or cruel to those who are perceived as different. Maturation through adolescence can be a perplexing process, but if it is successfully navigated, the adolescent develops the capacity to form strong commitments and fidelity to self and others.

Psychopathologies that can emerge during adolescence include eating disorders and schizophrenia, in addition to those mentioned above.

Late Adolescence to Early Adulthood (17–20 Years)

Among the developmental tasks of late adolescence that continue into early adulthood are finding purpose and meaning in life through work and other interests and forming long-term or lifelong romantic attachments and friendships. Erikson described the challenge of this time of life as *intimacy versus isolation*. Until they have established a stable and well-integrated self-identity, adolescents can be so self-absorbed that romantic relationships are mostly self-centered. Once an integrated identity is established, though, the late adolescent or young adult may be capable of achieving the genuine mutuality necessary for intimacy. If not, there is a risk of isolation. According to Erikson, the ultimate outcome is the attainment of mature love.

During this time of transition into adulthood, personality disorders may be identified.

Adulthood

In Eriksonian terms, the broad expanse between young adulthood and old adulthood is captured in the struggle between *generativity versus stagnation*. For some, a good measure of conventional adulthood may also involve continuing growth in the capacity for mature love as expressed in the tension between intimacy and isolation. But for most, this is a time of increasing capacity for mutuality, furthered by the necessities of parenting among those who choose to shoulder those responsibilities. Individuals' perceptions of themselves and their relationships with their partners change as their own children move from phase to phase in their development.

A second arena of focus in middle adulthood is career, which may involve pursuing a formal, well-defined, traditional profession; meeting the significant challenges of raising children; or striking out in entrepreneurial risk taking.

Whether in a relationship or a family or in the marketplace of employment, adults continue to build their lives, learning to express love that is other-centered, contributing to positions of commercial, civic, professional, religious, or societal responsibility. There may be children to raise and then to release into adulthood. Aging parents may introduce a necessity for role reversal, even as grandchildren oblige recognition of one's own advancing age. Successful adults survey the patterns of their lives and conclude that they have contributed to the world by being active and productive in their homes and communities. Those who feel that they have failed to achieve this assurance of having contributed will likely feel unproductive, disengaged, and perhaps threatened by the unyielding march of time.

Late Adulthood

Although no distinct boundary exists between middle and late adulthood, the chronologic age of 65 years is traditionally considered the entry point to this phase of the life cycle. Other terms for late adulthood that are commonly used in various contexts include *geriatric, elderly, older adult*, and *senior*; some terms are more acceptable than others. One accepted grouping of old age includes *young-old* (ages 65–74), *middle-old* (ages 75–84), and *oldest-old* (85 or older). Demographically, the oldest-old group is the fastest growing segment of the US population.

Individuals in late adulthood are diverse and cannot be treated alike simply because they are in the same age group. With people living longer and healthier, more differences exist between individuals as they get older. As in the early phase of human development, changes continue to occur in late adulthood in biologic, cognitive, emotional, social, and moral areas. However, changes in late life focus more predominantly on loss or decline, which leads to either adaptive or maladaptive adjustment.

- Clinically, autistic spectrum disorders, with markedly impaired social reciprocity, communication deficits, and related symptoms, tend to become apparent in the first year of life.
- Reactive attachment disorder may result from abusive or neglectful parenting that causes serious disruptions in separation-individuation, basic trust, and autonomy.
- Psychiatric disorders that could emerge in preschool-aged children include separation anxiety, oppositional defiant disorder, and attention-deficit/hyperactivity disorder.
- In the Eriksonian stage of *industry versus inferiority*, children begin the long effort to master the cognitive and social skills that will ultimately equip them for adult roles.
- Preadolescents tend to stress the value of shared rules in sustaining good social relationships and maintaining social order. Preadolescence is also a time when social media can exert profound influence. Difficult to monitor, instantly accessible, and seemingly irresistible, social media can enhance a sense of connectivity, but they can also have potentially devastating effects, such as cyberbullying.

- Psychopathologies that can emerge during adolescence include eating disorders and schizophrenia.

Psychological Tasks in Aging

When an older person experiences increased vulnerability in later life, such as impairment or disability, the person faces conflicts with the theme of integrity versus despair. The primary task in this stage is to maintain ego integrity while avoiding despair. Erikson's eighth stage, *integrity versus despair*, is the most well-known developmental stage in late life. As people grow older, they achieve a sense of *integrity*, characterized as a feeling of satisfaction as they reflect on their life, fulfilling relationships, work productivity, contribution to society, and an overall feeling of having had purpose or meaning in life. In contrast, if they do not achieve a sense of integrity, they may be stuck in *despair*, characterized by an overall discontent with life, filled with regret and disappointment, and a feeling of not having had any purpose or meaning in life.

Throughout the life cycle, an individual develops psychological defense mechanisms for psychological survival (see Table 36.1 in Chapter 36, "Principles of Psychiatry and Psychology"). Defense mechanisms have been conceptualized and categorized in different ways, although the most common are Vaillant's categories, which include pathologic, immature, neurotic, and mature defenses. Mature defenses, the healthiest defenses, allow an older person to cope and adapt to the challenges of aging. Examples of mature defenses are sublimation (conscious transformation of socially unacceptable impulses into socially acceptable behavior), humor (ability to look at oneself with humor and constructively deal with an otherwise painful or uncomfortable situation), suppression (conscious effort to restrict unwanted thoughts or feelings), and altruism (service to others that is rewarding and pleasurable). Even though successful adaptation depends on the defense mechanisms used throughout one's adult life, defense mechanisms are not static. Even in old age, mature defenses can be learned, and other maladaptive defenses minimized or extinguished. When Vaillant followed a group of Harvard freshmen into old age, he found that maladaptive coping mechanisms can decrease and adaptive coping mechanisms can increase over time; mature coping mechanisms were linked to success and fulfillment in old age.

Kohut developed the concept of self-psychology from the Freudian theory of the id, ego, and superego. However, Kohut focused on the development of the sense of self and the maintenance of self-esteem. Kohut's emphasis on narcissism applies to old age because it is commonly a season of life when a person must continually cope with narcissistic injury from multiple losses experienced in the process of aging. A major developmental task in old age is maintenance of self-esteem, which can be achieved with maintenance of emotional and physical functioning, adequate social support, mature coping, and economic security. Inability of an older person to maintain self-esteem results in depression, anxiety, anger, and dissatisfaction.

Levinson developed a theory of adult development that suggests that growth and development continue into adult years. According to Levinson, a transitional period occurs at age 60 to 65 years, when a person passes into late adulthood. A major event is retirement, but other turning points include physical decline, loss of loved ones, and a clearer sense of one's own mortality. An older person must struggle with losses and successfully navigate the transition in order to create a new life structure.

Psychosocial Aspects of Aging

Retirement

Retirement is a major life event in late adulthood that is generally anticipated with pleasure and planning. Retired persons look forward to leisure and freedom from employment responsibilities. While some continue to work, others pursue new or old hobbies, travel, engage in charity work, and stay connected with family and friends. However, retirement becomes stressful when unplanned or when accompanied by economic hardship. In a society that values productivity, retired persons may find themselves contending with low self-esteem, isolation, and loneliness and with feeling useless and unproductive.

Widowhood and Widowerhood

Death of a spouse is the most stressful of all life events and causes significant suffering among widows and widowers. Although their grief and mourning may last for years, most are able to cope. Women live longer than men, and the ratio of widows to widowers is 4 to 1. There are sex differences in coping with the death of a spouse. Widows cope better emotionally, are able to connect with a social network, and pursue new activities, although they experience more financial stress. Widowers, in contrast to widows, are more likely to remarry and are more prone to early death. In the United States, white widowers who are 85 years or older are at highest risk of suicide.

Sexuality

There is a myth that sexual activity stops in old age. The main challenge for widows and widowers is finding a new partner, particularly since women outnumber men in old age. In addition, societal negative attitudes about sexuality in late adulthood discourage older adults from being more open about sexuality. Sexual desire and the ability to enjoy sexual activity do not decrease in old age despite aging-related biologic changes that lead to decreased sexual performance, although advancing age may require a change in pace and approach.

Relationships

People now live longer and therefore develop longer relationships with family and friends. Older adults generally perceive relationships with grown children and with other older adults as positive. Grandparenting is a role that is also often viewed positively, allows an older person to find further meaning and purpose in life, and provides an opportunity to pass on values and wisdom to a younger generation. Having close friends and maintaining a social network help older adults maintain self-esteem, reduce isolation, and avoid depression.

Socioeconomics

Many older individuals live below the poverty level, and poor economic conditions adversely affect their psychological, physical, and social well-being. Retirement benefits from Social Security require a person to have worked 10 years. Despite the availability of Medicare and Medicaid, older adults may have limited access to health care, especially mental health care. Long-term care is costly—whether in a nursing home, assisted living facility, or other health care facility—and the expense is not covered by Medicare. Prescription medications are often expensive and prohibitive costs may contribute to treatment nonadherence.

Death and Dying

Thanatology is the study of the biopsychosocial aspects of death and dying. The concept of the irreversibility of death is understood by a person at around the age of 7. In late adulthood, people experience the deaths of loved ones and are faced with the eventuality of their own death. Those who feel that their lives have had meaning and purpose are more inclined to accept death peacefully and without fear. However, those who perceive their lives as not having had meaning often react negatively to death. Kübler-Ross

---

Box 37.1 • Kübler-Ross' 5 Stages of Grief

1. Denial
2. Anger
3. Bargaining
4. Depression
5. Acceptance

---

described 5 stages of grief when people face their own impending death: denial, anger, bargaining, depression, and acceptance (Box 37.1). There is no sequence to these reactions, nor do people progress through all stages. Individuals who have engaged in an active practice of faith—as opposed to occasional conformity to the external trappings of a religion—characteristically face death with a perspective that places material life in this world in a broader context and thereby often enables them to view death as a transition to a continuing but different reality. Some people benefit from the process of life review through reminiscing, reflecting on the meaning and purpose of their lives, and achieving greater peace. However, some people become stuck in the negative aspects of a personal life review and become increasingly anxious about impending death. Palliative and hospice programs can provide excellent care to persons at the end of life and assist the patient and family in maintaining the best possible quality of life.

- In a society that values productivity, retired persons may find themselves contending with low self-esteem, isolation, and loneliness and with feeling useless and unproductive.
- Having close friends and maintaining a social network help older adults maintain self-esteem, reduce isolation, and avoid depression.
- Kübler-Ross described 5 stages of grief when people face their own impending death: denial, anger, bargaining, depression, and acceptance.

Mood Disorders

SIMON KUNG, MD

Introduction

Mood disorders (depression and bipolar disorders) are the second most common set of psychiatric disorders, behind anxiety disorders. The lifetime prevalence of any mood disorder in US adults is approximately 20%, and the 12-month prevalence is approximately 10%.

Common mood disorders and their treatment are discussed below. Additional information on pharmacologic therapy and electroconvulsive therapy is covered in Chapter 45, "Pharmacologic Treatment of Psychiatric Disorders."

Depressive Disorders

Major Depressive Disorder

Epidemiology

Major depressive disorder (MDD) and dysthymia are the 2 main diagnoses describing patients with unipolar depressed mood. The lifetime prevalence of MDD in US adults is approximately 17%, and the 12-month prevalence is approximately 7%. The average age at onset is 32 years, with MDD affecting nearly twice as many women as men. MDD was the leading cause of disability in the Western world in 2010.

Clinical Features

The *Diagnostic and Statistical Manual of Mental Disorders* (Fifth Edition) criteria for a major depressive episode require a 2-week duration of a change in previous functioning in which at least 5 of 9 symptoms must occur on more days than not, and at least 1 of the symptoms must be either depressed mood or loss of interest or pleasure. In children and adolescents, irritability can substitute for depressed mood. The 9 symptoms include depressed mood in addition to 8 others, which can be remembered with the mnemonic *SIGECAPS* (Box 38.1). The symptoms must cause clinically significant distress or impairment in functioning and cannot be attributed to medications, underlying medical causes, or normal bereavement. Additional qualifiers indicate other features: occurrence (single [ie, first episode] or recurrent), severity, presence of psychotic symptoms, subtype (melancholic, atypical, or catatonic), and timing (postpartum onset or seasonal component).

Diagnosis

The diagnosis of MDD is based on the clinical interview. There are no diagnostic laboratory or imaging tests, but medical and neurologic contributors to depression (eg, thyroid abnormalities, brain tumors) must be ruled

---

Box 38.1 • Mnemonic for Symptoms of Major Depressive Disorder: SIGECAPS

*S*leep disturbance (insomnia or hypersomnia)
*I*nterest in activities decreased—anhedonia
*G*uilty feelings or feeling worthless
*E*nergy decreased—fatigue
*C*oncentration decreased or indecisiveness
*A*ppetite change (gain or loss of weight)
*P*sychomotor agitation or retardation
*S*uicidal thoughts

Abbreviations: MDD, major depressive disorder; PHQ-9, Patient Health Questionnaire; SSRI, selective serotonin reuptake inhibitor; STAR*D, Sequenced Treatment Alternatives to Relieve Depression; NOS, not otherwise specified; IPSRT, interpersonal and social rhythm therapy

out. Screening instruments can assist in the diagnosis. The Patient Health Questionnaire (PHQ-9) is commonly used, especially in primary care settings. The patient marks how often the 9 symptoms of depression are experienced: none of the time, less than half the time, more than half the time, or almost all the time. A score of more than 4 warrants further discussion with the patient. Differential diagnoses of MDD include the possibility of other mood, personality, or substance-use disorders, and diagnoses can be more difficult with concurrent medical illness when the symptoms of the illness overlap with the symptoms of depression.

Treatment

The treatment of MDD is guided by the biopsychosocial model, recognizing that biologic, psychological, and social factors all contribute to a patient's depression, and thus all domains need to be addressed. In mild to moderate depression, psychotherapy alone can be used, while in moderate to severe depression, medications are recommended. The best outcomes result when both medications and psychotherapies are used. Once MDD is in remission, the same medications should be continued at the same dosages for at least 9 to 12 months for the first episode of depression. For subsequent episodes, the duration of treatment extends to years.

Antidepressants are the mainstay of pharmacologic treatment, beginning with a first-line selective serotonin reuptake inhibitor (SSRI). If an antidepressant results in no benefit after an adequate duration (approximately 2 months) at a maximum or near-maximum dose, the medication should be switched to a different antidepressant. That next antidepressant can be from the same class or a different class, such as a serotonin-norepinephrine reuptake inhibitor, a tricyclic, a monoamine oxidase inhibitor, or another drug such as bupropion or mirtazapine. If an antidepressant results in partial benefit, it can be combined with another antidepressant or augmented with a nonantidepressant, such as a mood stabilizer (eg, lithium carbonate), an atypical antipsychotic (eg, aripiprazole, olanzapine, quetiapine), or others (eg, liothyronine). In general, the antidepressants have similar efficacy, and medication selections are guided by patient response, patient preference, the ability of the medication to treat other symptoms (such as pain), and side effects. With each successive medication trial, the chances of remission decrease. In the large National Institute of Mental Health–sponsored Sequenced Treatment Alternatives to Relieve Depression (STAR*D) study of MDD treatment, the initial remission rate with a first-line SSRI (citalopram) was about 30%. After a second antidepressant trial, the remission rate was approximately 21%, and after a third and fourth antidepressant trial, remission rates were 16% and 7%, respectively. However, the cumulative remission rate after these 4 medication trials was calculated to be approximately 50%. Note that remission (the absence of symptoms or the presence of only a few symptoms) is a more stringent measure than response (improvement of 50% from baseline).

Brain stimulation techniques such as electroconvulsive therapy, transcranial magnetic stimulation, and vagal nerve stimulation can be considered for treatment-resistant depression. Electroconvulsive therapy is discussed further in Chapter 45, "Pharmacologic Treatment of Psychiatric Disorders." Transcranial magnetic stimulation consists of outpatient stimulation of the left dorsolateral prefrontal cortex daily for 4 to 6 weeks; open-label studies have reported response rates of up to 56% and remission rates of up to 30%. Vagal nerve stimulation is also used in treatment-resistant epilepsy and involves implantation of a device, with a 9- to 12-month wait for a 30% response. Deep brain stimulation for depression is promising but still investigational.

In addition to biologic treatment of MDD, it is imperative to recommend psychosocial interventions. Psychological interventions include individual and group treatments. Cognitive behavioral therapy is the most common and has the most evidence of efficacy. Supportive psychotherapies help patients build on strengths and coping strategies. Improvement of patient social stresses, such as relationship conflicts, occupational stresses, and financial stresses, are also important.

Dysthymia

Dysthymia, or dysthymic disorder, is a low-grade chronic depression occurring most of the day for more days than not and lasting at least 2 years without more than 2 months of symptom remission. The depressed mood is accompanied by at least 2 of the following: sleep disturbance, appetite change, low energy, poor concentration or indecisiveness, low self-esteem, and hopelessness. In children and adolescents, the mood can be irritable instead of depressed, and the minimum duration is 1 year. The symptom severity does not reach the level of major depression in that patients can typically function and perform their life activities.

Dysthymia is not as well studied as MDD, and the differential diagnosis includes depressive personality. Patients can receive a diagnosis of both dysthymia and major depressive episode (ie, *double depression*). Treatment of dysthymia is the same as for MDD, with perhaps more emphasis on psychological interventions.

- The 9 symptoms of major depressive disorder (MDD) include depressed mood in addition to 8 others, which can be remembered with the mnemonic *SIGECAPS* (Box 38.1).
- Antidepressants are the mainstay of pharmacologic treatment of MDD, beginning with a first-line SSRI.
- In the large National Institute of Mental Health–sponsored STAR*D study of MDD treatment, the initial

remission rate with a first-line SSRI (citalopram) was about 30%; however, the cumulative remission rate after 4 medication trials improved to approximately 50%.

Bipolar Disorders

Overview

The hallmark of bipolar disorder (formerly known as manic-depressive disorder or bipolar affective disorder) is sustained elevated mood or extreme irritability different from baseline. Depressive episodes are also expected. The severity and duration of these mood episodes defines bipolar I disorder, bipolar II disorder, bipolar disorder–not otherwise specified (NOS), and cyclothymia.

Epidemiology

The lifetime prevalence of bipolar disorders in US adults is approximately 4%, and the 12-month prevalence is approximately 2.6%. The average age at onset is 25 years, with women and men affected about equally.

Clinical Features

Bipolar I Disorder

In bipolar I disorder, patients experience manic episodes in addition to major depressive episodes. For bipolar I disorder, a manic episode is defined by at least 7 days of euphoric mood or extreme irritability with at least 3 (4 if the mood is only irritable) of the symptoms in the mnemonic *DIGFAST* (Box 38.2). The 7-day duration criterion is not needed if psychiatric hospitalization results because of the manic behaviors. In these manic episodes, there might be psychotic symptoms. Depressive symptoms might also coexist with manic symptoms, such that the criteria for both manic episode and major depressive episode are satisfied. Such cases are *mixed episodes.*

Box 38.2 • Mnemonic for Symptoms of Bipolar I Disorder: *DIGFAST*

*D*istractibility

*I*nsomnia (decreased need for sleep)

*G*randiosity or inflated self-esteem

*F*light of ideas or racing thoughts

*A*ctivities (increased goal-directed activities) or *A*gitation (psychomotor agitation)

*S*peech (increased or pressured speech)

*T*houghtlessness (impulsivity such as spending sprees, sexual indiscretions, reckless driving)

Bipolar II Disorder

In bipolar II disorder, patients experience hypomanic episodes (defined as duration >4 days but <7 days of the same symptom criteria as for bipolar I disorder) and major depressive episodes. The hypomanic episodes of bipolar II disorder do not significantly impair functioning and cannot contain psychotic symptoms. Patients still perform their daily activities, but their symptoms differ from baseline and are noticed by others. The qualifier *rapid cycling* is used to describe bipolar I disorder and bipolar II disorder when there are more than 4 mood episodes (manic, hypomanic, or depressive) in 1 year.

Other

Bipolar disorder–NOS describes bipolar disorders that do not satisfy the criteria for bipolar I disorder or bipolar II disorder (eg, symptom criteria are met and there is definite mood cycling, but the duration is <4 days). *Cyclothymia* describes sustained cycling of mood in which there are hypomanic episodes, but the depressive episodes do not meet criteria for a major depressive episode.

Diagnosis

The diagnosis of bipolar disorder is made clinically since there are no laboratory or imaging tests to confirm the diagnosis. Manic episodes are easier to distinguish than subtler hypomanic episodes. If a manic or hypomanic episode occurs, but the patient has never had a depressive episode, a future depressive episode is considered inevitable, and bipolar disorder remains the diagnosis. Because most mood episodes in bipolar disorder are depressive episodes, differentiating a bipolar depressive episode from a unipolar depressive episode can be difficult. Factors that suggest bipolar disorder instead of major depression include earlier onset of symptoms (which can be in the teenaged years), postpartum depression, unexpected effects of antidepressants (eg, worsening of symptoms or induction of hypomania or mania), and family history of bipolar disorder.

Up to 50% of patients with bipolar disorder might have a comorbid substance use disorder, compared with approximately 33% of patients with unipolar depression. Other difficulties in diagnosing bipolar disorder are the overlap of symptoms: Racing thoughts, insomnia, irritability, and mood swings can also be seen in depressive disorders, anxiety disorders, or personality styles or disorders.

Treatment

Pharmacologic treatment of bipolar disorder must take into account the phase of illness, that is, whether the patient is manic, is having mixed episodes, is depressed, or is euthymic and needs maintenance therapy. Traditionally, mood stabilizers such as lithium and anticonvulsants (especially valproic acid) are used; in the medical literature, valproic acid is preferred to lithium for rapid cycling bipolar disorder. More recently, atypical antipsychotic monotherapy has been used for manic, mixed, and depressive phases, but there are concerns about metabolic side effects. The use of antidepressants in bipolar disorder is controversial because of the risk of a switch to mania. Generally, the use of antidepressants is avoided in bipolar I disorder, but their use is considered for other types of bipolar disorder. Lamotrigine has benefit for bipolar disorder maintenance and depression, but it is not an effective antimanic medication. There is more evidence of efficacy in bipolar disorders for anticonvulsants such as valproic acid, carbamazepine, oxcarbazepine, and lamotrigine than for gabapentin and topiramate. The combination of mood stabilizers and atypical antipsychotics can be more effective in cases that are more difficult to treat. Adherence to medical therapy is an important issue because of patients' desire to feel the elevations of hypomania and mania and to avoid medication side effects.

Despite perceptions that the main focus of treating bipolar disorders is medications, a biopsychosocial treatment approach is still the ideal. Cognitive behavioral therapy, psychoeducation (to help patients understand and accept their illness and the importance of medication adherence), family therapy (to engage family support), and interpersonal and social rhythm therapy (IPSRT) can all be used. IPSRT teaches the patient how to improve interpersonal relationships and communications and how to keep a regular schedule, including sleep, to minimize potential episode triggers. Elements of dialectical behavioral therapy are useful in nonmedication approaches to control mood swings and irritability. Comorbidities such as substance abuse must be treated, and sobriety must be ensured.

- For bipolar I disorder, a manic episode is defined by ≥7 days of euphoric mood or extreme irritability with ≥3 (4 if the mood is only irritable) of the symptoms in the mnemonic *DIGFAST* (Box 38.2).
- The hypomanic episodes of bipolar II disorder do not significantly impair functioning and cannot contain psychotic symptoms.
- Factors that suggest bipolar disorder instead of major depression include earlier onset of symptoms (which can be in the teenaged years), postpartum depression, unexpected effects of antidepressants (eg, worsening of symptoms or induction of hypomania or mania), and family history of bipolar disorder.

- Traditionally, bipolar disorder has been treated with mood stabilizers such as lithium and anticonvulsants (especially valproic acid); in the medical literature, valproic acid is preferred to lithium for rapid cycling bipolar disorder. More recently, atypical antipsychotic monotherapy has been used for manic, mixed, and depressive phases.

Mood Disorder Due to a General Medical Condition

When a medical condition (eg, stroke, hypothyroidism) physiologically affects mood symptoms (depressive or manic), the preferred diagnosis is mood disorder due to a general medical condition. When the medical condition resolves (if reversible), the mood disorder also resolves. In clinical practice, the diagnosis might be used more loosely, and differential diagnoses include adjustment disorders and full MDDs.

Treatment consists of optimizing therapy for the medical condition and using standard mood disorder treatments. Whenever possible, management strategies should be parsimonious with medications (eg, choosing antidepressants with pain benefit if pain is an issue) and avoid medications that might exacerbate medical conditions (eg, foregoing use of a medication that has the potential to cause weight gain in an already overweight patient).

Substance-Induced Mood Disorder

When mood symptoms occur within 1 month after substance use, intoxication, or withdrawal, the diagnosis of substance-induced mood disorder is appropriate. If sobriety can be achieved and maintained, and the mood symptoms then remit, the substance-induced diagnosis is confirmed. However, many patients have comorbidities and require separate diagnoses for a mood disorder and a substance use disorder (ie, *dual diagnosis*). Comorbidity of substance abuse is high among patients with depression (33%) or bipolar disorder (up to 50%).

The substances in this diagnosis are not limited to alcohol or illicit drugs. Medications such as prednisone can also induce mood symptoms and may be included in the diagnosis of substance-induced mood disorder.

39 Anxiety Disorders

MICHAEL M. REESE, MD

Introduction

Anxiety disorders are among the most frequent psychiatric ailments in US adults, with lifetime and 12-month prevalence rates of 29% and 18%, respectively. Nearly 30 million people are affected in the United States, with females affected nearly twice as frequently as males. Estimated annual costs related to anxiety disorders, including lost productivity, death, and treatment expenses, are more than $42 billion.

Anxiety disorders and their treatment are discussed in this chapter. Further discussion of pharmacologic agents used in anxiety disorders is found in Chapter 45, "Pharmacologic Treatment of Psychiatric Disorders."

- Anxiety disorders are among the most frequent psychiatric ailments in US adults, with lifetime and 12-month prevalence rates of 29% and 18%, respectively.

Panic Disorder

Epidemiology

The lifetime prevalence of panic disorder is reported to be 1.5% to 3.5%. Females are 2 to 3 times more likely to be affected than males. Onset can occur at any age, but panic disorder commonly arises in late adolescence to the mid 30s.

Etiology

Etiologic theories abound. Biologic underpinnings are suggested by the fact that intravenous sodium lactate or inhaled carbon dioxide can induce panic attacks in susceptible individuals. Brain imaging studies suggest amygdala hyperactivity and decreased prefrontal cortical regulation of fear circuitry. First-degree relatives of individuals with panic disorder are up to 8 times more likely to have this condition. Cognitive theorists note that individuals with panic disorder often show a strong propensity to misinterpret physical symptoms.

Clinical Features

The signature feature of panic disorder is recurrent, unexpected panic attacks. Panic attacks are discrete periods of intense fear or distress, cued or not. They have an abrupt onset, typically last 5 to 20 minutes, and are commonly associated with autonomic symptoms.

Although panic attacks can be isolated events, in panic disorder the onset of panic attacks is followed by at least 1 month of persistent concern about having another panic attack. In addition, the person is concerned about what the panic attacks may signify and adopts behavioral changes, including phobic avoidance, in an effort to cope with these attacks.

Panic disorder may or may not be associated with agoraphobia. Agoraphobia is characterized by intense anxiety about being in places or situations from which egress may be difficult or embarrassing, or in which assistance might be unavailable. Individuals with agoraphobia avoid the associated circumstances or endure the situations with great discomfort, worry about experiencing a panic attack, or require the presence of a companion.

Significant comorbidity exists between panic disorder and multiple medical conditions, including cardiac, endocrine, gastrointestinal, and pulmonary disorders. At the outset, a nonpsychiatric physician assesses most patients

Abbreviations: ASD, acute stress disorder; CBT, cognitive behavioral therapy; EMDR, eye movement desensitization and reprocessing; GABA, γ-aminobutyric acid; GAD, generalized anxiety disorder; OCD, obsessive-compulsive disorder; PTSD, posttraumatic stress disorder

with panic disorder. Individuals may receive extensive medical evaluations for various somatic symptoms. Rates of comorbid major depression in individuals with panic disorder range from 10% to 65%. Other anxiety disorders co-occur at rates ranging from 5% to 30%. Comorbid substance abuse occurs in approximately 15% of individuals with panic disorder.

Clinical Course and Prognosis

The course of panic disorder is often punctuated by periods of exacerbation and remission. Over the long-term course, approximately 30% to 40% of affected persons recover, 50% have limited impairment, and 10% to 20% have significant impairment. Predictors of worse prognosis are more severe initial panic attacks, presence of agoraphobia, longer duration of illness, comorbid depression, history of separation from a parent, high interpersonal sensitivity, and single marital status.

Treatment

Cognitive behavioral therapy (CBT) and exposure therapy can be effective alone or in conjunction with anxiolytic medications. CBT begins with psychoeducation regarding the CBT model of panic disorder.

- Panic attacks are discrete periods of intense fear or distress, cued or not. They have an abrupt onset, typically last 5–20 minutes, and are commonly associated with autonomic symptoms.
- Rates of comorbid major depression in individuals with panic disorder range from 10%-65%.

Obsessive-Compulsive Disorder

Epidemiology

The lifetime prevalence of obsessive-compulsive disorder (OCD) in the general population is estimated to be 2% to 3%. Among adults, OCD is slightly more frequent in woman, but among adolescents, males are more commonly affected. The mean age at onset is about 20 years, with two-thirds of cases beginning before age 25.

Etiology

OCD is believed to be a neurobiological illness tied in part to serotonergic dysregulation. From a neuroimmunologic standpoint, there may be an association between streptococcal infection and OCD. Positron emission tomography suggests increased activity in the frontal lobes and basal ganglia in individuals with OCD. Relatives of probands with OCD consistently have a 3-fold to 5-fold higher likelihood of having OCD or obsessive-compulsive features than families of control probands.

Clinical Features

More than 50% of individuals with OCD have a sudden onset of symptoms. In 50% to 70% of patients, the onset of symptoms occurs after a stressful event. There is often a delay of 5 to 10 years before an individual seeks psychiatric attention.

OCD is defined by recurrent obsessions or compulsions that are time-consuming (taking up >1 hour daily), cause marked distress, or significantly impair routine functioning. The individual recognizes that the obsessions or compulsions are unreasonable and typically avoids the objects or circumstances that provoke the obsessions or compulsions. Both obsessions and compulsions are present in 80% of individuals with OCD. Compulsive behaviors most often follow obsessional thinking. Acting on the compulsions is usually an attempt to reduce the angst associated with the obsession or prevent some dreaded event or situation. Common obsessions include repeated thoughts about contamination, repeated doubts, the need to have things in a specific order, aggressive impulses, and sexual imagery. Common compulsions include washing and cleaning, checking, or counting.

OCD is frequently comorbid with other mental illnesses. The lifetime prevalence for major depressive disorder in individuals with OCD is approximately 67%. The incidence of comorbid Tourette disorder is 5% to 7%. Other common comorbid psychiatric diagnoses include alcohol abuse, eating disorders, and other anxiety-spectrum disorders.

Clinical Course and Prognosis

The course of OCD is variable but almost never brief. About 20% to 30% of individuals have significant improvement in their symptoms; 40% to 50% have moderate symptoms, and 20% to 30% have either persistent illness or worsening symptoms. Factors associated with a good prognosis include obsessions without accompanying compulsions, abrupt onset, episodic rather than chronic symptoms, and overall good social and occupational functioning.

Treatment

A combination of a serotonergic agent and CBT is considered the most effective treatment. The behavioral treatment component of OCD includes exposure and response (ritual) prevention. Exposure is more beneficial in decreasing obsessions, whereas response prevention is more helpful in decreasing compulsive behavior. In individuals with marked chronic debility and treatment refractoriness, electroconvulsive therapy and psychosurgery are considerations. Although infrequent, the most commonly performed surgery is anterior cingulotomy. Nonablative surgical techniques (eg, deep brain stimulation) are under investigation.

- In 50%-70% of patients with obsessive compulsive disorder (OCD), the onset of symptoms occurs after a stressful event.
- For OCD, a combination of a serotonergic agent and CBT is considered the most effective treatment.

Acute Stress Disorder

Overview and Definition

Acute stress disorder (ASD) involves the development of physiologic and psychological responses that occur following exposure to 1 or more situations involving death, serious injury, or a threat to physical integrity. Events such as natural disasters, explosions, physical or sexual assaults, or motor vehicle accidents exemplify events that may lead to this disorder.

Epidemiology

The point prevalence of ASD following trauma exposure has been estimated at 5% to 20%, depending on the nature and severity of the event and the instrument used to measure the disorder. Rates of ASD after a motor vehicle crash are 13% to 21%; after assault, 16% to 19%; and after witnessing a mass shooting, 33%. The risk of ASD after a traumatic event is associated with the following characteristics: history of an antecedent psychiatric disorder, history of prior traumatic exposures, female sex, trauma severity, eroticism, lack of social supports, and avoidant coping.

Clinical Features

Characteristic symptoms of ASD include having 3 or more dissociative symptoms. These symptoms may include a subjective sense of numbing, detachment or absence of emotional responsiveness, derealization, depersonalization, and dissociative amnesia. Other features include persistently reexperiencing the traumatic event through recurrent dreams, images, thoughts, or flashbacks; marked avoidance of stimuli that bring recollections of the events; and severe symptoms of anxiety that may include irritability, sleep disturbance, restlessness, and hypervigilance. The symptoms must result in clinically significant distress and markedly interfere with normal functioning.

By definition, ASD occurs within 4 weeks following trauma exposure and lasts for a minimum of 2 days. Should the duration of symptoms exceed 1 month following trauma exposure, posttraumatic stress disorder (PTSD) is diagnosed. Retrospective studies have found that in 72% to 83% of individuals with ASD, PTSD develops 6 months after the trauma and that 63% to 80% of those with ASD meet criteria for PTSD 2 years after the trauma.

Treatment

Evidence suggests that exposure-based, trauma-focused CBT is efficacious in the early aftermath of a traumatic event. Psychological debriefing does not appear to be helpful in protecting against the development of PTSD and may have harmful effects.

- Acute stress disorder (ASD) involves the development of physiologic and psychological responses that occur following exposure to ≥1 situations involving death, serious injury, or a threat to physical integrity.
- The risk of ASD after a traumatic event is associated with the following characteristics: history of an antecedent psychiatric disorder, history of prior traumatic exposures, female sex, trauma severity, eroticism, lack of social supports, and avoidant coping.

Posttraumatic Stress Disorder

Overview

PTSD is defined by the development of symptoms after exposure to a traumatic event or events marked by actual or threatened death or serious injury or a threat to the integrity of self or others. Three cardinal features are hyperarousal, intrusive reexperiencing (flashbacks) of the initial trauma, and psychic numbing and avoidance of reminders of the trauma. Duration of symptoms is more than 1 month. The symptoms cause clinically significant distress or impairment in routine functioning. Individuals with PTSD may describe painful guilt feelings about surviving when others did not survive or about taking actions that were necessary to survive.

Epidemiology

The lifetime incidence of PTSD is estimated to be 9% to 15%. The lifetime prevalence in the general population is about 8%. Although approximately 38% of the general population is exposed to catastrophic stressors, PTSD develops in only a fraction of these individuals. PTSD can occur at any age, but it is most prevalent in young adulthood and is much more likely to occur in females. The likelihood of PTSD developing may increase as the intensity and physical proximity to the stressor increases. The highest rates are found among survivors of rape, military combat and captivity, and ethnically or politically motivated incarceration and genocide.

Clinical Features

Symptoms typically begin within 3 months after the trauma; however, sometimes symptoms are delayed months or even years. Complete recovery occurs within 3 months in nearly half of individuals, while others have a much more persistent course, with some experiencing a waxing and waning course over years. Symptom reactivation may occur in response to reminders of the original trauma, life stressors, or new traumatic events. The course is often confounded if the risk of the trauma is ongoing or if the individual attempts to mitigate symptoms through self-medication with alcohol or drugs. The prognosis is best for those with strong support networks, fewer comorbid diagnoses, a rapid onset of symptoms, and engagement in empirically validated treatments.

PTSD is rarely an isolated diagnosis: 50% to 88% of individuals have at least 1 other concomitant diagnosis. The most prevalent comorbid diagnoses are major depressive disorder, alcohol abuse, other anxiety spectrum disorders, and somatization disorder.

Treatment

The main target of early intervention is the prevention of chronic PTSD. Studies have established the efficacy of early, trauma-focused, exposure-based CBT in preventing chronic PTSD. For chronic PTSD, trauma-focused CBT is also recommended. A variant of trauma-focused CBT, eye movement desensitization and reprocessing (EMDR), has shown efficacy in several well-controlled studies.

- Three cardinal features of posttraumatic stress disorder (PTSD) are hyperarousal, intrusive reexperiencing (flashbacks) of the initial trauma, and psychic numbing and avoidance of reminders of the trauma.
- The most prevalent comorbid diagnoses with PTSD are major depressive disorder, alcohol abuse, other anxiety spectrum disorders, and somatization disorder.

Generalized Anxiety Disorder

Overview

Generalized anxiety disorder (GAD) is manifested by a constellation of symptoms associated with excessive anxiety and worry occurring more days than not during a time frame of at least 6 months. The anxiety centers on various circumstances or situations. Individuals find it difficult to control and manage their worries. Symptoms associated with GAD can include trembling, diaphoresis, muscle tension, disturbed sleep, irritability, restlessness, and impaired concentration. The symptoms result in functional impairment. To make the diagnosis, as is the case with other anxiety disorders, the disturbance is ascertained not to be due to the direct physiologic effects of a substance or a nonpsychiatric medical condition.

Epidemiology

Lifetime prevalence is estimated to range from 4% to 8%. The disorder frequently commences in late adolescence or early adulthood. It is reported to be twice as common in females as males.

Twin studies suggest that GAD is associated with moderate heritability. About 25% of first-degree relatives of patients with GAD are also affected. Other postulated biologic mechanisms include amygdala hypersensitivity, serotonergic dysregulation, noradrenergic activation, and aberrancies in the γ-aminobutyric acid (GABA)-benzodiazepine receptor. Cognitive theories suggest a connection to early cognitive schemas arising from negative experiences of the world as a dangerous place or insecure, anxious early attachments to significant caregivers.

Clinical Features

Many individuals with GAD describe feeling anxious and nervous all their lives. Such individuals commonly report that there has never been a time in their lives, as far back as they can recollect, that they were not anxious. GAD tends to be a chronic, relapsing condition with marked morbidity. GAD appears to account for a great degree of anxiety in late life and is frequently comorbid with medical ailments.

In clinical settings, GAD is commonly comorbid with major depression and other anxiety disorders. Abuse of alcohol and anxiolytic medications is common and can confound the clinical presentation. In the elderly, it is especially vital to distinguish GAD from other anxiety states that could be connected to delirium, dementia, psychosis, or depression or that may be manifestations of underlying medical conditions.

Treatment

Several studies support various psychotherapies as being helpful in treating GAD, including stress management and problem-solving techniques along with CBT. Mild forms of GAD may respond to simple psychological measures such as assurance, explanation of somatic symptoms, clarification of conflicts, and discussion of coping mechanisms.

- Generalized anxiety disorder (GAD) frequently commences in late adolescence or early adulthood. It is reported to be twice as common in females as males.
- In the elderly, it is especially vital to distinguish GAD from other anxiety states that could be connected to delirium, dementia, psychosis, or depression or that may be manifestations of underlying medical conditions.

Specific Phobia

Overview

Specific phobia is defined by a marked and persistent fear that is triggered by the presence or anticipation of a specific object or situation. Being subjected to the phobic stimulus almost inevitably results in an immediate anxiety response that may include a panic attack. The phobic circumstance is avoided or endured with intense anxiety or distress. The avoidance leads to functional impairment, or there is marked stress at having a phobia. In descending order of frequency, specific phobias include animals, storms, heights, illness, injury, and death.

Epidemiology and Etiology

Phobic disorders are among the most common of all mental disorders and have a lifetime prevalence of approximately 10% to 11%. The onset typically is in childhood or early adulthood, with a median age at onset of 15 years. Females are affected more than twice as often as males.

The suggested causes of specific phobia include those with psychodynamic, behavioral, and biologic underpinnings. Specific phobia tends to run in families.

The age at onset has a bimodal distribution. Animal phobia, natural environment phobia, and blood-injection-injury phobia peak in childhood. Other phobias, such as situational phobias (except for fear of heights), have a peak in early adulthood (mid 20s).

Clinical Course and Prognosis

Relatively little is known about the long-term course of phobic disorders. Available data suggest that most specific phobias that begin in childhood continue into adulthood and persist for many years. Phobias persisting into adulthood have a spontaneous remission rate of approximately 20%. Unlike the fluctuating course typically seen with other anxiety disorders, the severity of specific phobias is thought to remain relatively constant. Most individuals with specific phobias learn to "live around" the phobic object by simply avoiding the situations where they may be exposed to the phobic stimulus.

Treatment

Behavioral or cognitive behavioral therapies are the most effective treatment modalities for specific phobia. Behavioral therapy includes 3 components: exposure, systematic desensitization, and participant modeling. Other psychotherapies may include psychodynamic-oriented therapy, hypnotherapy, supportive therapy, and family therapy.

Social Phobia

Overview

Social phobia, also known as social anxiety disorder, is a common condition that includes concerns associated with excessive fears of scrutiny, embarrassment, and humiliation in social or performance situations leading to marked distress or impairment in functioning. There are 2 subtypes

of social phobia: generalized and nongeneralized. In the generalized variety, a person experiences distressing fears in most social situations. In the nongeneralized subtype, the distress is limited to 1 or a few social circumstances, such as speaking in public, eating in public, or using public lavatories. In social phobia, the social situations are avoided or endured with dread and severe anxiety. Exposure to the triggering situations may lead to a panic attack.

Epidemiology

Social phobia typically manifests itself between ages 11 and 15 years. Although lifetime prevalence is reported to range from 5% to 7%, it is often unrecognized and undertreated. Only about 3% of individuals receive treatment. It is somewhat more common in females than males. In the general population, most individuals with social phobia fear public speaking.

A strong familial risk for social phobia has been identified, likely reflecting both heritable and environmental factors. Social phobia often evolves out of childhood traits of shyness and behavioral inhibition and a tendency to avoid novel people and experiences. Evidence exists for hyperactivity of the amygdala and associated fear circuitry in response to social threats.

Clinical Course and Prognosis

The course of social phobia tends to be chronic. The onset may abruptly follow a stressful or humiliating experience, or it may be insidious. The duration is often lifelong; however, the condition may diminish in severity or remit during adulthood.

Social phobia is associated with a 3- to 6-fold higher risk of major depressive disorder, dysthymic disorder, and bipolar disorder. Social phobia can be complicated by the use of alcohol or other substances in an effort at self-medication.

Treatment

Empirically validated psychosocial interventions for social phobia have primarily emanated from CBT. They encompass 4 main treatment approaches: exposure-based strategies, cognitive therapy, social skills training, and applied relaxation.

- For social phobia, evidence exists for hyperactivity of the amygdala and associated fear circuitry in response to social threats.

Anxiety Disorder Secondary to a General Medical Condition

To ascertain whether anxiety symptoms are a result of a medical condition, the clinician must first identify the presence of a medical illness and then establish that the symptoms are linked etiologically to the medical condition by a physiologic mechanism. In reaching this diagnosis, a thoughtful and comprehensive evaluation of multiple factors is required. Although no fool-proof guidelines exist for definitively concluding that the nexus between the anxiety symptoms and the medical condition is causative, several points provide direction in this endeavor: the presence of a temporal connection between onset, exacerbation, or remission of the general medical ailment and the anxiety symptoms; existence of features that are uncharacteristic of a primary anxiety disorder (eg, atypical age at onset or atypical course); and judgment by the clinician that the disturbance is not better accounted for by a primary anxiety disorder.

Nonpsychiatric medical causes of anxiety are legion and include cardiopulmonary, endocrine, neurologic, autoimmune, and toxic or metabolic disorders.

Substance-Induced Anxiety Disorder

In substance-induced anxiety disorder, patients present with panic, worry, phobias, or obsessions in the context of the use of either prescribed or nonprescribed substances, illicit substances, or exposure to heavy metals and toxins.

Reaching this diagnosis requires performing a physical examination and obtaining a comprehensive medical history that includes attention to all prescribed and nonprescribed pharmaceuticals the person is taking. In addition, a history of the individual's use of alcohol, tobacco, caffeine, and recreational drugs is necessary.

Appropriate laboratory screening may be useful and could include blood or urine specimens (or both) for drugs. The onset of this disorder can occur in the context of substance intoxication or substance withdrawal.

Psychotic Disorders

40

KEITH G. RASMUSSEN, MD

Introduction

Common psychotic disorders and their treatment are reviewed in this chapter. Additional information on pharmacologic treatment of psychotic disorders is found in Chapter 45, "Pharmacologic Treatment of Psychiatric Disorders."

Schizophrenia

Epidemiology

The prevalence of schizophrenia is approximately 1%, a figure strikingly similar across countries and cultures. Mean age at onset for males is typically in the early 20s, but for females it is in the late 20s. Schizophrenia only rarely remits entirely and is most often a chronic, disabling disorder characterized by exacerbations and partial remissions. It is associated with profound financial costs in terms of chronic needs for all aspects of functioning, including housing, medication, and medical care. Most schizophrenic patients lack gainful employment and receive government-sponsored disability payments.

First-degree relatives of a proband with schizophrenia have an approximately 10-fold higher risk of schizophrenia developing than the population at large. Additionally, twin and adoption studies show a much higher risk among biologic siblings of probands with schizophrenia.

Pathophysiology

The pathophysiology of schizophrenia is unknown but is thought to involve a disturbance in neurodevelopment. Structural brain studies have consistently found increased size of the lateral ventricles and decreased cortical thickness, although neither of these findings is sufficiently sensitive to be diagnostic of the disorder. Functional brain imaging studies of schizophrenic patients have shown decreased blood flow in the frontal lobes. Abnormalities of brain lateralization have also been found in electrophysiologic and brain imaging studies, as have alterations in smooth pursuit and saccadic eye movements. The neurotransmitter dopamine has been implicated in schizophrenia pathophysiology for decades, although no specific diagnostic test of dopamine function has emerged. In neuroimaging studies, a consistent finding has been excessive presynaptic dopaminergic function, while a less consistent finding has been excessive density of postsynaptic dopamine type 2 receptors. A newer avenue of investigation has focused on the glutamatergic receptor system, with 1 theory being that schizophrenia may represent hypofunction at N-methyl-D-aspartate (NMDA) receptors.

Clinical Features and Diagnostic Criteria

The generally accepted criteria for schizophrenia include 5 broad areas. Criterion A consists of *active-phase* symptoms of schizophrenia (Box 40.1). These include 1) delusions or hallucinations, 2) disorganized speech (reflecting disordered thought processes, such as loose associations or frank derailment), 3) disorganized behavior (ie, markedly odd, dysfunctional behavioral patterns), 4) catatonic signs, and 5) negative symptoms (eg, blunted affect, poverty of speech, social withdrawal, avolition). Criterion A is met if 2 of these 5 are present and the duration is at least 1 month (or shorter if treatment began within a month of onset). In some cases, only 1 of these is needed if the delusions are bizarre (eg, delusions of thought insertion, thought broadcasting, or thought withdrawal) or if the hallucinations are auditory and consist of 1 voice

---

Abbreviations: ASD, autistic spectrum disorder; NMDA, N-methyl-D-aspartate

> **Box 40.1 • Active-Phase Symptoms (Criterion A) of Schizophrenia**
>
> Delusions, hallucinations
> Disorganized speech
> Disorganized behavior
> Catatonic signs
> Negative symptoms (eg, blunted affect, social withdrawal)

commenting on ongoing behavior or 2 or more voices referring to the patient in the third person. Catatonic signs include disturbances of motor function, such as mutism, stupor, waxy flexibility, posturing, verbal perseverations, or strange facial expressions.

Criterion B describes significant social, occupational, self-care, or educational dysfunction as the result of the symptoms and signs of the disorder. Criterion C describes the duration requirements for schizophrenia: the active-phase symptoms must last at least 1 month (or less if being treated), but the total duration of illness, including prodromal and residual symptoms, must be at least 6 months. Prodromal symptoms occur before the classic active-phase symptoms of schizophrenia and typically consist of odd ideations (eg, ideas of reference, vague feelings of suspiciousness without blatant delusional belief), odd behavior (eg, whispering to oneself), or odd speech that is not severe enough to meet criterion A. Prodromal signs are often gradual in onset and subtle in nature; they may be appreciated as prodromal only after the subsequent onset of active-phase symptoms. Similarly, upon resolution of active-phase symptoms, whether spontaneously or with treatment, the patient typically has residual symptoms that, like prodromal symptoms, represent attenuated forms of the active phase of illness.

Criteria D, E, and F describe the features differentiating schizophrenia from schizoaffective disorder (see below), psychoses resulting from substances or medical conditions (see below), and autistic spectrum disorders (ASDs). In ASDs, if a previously existing pervasive developmental disorder is present, delusions or hallucinations must also be present for a diagnosis of schizophrenia to be rendered because patients with ASD often have oddities of behavior or speech and avolition.

Schizophrenia also has longitudinal course specifiers. These include *episodic with interepisode residual symptoms* (ie, ≥2 episodes of active-phase symptoms have occurred, with residual symptoms in between); *episodic with no interepisode residual symptoms* if active-phase symptoms completely resolve between episodes; *continuous*; and *single episode* with either partial or full remission. The additional specifier *with prominent negative symptoms* can be applied if blunted affect, alogia, or avolition is present.

Subcategories

Schizophrenia can be subcategorized into *disorganized, paranoid, catatonic, undifferentiated*, and *residual* types (Table 40.1).

Schizophreniform Disorder

Schizophreniform disorder has the essential clinical features of schizophrenia, which include prodromal, active-phase, and residual symptoms, lasting at least 1 month but no more than 6 months. Functional decline is also not required for a diagnosis of schizophreniform disorder. The specifier *with good prognostic features* indicates the presence of at least 2 of the following: less than 4 weeks elapse between the earliest departure from normal behavior to the onset of clearly psychotic symptoms; good premorbid functioning; the presence of confusion or perplexity (the so-called oneiroid state) when psychotic; and the absence of a flat or blunted affect. If fewer than 2 of these are present, the specifier *without good prognostic features* is used. The schizophreniform disorder diagnosis is used when a patient had a psychotic course exceeding 1 month but full recovery in less than 6 months or when a patient has not been psychotic for 6 months but is still ill, in which case the specifier *provisional* is used.

The mainstay of schizophrenia treatment is antipsychotic medications, which are reviewed in detail in Chapter 45, "Pharmacologic Treatment of Psychiatric Disorders." Electroconvulsive therapy is used less commonly for schizophrenia than in past decades, but it can be highly effective for patients with fulminant positive signs or catatonia. Additionally, rehabilitative efforts are usually undertaken to attempt to teach daily life or simple work skills to patients who have chronic schizophrenia. Most

Table 40.1 • Subtypes of Schizophrenia

Subtype	Description
Disorganized	Presence of disorganized speech and behavior along with flat or inappropriate affect and absence of catatonic signs
Paranoid	Presence of ≥1 delusions or auditory hallucinations in the absence of significant other active-phase symptoms
Catatonic	Presence of ≥1 prominent catatonic signs
Undifferentiated	Presence of active-phase symptoms that do not meet criteria for any of the other 3 types above
Residual	Attenuated psychotic signs or negative symptoms that do not meet criterion A

schizophrenic patients live with parents or in a group home and require intense case management and social work interventions to manage daily life.

- First-degree relatives of a proband with schizophrenia have an approximately 10-fold higher risk of schizophrenia developing than the population at large.
- Functional brain imaging studies of schizophrenic patients have shown decreased blood flow in the frontal lobes.
- *Active-phase* symptoms of schizophrenia include 1) delusions or hallucinations, 2) disorganized speech (reflecting disordered thought processes, such as loose associations or frank derailment), 3) disorganized behavior (ie, markedly odd, dysfunctional behavioral patterns), 4) catatonic signs, and 5) negative symptoms (eg, blunted affect, poverty of speech, social withdrawal, avolition).
- Schizophreniform disorder has the essential clinical features of schizophrenia, which include prodromal, active-phase, and residual symptoms, lasting ≥1 month but ≤6 months.
- Electroconvulsive therapy is used less commonly for schizophrenia than in past decades, but it can be highly effective for patients with fulminant positive signs or catatonia.

Schizoaffective Disorder

Epidemiology

Schizoaffective disorder is somewhat more common in women than men, predominantly because of the increased incidence of depressive episodes in women who have psychotic rather than manic or mixed states. Age at onset and longitudinal course tend to be intermediate between those for patients with bipolar disorder or schizophrenia. That is, schizoaffective disorder usually manifests in young adulthood but is more likely than schizophrenia to manifest first in middle age. It may be a chronic disabling condition but is more likely than schizophrenia to remit.

Clinical Features and Diagnostic Criteria

It has long been recognized that some patients do not fit into a classic schizophrenia category because they have significant bouts of either depression or mania (or both) but do not have a primary mood disorder. The concept of schizoaffective disorder covers patients who, during an illness, meet criteria for a major depressive or manic episode and also meet criterion A for schizophrenia concomitantly with the mood episode, but who have delusions or hallucinations without mood symptoms for at least 2 weeks. The period of psychosis without mood symptoms may precede

the mood episode or occur after its resolution (or both, which is a fairly typical pattern). If the mood episode is depressive, *depressive type* is the appropriate specifier, while *bipolar type* is used if there has been a manic or mixed-mood episode. Of note, there are no particular diagnostic tests that help distinguish schizoaffective disorder from other psychotic disorders, nor is the pathophysiology of this disorder known.

Treatment

The treatment of schizoaffective disorder during acute episodes usually involves at least an antipsychotic agent; second-generation compounds are the first choice. The decision to add an antidepressant or mood-stabilizing drug (in the instance of mania) depends on the response to antipsychotic medication alone. Most psychiatrists advise against the use of an antidepressant medication during the fulminant psychotic phase of the illness because the medication may worsen the psychosis. If the clinician is certain that the episode is a psychotic depression that is a component of major depressive or bipolar disorder, concomitant antidepressant and antipsychotic medication is the pharmacologic standard. After an appropriate period of single-therapy antipsychotic medication, however, if the psychosis has resolved but the depressive symptoms persist, addition of an antidepressant is indicated. For manic or mixed episodes, an antipsychotic agent alone usually quells the symptoms sufficiently along with the psychosis; addition of an antimanic drug is needed only if there is incomplete resolution of the mania or if a prophylactic regimen is needed later.

- The concept of schizoaffective disorder covers patients who, during an illness, meet criteria for a major depressive or manic episode and also meet criterion A for schizophrenia concomitantly with the mood episode, but who have delusions or hallucinations without mood symptoms for ≥2 weeks.

Brief Psychotic Disorder

Epidemiology

Since brief psychotic disorder rarely comes to the attention of medical or mental health practitioners, data on the prevalence, sex ratio, and pathophysiology are extremely scarce.

Clinical Features

Brief psychotic disorder is a syndrome of psychosis that lasts at least 1 day but no more than 1 month and is not caused by a substance or general medical condition. The symptoms include at least 1 of the following: delusions, hallucinations, disorganized speech, or grossly disorganized or catatonic behavior. These symptoms must not be considered a normal part of the person's sociocultural context. For example, in some cultures it is considered normal for a grieving person to hear the voice of the recently deceased spouse, and this would not qualify for the diagnosis of a brief psychotic disorder. The specifiers *with marked stressors* or *without marked stressors* may be used to denote whether a precipitating life stressor preceded the psychosis, and *with postpartum onset* can be specified if the psychosis occurs within 4 weeks of the patient giving birth. In that case, the symptoms cannot meet criteria for another type of psychosis, such as mania or depression with psychotic features.

- Brief psychotic disorder is a syndrome of psychosis that lasts ≥1 day but ≤1 month and is not caused by a substance or general medical condition.

Delusional Disorder

Epidemiology

People with delusional disorder do not usually seek psychiatric help, so precise data on the average age at onset, longitudinal course, and treatment outcomes are scarce. In samples of patients clinically treated in outpatient settings, there is a female preponderance, while in forensic settings (eg, jails, prisons, referrals from courts) there is a male preponderance.

Clinical Features

Delusional disorder is characterized by the presence of delusions without hallucinations, thought or behavioral disorganization, catatonia, or negative symptoms. The delusions must not be "bizarre" in the sense that the beliefs are events that could plausibly occur. For example, if a man believes that the Federal Bureau of Investigation is investigating him, even in the face of contradictory evidence, such investigations do occur. However, if he believes that electrodes have been placed in his brain to monitor his thoughts, that would constitute a bizarre delusion and the diagnosis would more likely be another psychotic disorder such as schizophrenia.

From a distance, people with delusional disorder appear to be normal. They do not exhibit overtly odd behavior, although they tend to be loners. The syndrome is chronic and may, over many years or decades, progressively worsen to the point that the person exhibits sufficiently disruptive behavior (like complaining to the authorities or to families) or enough emotional distress to be brought to a mental health professional's attention. Even then, however, patients usually deny having any problems and refuse treatment.

Subtypes of Delusional Disorder

There are 7 generally recognized subtypes of delusional disorder (Table 40.2).

Table 40.2 • Subtypes of Delusional Disorder

Subtype	Characteristics
Erotomanic	• Patient has delusion that somebody, usually of higher social status, is in love with the patient • Patient may stalk, pursue, or otherwise harass the perceived lover and even cause violence if the affection is unrequited
Jealous	• The patient believes that the spouse or partner is being unfaithful, in spite of clear evidence to the contrary • The delusional patient may undertake extreme measures to try to prove the presumed infidelity (eg, bugging telephones, hiring private detectives) and possibly use violence
Grandiose	• Patients have grandiose beliefs in their power, talent, skills, or accomplishments (mania must be ruled out)
Somatic	• Patients have delusions about bodily function • Patients are highly likely to consult with a physician—not with psychiatric concerns but rather with bodily complaints • Somatic delusions must be differentiated from the somatocentric worry and rumination of depressed, anxious, or somatoform patients
Persecutory	• Patients believe that some type of harassment or mistreatment is directed at them • Violence against the perceived persecutors is a real possibility
Mixed	• Patient has >1 of the above types of delusion
Unspecified	• Patients have delusions that cannot be further characterized

Treatment

If a delusional disorder patient agrees to treatment, antipsychotic medication would be the first choice. Most patients with delusional disorder, however, refuse treatment. Nothing is known of the pathophysiology of delusional disorder. Pharmacologic treatment may attenuate the intensity of the delusional conviction and consequent behaviors, but it almost never eliminates the delusion.

- Delusional disorder is characterized by the presence of delusions without hallucinations, thought or behavioral disorganization, catatonia, or negative symptoms.

Psychotic Disorder Due to a General Medical Condition

If prominent hallucinations or delusions result directly from a medical condition, the diagnosis is psychotic disorder due to a general medical condition. Numerous medical and neurologic conditions can be associated with the onset of psychosis. Treatment logically involves controlling the underlying medical disorder but may also require antipsychotic medication. In some cases, as soon as the underlying medical condition abates, so does the psychosis. In other cases, the psychosis may persist even after the medical condition has resolved. Psychoses due to general medical conditions are heterogeneous: Hallucinations may be visual, auditory, olfactory, gustatory, or tactile. Onset is usually fairly abrupt. The differential diagnosis commonly includes delirium since many medical conditions cause not only psychosis but also impairments in the level of consciousness as well as other cognitive dysfunctions.

Substance-Induced Psychotic Disorder

Delusions or hallucinations may be caused by substances, including drugs of abuse, prescription medications, or environmental toxins (eg, mercury poisoning). Onset of the psychosis may occur during intoxication, withdrawal (eg, with alcohol and benzodiazepines), or after prolonged exposure (eg, a delusional state after years of amphetamine abuse). The psychosis usually resolves with abstinence from the offending agent, but this may require more time than the half-life of the substance might suggest; occasionally, the psychosis is permanent. Treatment with antipsychotic medication is usually necessary for acute psychosis, but long-term treatment may be needed in some cases. Additional details are provided in Chapter 44, "Substance Use Disorders."

Personality and Illness

BRIAN A. PALMER, MD

Introduction

Definition and Overview

A personality disorder (PD), as defined in the *Diagnostic and Statistical Manual of Mental Disorders* (Fifth Edition) (*DSM-V*), is "an enduring pattern of inner experience and behavior that deviates markedly from the expectations of the individual's culture, is pervasive and inflexible, has an onset in adolescence or early adulthood, is stable over time, and leads to distress or impairment." *DSM-V* has revised PDs as individual disorders, so that they are no longer reported on Axis II; *DSM-V*, unlike previous editions, does not use the axis system.

The PDs are divided into 3 clusters by their descriptive similarities. Cluster A reflects odd or eccentric character structure; Cluster B reflects dramatic, emotional, or erratic character structure; and Cluster C reflects anxious or fearful character structure. Further details on diagnosis, etiology, and treatment issues follow. Accurate identification and optimal treatment of PDs can help improve outcomes of other psychiatric and medical illness.

Diagnosis and Outcome

While classic teaching is that PDs are always enduring and inflexible, current evidence has called this into question. Borderline PD (BPD) improves dramatically, with 80% of patients no longer meeting full criteria within 10 years after the diagnosis (although social and occupational impairments persist).

That said, inflexibility is a hallmark of PDs—inflexibility of behavioral responses, emotional responses, thought patterns, or interpersonal relationships typify PDs. In addition to pervasiveness, inflexibility may be the most useful clinical guide to determining when a patient's response reflects a PD. For example, patients with avoidant PD may so fear criticism that they are deeply lonely because of their isolation yet remain inflexible in the avoidance, despite its consequences.

PDs are, by definition, accompanied by functional impairment in work or school, social relationships, or leisure. PDs are seen in 12% of the population and are frequently encountered clinically.

Comorbidity

The presence of a comorbid PD often complicates treatment of other psychiatric disorders and medical illnesses. The frequency of comorbidity is high. Among patients with major depressive disorder, as many as 50% have a Cluster B or Cluster C personality disorder. The comorbidity between anxiety disorders and Cluster C PDs is 25%. Substance use disorders are associated with a comorbid Cluster B PD more than 50% of the time. Understanding the interplay between personality structure or disorder and psychiatric and medical illnesses can enhance treatment effectiveness.

- A PD, as defined in the *DSM-V*, is "an enduring pattern of inner experience and behavior that deviates markedly from the expectations of the individual's culture, is pervasive and inflexible, has an onset in adolescence or early adulthood, is stable over time, and leads to distress or impairment."
- Among patients with major depressive disorder, as many as 50% have a Cluster B or Cluster C personality disorder.

Abbreviations: BPD, borderline personality disorder; DBT, dialectical behavioral therapy; *DSM-V, Diagnostic and Statistical Manual of Mental Disorders* (Fifth Edition); PD, personality disorder

Cluster A PDs

Cluster A PDs are summarized in Table 41.1.

Paranoid PD

Paranoid PD is seen in approximately 1% of the population and is more common among men.

It is characterized by pervasive, persistent, and inappropriate mistrust of others' motives, leading patients with this disorder to persistently question the loyalty of friends, the trustworthiness of associates, and the intentions of their physicians. They are vigilant, scanning the environment for the next source of possible attack, and in response to perceived threats, they react quickly with anger and counterattacking behavior. They hold long-term grudges and are litigious, frequently amassing documentation to support their preconceived idea that others are hostile to them. These features lead to difficulties with workplace and intimate relationships, frequently resulting in social isolation.

Paranoid PD can coexist with psychotic disorders and can exist before the development of schizophrenia. That said, the suspiciousness of paranoid PD does not include prominent and persistent delusions as would be seen in paranoid schizophrenia or delusional disorder, persecutory subtype. It is further differentiated from paranoid schizophrenia by the lack of perceptual disturbances and from schizotypal PD by the lack of magical thinking.

Because of their mistrust, patients with PD rarely seek psychiatric treatment, although they will inevitably be cared for in the rest of the medical system. An exceptionally respectful, honest, straightforward style can be helpful, with direct apologies when indicated. Antipsychotic medications have been poorly studied in this population but may offer relief during more severe paranoid decompensations.

Schizoid PD

Seen in less than 1% of the population, schizoid PD is more common among men than women.

This disorder is characterized by a detachment from social relationships and a restricted range of emotional expression in interpersonal settings. People with schizoid PD neither desire nor enjoy close relationships and instead choose solitary activities, such as computer games. They appear detached and experience little pleasure in social enterprises.

Despite this social withdrawal, schizoid PD actually has less association with schizophrenia than does schizotypal PD. Patients with avoidant PD (in Cluster C) have few close relationships because of their fears of rejection rather than a diminished interest or need for closeness as is seen in schizoid PD. Schizoid PD should be differentiated from higher-functioning autistic disorders (autism spectrum disorder) by the lack of stereotyped behaviors and by the indifference to—rather than the inability to form—social relations.

Patients with schizoid PD rarely seek psychiatric treatment (although supportive, dynamic, and dialectical behavioral therapy [DBT] approaches can help), and in medical settings they may do well with a straightforward, problem-focused approach.

Schizotypal PD

Schizotypal PD is seen in approximately 1% of the population, and it is the PD most closely linked to schizophrenia.

People with schizotypal PD have nondelusional ideas of reference, odd beliefs or magical thinking (such as belief in telepathic powers), odd thinking or speech patterns, and social anxiety or isolation. It is differentiated from the other Cluster A PDs by its peculiarity and odd beliefs. It does not have the enduring periods of active psychosis and the decline in social or occupational functioning typical of schizophrenia.

Data suggest that schizotypal PD should be considered part of the schizophrenia spectrum, and treatment with antipsychotic medications (generally at low doses) and social skills training can be helpful.

Table 41.1 • Cluster A Personality Disorders (Odd or Eccentric Character Structure)

Personality Disorder	Prevalence		Clinical Features	Other
	%	Sex Predilection		
Paranoid	1–1.5	Men	Distrust of others' motives Fear of next attack against them Often litigious	Rule out schizophrenia and delusional disorder Rarely seek treatment because of mistrust
Schizoid	<1	Men	Restricted social relationships and emotional expression Preference for solitary activities (eg, computer games) Little pleasure in social activities	Rarely seek treatment
Schizotypal	1	. . .	Odd beliefs or magical thinking Social anxiety or isolation	Considered part of schizophrenia spectrum

- Schizoid PD should be differentiated from higher-functioning autistic disorders (autism spectrum disorder) by the lack of stereotyped behaviors and by the indifference to—rather than the inability to form—social relations.
- Data suggest that schizotypal PD should be considered part of the schizophrenia spectrum, and treatment with antipsychotic medications (generally at low doses) and social skills training can be helpful.

Cluster B PDs

Cluster B PDs are summarized in Table 41.2.

Antisocial PD

Antisocial PD is seen in 1.7% of the population and is considerably more common in men than women.

Antisocial PD has substantial heritability, and the environmental contributions of absent or abusive parenting also likely have a role. Brain changes in antisocial PD include reduced temporal lobe and whole brain volume, with differential limbic or prefrontal fear conditioning.

Antisocial PD is characterized by a long-standing pattern of disregard for the rights of others (or, more rarely, enjoying harming others). It is highly prevalent among prisoners and is highly associated with substance use disorders. It requires diagnosis in adulthood and also requires evidence of conduct disorder before age 15. It is differentiated from narcissism by the lack of impulsivity and recklessness in narcissism and the functions of exploitation or disregard in each disorder (ie, regulation of self-esteem in narcissism contrasted with the monetary or power motives more common in antisocial PD).

Antisocial PD is poorly treated by contemporary approaches, most likely because people with the disorder have no regard for negative consequences. No medications have been shown to be effective, although treatment of comorbid substance use disorders is warranted. Antisocial PD does decrease in prevalence over time, and there is at least indirect evidence that social learning (including in prisons) may offer some benefit.

Borderline PD

BPD is common, seen in 2% to 3% of the general population (although the largest epidemiologic study reported a prevalence of 5.9%), and unlike patients with many personality disorders, patients with BPD are more likely to seek treatment. In clinical populations, it is much more common (75%) in women, although in community samples the prevalence differences between the sexes is close to zero. BPD is highly heritable, with evidence for increased activation of the amygdala or limbic system and decreased cortical control, particularly with interpersonal stressors. Adverse childhood events are overrepresented in patients with BPD.

BPD is characterized by insecure attachments, with undue reliance on an idealized other for stabilization of self and emotions—an exclusivity that inevitably fails, leading to problems with anger and impulsive behaviors, including self-injury and recurrent suicide attempts. During periods of severe stress, transient psychotic symptoms may emerge (eg, paranoia and dissociation).

BPD is distinguished from bipolar disorder by its abandonment sensitivity and self-harm as well as by the lack of elation and sleep-deprived energy enhancement seen in bipolar disorder. BPD has some overlap (>25%) with features of the other Cluster B disorders, and it very commonly co-occurs with major depression, a disorder that is likely to persist until the BPD symptoms remit.

Fortunately, 50% of patients with BPD no longer meet full criteria within 2 years, a finding that increases to 80% within 10 years, although functional impairments typically persist.

Table 41.2 • Cluster B Personality Disorders (Dramatic, Emotional, or Erratic Character Structure)

Personality Disorder	Prevalence		Clinical Features	Other
	%	Sex Predilection		
Antisocial	1.7	Men	Long-standing disregard for rights of others (conduct disorder present in youth)	Substantial heritability Common in prisoners Poorly treatable
Borderline	2–3	Women	Insecure attachments Reliance on an idealized other for stabilization of self and emotions, leading to anger and impulsiveness	Highly treatable
Histrionic	2	Women	Overly concerned with receiving attention Exaggerated emotionality and dramatic behavior	May respond to dynamic treatment
Narcissistic	0.5	Men	Difficulty regulating self-esteem Grandiose sense of self	. . .

BPD is one of the most treatable PDs. Medications may be helpful with the cognitive, behavioral, and affective symptom components, although benzodiazepines have not been shown to offer benefit and have (in the case of alprazolam) been shown to worsen the course. Data support the use of selective serotonin reuptake inhibitor antidepressants, atypical antipsychotics, and anticonvulsant mood stabilizers, but no data support the commonly used polypharmacy approaches for these patients.

Psychosocial treatment of BPD includes 6 empirically validated treatments, each with its own theoretical orientation and purported mechanism of change. DBT is the most widely available of these. Common features of effective treatment include structure and goals, an active (but not reactive) therapist stance, a real relationship with a therapist, and an emphasis on making sense of experiences (thoughts and feelings) that lead to impulsivity, dissociation, or uncontrollable anger.

In studies of medical outcomes, patients with BPD have fewer proactive health behaviors and a greater tendency to use emergency services, leading to poorer control of chronic health conditions and (of note for readers of this text) unfavorable control of migraine headache.

Histrionic PD

Histrionic PD occurs in 2% of the general population, more frequently in women than men.

People with this disorder are overly concerned with receiving attention through dramatic behavior, flirtation, and exaggerated emotionality and theatricality. Physical appearance is used to enhance self-attention. Unlike people with dependent PD, people with histrionic PD can be quite autonomous (particularly when such an approach effectively elicits attention). They do not have the rage or self-injury of BPD, and while people with narcissistic PD do regulate self-esteem through attention, admiration is more central to narcissistic PD than to histrionic PD.

Dynamic treatment can help patients enhance the depth of their relationships and broaden their skill set for connecting with others.

Narcissistic PD

Narcissistic PD is rarer than most PDs (prevalence, 0.5%) and is more common among men than women.

The core feature is difficulty regulating self-esteem; people with the disorder have a grandiose sense of self-importance and are preoccupied with fantasies of unlimited power, brilliance, and beauty and require excessive admiration from others and lack empathy. When self-esteem inevitably plummets with a small slight or criticism, the injury results in significant hurt or anger.

Unlike those with antisocial PD, people with narcissistic PD rationalize their exploitation of others on the basis of their personal virtues. Adjustment disorders can

manifest with narcissistic features, and mania can share the grandiosity of narcissistic PD.

Individual psychodynamic psychotherapy can help patients change over time.

- Brain changes in antisocial PD include reduced temporal lobe and whole brain volume, with differential limbic or prefrontal fear conditioning.
- Fortunately, 50% of patients with BPD no longer meet full criteria within 2 years, a finding that increases to 80% within 10 years, although functional impairments typically persist.
- BPD is one of the most treatable PDs.
- DBT is the most widely available psychosocial treatment of BPD.
- Unlike those with antisocial PD, people with narcissistic PD rationalize their exploitation of others on the basis of their personal virtues.

Cluster C PDs

Cluster C PDs are summarized in Table 41.3.

Avoidant PD

Avoidant PD is seen in 1.5% to 3% of people, more commonly among women than men.

People with avoidant PD deeply fear criticism and rejection and avoid intimacy, occupations with interpersonal contact, social settings where being liked is uncertain, and other personal risks. While people with schizoid PD are socially isolated, people with avoidant PD want to have relationships but avoid them out of fear. Unlike social phobia (with which there is overlap), avoidant PD reflects a pattern of interpersonal relations that impact functioning, rather than a specific fear of a particular aspect of a social interaction (eg, speaking to a group).

Cognitive therapy (challenging patients' distorted assumptions), dynamic therapy, and social skills training may prove useful, and antidepressants and anxiolytics can help relieve some symptoms.

Dependent PD

Dependent PD is seen in 1% to 1.5% of the population and is considerably more common among women than men.

People with the disorder require undue advice and reassurance before making everyday decisions, and they rely on others to make most of their life decisions. These people have unrealistic fears of disapproval and have difficulty disagreeing, feeling unrealistically preoccupied with fears of having to take care of themselves. While those with BPD desire ongoing support and fear aloneness, people with dependent PD desire much more control by the other and are quick to apologize or appease rather than

Table 41.3 • Cluster C Personality Disorders (Anxious or Fearful Character Structure)

Personality Disorder	Prevalence %	Sex Predilection	Clinical Features	Other
Avoidant	1.5–3	Women	Fear criticism and rejection and avoid social situations	Cognitive, dynamic, and social skills training Antianxiety or antidepressive medications may help some symptoms
Dependent	1–1.5	Women	Require excessive reassurance and advice in everyday decisions Fear disapproval	Cognitive therapy
Obsessive-compulsive	2	Men	Preoccupied with perfectionism, control, orderliness	Distinguish from obsessive-compulsive disorder (the personality disorder does not have obsessional thoughts or repetitive behaviors that relieve the obsession)

become rageful when abandonment threatens. Unlike those with avoidant PD, people with dependent PD seek out relationships.

Treatment is primarily psychotherapeutic, with evidence supporting psychodynamic, cognitive behavior, couples, family, and group psychotherapies.

Obsessive-Compulsive PD

Obsessive-compulsive PD is seen in approximately 2% of the population and is more common in men than in women. Developmental contributions appear to be important in its development.

People with the disorder are preoccupied with orderliness, perfectionism, and mental or interpersonal control to such a degree that it impairs their ability to complete tasks or participate in life's social and occupational demands. Rigid and stubborn, people with obsessive-compulsive PD may hoard money or objects to foster a sense of protection from future disaster. Unlike those with obsessive-compulsive disorder (which can be comorbid), people with obsessive-compulsive PD do not have obsessional thoughts or repetitive behaviors that relieve the obsession.

Psychodynamic or psychoanalytic therapy with a strong focus on experiencing the emotions (such as fear) that are managed by the PD can be helpful. Similarly, cognitive therapies can help reduce the distorted beliefs that fuel the need to control and bring excessive order.

- While people with schizoid PD are socially isolated, people with avoidant PD want to have relationships but avoid them out of fear.
- Unlike those with obsessive-compulsive disorder (which can be comorbid), people with obsessive-compulsive PD do not have obsessional thoughts or repetitive behaviors that relieve the obsession.

42 Miscellaneous Psychiatric Disorders[a]

KARI A. MARTIN, MD

Introduction

With a number of psychiatric disorders, patients present with medical and psychological symptoms not well explained by medical conditions or substance use. Core clinical features of some of the disorders are compared in Table 42.1. This chapter reviews those disorders in addition to dissociative disorders, sexual disorders, and adjustment disorders.

Somatic Symptom Disorders

Definition and Epidemiology

Somatic symptom disorders have lifetime prevalence rates of 0.2% to 2% for women and less than 0.2% for men. The onset is before the age of 30, and symptoms persist for many years. The cost to the US health care system is estimated at $100 billion annually.

These disorders exist at the interface between psychiatry and neurology and include medically unexplained symptoms. That is, the multiple somatic complaints cannot be explained by any known general medical condition or by the direct effect of a substance.

Pathophysiology

Functional imaging studies of the brain show increased activity in limbic areas in response to painful stimuli in patients who have somatic symptom disorders compared with those who do not. In addition, patients who have somatic symptom disorders may have a generalized decrease in gray matter density.

Clinical Features

The diagnosis of a somatic symptom disorder requires the presence of physical symptoms suggestive of a general medical condition, but the symptoms cannot be fully explained by the general medical condition. Physical examination findings are often inconsistent or incongruous with known neurologic disease. Somatic symptoms and cognitive distortions are core features of these disorders. At present, no conceptual framework adequately explains the disorders, but advanced functional imaging techniques suggest a dysfunction of the nervous system.

Patients with somatic symptom disorders have symptoms that cause clinical distress or impairment in social, occupational, or other areas of functioning. In contrast to patients with factitious disorders or malingering, patients with somatic symptom disorder have physical symptoms that are not intentional or voluntary.

When a comorbid general medical condition exists, somatic symptom disorder can be difficult to diagnose. However, if the physical complaints or resulting social or occupational impairment are in excess of what would be expected from the overall assessment (history, physical examination, and laboratory tests), a diagnosis of somatic symptom disorder may still be entertained.

Diagnosis

Criteria for somatic symptom disorder in the *Diagnostic and Statistical Manual of Mental Disorders* (Fifth Edition) require that 1 or more somatic symptoms result in significant disruption of daily life and persist for at least 6 months. Patients may have excessive thoughts, feelings,

---

[a] Portions previously published in Weber S. Dissociative symptom disorders in advanced nursing practice: background, treatment, and instrumentation to assess symptoms. Issues Ment Health Nurs. 2007 Sep;28(9):997–1018; Cole BE. Pain management: classifying, understanding, and treating pain. Hosp Physician. 2002 Jun;38(6):23–30; and LoPiccolo CJ, Goodkin K, Baldewicz TT. Current issues in the diagnosis and management of malingering. Ann Med. 1999 Jun;31(3):166–74. Used with permission.

Table 42.1 • Select Disorders With Medical or Psychological Symptoms Unexplained by Medical Conditions or Substance Use

Disorder	Brief Description
Somatic symptom disorders	Multiple somatic complaints not fully explained by a medical condition or substance use
Conversion disorder	Voluntary but unconscious motor or sensory function deficits that suggest a general medical or neurologic condition Symptoms do not fit known physiologic mechanisms
Hypochondriasis	Preoccupation with having or acquiring a serious illness
Factitious disorders	Physical or psychological symptoms that are purposely feigned to achieve the sick role (the primary gain) with potential personal benefits (the secondary gain)
Malingering	Physical or psychological symptoms purposely feigned and consciously motivated by an external incentive (the primary gain is receiving compensation, avoiding prosecution, or receiving another personal benefit)

or behaviors related to the somatic symptoms as manifested by disproportionate and persistent thoughts about the seriousness of the symptoms, a persistently high level of anxiety about health or symptoms, and excessive time and energy devoted to health symptoms.

Clinical Course and Treatment

Somatic symptom disorder is generally a chronic condition that fluctuates over time. It rarely completely resolves.

Cognitive behavior therapy is the most useful treatment of somatic symptom disorder. Other considerations include use of antidepressants and supportive psychotherapy. A consultation letter to the primary care physician can be effective and may decrease further unnecessary diagnostic or treatment interventions.

Undifferentiated Somatic Symptom Disorder

Undifferentiated somatic symptom disorder is a category of somatic symptom presentations that do not meet the full criteria for one of the specific somatic symptom disorders. The important criterion for this diagnosis is that 1 or more physical complaints persist for 6 months or longer. Common complaints include chronic fatigue, loss of appetite, or gastrointestinal or genitourinary tract symptoms. General medical conditions do not fully explain the symptoms, and the symptoms are not direct effects of substance use or medication side effects. The symptoms are not

feigned, and they cause clinically significant distress or impairment in important areas of functioning.

- Patients who have somatic symptom disorders may have a generalized decrease in gray matter density.
- The diagnosis of a somatic symptom disorder requires the presence of physical symptoms suggestive of a general medical condition, but the symptoms cannot be fully explained by the general medical condition.
- Patients with somatic symptom disorders have symptoms that cause clinical distress or impairment in social, occupational, or other areas of functioning. In contrast to patients with factitious disorders or malingering, patients with somatic symptom disorder have physical symptoms that are not intentional or voluntary.

Conversion Disorder

Epidemiology

Conversion disorder affects women more often than men, and a history of sexual and physical abuse may be reported. Patients present in their teens or early 20s and have elevated rates of other psychiatric comorbidities.

Pathophysiology

Functional brain imaging has suggested that the perigenual anterior cingulate and the posterior parietal cortices may be important in a functional unawareness circuit that is the neurologic basis of conversion disorder.

Clinical Features

Historically, conversion disorder was known as *hysteria*. Reclassification of hysteria as a psychiatric disorder began with the writings of Sigmund Freud. In conversion disorder, psychological factors are judged to be associated with voluntary but unconscious motor or sensory function deficits that suggest a neurologic or other general medical condition. The symptoms are not intentionally produced. As part of the criteria, these symptoms cannot be fully explained by neurologic or other conditions, by the direct effects of a substance, or by a culturally sanctioned behavior.

Conversion symptoms do not fit known physiologic mechanisms. Neurologic examination findings may show contradictory patterns of weakness or reflexes that do not conform to what one might expect anatomically. For example, patients with hemiplegia have weakness in flexor muscle groups rather than in extensor muscle groups. In patients with functional tremor, the patient's tremor is often distractible and may stop or change frequency during rapid movements of the unaffected hand.

The onset of conversion disorder is generally sudden, with a short duration and frequent recurrences. A patient's affective response to the condition may vary from an unusually calm demeanor (la belle indifférence) to one that is highly emotional.

The treating psychiatrist and the neurologist should maintain a strong liaison.

- In conversion disorder, psychological factors are judged to be associated with voluntary but unconscious motor or sensory function deficits that suggest a neurologic or other general medical condition.
- Conversion symptoms do not fit known physiologic mechanisms.

Pain Disorder

For patients with pain disorder, pain is the essential feature and important focus of the clinical presentation. Criteria suggest that the pain is significant enough to cause marked distress or impairment in social, occupational, or other important areas of functioning. Psychological factors have a role in the onset, severity, exacerbation, or maintenance of the pain. The pain is not intentionally produced or feigned, and it is not better accounted for by a mood, anxiety, or psychotic disorder or dyspareunia.

Pain disorders can be further categorized by the duration of pain: *acute* if the pain is less than 6 months and *chronic* if the duration of the pain is 6 months or longer. Pain disorder is further subtyped according to the factors involved in the cause and maintenance of the pain: 1) pain disorder associated with psychological factors, 2) pain disorder associated with both psychological factors and a general medical condition, and 3) pain disorder associated with a general medical condition. Pain disorder associated with a general medical condition is not considered a mental disorder.

Hypochondriasis

Epidemiology

The prevalence of hypochondriasis in the general population is 1% to 5%.

Clinical Features

The important feature of hypochondriasis is the patient's preoccupation with having or acquiring a serious illness. Bodily signs and symptoms are often misinterpreted to support the illness conviction. A general medical condition, if present, does not fully account for the person's concerns about disease or the physical signs or symptoms. Fear of disease persists despite medical reassurance.

Patients are not delusional, and they can acknowledge the possibility that they may be exaggerating the extent of the feared disease or that there may be no disease at all.

Treatment

Selective serotonin reuptake inhibitors can be effective in the treatment of hypochondriasis. Regular visits with a trusted primary care physician can often alleviate some of the health anxiety.

- The important feature of hypochondriasis is the patient's preoccupation with having or acquiring a serious illness.

Factitious Disorders

Epidemiology

Prevalence rates of 0.08% have been reported for factitious disorders in referrals to consultation-liaison services.

Clinical Features

Factitious disorders are characterized by physical or psychological symptoms that are purposely produced or feigned to achieve the sick role (the primary gain). Symptoms are judged to be intentionally produced by the production of direct evidence or by excluding other causes of the symptoms. Patients often engage in pathologic lying. Symptom description may be vague and inconsistent. Repeated hospitalizations may take patients to numerous health care institutions across the country. These patients typically have poor social support. They may also be fairly well versed in medical terminology or have limited medical training themselves.

Factitious disorders can be further subdivided according to the predominant symptoms: 1) Psychological signs and symptoms may predominate. For example, patients may ingest psychoactive substances to feign a mental disorder (eg, hypnotic consumption to induce lethargy). 2) Physical signs and symptoms of a general medical condition may predominate. For example, patients may surreptitiously inject insulin to induce hypoglycemia, or they may consume anticoagulants to cause hematuria.

Munchausen syndrome is the most severe and chronic form of factitious disorder. It is characterized by recurrent hospitalization, peregrination (traveling), and pseudologia fantastica (pathologic lying).

Outcome

Patients with factitious disorders have high mortality and morbidity rates. The primary (unconscious) gain is to achieve the sick role, but a secondary (conscious) gain is also common (eg, attaining a financial advantage, attempting to avoid an untoward legal outcome, or seeking personal attention).

- Factitious disorders are characterized by physical or psychological symptoms that are purposely produced or feigned to achieve the sick role (the primary gain).

Malingering

Malingering differs from factitious disorder in that a malingering patient is consciously motivated by an external incentive. This motivation may be more obvious and recognizable when other circumstances are known. The malingering patient's motivation is to receive compensation, avoid prosecution, obtain shelter, or in some other way obtain a personal benefit. The malingering patient's feigned medical symptoms disappear when the symptoms are no longer useful.

- Malingering differs from factitious disorder in that a malingering patient is consciously motivated by an external incentive. This motivation may be more obvious and recognizable when other circumstances are known.

Dissociative Disorders

Overview

The core component of dissociative disorders is a disruption in the integrated functions of consciousness, memory, identity, or perception (Table 42.2). Onset and course of the disturbance may be sudden or gradual, transient or chronic. Patients have high scores for hypnotizability as measured by standardized testing.

Table 42.2 • Dissociative Disorders

Disorder	Brief Description
Dissociative amnesia	Inability to recall important personal information
Dissociative fugue	Sudden, unexpected travel away from one's usual residence with an inability to recall the past and confusion about one's identity
Dissociative identity disorder	Presence of ≥2 distinct identities that control the behavior
Depersonalization disorder	Persistent or recurrent episodes of depersonalization (feeling of detachment)

Dissociative Amnesia

The inability to recall important personal information, particularly traumatic or stressful information, is the key characteristic of dissociative amnesia. This is generally information that is too extensive to be explained by ordinary forgetfulness. Patients can present at any age, and the main manifestation is a retrospective gap in memory. Acute amnesia may resolve without treatment after the patient is removed from the traumatic circumstances with which the amnesia was associated.

Dissociative Fugue

Dissociative fugue is often defined by sudden, unexpected travel away from one's home or one's customary place of work, accompanied by an inability to recall one's past and confusion about personal identity or the assumption of a new identity. Patients are generally brought to clinical attention because of amnesia for recent events or lack of awareness of personal identity. When patients return to the prefugue state, they may have no memory of events that occurred during the fugue.

Dissociative Identity Disorder

Dissociative identity disorder (also called multiple personality disorder) is characterized by the presence of 2 or more distinct identities or personality states that recurrently control the person's behavior and by an inability to recall important personal information that is too extensive to be explained by ordinary forgetfulness. Identity fragmentation is the key feature. The identity states may vary in sex, age, and physiologic function, including hand dominance, pain tolerance, visual acuity, symptoms of asthma, sensitivity to allergens, and response of blood glucose to insulin. A history of severe sexual or physical abuse is often present. The disorder also significantly overlaps with borderline personality disorder. Treatment often focuses on integrating the identities.

Depersonalization Disorder

Depersonalization disorder is characterized by persistent or recurrent episodes of depersonalization characterized by a feeling of detachment or estrangement from one's self. Patients often describe feeling that they are living in a dream or a movie. They may also describe automation, or feeling like an outside observer of their body or mental processes. *Derealization*, a sense that the external world is strange or unreal, often accompanies the depersonalization. Patients maintain intact reality testing.

Brief periods of depersonalization are common, and the diagnosis is made only if the symptoms are sufficiently severe to cause marked distress or impaired functioning.

Dissociative Disorder Not Otherwise Specified

Dissociative disorder not otherwise specified is a residual category for disorders in which the predominant feature is a dissociative symptom, but criteria for a specific dissociative disorder are not met. Dissociative trance states, dissociation due to brainwashing, and derealization unaccompanied by depersonalization are in this category.

- The inability to recall important personal information, particularly traumatic or stressful information, is the key characteristic of dissociative amnesia. This is generally information that is too extensive to be explained by ordinary forgetfulness.

Sexual Disorders

Overview

Sexual dysfunction is defined by a distortion in the normal sexual response cycle or by pain associated with sexual intercourse. The sexual response cycle is commonly divided into the stages of desire, excitement, orgasm, and resolution.

Sexual Pain Disorders Including Dyspareunia and Vaginismus

Dyspareunia is genital pain associated with sexual intercourse and can occur in both males and females. Female patients may describe the pain during intromission or during penile thrusting. To qualify for this disorder, the pain cannot be caused by vaginismus only or from a lack of lubrication. In addition, it is not due to the effects of a medication or to a general medical condition alone.

Vaginismus is the recurrent or persistent involuntary contraction of the perineal muscles surrounding the outer third of the vagina when the vagina is penetrated with penis, finger, tampon, or speculum. The condition must cause marked distress or interpersonal difficulty and cannot be better accounted for by another psychiatric disorder or a general medical condition. Vaginismus can be lifelong or acquired suddenly in response to sexual trauma.

Sexual Dysfunction Due to a General Medical Condition

In sexual dysfunction due to a general medical condition, the presence of clinically significant sexual dysfunction is judged to be due exclusively to the direct physiologic effects of a general medical condition. The sexual dysfunction can involve pain with intercourse, hypoactive sexual desire, male erectile dysfunction, and other aberrations with the normal sexual response cycle. Sexual dysfunction may be associated with some neurologic conditions, including multiple sclerosis, spinal cord lesions, neuropathy, and temporal lobe lesions.

Eating Disorders

Overview

Eating disorders are characterized by severe disturbances in eating behavior.

Anorexia Nervosa

Patients with anorexia nervosa refuse to maintain a minimally normal body weight (ie, 85% of the expected body weight) and are intensely afraid of gaining weight. Associated features of anorexia include amenorrhea, laguno, electrolyte imbalances, and a predisposition to cardiac arrhythmias, which can be fatal. Among persons with anorexia, the overall mortality is 10%.

Anorexic patients are often characterized by inflexible thinking and a strong need to control their environment. Obsessive-compulsive features are prominent.

Anorexia nervosa is categorized as *restricting* or as *binge-eating/purging*. The restricting type is a disorder in which weight loss is accompanied by dieting, fasting, or excessive exercise. The binge-eating/purging type is a disorder of patients who have regularly engaged in binge eating or purging (or both) during the current episode.

Treatment is difficult and is generally best done in a residential eating disorder center where appropriate medical and psychiatric interventions can be attempted.

Bulimia Nervosa

The lifetime prevalence of bulimia nervosa is 1% to 3% among women.

In contrast to patients who have anorexia nervosa, patients with bulimia nervosa have a normal weight and are frequently overweight. The essential feature of bulimia nervosa is binge eating and inappropriate compensatory methods to prevent weight gain. The diagnostic criteria require that binge eating and inappropriate compensatory behaviors occur at least twice weekly for 3 months. Compared with patients who have the restricting type of anorexia nervosa, patients with bulimia nervosa are more likely to have problems with impulse control and substance abuse and to be sexually active. Personality disorders are common in patients with anorexia nervosa or bulimia nervosa.

- Anorexic patients are often characterized by inflexible thinking and a strong need to control their environment. Obsessive-compulsive features are prominent.
- The essential feature of bulimia nervosa is binge eating and inappropriate compensatory methods to prevent weight gain.

Adjustment Disorders

Adjustment disorders are a residual category used to describe disorders that result from an identifiable stressor and do not meet criteria for another psychiatric disorder. The symptoms must develop within 3 months after the onset of the stressor. The reaction is in excess of what would be expected from the nature of the stressor. Adjustment disorders are currently coded according to the subtype that characterizes the predominant symptoms: 1) adjustment disorder with depressed mood, 2) adjustment disorder with anxiety, 3) adjustment disorder with mixed anxiety and depressed mood, 4) adjustment disorder with disturbance of conduct, 5) adjustment disorder with mixed disturbance of emotions and conduct, and 6) adjustment disorder, unspecified. The adjustment disorder can be described as *acute* if the symptoms have persisted for less than 6 months or as *chronic* if the symptoms have persisted for 6 months or more.

Adjustment disorders generally resolve or progress to a more severe mood disorder, such as major depression.

43

Psychiatric Disorders Associated With Infancy, Childhood, and Adolescence

JYOTI BHAGIA, MD

Introduction

This chapter covers key psychiatric disorders of infancy, childhood, and adolescence. In some instances, the disorders are briefly mentioned here and covered in more detail in other chapters as indicated.

Attention-Deficit/Hyperactivity Disorder

Epidemiology

Attention-deficit/hyperactivity disorder (ADHD) is a neurobiological disorder that is present in 4% to 7% of school-aged children and is 4 times more common in boys than in girls. Some symptoms must be present before age 7 years, although for many children, ADHD is not diagnosed until after age 7 years.

Pathophysiology

The causes of ADHD are unknown. However, several factors that likely mediate expression of ADHD have been suggested, including prenatal toxin exposure, mechanical insults to the nervous system, and natal stress. Additionally, work with dopamine and norepinephrine receptors and transporters suggests dysfunction in the brain's distributed network organization.

ADHD is considered a polygenetic disorder. Evidence of a genetic contribution is indicated by greater concordance in monozygotic twins than in dizygotic twins. Moreover, first-degree relatives have a 10% to 35% higher incidence of ADHD, and children of parents with ADHD may have a 50% higher incidence.

Clinical Features

Symptoms often consist of a persistent pattern of inattention or hyperactive and impulsive behavior (or both) at home and at school. For a diagnosis of ADHD, 6 out of 9 symptoms of inattention and 6 out of 9 symptoms of hyperactive and impulsive behavior must be present for at least 6 months (Box 43.1). These symptoms cause significant impairment in social, academic, and extracurricular activities.

There are 3 types of ADHD: *inattentive type*, primarily with symptoms of inattention; *hyperactive-impulsive type*, primarily with symptoms of hyperactivity and impulsivity; and *combined type*, which is the most common.

Diagnosis and Treatment

ADHD diagnosis is based on a clinical interview along with ADHD rating scales from parents and teachers. ADHD often coexists with oppositional defiant disorder, learning disorders, tic disorders, anxiety disorders, and mood disorders. It is important to rule out medical conditions that could mimic ADHD symptoms, including hearing problems, thyroid disorders, and absence seizures.

Once ADHD is diagnosed, treatment consists of medication, cognitive behavior or other therapy, parent management training, social skills training, or a combination of these. Medication is effective in 70% of patients treated with stimulants. Combined treatment is especially useful in patients with ADHD complicated by behavior disorders.

Abbreviations: ADHD, attention-deficit/hyperactivity disorder; ADOS, Autism Diagnostic Observation Schedule; ASD, autism spectrum disorder; IEP, Individualized Education Program; PDD-NOS, pervasive developmental disorder, not otherwise specified

Box 43.1 • Clinical Symptoms and Features of Attention-Deficit/Hyperactivity Disorder

Inattention

Poor attention to details

Difficulty focusing attention on task

Distracted (does not listen when directly spoken to)

Fails to complete schoolwork or chores

Difficulty organizing tasks

Reluctant to engage in tasks requiring sustained attention

Loses things needed for tasks

Distracted by extraneous stimuli

Forgetful in daily activities

Hyperactive and Impulsive Behavior

Fidgets or taps hands or feet

Leaves seat when expected to remain seated

Runs or climbs in inappropriate situations

Unable to play or engage in leisure activities quietly

"On the go" and difficult to keep up with

Often talks excessively

Blurts out answer before question is completed, and inappropriately intrudes in conversations

Difficulty waiting for a turn

Interrupts or intrudes in others' conversations and activities

Adapted from American Psychiatric Association. Diagnostic and statistical manual of mental disorders: DSM-5. 5th ed. Arlington (VA): American Psychiatric Association; c2013. p. 59–60. Used with permission.

Dopamine and norepinephrine are the 2 neurotransmitters linked most closely with ADHD. Stimulants (eg, methylphenidate and dextroamphetamine) and nonstimulants (eg, atomoxetine and bupropion) that work on these neurotransmitters are the most effective ADHD medications.

Clinical Course and Prognosis

The course of ADHD is variable, and symptoms may persist into adolescence and adulthood. Symptoms of hyperactivity may decrease in adolescence, although inattention will remain. The prognosis is improved with treatment and behavior management.

- ADHD is 4 times more common in boys than in girls.
- For a diagnosis of ADHD, 6 out of 9 symptoms of inattention and 6 out of 9 symptoms of hyperactive and impulsive behavior must be present for ≥6 months (Box 43.1).

- It is important to rule out medical conditions that could mimic ADHD symptoms, including hearing problems, thyroid disorders, and absence seizures.

Learning Disorders

Overview and Epidemiology

Children with a learning disorder are unable to acquire sufficient skills in reading, writing, or mathematics compared with other children of similar age and intelligence. Learning disorders are prevalent in 5% of school-aged children. These disorders include reading disorder, mathematics disorder, disorder of written expression, and learning disorder, not otherwise specified.

Clinical Features

Reading disorder is also known as dyslexia. It affects 4% of school-aged children and causes impairment in recognizing words, reading comprehension, and reading ability. Furthermore, reading disorder is common in children with ADHD.

Mathematics disorder is present in approximately 1% of school-aged children. These children experience difficulty in learning and remembering basic numerical facts. Children with mathematics disorder often have reading and writing disorders as well.

Disorder of written expression, found in 4% of children, is characterized by a significantly lower level of writing skills, including poor grammar, spelling, and handwriting. Psychological testing, including IQ and academic achievement testing, is done to confirm the diagnosis of a learning disorder. Extra academic help with an Individualized Education Program (IEP) is recommended for skill improvement.

Autism Spectrum Disorder

Overview

Pervasive developmental disorders include a spectrum of disorders in which there is a delay in the development of social skills, language and development, and stereotypical behavior and movements. These include autism, Rett disorder, childhood disintegrative disorder, Asperger syndrome, and pervasive developmental disorder, not otherwise specified (PDD-NOS).

Epidemiology

About 1 in 88 children have been identified with an autism spectrum disorder (ASD). Autism is a developmental disorder that presents in the first 3 years of life and is 4 to 5 times more common in boys than in girls.

Pathophysiology

The high rate of intellectual disability and associated seizure disorder suggest a biologic basis for ASD. Discrete causal factors have proved elusive. Increased paternal age (>40 years) increases ASD risk. Several teratogens, including medications and immunizations, have been potentially associated with ASD, but no definite linkage has been established. Genetic susceptibility appears to be important. Identical twins are much more likely than fraternal twins to have autism. Other causes have been suspected but not proved.

Clinical Features

Children with autism are very sensitive to loud noises, light, touch, and changes in routine. They may also have a heightened response to pain. Of the children with this disorder, 75% have intellectual disability, one-third of whom have mild to moderate disability and close to half are severely disabled.

Fragile X syndrome is present in 1% of autistic children. Tuberous sclerosis, another genetic disorder, may affect up to 2% of autistic children. Other neurologic disorders commonly associated with autism include congenital rubella and phenylketonuria.

Diagnosis

The diagnosis of autism is made through a clinical interview and examination, and psychological testing with the Autism Diagnostic Observation Schedule (ADOS), a standardized screening tool. Most children with ASD do not receive a diagnosis until they are late preschoolers.

Other Pervasive Developmental Disorders

Other pervasive developmental disorders include Asperger syndrome, which is clinically similar to autism except for normal language development. Rett disorder, more commonly found in females, is a condition in which the child has normal development until 6 months, but between age 6 months and 2 years, there is progressive encephalopathy. Childhood disintegrative disorder is a rare condition characterized by a child appropriately learning skills but then losing them by age 10.

All other disorders that do not meet the criteria for the disorders mentioned above are considered under the category of PDD-NOS (also called atypical autism).

Treatment

Treatment of pervasive developmental disorders includes a combination of the following: applied behavior analysis, medications, occupational therapy, physical therapy, speech-language therapy, and sensory integration. Constructive adaptation can help ameliorate symptoms and improve overall quality of life.

- Pervasive developmental disorders include a spectrum of disorders in which there is a delay in the development of social skills, language and development, and stereotypical behavior and movements.
- About 1 in 88 children have been identified with an ASD.
- Several teratogens, including medications and immunizations, have been potentially associated with ASD, but no definite linkage has been established.

Mental Retardation

Mental retardation is a developmental disability characterized by significant impairment in intellectual and adaptive functioning. With standardized testing, an IQ of 70 or less is considered mental retardation; the prevalence is approximately 1% in the US population. Mental retardation is further categorized into mild (IQ, 50–55 to 70), moderate (IQ, 35–40 to 50–55), severe (IQ, 20–25 to 35–40), and profound (IQ, <20–25).

The cause of mental retardation can be genetic or acquired or a combination of both. Mental retardation is commonly seen in patients with Down syndrome, fragile X syndrome, phenylketonuria, and multiple other metabolic syndromes. A careful genetic evaluation, chromosomal studies, urine and blood analysis, and a thorough physical examination are important parts of the diagnostic evaluation of possible mental retardation. Psychosocial treatment, pharmacotherapy, and family education may all have a role in management options. For details, see Volume 2, Chapter 71, "Neurological Development and Developmental Disabilities."

- Mental retardation is a developmental disability characterized by significant impairment in intellectual and adaptive functioning.

Tic Disorders

Tics are involuntary, repetitive muscle movements or vocalizations. Tic disorders are neuropsychiatric disorders that usually begin in childhood and continue to wax and wane throughout life. Tic disorders include chronic motor or vocal tic disorder, Tourette syndrome, transient tic disorder, and tic disorder, not otherwise specified. For details, see Volume 2, Chapter 27, "Movement Disorders in Childhood."

Motor Skills Disorder

Motor skills disorder, also known as developmental coordination disorder, is a condition characterized by delay in achieving motor milestones. Both fine and gross motor skills may be affected in this disorder. It is present in 5% of school-aged children, and its causes may be organic or developmental. The disorder must be differentiated from medical conditions such as cerebral palsy and muscular dystrophy. Treatment includes sensory integration therapy by an occupational therapist and modified physical education.

Communication Disorders

Epidemiology

The prevalence of all communication disorders is approximately 3% to 5% of children. Communication disorders are 2 to 3 times more common in boys than in girls.

Description and Clinical Features

A communication disorder is a speech or language impairment that may include disruptions in the ability to either send or receive conventional elements of communication, whether verbal, nonverbal, or graphic, with or without an inability to comprehend or process those elements. The 2 types of communication disorders are language disorders and speech disorders.

Language disorders include expressive language disorder and mixed receptive-expressive language disorder. People with *expressive language disorder* have difficulty expressing themselves beyond simple sentences and have a vocabulary that is smaller than expected for their age; the disorder is confirmed with standardized testing. By definition, the diagnosis also requires that the language difficulties are sufficient to interfere with expected academic, occupational, or social function. However, language comprehension in children with expressive language disorder is within normal limits.

In *mixed receptive-expressive language disorder*, both the comprehension and the expression of language are impaired. Children with developmental language disorders often have limited speech and a limited range of vocabulary, and they use short sentences, simplistic grammar, and idiosyncratic ordering of words.

Speech disorders include phonologic disorder and stuttering. Phonologic disorder is characterized by poor sound production as well as omissions and substitutions of sounds. Affected children do not produce developmentally expected speech sounds, especially consonants. Although there may be an identifiable physical reason for the problem (eg, neuromuscular impairments, structural defects, hearing impairment), most children with phonologic difficulties do not have an underlying physical cause.

Fluency disorders (ie, stuttering) can be either neurogenic or developmental in origin, although neurogenic causes are rare. Developmental stuttering is characterized by a break in fluency with particular sounds, syllables, or words being repeated or unduly prolonged. The cause of stuttering is unclear, but there appears to be a genetic-environmental interaction that capitalizes on predisposed individuals, particularly boys and those with a family history of stuttering.

Diagnosis

The diagnosis of communication disorders requires a thorough medical examination, including a hearing assessment followed by a complete speech and language assessment by a qualified expert. The assessment is likely to include observation, standardized evaluations, and perhaps quantitative observation.

Treatment

Therapeutic intervention and management depend on etiologic determinations, the age of the child, and the degree of impairment. Individual or group speech and language therapy can be very effective; as a general rule, early intervention is favored, although each child's situation deserves individual assessment.

- A communication disorder is a speech or language impairment that may include disruptions in the ability to either send or receive conventional elements of communication, whether verbal, nonverbal, or graphic, with or without an inability to comprehend or process those elements.

Elimination Disorders

Enuresis

Enuresis is the repeated, unwanted voiding of urine with a frequency of at least twice a week for at least 3 months and occurring in the absence of the physiologic effect of a substance or a general medical condition in a child who is at least 5 years old. The overall prevalence by age 10 is 10%. The majority of children have monosymptomatic enuresis (ie, there are no other lower urinary tract symptoms), and 80% of these have primary enuresis (ie, they have never known a sustained capacity for remaining dry overnight). Secondary enuresis is the development of enuresis after a child has achieved the ability to sleep through the night without voiding in bed for at least 6 months. Secondary enuresis often appears to be precipitated by life stressors. Primary monosymptomatic enuresis is usually a self-limited illness.

Treatment includes behavior therapy with classic conditioning, medications, and psychotherapy. Children with nonmonosymptomatic enuresis, of whom about 20% also have daytime symptoms, need a medical evaluation for possible urologic or neurologic contributions.

Encopresis

Encopresis is the repeated, unwanted passage of feces with at least 1 event per month for 3 months in children who are at least 4 years old and in whom the behavior is not related to the physiologic effects of a substance or a general medical condition. By age 7 to 8 years, encopresis is prevalent in 1.5% of boys and 0.5% of girls. There is some overlap between the elimination disorders—about 15% of children with enuresis also have difficulties with encopresis. Behavior therapy, medications, supportive psychotherapy, and relaxation techniques can be very useful in treatment.

Substance Use Disorders

44

TAMARA J. DOLENC, MD

Introduction

Substance dependence is a chronic, relapsing illness. Episodes of intoxication are common, along with significant medical and social consequences. Substance dependence is accompanied by loss of control over the amount used, continued use despite negative consequences, preoccupation with use, and dysphoria during abstinence. In heavy and long-term users, abrupt cessation or reduction in substance use results in withdrawal syndrome.

Risk of substance dependence is influenced by genetic, psychosocial, and environmental factors. Patients with substance use disorders come from all age groups and from all ethnic, cultural, and socioeconomic backgrounds. Thus, a history of substance use should be obtained from every patient. The majority of patients with serious mental illness abuse alcohol or drugs, and most patients with alcohol and drug use disorders have another psychiatric disorder.

Substances of abuse are thought to exert their rewarding effects through dopamine and the brain reward system involving the nucleus accumbens, ventral tegmental area, and amygdala.

Diagnostic criteria for substance abuse and substance dependence are shown in Boxes 44.1 and 44.2 respectively. Drug screen testing is common when patients present with symptoms of intoxication or withdrawal. Substances can be detected in urine for various lengths of time, as shown in Table 44.1.

This chapter emphasizes the identification and treatment of substance abuse disorders; further discussion of intoxication and withdrawal syndromes is included in Volume 2, Chapter 81, "Intoxications and Nontraumatic Neurologic Injury."

Substances

Alcohol

The lifetime prevalence of alcohol use disorders is estimated to be 30% and the lifetime prevalence of alcohol dependence, 12% to 15%. Problematic drinking is 2 to 3 times less likely among women than men, but women experience adverse consequences earlier than men.

Patients with alcohol use disorders are more likely to have another substance use disorder, anxiety disorder, depression, bipolar disorder, schizophrenia, or antisocial personality disorder. It is estimated that alcohol is involved in up to 50% of suicides.

Several screening instruments have been successfully used in identifying problematic drinking. The most commonly used is the CAGE questionnaire (Box 44.3). A CAGE questionnaire score of 2 or more is considered

---

Box 44.1 • Criteria for the Diagnosis of Substance Abuse

One or more of the following criteria must be present at any time in the same 12-month period:

1. Substance use results in failure to fulfill major obligations
2. Recurrent substance use in physically dangerous situations
3. Recurrent substance-related legal problems
4. Continued substance use despite recurrent social or interpersonal problems
5. Patient has never met criteria for dependence with this substance

---

Abbreviations: CNS, central nervous system; GABA, γ-aminobutyric acid; GHB, γ-hydroxybutyric acid; LSD, lysergic acid diethylamide; MDMA, 3,4-methylenedioxymethamphetamine; PCP, phencyclidine

Box 44.2 • Criteria for the Diagnosis of Substance Dependence

Three or more of the following criteria must be present at any time in the same 12-month period:

1. Tolerance: increased amounts of the subtance are needed to achieve intoxication or the desired effect, and there is a markedly diminished effect with continued use of the same amount of substance
2. Clinical withdrawal symptoms
3. Substance is often taken in larger amounts or for longer periods than intended
4. Persistent desire or unsuccessful efforts to cut down or control use of the substance
5. Significant amount of time is spent obtaining the substance, using the substance, or recovering from its effects
6. Important activities are given up or reduced because of substance use
7. Continued substance use despite adverse consequences

Table 44.1 • Length of Time That Selected Substances Can Be Detected in Urine

Substance	Duration of Detectable Presence in Urine
Alcohol	7–12 h
Amphetamines and methamphetamines	2 d
Cannabis Single use Heavy long-term use	3 d 30 d
Cocaine	2–4 d
Diazepam	30 d
Heroin	2 d
Lorazepam	3 d
Morphine	3 d
Phencyclidine (PCP)	8 d

clinically significant, suggesting clearly problematic alcohol use.

The effects of alcohol are primarily mediated through activation of γ-aminobutyric acid (GABA) type A receptors. Opioid peptides, dopamine, serotonin, and glutamate have also been implicated. Acute alcoholic hallucinosis occurs with abrupt discontinuation of alcohol use or during intoxication. Unlike in delirium, the sensorium is clear, hallucinations are most often auditory and paranoid in nature, and there is no tremor or autonomic hyperarousal.

Alcohol withdrawal symptoms occur with abrupt cessation of alcohol use or with diminishing alcohol blood levels in dependent patients. Symptoms usually start about 8 hours after the last drink, tend to peak within 24 hours, and resolve in a week. They can include sweating, insomnia, headache, tremor, anxiety, anorexia, nausea, and vomiting. The most severe form of alcohol withdrawal is delirium tremens, which usually starts 48 to 72 hours after the last drink, and is characterized by delirium, tremor, autonomic hyperactivity, fever, restlessness, and frightening visual hallucinations. Patients may also experience auditory and tactile hallucinations.

Relapse prevention treatment should be individualized to the patient's needs. The strategies include self-help programs, such as Alcoholics Anonymous, motivational enhancement, and cognitive behavior therapy. Naltrexone, acamprosate, and disulfiram are used to reduce cravings, to decrease the amount of alcohol used, and to promote abstinence.

Cocaine, Methamphetamine, and Prescription Stimulants

Cocaine and methamphetamines are central nervous system (CNS) stimulants, as are stimulant medications (methylphenidate, amphetamine salts, modafinil), pseudoephedrine, and 3,4-methylenedioxymethamphetamine (MDMA) (popularly called ecstasy or molly). While cocaine blocks synaptic reuptake of dopamine, methamphetamine blocks dopamine reuptake and promotes its release.

Acute effects of stimulants include sympathetic arousal, high energy, euphoria (the sense of a high), inflated self-esteem, increased sex drive, accentuated alertness, and decreased appetite. Stimulant use may cause anxiety, irritability, panic attacks, mania, and aggressive behaviors.

Long-term use of a CNS stimulant may result in weight loss, respiratory effects, arrhythmias, arterial vasospasm, myocardial infarction, stroke, nasal septum necrosis (with intranasal use), dental problems, and seizures. Patients may experience tactile hallucinations that may result in

Box 44.3 • CAGE Questionnaire[a]

Have you ever felt you should *cut* down on your drinking?

Have people *annoyed* you by criticizing your drinking?

Have you felt bad or *guilty* about your drinking?

Have you ever had a drink first thing in the morning to steady your nerves or get rid of a hangover (*eye-opener*)?

[a] Each "yes" answer earns 1 point. The maximum score is 4 points, and a score of 2 or more points suggests problematic alcohol use.

skin manipulation and infections. Long-term CNS stimulant use has also been associated with depression, psychosis, and cognitive impairment.

Intravenous drug use can cause cellulitis, local and solid organ abscesses, vasculitis, endocarditis, hepatitis B and C infection, human immunodeficiency virus infection, pulmonary emboli, and sepsis.

Stimulant withdrawal occurs within hours to days of the last use in dependent patients. It is characterized by mood dysphoria, fatigue, insomnia or hypersomnia, increased appetite, psychomotor changes, and bothersome dreams.

Relapse prevention strategies include self-help groups and cognitive behavior therapy. There are no US Food and Drug Administration–approved treatments for stimulant abuse.

Opiates

Prescription opioid abuse is a major public health problem. A large majority of opioid-dependent patients have comorbid depression, posttraumatic stress disorder, or antisocial personality disorder. Eating foods with poppy seeds can result in a positive urine drug test because of their morphine and codeine content.

Opiates bind to opioid receptors in the brain, gastrointestinal tract, and autonomic nervous system. Effects of opiate use include a sense of calm, pain relief, cough suppression, miosis, respiratory depression, constipation, and urinary retention. Opiates can cause nausea or vomiting.

Opioid withdrawal occurs with abrupt cessation or decreased opioid use in dependent patients or with administration of an opioid antagonist in long-term heavy users. Symptoms include dysphoria, nausea, vomiting, diarrhea, myalgias, lacrimation, rhinorrhea, yawning, sweating, piloerection (the source of the term *cold turkey*), mydriasis, and sometimes fever. Untreated opioid withdrawal during pregnancy can pose significant risk to the mother and unborn child. Methadone, buprenorphine and naloxone, and clonidine are used in detoxification.

For maintenance treatment of opioid dependence, methadone and the combination of buprenorphine and naloxone are commonly prescribed. Buprenorphine is a partial opioid agonist, and naloxone is an opioid antagonist. Naloxone is not active orally and becomes active only if it is administered intravenously; when combined with buprenorphine, it can precipitate opioid withdrawal and thereby deter patients from inappropriate use. Additional treatment options include psychosocial treatments, including cognitive behavior therapy, behavioral approaches, family and group therapies as well as Narcotics Anonymous self-help groups, and long-term therapeutic communities.

Sedatives, Anxiolytics, and Hypnotics

Benzodiazepines and barbiturates are commonly misused and abused. Like alcohol, they are CNS depressants. Therefore, symptoms of withdrawal are similar to those associated with alcohol and may include seizures and delirium. The half-life of a substance determines the timing of the onset of withdrawal. With short-acting agents (eg, lorazepam, alprazolam), symptoms start within hours after the last use; with longer-acting agents (eg, clonazepam, diazepam, chlordiazepoxide), withdrawal symptoms may not emerge until several days after the last use.

Hallucinogens

Hallucinogens, a diverse group of substances, include lysergic acid diethylamide (LSD), psilocybin, mescaline, designer drugs (MDMA and γ-hydroxybutyric acid [GHB]), and the dissociative anesthetics phencyclidine (PCP) and ketamine.

Acute effects of hallucinogens include more intense perceptions, perceptual distortions (light trails behind moving objects, macropsia, micropsia, and synesthesias), as well as existential experiences, hallucinations, and paranoia. Flashbacks, the unexpected reexperiencing of perceptual disturbance, may occur for up to a year (rarely, later) after use. PCP can cause extremely dangerous and violent behavior. Long-term hallucinogen use can lead to depression, anxiety, and psychosis.

Cannabis

Cannabis is the most widely used illicit substance. Its acute effects include a sense of relaxation, mild euphoria, perceptual distortions, and amplifications of regular life experiences (eating, music, sex). In some users, cannabis causes dysphoric mood, anxiety, panic attacks, and paranoia.

Inhalants

Inhalants are a large group of volatile hydrocarbons that are used in many household products, such as glue, shoe polish, spray paint, and gasoline. Inhalant use is particularly common among adolescents. Long-term use of inhalants may lead to white matter changes, cerebral atrophy, and cognitive impairment.

- A CAGE questionnaire score of ≥2 is considered clinically significant, suggesting clearly problematic alcohol use.
- Symptoms of alcohol withdrawal usually start about 8 hours after the last drink, tend to peak within 24 hours, and resolve in a week.
- Long-term use of a CNS stimulant may result in weight loss, respiratory effects, arrhythmias, arterial vasospasm, myocardial infarction, stroke, nasal septum necrosis (with intranasal use), dental problems, and seizures.
- For maintenance treatment of opioid dependence, methadone and the combination of buprenorphine and naloxone are commonly prescribed.
- Long-term use of inhalants may lead to white matter changes, cerebral atrophy, and cognitive impairment.

45 Pharmacologic Treatment of Psychiatric Disorders

OSAMA A. ABULSEOUD, MD

Introduction

Human behaviors, including thinking, feeling, and action, can be viewed as products of the interactions between brain circuits, neurotransmitters, and oscillations that are influenced to a certain extent by inherited genes, acquired values, and social norms. A psychiatric disorder reflects a dysfunctional brain, and one way to treat such a disorder is through the use of pharmacologic compounds that can help restore order in disorderly brains.

This chapter reviews the 4 main classes of drugs used to treat major mental illnesses: antidepressants, mood stabilizers, sedative hypnotics, and antipsychotics, followed by brief comments on a few drugs used to treat alcohol, opiate, and nicotine dependence. A short account on the use of electroconvulsive therapy (ECT) for difficult-to-treat conditions concludes the chapter.

Antidepressants

Tricyclic Antidepressants

Overview and Classification

Tricyclic antidepressants (TCAs) share a basic tricyclic (or heterocyclic) structure, mechanism of action, and many side effects. Their use introduced important observations, such as drug action involving norepinephrine and serotonin neurotransmitters, the need for adequate dose and duration during short-term treatment, the importance of continuation treatment of chronic depression, and the concepts of polymorphisms in the cytochrome P450 (CYP) isoenzymes and drug-drug interactions.

TCAs are classified as *tertiary amines* (eg, amitriptyline, clomipramine, doxepin, and imipramine), *secondary amines* (eg, desipramine, nortriptyline, and protriptyline), and *tetracyclics* (eg, amoxapine and maprotiline). Tertiary amines have greater affinity for the serotonin transporter, and secondary amines are relatively more potent at the norepinephrine transporter. However, tertiary amines are demethylated to secondary amines during hepatic metabolism.

Mechanism of Action

Tertiary TCAs block serotonin transporters and inhibit the uptake of serotonin, leading to an increase in synaptic serotonin levels. High synaptic serotonin levels stimulate the presynaptic somatodendritic serotonin 1A (5-hydroxytryptamine 1A [5-HT$_{1A}$]) autoreceptor, which results in a decrease in the firing rate of the presynaptic serotonin neuron. Presynaptic autoreceptors are desensitized in 10 to 14 days with subsequent enhancement of serotonin transmission.

Secondary TCAs block norepinephrine transporters and inhibit the uptake of norepinephrine, leading to an increase in synaptic norepinephrine levels. High synaptic norepinephrine levels stimulate the presynaptic somatodendritic α-2 noradrenergic autoreceptor, which results in a decreased firing rate of the presynaptic noradrenergic

Abbreviations: CYP, cytochrome P450; ECT, electroconvulsive therapy; FDA, US Food and Drug Administration; GABA, γ-aminobutyric acid; H$_1$, histamine$_1$; 5-HT$_1$, serotonin 1 (5-hydroxytryptamine 1); 5-HT$_{1A}$, serotonin 1A (5-hydroxytryptamine 1A); 5-HT$_2$, serotonin 2 (5-hydroxytryptamine 2); MAO, monoamine oxidase; MAOI, monoamine oxidase inhibitor; SNRI, selective serotonin-norepinephrine reuptake inhibitor; SSRI, selective serotonin reuptake inhibitor; TCA, tricyclic antidepressant

neuron. In contrast to the serotonergic system, the firing rate of noradrenergic neurons remains inhibited with long-term treatment, suggesting that somatodendritic α-2 receptors do not desensitize.

Dosing

Approximately 5% to 10% of whites are homozygous for the autosomal recessive CYP2D6 trait, resulting in deficient hydroxylation of desipramine and nortriptyline (ie, they are poor metabolizers). About 20% of Asians have a genetic polymorphism resulting in deficient CYP2C19 metabolism. The relationship between plasma level and response has been clarified for the tricyclics, rendering serum levels a helpful tool in assessing the adequacy of a therapeutic trial.

Clinical Uses

TCAs are used for major depression, psychotic depression, obsessive-compulsive disorder, panic disorders, and pain syndromes. Specific TCAs may be indicated for individual diagnoses (Table 45.1).

TCAs generally are not recommended for treating bipolar depression since TCAs are more likely than other agents to induce a manic switch. In addition, they are not recommended for treating depression in children because of a lack of efficacy and reported serious side effects. However, imipramine (25–50 mg at bedtime) has US Food and Drug Administration (FDA) approval for treatment of nocturnal enuresis in children.

Side Effects

The tricyclic and tetracyclic compounds have various adverse actions mediated by other receptors. Blocking muscarinic receptors results in anticholinergic side effects, such as dry mouth, constipation, and urinary retention. Amitriptyline is the most anticholinergic, while desipramine is the least anticholinergic in this class. Blocking histamine$_1$ (H$_1$) receptors leads to sedation. Doxepin is the most potent H$_1$ antagonist among TCAs. Tricyclics act on fast sodium channels and can cause adverse effects such as orthostatic hypotension, tachycardia, and cardiac conduction problems. Other side effects include sexual dysfunction, increased sweating, headache, carbohydrate craving and weight gain, fine rapid tremors, and delirium.

Serious side effects include cardiac arrhythmias. An overdose can be fatal, with death most commonly occurring as a result of cardiac arrhythmia.

Interactions

There are many potential interactions with TCAs. Not all are listed here. One of the most concerning is interaction with monoamine oxidase (MAO) inhibitors (MAOIs). This can result in a sudden catecholamine increase and a potentially fatal hypertensive reaction. However, TCAs and MAOIs are used together to treat patients with refractory depression. Treatment is begun with lower doses, and either the 2 compounds are started together or the TCA is started first and followed by cautious addition of the MAOI (TCAs should not be added if the patient is already taking an MAOI).

Tricyclics also may interact with quinidine and can increase TCA levels (quinidine is a potent CYP2D6 inhibitor) and cause greater cardiac conduction delay. Nicotine induces the CYP1A2 pathway and may lower concentrations of the tertiary tricyclics, but the secondary tricyclics (eg, desipramine, nortriptyline) appear to be less affected. The tertiary tricyclics compete with warfarin for some metabolic enzymes (eg, CYP1A2) and may increase warfarin levels.

Monoamine Oxidase Inhibitors

Overview

Two isoenzymes (MAO-A and MAO-B) have been identified. The gene for both enzymes is located on the short arm of the X chromosome, while the enzymes themselves are widespread in the subcortical regions of the brain, especially in the glia and outer mitochondrial membrane of the dopaminergic and noradrenergic neurons for MAO-A and serotonergic neurons for MAO-B isoenzymes. Tranylcypromine, phenelzine, and isocarboxazid are all nonselective irreversible MAOIs. Moclobemide is a selective, reversible MAO-A inhibitor, and L-deprenyl (selegiline hydrochloride) is an irreversible but selective MAO-B inhibitor.

Mechanism of Action

MAO enzymes are bound to the outer mitochondrial surface and maintain a low cytoplasmic concentration of

Table 45.1 • Selected TCAs

Drug	Class	Common Uses	Notable Adverse Effects of TCAs
Amitriptyline	Tertiary amine	Chronic pain, depression	Antimuscarinic effects (dry mouth, constipation, urinary retention); antihistaminergic effects (sedation); rarely, cardiac conduction abnormalities
Clomipramine	Tertiary amine	Obsessive-compulsive disorder	
Imipramine	Tertiary amine	Nocturnal enuresis, panic disorder	
Nortriptyline	Secondary amine	Chronic pain, depression	

Abbreviation: TCA, tricyclic antidepressant.

amines within the cytoplasm only (not in vesicles). MAOIs increase the amine content in the cytoplasm. Initial use leads to an increase in synaptic catecholamine (serotonin, dopamine, and norepinephrine) levels. High synaptic norepinephrine levels stimulate the presynaptic somatodendritic α-2 noradrenergic autoreceptor, which results in a decreased firing rate of the presynaptic noradrenergic neuron. Long-term treatment with MAOIs leads to downregulation of α-adrenoreceptors and serotonin 1 (5-HT$_1$) and serotonin 2 (5-HT$_2$) receptors, with a subsequent antidepressant response.

Clinical Uses

Clinical uses of MAOIs include treatment of major and atypical depression (*atypical depression* is characterized by mood reactivity, hyperphagia, hypersomnia, severe fatigue, and rejection sensitivity); panic disorder and social phobia (phenelzine, tranylcypromine, and moclobemide are all effective); posttraumatic stress disorder (phenelzine has proved effective); and bulimia nervosa (phenelzine and isocarboxazid have been shown to be effective in treating some symptoms).

Side Effects

In general, MAOIs have more severe or frequent side effects than other antidepressants. The most common side effect is orthostatic hypotension. Other frequent side effects include dizziness, headache, dry mouth, insomnia, constipation, blurred vision, nausea, peripheral edema, forgetfulness, fainting spells, hesitancy of urination, weakness, and myoclonic jerks.

Long-term side effects include weight gain (more so with phenelzine than with tranylcypromine), edema (also more so with phenelzine than with tranylcypromine), muscle cramps, carbohydrate craving, sexual dysfunction,

pyridoxine deficiency, hypoglycemia, hypomania, urinary retention, and disorientation.

Interactions

Several food items can interact with MAOIs. These include foods containing high tyramine levels, such as aged cheese, cream cheese, cottage cheese, red wine, banana peel, bean curd, fava beans, sausage, pepperoni, salami, and sauerkraut. In addition, large amounts of caffeine, chocolate, nuts, and soy sauce should be used only with caution.

MAOIs also interact with several medications, including some nonprescription medications. Drugs that should be avoided during the use of MAOIs and for 3 to 4 weeks afterward include those that increase serotonin, norepinephrine, or dopamine levels, such as selective serotonin reuptake inhibitors (SSRIs), selective serotonin-norepinephrine reuptake inhibitors (SNRIs), TCAs, dextromethorphan (in cough syrup), amphetamines and all stimulants, ephedrine (in decongestants), and norepinephrine (in local anesthetics).

SSRIs and SNRIs

Overview

The ubiquity of SSRIs derives from their safety, efficacy, and favorable side-effect profile (Table 45.2). SSRIs currently available in the United States include fluoxetine, paroxetine, sertraline, citalopram, and escitalopram. In 1993, venlafaxine was introduced, the first of the SNRIs. Duloxetine, desvenlafaxine, and milnacipran have followed, although milnacipran has FDA approval for use only in fibromyalgia.

Mechanism of Action

Abnormalities in central serotonin function have been hypothesized to underlie disturbances in mood, anxiety,

---

Table 45.2 • Selected SSRIs and SNRIs

Drug	Class	Common Uses	Notable Adverse Effects
Fluoxetine	SSRI	Depression, anxiety, OCD	Diarrhea, anorgasmia, suicidality, rarely serotonin syndrome (rigidity, akathisia, delirium, abdominal pain, nausea, diaphoresis, tachycardia, occasionally hyperpyrexia)[a]
Paroxetine	SSRI	Depression, anxiety, OCD	
Sertraline	SSRI	Depression, anxiety, OCD	
Citalopram	SSRI	Depression, anxiety, OCD	
Escitalopram	SSRI	Depression, anxiety, OCD	
Venlafaxine	SNRI	Depression, anxiety	Hypertension
Duloxetine	SNRI	Chronic pain	Sweating
Desvenlafaxine	SNRI	Depression, anxiety	Hypertension
Milnacipran	SNRI	Fibromyalgia	Hypertension

Abbreviations: OCD, obsessive-compulsive disorder; SNRI, selective serotonin-norepinephrine reuptake inhibitor; SSRI, selective serotonin reuptake inhibitor.

[a] These adverse effects are applicable to all the SSRIs listed in this table.

satiety, cognition, aggression, and sexual drive. SSRIs block serotonin reuptake, leading to an acute increase in synaptic serotonin. Elevated synaptic serotonin levels activate somatodendritic autoreceptors (decreased firing) and terminal serotonin autoreceptors (decreased release), which eventually decrease synaptic serotonin levels. Long-term administration leads to downregulation of 5-HT$_{1A}$ receptors and reestablishes a normal rate of firing, despite sustained reuptake blockade, resulting in increased synaptic serotonin concentration. The SNRIs add potent uptake inhibition of norepinephrine; this occurs only with venlafaxine doses in excess of 150 mg daily, although duloxetine has an equal affinity for norepinephrine and serotonin, regardless of the dose.

Clinical Uses

Clinical uses for SSRIs are listed in Box 45.1.

Side Effects

Enhancement of serotonin within the central nervous system can lead to agitation, anxiety, sleep disturbance,

---

> **Box 45.1 • Clinical Uses for Selective Serotonin Reuptake Inhibitors**
>
> *Depression*
>
> Major depression
> Anxious depression
> Premenstrual dysphoric disorder
>
> *Anxiety*
>
> Generalized anxiety
> OCD
> OCD spectrum disorders (skin picking, panic disorder, body dysmorphic disorder, PTSD)
>
> *Eating disorders*
>
> Binge eating
>
> *Pain disorders*
>
> Fibromyalgia
> Chronic pain syndrome
> Hot flashes associated with menopause
> Migraine
>
> *Other*
>
> Anger or aggression
> Premature ejaculation
>
> Abbreviations: OCD, obsessive-compulsive disorder; PTSD, posttraumatic stress disorder.

---

tremor, sexual dysfunction (primarily anorgasmia), or headache. Enhancement of serotonin within the gastrointestinal tract can provoke nausea and diarrhea.

Autonomic side effects include dry mouth and diaphoresis. Sleep-related side effects are decreased rapid eye movement sleep and increased non–rapid eye movement sleep. Rare side effects include arthralgia, lymphadenopathy, the syndrome of inappropriate secretion of antidiuretic hormone, agranulocytosis, and hypoglycemia. Venlafaxine and desvenlafaxine may provoke sustained, dose-related elevations in blood pressure.

An FDA boxed warning exists for SSRIs and suicidality. In most cases, the therapeutic benefit of SSRIs or SNRIs outweighs the risk of increased suicidal thoughts or behaviors. However, particular caution is required when prescribing SSRIs or SNRIs to children, adolescents, and adults through age 25 years.

Another serious side effect includes the serotonin syndrome. Progressive symptoms may include akathisia, tremor, delirium, clonus, and muscular rigidity. Abdominal pain, hyperactive bowel sounds, nausea, diarrhea, diaphoresis, and tachycardia are common. Severe manifestations may include hyperpyrexia, hypertension, or cardiovascular shock and death. (See also Volume 2, Chapter 8, "Neuromuscular Disease in the Neuroscience Intensive Care Unit.")

SSRI and SNRI discontinuation symptoms occur most frequently with agents that have a short elimination half-life and no active metabolite. The most common symptoms are dizziness, nausea, vomiting, fatigue, lethargy, flulike symptoms, and sensory and sleep disturbances. The psychological symptoms most commonly reported are anxiety, irritability, and crying spells.

Interactions

SSRIs are both substrates for and inhibitors of oxidation through CYP2D6 (paroxetine and fluoxetine are the principal offenders—the effects of the others are much less clinically relevant). Through inhibition of CYP2D6, fluoxetine and paroxetine increase the concentration of concomitantly administered drugs that rely on this enzyme for metabolism. This has particular clinical relevance when the second agent has a narrow therapeutic index. Examples of such agents include flecainide, quinidine, carbamazepine, propafenone, TCAs, and several antipsychotics. The clinical consequence is that efficacy may be enhanced or impaired or the adverse-event profile may be heightened (or both efficacy and the adverse-event profile may be affected).

- Tertiary TCAs block serotonin transporters and inhibit the uptake of serotonin, leading to an increase in synaptic serotonin levels.
- Secondary TCAs block norepinephrine transporters and inhibit the uptake of norepinephrine, leading to an increase in synaptic norepinephrine levels.

- Approximately 5%-10% of whites are homozygous for the autosomal recessive CYP2D6 trait, resulting in deficient hydroxylation of desipramine and nortriptyline (ie, they are poor metabolizers).
- MAOIs increase the amine content in the cytoplasm. Initial use leads to an increase in synaptic catecholamine (serotonin, dopamine, and norepinephrine) levels.
- The most common side effect of MAOIs is orthostatic hypotension.
- Several food items can interact with MAOIs.
- An FDA boxed warning exists for SSRIs and suicidality.
- SSRIs are both substrates for and inhibitors of oxidation through CYP2D6.
- The inhibition of CYP2D6 (eg, by fluoxetine or paroxetine) increases the concentration of drugs that rely on CYP2D6 for metabolism. This has particular clinical relevance when the second agent has a narrow therapeutic index (eg, flecainide, quinidine, carbamazepine, propafenone, TCAs, and several antipsychotics). The clinical consequence is that efficacy may be enhanced or impaired or the adverse-event profile may be heightened (or both efficacy and the adverse-event profile may be affected).

Mood Stabilizers

Lithium

Lithium is still the gold standard for treatment of bipolar disorder and particularly for mania. Its efficacy is well documented even though its mechanism of action is largely unknown.

Indications

In addition to its use for acute mania, lithium is indicated for long-term bipolar disorder prophylaxis and as an augmenting agent for antidepressants in refractory unipolar depression. Lithium and clozapine are the only 2 psychotropic medications known to reduce suicidality.

Dosing

Acute mania requires serum levels ranging from 0.8 to 1.2 mEq/L, while lower serum levels (0.6–1.0 mEq/L) are typically sufficient during maintenance treatment. In addition to lithium plasma levels, renal and thyroid function should be monitored during lithium treatment every 3 to 6 months initially and then annually in psychiatrically stable patients.

Side Effects

Side effects of lithium are listed in Table 45.3.

Interactions

Concomitant use of nonsteroidal antiinflammatory drugs, angiotensin-converting enzyme inhibitors, spironolactone, or thiazide diuretics typically increases serum lithium levels.

Valproate

Overview

Valproate has been used effectively as an anticonvulsant and as a mood stabilizer in the United States. Valproate is available in oral and intravenous forms.

Clinical Uses

Valproate is indicated as monotherapy for acute mania or as an adjunct to other antimanic agents, such as lithium, in maintenance treatment of bipolar disorder. However, unlike lithium, valproate is effective in treating mixed mania, rapid cycling bipolar disorder, and comorbid substance use, particularly alcohol dependence.

Side Effects

Gastrointestinal tract disturbances include nausea, vomiting, diarrhea, anorexia, and weight gain.

Table 45.3 • Side Effects of Lithium

System or Organ	Side Effect	Monitoring
Digestive system	Nausea, vomiting, metallic taste, dry mouth	...
Heart	Sinus bradycardia, sinus node dysfunction, T-wave changes	Electrocardiogram before treatment, especially if patient is older than 50 y or has a cardiac condition
Nervous system	Headache, generalized weakness, dizziness, confusion, ataxia, tremors, slow cognition	Lithium serum level
Kidney	Polyuria, polydipsia, impaired urine concentration capacity Acute renal failure (from long-term use or toxic levels)	Lithium serum level Renal function tests
Endocrine system	Hypothyroidism, hyperparathyroidism, hypercalcemia, diabetes insipidus	Thyroid function

Serious side effects of valproate may include hepato-toxicity, pancreatitis, and nonhepatic hyperammonemia. Hepatotoxicity is a rare side effect, but checking liver enzymes at baseline and at intervals of 6 to 12 months during treatment is indicated. Occasionally, hyperammone-mic encephalopathy develops with normal transaminases. Pancreatitis is another rare but serious potential side effect of valproate treatment. Symptoms of acute abdominal pain, persistent vomiting, and elevated serum amylase concentrations necessitate stopping the use of valproate.

Interactions

Protein-bound drugs such as aspirin can displace valproate from its binding sites and elevate free valproate serum levels. In turn, valproate can displace lamotrigine, phenytoin, or phenobarbital from their binding sites, increasing their levels. Valproate also competes with hepatic lamotrigine glucuronidation, resulting in increased lamotrigine levels.

Lamotrigine

Overview

Lamotrigine is another anticonvulsant with mood-stabilizing properties. It appears to regulate glutamatergic neurotransmission at key brain regions involved in mood regulation, such as the anterior cingulate and prefrontal cortex.

Clinical Uses

Although lamotrigine is FDA approved for maintenance therapy in bipolar I disorder, it is more commonly used in averting depressive episodes in patients with bipolar II disorder.

Side Effects

Adverse effects may include nausea, headache, dizziness, diplopia, and ataxia. Rash may also occur.

The most serious potential side effect of lamotrigine is Stevens-Johnson syndrome. Patients with Stevens-Johnson syndrome present with a progressive, pruritic, tender rash that involves the eyes, lips, or mouth and is associated with fever, malaise, pharyngitis, and anorexia. Although Stevens-Johnson syndrome is rare (1–3 in 1,000 patients), children, and patients taking valproate or those who receive rapid titration or high lamotrigine doses are at higher risk. If Stevens-Johnson syndrome develops, the patient should stop taking lamotrigine and should be hospitalized. Rechallenge with lamotrigine after recovery from Stevens-Johnson syndrome is not recommended.

Interactions

Initiating use of lamotrigine while a patient is already receiving valproate treatment requires extra caution: The initial lamotrigine dosage should be 25 mg every other day, with a very gradual upward titration.

- In addition to lithium plasma levels, renal and thyroid function should be monitored during lithium treatment every 3–6 months initially and then annually in psychiatrically stable patients.
- Valproate is indicated as monotherapy for acute mania or as an adjunct to other antimanic agents, such as lithium, in maintenance treatment of bipolar disorder.
- Serious side effects of valproate may include hepatotoxicity, pancreatitis, and nonhepatic hyperammonemia.

Sedative Hypnotics

Benzodiazepines

Overview

All benzodiazepines are effective in reducing anxiety. They bind to an allosteric site in the γ-aminobutyric acid (GABA) A receptor, opening chloride channels and causing hyperpolarization of the neurons.

Clinical Uses

Benzodiazepines are indicated for panic disorder, generalized anxiety, and insomnia. They are also used effectively as muscle relaxants and anticonvulsants, especially for patients with alcohol withdrawal.

The most important differences among the multiple benzodiazepines are potency and elimination half-life. Compounds with a long half-life tend to accumulate with repeated doses and cause more sedation and cognitive side effects. Although all benzodiazepines carry the risk of dependence and withdrawal symptoms, this is most problematic with high-potency agents.

For comparison, 1 mg of lorazepam is equivalent to 0.25 mg of alprazolam, 0.5 mg of clonazepam, 5 mg of diazepam, 5 mg of temazepam, or 10 mg of chlordiazepoxide.

Side Effects

Sedation, relative inattention, mild forgetfulness, and retrograde amnesia are not uncommon. Benzodiazepines increase the risk of falls, especially among the elderly, so their use is limited in the geriatric population.

Overdose can be fatal because of respiratory depression, especially if combined with alcohol; flumazenil, a benzodiazepine antagonist, is used to reverse the effect of benzodiazepines.

- Benzodiazepines increase the risk of falls, especially among the elderly, so their use is limited in the geriatric population.

Antipsychotics

Overview

The introduction of chlorpromazine in 1952 was a breakthrough in the development of modern psychopharmacology. It brought tranquility to the loud mental asylums and was followed by the production of several similar compounds: phenothiazines, butyrophenones, thioxanthenes, indoles, and benzamide. Collectively, they were called major tranquilizers or neuroleptics when extrapyramidal side effects were later observed. The principal pharmacologic activity is dopaminergic D_2 receptor blockade with variable activities at H_1, muscarinic M_1, and α_1-adrenergic receptors. Newer atypical antipsychotics include risperidone, quetiapine, clozapine, olanzapine, ziprasidone, and aripiprazole.

Mechanism of Action

The clinical efficacy of antipsychotics correlates with dopamine D_2 receptor blockade. The dopaminergic system consists of dopamine-producing neurons, dopaminergic circuits, and dopaminergic receptors.

The dopamine-producing neurons are present at 3 major locations:

1. Ventral tegmental area—immediately medial to the substantia nigra and containing dopaminergic neurons that are smaller and less densely packed than those in the substantia nigra pars compacta
2. Retrorubral area—in the caudal midbrain at the level of the medial lemniscus
3. Several hypothalamic nuclei—eg, arcuate, periventricular, paraventricular, and supraoptic nuclei

Dopamine is synthesized inside these neurons, through the conversion of L-tyrosine to L-dopa (L-dihydroxyphenylalanine) by the enzyme tyrosine hydroxylase; L-dopa is converted to dopamine by the enzyme L-aromatic amino acid decarboxylase. Released dopamine is taken up by the dopamine transporter located at the somatodendritic junction and on dopaminergic nerve terminals.

Four major dopaminergic circuits have been delineated: the nigrostriatal, mesolimbic, mesocortical, and tuberoinfundibular circuits. The nigrostriatal circuitry has critical roles in maintaining normal motor activity and reward pathways. The mesolimbic circuit is critical for motivation, selection, and orchestration of goal-directed behaviors, motor activity, and reward pathways. The mesocortical circuit has an integral role in cognition. The tuberoinfundibular circuit inhibits prolactin release in the pituitary.

The dopaminergic receptors can be divided into the D_1 family, containing the D_1 and D_5 receptors, and the D_2 family containing the D_2, D_3, and D_4 receptors. The D_1 receptors are important in higher cognitive function and perhaps in the actions of medications like methylphenidate. The D_2 receptors have long been implicated in the pathophysiology and treatment of schizophrenia. The highest density of D_3 receptors is in the nucleus accumbens, while the D_4 and D_5 receptors are not as highly expressed in the brain.

Clinical Uses

Antipsychotics are used in the treatment of schizophrenia, schizoaffective disorders, substance-induced psychosis, major depression with psychotic features, and mania (Table 45.4). They are also used effectively to treat conditions such as Tourette syndrome, psychosis associated with Huntington disease, nausea, emesis, and hiccups.

Side Effects

Extrapyramidal side effects include muscle rigidity, dystonia, bradykinesia, akathisia, tremors, and tardive dyskinesia. In general, the newer atypical antipsychotics cause fewer extrapyramidal effects. Photosensitivity, orthostatic hypotension, sedation, weight gain, prolongation of the corrected QT interval, and anticholinergic side effects such

Table 45.4 • Selected Antipsychotics

Drug	Class	Common Uses	Notable Adverse Effects
Chlorpromazine	Conventional	Psychosis, hiccups	Parkinsonism (bradykinesia, rigidity, tremor), neuroleptic malignant syndrome (delirium, hyperprolactinemia and galactorrhea, hyperpyrexia, rigidity, rhabdomyolysis), tardive dyskinesia
Haloperidol	Conventional	Psychosis	
Risperidone	Atypical	Psychosis, mood stabilization	. . .
Quetiapine	Atypical	Psychosis, mood stabilization	Prolongation of corrected QT interval
Clozapine	Atypical	Psychosis, mood stabilization	Agranulocytosis
Olanzapine	Atypical	Psychosis, mood stabilization	. . .
Ziprasidone	Atypical	Psychosis, mood stabilization	. . .
Aripiprazole	Atypical	Psychosis, mood stabilization	. . .

as dry mouth, constipation, and blurred vision also occur. These side effects are more common with low-potency agents. Antipsychotic-induced prolactin elevation can cause sexual dysfunction, amenorrhea, gynecomastia, galactorrhea, or hypoestrogenism and osteopenia.

Serious side effects of antipsychotics are rare but include neuroleptic malignant syndrome and agranulocytosis; elderly patients treated for delirium may have increased mortality. Neuroleptic malignant syndrome is a medical emergency. Patients present with delirium associated with fever, muscle rigidity, autonomic instability, and variable elevations in the creatine kinase level. (See also Volume 2, Chapter 8, "Neuromuscular Disease in the Neuroscience Intensive Care Unit."). Many antipsychotics can cause agranulocytosis, but only the use of clozapine requires a pretreatment white blood cell count with a differential count for absolute neutrophils.

Clozapine should not be prescribed for patients who have low neutrophil counts or who are receiving other drugs that can cause granulocytopenia. A complete blood cell count with a differential leukocyte count should be done weekly for the first 6 months, biweekly for the second 6 months, and then every 4 weeks throughout the duration of treatment. Patients who require high-dose clozapine (>600 mg daily) are frequently prescribed a prophylactic anticonvulsant owing to increased seizure risk.

Use of antipsychotics to treat delirium or agitation in elderly patients has been associated with an increase in mortality.

Interactions

Conventional antipsychotics are highly protein bound and can displace other protein-bound drugs such as warfarin, digoxin, and valproate, leading to elevations in the serum levels of these medications. Many of the conventional antipsychotics are metabolized hepatically through the CYP2D6 and CYP3A4 isoenzymes; at the same time, they also potently inhibit the CYP2D6 isoenzyme. Other medications metabolized through the CYP2D6 isoenzyme, such as quinidine, paroxetine, and fluoxetine, should be used carefully in patients receiving conventional antipsychotics.

- The clinical efficacy of antipsychotics correlates with dopamine D_2 receptor blockade.
- Antipsychotics are used in the treatment of schizophrenia, schizoaffective disorders, substance-induced psychosis, major depression with psychotic features, and mania.
- Serious side effects of antipsychotics are rare but include neuroleptic malignant syndrome and agranulocytosis; elderly patients treated for delirium may have increased mortality.

Pharmacotherapy for Chemical Dependency

Drug Treatment of Alcohol Use Disorder

Disulfiram is an aversive medication that binds irreversibly to the aldehyde dehydrogenase enzyme, resulting in an abrupt accumulation of acetaldehyde when alcohol is consumed, with the noxious results of flushing, nausea, vomiting, throbbing headache, and mild confusion. Efficacy is modest. The side effect profile includes drowsiness, lethargy, fatigue, hepatotoxicity, optic neuritis, and peripheral neuropathy.

Naltrexone, an orally bioavailable opioid antagonist, reduces the rewarding effect of alcohol by blocking the μ opioid receptors. Naltrexone is associated with less craving, increased rate of abstinence, and fewer drinking days. Initiation of naltrexone is delayed until after symptoms of withdrawal have resolved. Common side effects include nausea, headache, light-headedness, weakness, and, rarely, flulike symptoms. The FDA has issued a boxed warning for hepatotoxicity.

An injectable depot formulation of naltrexone produces detectable plasma concentrations for 30 days. Depot naltrexone was shown to significantly delay the onset to any drinking and increase the total number of abstinent days, but it did not reduce the risk of heavy drinking.

Acamprosate, a glutamate receptor modulator, increases GABA neurotransmission. European studies provided the basis for FDA approval in the United States since 2 large US studies did not show an advantage of acamprosate over placebo. The most common side effects include diarrhea, bloating, and pruritus. Since acamprosate is excreted (unmetabolized) through the kidney, use of acamprosate in patients with renal failure should be avoided.

Drug Treatment of Opioid Use Disorder

Naloxone is a short-acting μ-opioid receptor antagonist (high affinity) and a κ- and δ-opioid receptor antagonist (lower affinity) used to treat life-threatening opioid overdose. Naloxone induces opioid withdrawal in opioid-dependent patients who are actively using opioids.

Naltrexone is a long-acting competitive opioid antagonist that blocks the subjective effects of opiates. It also induces opioid withdrawal in opioid-dependent patients who are actively using opioids. Naltrexone is best for motivated health care professionals, business executives, or those under probation; in the general population, treatment-retention rates are low because naltrexone does not block cravings. Common side effects include transient nausea and gastrointestinal tract upset.

Methadone is a long-acting opioid agonist that is widely used as a maintenance treatment of opioid dependence but only in a methadone-licensed facility. Methadone has the benefits of good treatment retention rates, improved psychosocial adjustment, and reduced criminal activity. The main side effects include constipation, excessive sweating, drowsiness, and decreased sexual interest and performance.

Buprenorphine is a μ-opioid receptor partial agonist (high affinity) and a κ-opioid receptor antagonist (lower affinity) that is used as an office-based treatment of opioid dependence. Buprenorphine allows for accelerated withdrawal without significant distress.

Clonidine is a centrally acting α-adrenergic agonist that is used off-label to treat opioid withdrawal. It is most effective for suppression of autonomic signs and symptoms of opioid withdrawal; it is less effective for subjective withdrawal symptoms.

Drug Treatment of Nicotine Use Disorder

Nicotine replacement therapy includes gum, patch, inhaler, nasal spray, and lozenge delivery of nicotine. Compared with placebo, nicotine replacement therapy doubles the odds of tobacco abstinence because of its effect on reducing tobacco withdrawal, blocking reinforcing effects, managing negative mood states, and providing the opportunity to engage cognitive and behavioral strategies to change smoking behavior.

Bupropion is an antidepressant that inhibits reuptake of norepinephrine and dopamine and attenuates weight gain in abstinent smokers.

Varenicline is an α4β2 nicotinic acetylcholine receptor partial agonist that decreases nicotine craving and withdrawal and blocks the reinforcement associated with smoking. Its use in patients with prior suicidal ideation or action should be approached with caution.

Electroconvulsive Therapy

Overview

ECT is the induction of a generalized seizure under general anesthesia for therapeutic purposes. ECT was first used to treat a patient with catatonia in 1938. Currently about 100,000 patients annually receive ECT in the United States.

Three major issues should be addressed when ECT is considered:

1. Is ECT indicated? That is, does the patient have an ECT-responsive illness?

2. What are the risks associated with ECT? Does the patient have any medical conditions that increase the risk or require modifications of ECT technique?

3. Does the patient have the capacity to give informed consent for the procedure?

Indications

The principal indications for ECT are major depressive episode (unipolar or bipolar), acute mania, mixed affective state, and catatonia. ECT is the most effective short-term treatment of major depression; remission rates are more than 80% when ECT is used as a first-line treatment or for patients who have received inadequate pharmacotherapy. Patients who have no response to an adequate medication trial have lower response rates to ECT (50%-60%). Other predictors of good outcome with ECT include age older than 50 years, psychotic depression, severe vegetative signs, acute suicide risk, catatonia, and a previous, good response to ECT. In contrast, predictors of a poor outcome with ECT include personality disorders, somatization, comorbid alcohol or substance use disorders, and lack of response to TCAs.

Risks and Side Effects

ECT is a safe procedure performed under general anesthesia with a very low mortality rate (≤0.002%). Morbidity results from anesthesia or from the physiologic consequences of the induced seizure, causing transient blood pressure fluctuation, heart rate changes, and arrhythmias. Common, milder side effects include headache, nausea, and muscle aches.

The cognitive effects of ECT are mild and generally acceptable to the majority of patients. Three types of memory disturbance are associated with ECT:

1. An acute confusional state lasting up to an hour after each treatment—this may be more prolonged with advanced age

2. Retrograde amnesia that affects memories of events from the period of the illness and treatment

3. Anterograde amnesia with impairment in retaining new memories after ECT—this typically resolves within 1–3 weeks after a course of ECT
   - The principal indications for ECT are major depressive episode (unipolar or bipolar), acute mania, mixed affective state, and catatonia.
   - The cognitive effects of ECT are mild and generally acceptable to the majority of patients.

46 Nonpharmacologic Treatment of Psychiatric Disorders

JARROD M. LEFFLER, PHD, LP

Introduction

Nonpharmacologic therapies often complement pharmacologic therapies in the treatment of psychiatric disease. An overview of the theory and practice of psychotherapy and interventions is provided in this chapter.

Psychotherapy

Psychodynamic or Psychoanalytic

Psychodynamic or psychoanalytic psychotherapy, developed by Sigmund Freud, has influenced many forms of psychotherapy. The underlying framework of psychoanalytic theory holds that a majority of our psychological experiences are unconscious. Early life experiences influence the development of our personality and interpersonal styles. Our view of self, others, and our relationships affects how we experience psychological distress. The development of personality includes moving from an immature state to a mature state of independence with the ability to regulate aggressive and sexual urges. Freud's theory recognizes 5 stages of psychosexual development, which are listed in Table 46.1. (See also Chapter 37, "Psychological Development Through the Life Cycle.")

Freud also focused on the structure of the individual's psychic apparatus. He postulated that there are 3 structures. The *id* consists of instinctual experiences usually related to sexual and aggressive impulses. The *ego* represents organized functions that guide the relationship between internal demands and the external world. The *superego*—which begins to emerge around age 5 years—is our internal gauge of moral standards that provides rules and guidelines for decisions and behaviors.

Psychoanalysis uses free association. This technique allows patients to be co-observers of their experiences with their analyst, who encourages the patients to share ideas and experiences as well as reactions. Interpretations are implemented to help guide the patients and to put into context the content of their free associations.

The act of transferring feelings, beliefs, and interpersonal experiences to the therapist is known as *transference* and can be seen as a therapeutic experience that affects the outcome of the intervention. The transferring of feelings, beliefs, and interpersonal experiences from the therapist to the patient is known as *countertransference*. This experience could have a negative impact on the therapeutic relationship. Freud believed that *transference neurosis*—that is, the experience of the patient viewing the relationship with the analyst as similar to the parental relationship—is a necessary component of successful treatment progression.

Table 46.1 • Freud's Stages of Psychosexual Development

Stage	Age
Oral	0–18 mo
Anal	18 mo to 3 y
Phallic	3–6 y
Latency	6 y to puberty
Genital	Puberty to adulthood

Adapted from Feldman RS. Child development: a topical approach. Upper Saddle River (NJ): Prentice Hall; c1999. 575 p. Used with permission.

Therapy consists of 4 phases: The first is the *opening phase*, in which the analyst learns more about the patient and pays attention to everything the patient says and does. In the second phase, *development of transference*, the patient identifies the analyst as a significant person in the patient's life. The third phase, *working through*, occurs simultaneously with the second phase and extends beyond it, taking the emotions and memories evoked in the patient through transference and using them to foster a sense of recall and recognition of past events with the use of interpretation. The final phase, *resolution of transference*, is the termination phase at the end of treatment, which is determined by the patient's work to recognize and understand the transference.

Cognitive

Cognitive therapy is based on the belief that patients' thoughts affect their feelings and resulting behaviors. Therapy is focused on addressing inaccurate information processing. Techniques are implemented to help the patient modify unhealthy assumptions that foster and support maladaptive emotions and behaviors. The overall goal is to ameliorate biases or distortions in thinking. Cognitive therapy is a structured intervention that is likely to be completed in 12 to 24 weeks.

Fundamental aspects of the theory include schemas, voluntary and automatic thoughts, social learning, and cognitive distortions. *Schemas*, which are core beliefs, are cognitions that develop from early experiences and include the individual's beliefs and assumptions. This process involves forging perspectives about self, others, and the world. Further experiences and outcomes support maladaptive and healthy schemas. *Automatic thoughts* are influenced by faulty assumptions. These thoughts are paired with emotions and appear accurate to the individual but often have limited or contrary support. *Social learning* is a mechanism by which individuals develop and reinforce thoughts and experiences. *Cognitive distortions* are inaccuracies in reasoning, which can be specific or general, and include overgeneralization, mind reading, and dichotomous thinking.

In the therapeutic process, the therapist encourages and assists with thought exploration. The patient decides to accept or reject the therapist's description and hypothesis testing of thoughts. Therapy progresses to challenging maladaptive thoughts and developing more healthy and supportive beliefs. This change fosters improvement in emotions and behaviors. Key concepts of cognitive therapy include collaborative empiricism, Socratic dialogue, and guided discovery. *Collaborative empiricism* indicates that the patient and therapist work together to identify treatment goals and test hypotheses about the patient's thinking and experience. There is also a focus on empirical evidence to assess the accuracy of cognitions. The use of questioning in *Socratic dialogue* is critical in this intervention and consists of the therapist facilitating the patient's exploration of thoughts to arrive at a more accurate interpretation of information. The therapist assists the patient in identifying healthy ways of thinking through the use of *guided discovery*, which includes providing the patient with experiences to test and challenge faulty thoughts. The first sessions include getting an accurate and detailed understanding of the patient's maladaptive and impairing experiences along with the thoughts associated with them. The middle and closing stages of therapy include focusing on the relationship of the patient's thoughts, feelings, and behaviors.

Supportive

Person-centered therapy, developed by Carl Rogers, focuses on supporting the individual in attaining self-actualization. Trust, congruence, unconditional positive regard, and empathy are key techniques implemented to assist the patient in achieving insights to facilitate therapeutic growth. Patients who have received this therapy have shown improvement in self-concepts and self-expression, and they have responded more successfully to stress.

Therapy is facilitated by the relationship between the patient and the therapist. Patients often experience incongruence between their experience and awareness and seek out therapy because they feel vulnerable. The therapist demonstrates unconditional positive regard and accepts the patient without judgment. The therapist's congruence signals genuineness to the patient, and through empathy the therapist can relate and appreciate the patient's experiences.

Therapy begins at the first session, with the therapist allowing the patient to proceed as the patient feels comfortable. The therapist allows the patient to recognize the patient's needs and does not offer suggestions or interpretations. In person-centered therapy, the patient sets the agenda and determines the topics to be discussed and the goals of treatment. By allowing patients to experience emotions in therapy and recognize and accept elements of themselves not fully realized before, self-actualization occurs and allows for a return to congruence and decreased vulnerability.

Crisis Intervention

Psychological crises take on many forms. Gerald Caplan identified a 4-stage crisis reaction model. In this model, there is 1) an initial rise of tensions due to precrisis events, 2) disruption and impairment in functioning due to being unable to resolve the crisis, 3) an increase in stress due to failure to resolve the crisis, and finally 4) either a modest resolution by implementing new problem-solving techniques or an eventual psychological decline.

Albert Roberts developed a 7-stage crisis intervention model to facilitate care to individuals who experience a crisis (Table 46.2). The 7 stages are 1) conducting an

Table 46.2 • Roberts' 7-Stage Crisis Intervention Model

Stage	Description
Conducting an assessment	The assessment needs to be quick but include the patient's supports, stressors, medical needs, and coping resources
Developing a collaborative relationship	The crisis worker facilitates rapport and implements strengths to foster trust and confidence
Identifying the problems	The crisis worker inquires about events that led up to the crisis or occurred before the crisis and prioritizes the concerns to address first
Exploring emotions	The patient's feelings are expressed, and the crisis worker must skillfully incorporate challenging and clarifying responses into the dialogue
Identifying coping strategies	The crisis worker identifies how the patient has coped or used problem-solving strategies in the past; the crisis worker and the patient can also brainstorm new coping strategies
Implementing an action plan	The crisis worker and the patient identify ways to successfully cope with and address the crisis and work through the meaning of the event
Planning for follow-up	The crisis worker plans to assess how the patient is functioning after the crisis and working to resolve the crisis, with areas of possible follow-up including social-emotional functioning and the need for additional follow-up or referral services

Adapted from Roberts AR. Crisis intervention handbook: assessment, treatment, and research. 3rd ed. Oxford (UK): Oxford University Press; c2005. 845 p. Used with permission.

assessment, 2) developing a collaborative relationship, 3) identifying the problems, 4) exploring emotions, 5) identifying coping strategies, 6) implementing an action plan, and 7) planning for follow-up.

- Freud postulated that there are 3 structures. The *id* consists of instinctual experiences usually related to sexual and aggressive impulses. The *ego* represents organized functions that guide the relationship between internal demands and the external world. The *superego*—which begins to emerge around age 5 years—is our internal gauge of moral standards that provides rules and guidelines for decisions and behaviors.
- Cognitive therapy is based on the belief that patients' thoughts affect their feelings and resulting behaviors. Therapy is focused on addressing inaccurate information processing.
- Person-centered therapy, developed by Carl Rogers, focuses on supporting the individual in attaining self-actualization.
- In person-centered therapy, the patient sets the agenda and determines the topics to be discussed and the goals of treatment.

Psychosocial Interventions

Relapse Prevention

Substance abuse relapse consists of 3 stages: emotional relapse, mental relapse, and physical relapse. *Emotional*

relapse includes experiencing feelings that promote the possibility of future use. *Mental relapse* includes recalling past use, denying its impact, considering use of the substance, and socializing with individuals who were associated with past use. The final stage, *physical relapse*, can occur quickly once a person engages in mental relapse. For relapse prevention, patients must recognize their emotions and work to alter their behaviors to avoid mental relapse.

The goal of relapse prevention is to educate the patient about these stages and develop strategies and skills to respond in a healthy way when faced with these challenges. Specific coping skills might include managing emotional states, interpersonal conflict, and social pressure; coping with urges; and developing a balanced lifestyle.

Self-help Groups

Alcoholics Anonymous and Narcotics Anonymous are self-help groups founded on the 12-step model. This model includes the use of open and closed meetings, specific types of meetings (eg, speaker meeting, speaker discussion), and a sponsor who is a veteran of the 12-step program. There is a strong emphasis on sharing experiences in a supportive environment.

Harm Reduction

Substance abuse is developed and maintained by an interaction of biopsychosocial factors. Harm reduction psychotherapy postulates that addressing substance use issues while focusing on social, emotional, psychological, and functional concerns is necessary to decrease substance use. The philosophy associated with harm reduction therapy is that drug use will continue, but specific measures can make it less injurious or destructive. Examples include supervised injection facilities, drug replacement and maintenance therapy, and syringe access programs.

- Substance abuse relapse consists of 3 stages: emotional relapse, mental relapse, and physical relapse.
- Self-help groups and harm reduction psychotherapy may be used in substance abuse treatment programs.

Questions and Answers

Questions

Multiple Choice (choose the best answer)

VII.1. Which of the following is most consistent with a diagnosis of anorexia nervosa, restricting type?
- a. Refusal to maintain body weight at or above minimal normal weight for age and height
- b. Intense fear of gaining weight except when underweight
- c. Dysmenorrhea in postmenarcheal females
- d. Depressed level of brain-derived neurotrophic factor
- e. Obsessive-compulsive features are absent

VII.2. The typical symptoms of alcohol withdrawal are:
- a. Fatigue, increased appetite, insomnia, and depressed mood
- b. Myalgias, diarrhea, piloerection, lacrimation, and sweating
- c. Insomnia, anxiety, sweating, tremors, nausea, and sympathetic arousal
- d. Hypotension, decreased respiratory rate, and myosis
- e. Dry mouth, flushed skin, constipation, confusion, and tachycardia

VII.3. Dissociative identity disorder is associated most strongly with:
- a. Borderline personality disorder
- b. Paranoid personality disorder
- c. Avoidant personality disorder
- d. Schizoid personality disorder
- e. Narcissistic personality disorder

VII.4. What is the prevalence of attention-deficit/hyperactivity disorder in school-aged children?
- a. 1% to 2%
- b. 4% to 7%
- c. 9% to 14%
- d. 16% to 22%
- e. 24% to 31%

VII.5. A 56-year-old practicing neurologist has the acute onset of auditory hallucinations in which multiple male voices are telling him they will kill him. Which of the following diagnoses is the most likely explanation for these symptoms?
- a. Schizophrenia
- b. Delusional disorder
- c. Capgras syndrome
- d. Alcohol-induced psychotic disorder
- e. Folie à deux

VII.6. Which of the following describes Erik Erikson's stage of late adulthood?
- a. Striving to contribute to society and accomplish things that benefit others versus being disengaged and uninvolved
- b. Developing a sense of personal control and independence versus feeling inadequate and insecure

- c. Forming loving and strong relationships versus inability to form intimate relationships leading to loneliness and depression
- d. Continually coping with narcissistic injury from physical, emotional, and social losses with adaptive versus maladaptive defense mechanisms
- e. Looking back on life lived with either a sense of satisfaction from a life filled with meaning and purpose versus a sense of regret and bitterness that life has been wasted

VII.7. Tourette syndrome is defined as childhood onset of:
- a. Vocal tics for a total period of 3 months
- b. Vocal and motor tics for a total period of 3 months
- c. Vocal and motor tics for more than 1 year
- d. Motor tics for more than 1 year
- e. Vocal or motor tics for at least 6 months

VII.8. Alcohol withdrawal develops in a 63-year-old man with chronic cognitive impairment and liver cirrhosis. Which medication is the best choice to treat alcohol withdrawal symptoms?
- a. Carbamazepine
- b. Diazepam
- c. Loratadine
- d. Lorazepam
- e. Propranolol

VII.9. Person-centered therapy focuses on:
- a. Interpreting dream meaning
- b. Childhood free associations
- c. Behavior activation plans
- d. Self-actualization
- e. Distress tolerance

VII.10. Which of the following antidepressants is most likely to cause akathisia or parkinsonism?
- a. Amoxapine
- b. Citalopram
- c. Mirtazapine
- d. Sertraline
- e. Vilazodone

VII.11. Which of the following statements about development in the preschool period is most true?
- a. In Freud's psychosexual theory of development, preschoolers are in the oral stage
- b. According to Erikson, the developmental challenge during the preschool period is autonomy versus shame and doubt
- c. Successfully meeting the developmental challenges of the preschool years typically leads to a firm sense of purpose as children move onto the school years
- d. The morality of preschoolers is preconventional in that they tend to follow rules only when a reward is offered

e. Play is an unimportant vehicle for enhancing motor, communication, cognitive, and social skills

VII.12. In Erikson's theory of ego development, the risk or challenge for the school-aged child is industry versus:
a. Inferiority
b. Shame and doubt
c. Indolence
d. Guilt
e. Role confusion

VII.13. A 25-year-old single man with a normal mood believes he is the incarnation of a great religious leader. Which of the following is a likely diagnosis?
a. Schizophrenia
b. Schizoaffective disorder
c. Delusional disorder
d. Answer choices *a* and *b*
e. Answer choices *a* and *c*

VII.14. A new neurology resident is finding an outpatient rotation increasingly difficult. Multiple patients have been late, compressing her schedule; she chose nonneurology rotations during her fourth year of medical school and internship to broaden her experience base, but now her neurology knowledge base is weak; and she worries she will be placed on academic probation. She files a complaint with her program director stating that she is being singled out, although her colleagues have a similar schedule and responsibilities. This action may reflect which of the following defense mechanisms?
a. Acting out
b. Displacement
c. Projection
d. Reaction formation
e. Splitting

VII.15. Which of the following personality disorders may benefit from the prescription of atypical antipsychotic medications?
a. Antisocial
b. Obsessive-compulsive
c. Dependent
d. Schizoid
e. Schizotypal

VII.16. In the course of evaluating and treating a particularly challenging patient with refractory headaches, which of the following is most likely to represent countertransference on the part of the neurologist?
a. Referral to another physician when the patient threatens violence
b. Consistently allowing extra time in clinic visits
c. Addressing the patient formally by name
d. Reviewing prior clinic notes during the patient's appointments
e. Ordering frequent screens for drugs of abuse

VII.17. Which of the following statements regarding bipolar disorder and major depression is true?
a. The female:male ratio in bipolar disorder is approximately equal to that in major depression
b. The average age at onset for bipolar disorder is slightly older than that for major depression
c. The lifetime prevalence of bipolar disorder in the United States is one-fourth that of major depression
d. Persons with major depression are more likely to also have a substance use disorder than those with bipolar disorder
e. Postpartum depression is more likely to occur in persons with major depression than in those with bipolar disorder

VII.18. In cognitive therapies, schemas are:
a. The meaning of one's interpersonal relationships
b. Core beliefs
c. Interventions to shape behaviors

d. Dysfunctional cognitions
e. A term used to describe the therapeutic process

VII.19. You are evaluating a patient for migraine headaches. Despite your recommendation for a prophylactic approach and a carefully controlled abortive regimen, she frequently goes to the emergency department for opioid pain relief and does not seem to improve from your work with her. When you ask her about her use of treatment, she becomes enraged and threatens you. She has a history of cutting herself and reports frequent, several-day periods of depression. Which of the following treatment options may be of help?
a. Referral to a dialectal behavioral therapy program
b. Prescription of a short-acting benzodiazepine to lower anxiety
c. Termination of care
d. Referral for psychoanalysis
e. Performing electroencephalography to exclude seizures

VII.20. Which of the following psychotropic medications is known to reduce the risk of suicidality?
a. Aripiprazole
b. Bupropion
c. Lithium
d. Phenelzine
e. Valproate

Answers

VII.1. **Answer a.**
Devlin MJ, Jahraus JP, DiMarco ID. Eating disorders. In: Levenson JL, editor. The American Psychiatric Publishing textbook of psychosomatic medicine: psychiatric care of the medically ill. 2nd ed. Washington (DC): American Psychiatric Publishing; c2011. p. 305–34.

VII.2. **Answer c.**
Kelly JF, Renner JA. Alcohol-related disorders. In: Stern TA, Rosenbaum JF, Fava M, Biederman J, Rauch SL, editors. Massachusetts General Hospital comprehensive clinical psychiatry. 1st ed. Philadelphia (PA): Mosby/Elsevier; c2008. p. 337–54.

VII.3. **Answer a.**
American Psychiatric Association. Diagnostic and statistical manual of mental disorders. 4th ed. Text Revision. Washington (DC): The Association; c2000. 370 p.

VII.4. **Answer b.**
Martin A, Volkmar FR, editors. Lewis's child and adolescent psychiatry: a comprehensive textbook. 4th ed. Philadelphia (PA): Wolters Kluwer Health/Lippincott Williams & Wilkins; c2007. 1062 p.

VII.5. **Answer d.**
Lishman WA. Organic psychiatry: the psychological consequences of cerebral disorder. 3rd ed. Oxford (UK): Blackwell Science; c1998. 922 p.

VII.6. **Answer e.**
Berk LE. Development through the lifespan. 5th ed. Boston (MA): Allyn & Bacon, c2010. 667 p.

VII.7. **Answer c.**
Dulcan MK, editor. Dulcan's textbook of child and adolescent psychiatry. 1st ed. Washington (DC): American Psychiatric Publishing; c2010. 1074 p.

VII.8. **Answer d.**
Galanter M, Kleber HD, editors. The American Psychiatric Publishing textbook of substance abuse treatment. 4th ed. Washington (DC): American Psychiatric Publishing; c2008. 752 p.

VII.9. **Answer d.**
Rogers CR. Client-centered therapy: its current practice, implications and theory. London (UK): Constable; c2003. 560 p.

VII.10. Answer a.

Schatzberg AF, Nemeroff CB, editors. The American Psychiatric Publishing textbook of psychopharmacology. 4th ed. Washington (DC): American Psychiatric Publishing; c2009. 1616 p.

VII.11. Answer b.

Southwick SM, Litz BT, Charney D, Friedman MJ, editors. Resilience and mental health: challenges across the lifespan. Cambridge (England): Cambridge University Press; c2011. 366 p.

VII.12. Answer a.

Erikson EH. Childhood and society. 2nd ed. New York (NY): W. W. Norton & Company; c1963. 445 p.

VII.13. Answer e.

Freudenreich O. Psychotic disorders: a practical guide. Philadelphia (PA): Wolters Kluwer Health/Lippincott Williams & Wilkins; c2008. 274 p.

VII.14. Answer c.

Vaillant GE. Adaptation to life. 1st ed. Boston (MA): Little, Brown; c1977. 396 p.

VII.15. Answer e.

Skodol AE, Gunderson JG. Personality disorders. In: Hales RE, Yudofsky SC, Gabbard GO, editors. The American Psychiatric Publishing textbook of psychiatry. 5th ed. Washington (DC): American Psychiatric Publishing; c2008. p. 821–60.

VII.16. Answer e.

Gabbard GO, Beck JS, Holmes J, editors. Oxford textbook of psychotherapy. New York (NY): Oxford University Press; c2005. 534 p.

VII.17. Answer c.

Sher L, Kahn DA, Oquendo MA. Mood disorders. In: Cutler JL, Marcus ER, editors. Psychiatry. 2nd ed. New York (NY): Oxford University Press; c2010. p. 53–100.

VII.18. Answer b.

Beck JS. Cognitive behavior therapy: basics and beyond. 2nd ed. New York (NY): Guilford Press; c2011. 391 p.

VII.19. Answer a.

Gunderson JG. Clinical practice: borderline personality disorder. N Engl J Med. 2011 May 26;364(21):2037–42.

VII.20. Answer c.

Stahl SM. Stahl's essential psychopharmacology: the prescriber's guide. 4th ed. Cambridge (UK): Cambridge University Press; c2011. 709 p.

SUGGESTED READING

Abbey SE, Wulsin L, Levenson JL. Somatization and somatoform disorders. In: Levenson JL, editor. The American Psychiatric Publishing textbook of psychosomatic medicine: psychiatric care of the medically ill. 2nd ed. Washington (DC): American Psychiatric Publishing; c2011. p. 261–90.

American Psychiatric Association. Diagnostic and statistical manual of mental disorders. 4th ed. Text Revision. Washington (DC): The Association; c2000. 370 p.

American Psychiatric Association. Diagnostic and statistical manual of mental disorders: DSM-5. 5th ed. Arlington (VA): American Psychiatric Association; c2013. 947 p.

Beck JS. Cognitive behavior therapy: basics and beyond. 2nd ed. New York (NY): Guilford Press; c2011. 391 p.

Berk LE. Development through the lifespan. 5th ed. Boston (MA): Allyn & Bacon, c2010. 667 p.

Crain WC. Theories of development: concepts and applications. 6th ed. Boston (MA): Prentice Hall; c2011. 432 p.

Davies D. Child development: a practitioner's guide. 2nd ed. New York (NY): Guilford Press; c2004. 478 p.

Devlin MJ, Jahraus JP, DiMarco ID. Eating disorders. In: Levenson JL, editor. The American Psychiatric Publishing textbook of psychosomatic medicine: psychiatric care of the medically ill. 2nd ed. Washington (DC): American Psychiatric Publishing; c2011. p. 305–34.

Dulcan MK, editor. Dulcan's textbook of child and adolescent psychiatry. 1st ed. Washington (DC): American Psychiatric Publishing; c2010. 1074 p.

Erikson EH. Childhood and society. 2nd ed. New York (NY): W. W. Norton & Company; c1963. 445 p.

Ewing JA. Detecting alcoholism: the CAGE questionnaire. JAMA. 1984 Oct 12;252(14):1905–7.

Feinberg TE, Farah MJ, editors. Behavioral neurology and neuropsychology. 2nd ed. New York (NY): McGraw-Hill Medical Publisher; c2003. 910 p.

Ferrando SJ, Levenson JL, Owen JA, editors. Clinical manual of psychopharmacology in the medically ill. 1st ed. Washington (DC): American Psychiatric Publishing; c2010. 610 p.

Freudenreich O. Psychotic disorders: a practical guide. Philadelphia (PA): Wolters Kluwer Health/Lippincott Williams & Wilkins; c2008. 274 p.

Gabbard GO. Psychodynamic psychiatry in clinical practice. 4th ed. Washington (DC): American Psychiatric Publishing; c2005. 629 p.

Gabbard GO, Beck JS, Holmes J, editors. Oxford textbook of psychotherapy. New York (NY): Oxford University Press; c2005. 534 p.

Galanter M, Kleber HD, editors. The American Psychiatric Publishing textbook of substance abuse treatment. 4th ed. Washington (DC): American Psychiatric Publishing; c2008. 752 p.

Gunderson JG. Clinical practice: borderline personality disorder. N Engl J Med. 2011 May 26;364(21):2037–42.

Heilman KM, Valenstein E, editors. Clinical neuropsychology. 5th ed. New York (NY): Oxford University Press; c2011. 690 p.

Huprich SK. Psychodynamic therapy: conceptual and empirical foundations. New York (NY): Routledge; c2009. 273 p.

Kelly JF, Renner JA. Alcohol-related disorders. In: Stern TA, Rosenbaum JF, Fava M, Biederman J, Rauch SL, editors. Massachusetts General Hospital comprehensive clinical psychiatry. 1st ed. Philadelphia (PA): Mosby/Elsevier; c2008. p. 337–54.

Lezak MD, Howieson DB, Bigler ED, Tranel D. Neuropsychological assessment. 5th ed. New York (NY): Oxford University Press; c2012. 1161 p.

Lieberman JA, Stroup TS, Perkins DO, editors. The American Psychiatric Publishing textbook of schizophrenia. 1st ed. Washington (DC): American Psychiatric Publishing; c2006; 435 p.

Lishman WA. Organic psychiatry: the psychological consequences of cerebral disorder. 3rd ed. Oxford (UK): Blackwell Science; c1998. 922 p.

Martin A, Volkmar FR, editors. Lewis's child and adolescent psychiatry: a comprehensive textbook. 4th ed. Philadelphia (PA): Wolters Kluwer Health/Lippincott Williams & Wilkins; c2007. 1062 p.

McVoy M, Findling RL, editors. Clinical manual of child and adolescent psychopharmacology. 2nd ed. Washington (DC): American Psychiatric Publishing; c2013. 458 p.

Moeller KE, Lee KC, Kissack JC. Urine drug screening: practical guide for clinicians. Mayo Clin Proc. 2008 Jan;83(1):66–76. Erratum in: Mayo Clin Proc. 2008 Jul;83(7):851.

Morgan JE, Ricker JH, editors. Textbook of clinical neuropsychology. New York (NY): Taylor & Francis; c2008. 1027 p.

National Institute of Mental Health [Internet]. Washington (DC): National Institutes of Health. [cited 2012 Nov 15]. Available from: http://www.nimh.nih.gov/index_shtml.

Oldham JM, Skodol AE, Bender DS, editors. The American Psychiatric Publishing textbook of personality disorders. 1st ed. Washington (DC): American Psychiatric Publishing; c2005. 708 p.

Potuzak M, Ravichandran C, Lewandowski KE, Ongur D, Cohen BM. Categorical vs dimensional classifications of psychotic disorders. Compr Psychiatry. 2012 Nov;53(8):1118–29. Epub 2012 Jun 7.

Renner JA, Ward EN. Drug addiction. In: Stern TA, Rosenbaum JF, Fava M, Biederman J, Rauch SL, editors. Massachusetts General Hospital comprehensive clinical psychiatry. 1st ed. Philadelphia (PA): Mosby/Elsevier; c2008. p. 355–69.

Rogers CR. Client-centered therapy: its current practice, implications and theory. London (UK): Constable; c2003. 560 p.

Sacks MH, Sledge WH, Warren C, editors. Core readings in psychiatry: an annotated guide to the literature. 2nd ed. Washington (DC): American Psychiatric Press; c1995. p. 688–90.

Sadock BJ, Sadock VA, Ruiz P, editors. Kaplan & Sadock's comprehensive textbook of psychiatry. 9th ed. Philadelphia (PA): Wolters Kluwer Health/Lippincott Williams & Wilkins; c2009. 4520 p.

Schatzberg AF, Nemeroff CB, editors. The American Psychiatric Publishing textbook of psychopharmacology. 4th ed. Washington (DC): American Psychiatric Publishing; c2009. 1616 p.

Schneier FR, Vidair HB, Vogel LR, Muskin PR. Anxiety disorders. In: Cutler JL, Marcus ER, editors. Psychiatry. 2nd ed. New York (NY): Oxford University Press; c2010. p. 170–209.

Shafer LC. Sexual disorders and sexual dysfunction. In: Stern TA, Fricchione GL, Cassem NH, Jellinek MS, Rosenbaum JF, editors. Massachusetts General Hospital handbook of general hospital psychiatry. 6th ed. Philadelphia (PA): Saunders/Elsevier; c2010. p. 323–35.

Shaffer DR. Developmental psychology: childhood and adolescence. 6th ed. Australia and Belmont (CA): Wadsworth Thomson Learning; c2002.

Shapiro D. Dynamics of character: self-regulation in psychopathology. New York (NY): Basic Books; c2000. 172 p.

Sher L, Kahn DA, Oquendo MA. Mood disorders. In: Cutler JL, Marcus ER, editors. Psychiatry. 2nd ed. New York (NY): Oxford University Press; c2010. p. 53–100.

Skodol AE, Gunderson JG. Personality disorders. In: Hales RE, Yudofsky SC, Gabbard GO, editors. The American Psychiatric Publishing textbook of psychiatry. 5th ed. Washington (DC): American Psychiatric Publishing; c2008. p. 821–60.

Snyder PJ, Nussbaum PD, Robins DL, editors. Clinical neuropsychology: a pocket handbook for assessment. 2nd ed. Washington (DC): American Psychological Association; c2006. 769 p.

Southwick SM, Litz BT, Charney D, Friedman MJ, editors. Resilience and mental health: challenges across the lifespan. Cambridge (UK): Cambridge University Press; c2011. 366 p.

Stahl SM. Stahl's essential psychopharmacology: the prescriber's guide. 4th ed. Cambridge (UK): Cambridge University Press; c2011. 709 p.

Summers RF, Barber JP. Psychodynamic therapy: a guide to evidence-based practice. New York (NY): Guilford Press; c2010. 355 p.

Vaillant GE. Adaptation to life. 1st ed. Boston (MA): Little, Brown; c1977. 396 p.

Vaillant GE. Triumphs of experience: the men of the Harvard Grant Study. Cambridge (MA): Belknap Press of Harvard University Press; c2012. 457 p.

Virani AS, Bezchlibnyk-Butler KZ, Jeffries JJ, Procyshyn RM, editors. Clinical handbook of psychotropic drugs. 19th ed. Ashland (OH): Hogrefe Publishing; c2012.

Wenar C, Kerig P. Developmental psychopathology: from infancy through adolescence. 5th ed. Boston (MA): McGraw-Hill; c2006. 557 p.

Wynn GH, Oesterheld JR, Cozza KL, Armstrong SC. Clinical manual of drug interaction: principles for medical practice. 1st ed. Washington (DC): American Psychiatric Publishing, c2009. 594 p.

Index